Principles and Practice of Urooncology

Gokhan Ozyigit • Ugur Selek
Editors

Principles and Practice of Urooncology

Radiotherapy, Surgery and Systemic Therapy

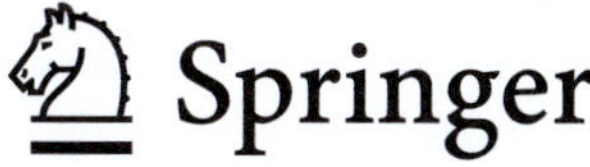

Editors
Gokhan Ozyigit
Chair and Professor
Department of Radiation Oncology
Hacettepe University
Ankara
Turkey

Ugur Selek
Chair and Professor
Department of Radiation Oncology
Koc University
Istanbul
Turkey

Adjunct Professor
Department of Radiation Oncology
The University of Texas MD Anderson
Cancer Center
Houston, TX
USA

ISBN 978-3-319-56113-4 ISBN 978-3-319-56114-1 (eBook)
DOI 10.1007/978-3-319-56114-1

Library of Congress Control Number: 2017948435

Printed on acid-free paper

This Springer imprint is published by Springer Nature
The registered company is Springer International Publishing AG
The registered company address is: Gewerbestrasse 11, 6330 Cham, Switzerland

To our families "Eda, Defne, Ipek" and "Ozlem, Melis, Burce," whose supports have made this book possible.
To our patients from whom we have learned to excel.

Preface

This evidence-based guide on lower genitourinary system (GUS) cancers is aiming to be a reference and first-aid book to enable practicing urooncologists to achieve the current management in the multidisciplinary setting of patient selection and cutting-edge treatment finalization.

This guide includes a surgical urooncology perspective with advanced technology to understand the competing surgical approaches, in addition to a medical oncology perspective in multidisciplinary tumor board.

The illustrative spectrum starting from delineation of tumor volumes and organs at risk based on CT simulation and ending at different definitive approaches of stereotactic body radiotherapy (SBRT), intensity-modulated radiation therapy (IMRT), tomotherapy, volumetric modulated arc therapy (VMAT), and proton therapy will highlight the practical tips to ease the management of everyday challenging cases and also provide a comparison of robotic radiosurgical techniques as CyberKnife and LINAC-based techniques.

Each related chapter will display an academic expert view of everyday cases at different stages including case presentations, contouring, treatment planning, and treatment delivery based on illustrations of slice-by-slice delineations on planning CT images and finalization of plan on detailed acceptance criteria. The book will be of value for practicing oncologists as well as other oncology fellows and residents interested in urooncology to facilitate the decision making in the management of patients with lower GUS cancers and will aid encountering daily challenges in clinical practice.

We hope *Principles and Practice of Urooncology* will meet the need for a practical and up-to-date review of lower genitourinary tumors for residents, fellows, and clinicians of radiation and medical and urological oncology, as well as for medical students, physicians, and medical physicists interested in lower genitourinary system malignancies.

Ankara, Turkey — Gokhan Ozyigit, M.D.
Istanbul, Turkey — Ugur Selek, M.D.

Acknowledgments

The editors are indebted to Corinna Hauser and Wilma McHugh from Springer DE and Abha Krishnan and Sivakumar Krishnamoorthy from SPi Global/Springer Nature for their assistance in preparing *Principles and Practice of Urooncology: Radiotherapy, Surgery, and Systemic Therapy*. We extend our most sincere gratitude to our colleagues and friends at Hacettepe University, Koc University, Başkent University, and University of Texas MD Anderson Cancer Center, as well as our families.

Contents

List of Contributors

Omer Acar, M.D. Department of Urology, School of Medicine, Koc University, Istanbul, Turkey

Bülent Akdoğan, M.D. Department of Urology, Hacettepe University, Ankara, Turkey

Sercan Aksoy, M.D. Department of Medical Oncology, Hacettepe University Cancer Institute, Ankara, Turkey

Fadıl Akyol, M.D. Department of Radiation Oncology, Hacettepe University, Ankara, Turkey

Vildan Alpan, M.Sc. Department of Radiation Oncology, American Hospital Texas MD Anderson Cancer Center, Istanbul, Turkey

Mesut Altan, M.D. Department of Urology, Hacettepe University, Ankara, Turkey

Sevil Bavbek, M.D. Department of Medical Oncology, American Hospital, Istanbul, Turkey

Yasemin Bolukbasi, M.D. Department of Radiation Oncology, Koc University, Istanbul, Turkey

Department of Radiation Oncology, The University of Texas MD Anderson Cancer Center, Houston, TX, USA

Seungtaek Choi, M.D. Department of Radiation Oncology, The University of Texas MD Anderson Cancer Center, Houston, TX, USA

Tarık Esen, M.D. Department of Urology, School of Medicine, Koc University, Istanbul, Turkey

Department of Urology, VKF American Hospital, Istanbul, Turkey

Ozan Cem Guler, M.D. Department of Radiation Oncology, Karadeniz Technical University, Trabzon, Turkey

Melis Gultekin, M.D. Department of Radiation Oncology, Hacettepe University, Ankara, Turkey

Pervin Hurmuz, M.D. Department of Radiation Oncology, Hacettepe University, Ankara, Turkey

Muşturay Karçaaltıncaba, M.D. Department of Radiology, Hacettepe University, Ankara, Turkey

Steven Kirsner, Ph.D. Department of Radiation Oncology, The University of Texas MD Anderson Cancer Center, Houston, TX, USA

Deborah A. Kuban, M.D., F.A.C.R., F.A.S.T.R.O. Department of Radiation Oncology, The University of Texas MD Anderson Cancer Center, Houston, TX, USA

Nil Molinas Mandel, M.D. Department of Medical Oncology, VKF Amerikan Hospital, Istanbul, Turkey

Selen Mandel Bezmialem School of Medicine, Istanbul, Turkey

Aydin Mungan, M.D. Department of Urology, Bulent Ecevit University, Zonguldak, Turkey

Cem Onal, M.D. Department of Radiation Oncology, Başkent University, Adana, Turkey

Mehmet Ruhi Onur, M.D. Department of Radiology, Hacettepe University, Ankara, Turkey

Haluk Ozen, M.D. Department of Urology, Hacettepe University, Ankara, Turkey

Gokhan Ozyigit, M.D. Department of Radiation Oncology, Hacettepe University, Ankara, Turkey

Yücel Sağlam, M.Sc. Department of Radiation Oncology, American Hospital Texas MD Anderson Cancer Center, Istanbul, Turkey

Sezin Yuce Sari, M.D. Department of Radiation Oncology, Hacettepe University, Ankara, Turkey

Ugur Selek, M.D. Department of Radiation Oncology, Koc University, Istanbul, Turkey

Department of Radiation Oncology, The University of Texas MD Anderson Cancer Center, Houston, TX, USA

Mehmet Ali Nahit Şendur, M.D. Department of Medical Oncology, Ankara Yıldırım Beyazıt University, Ankara, Turkey

Duygu Sezen, M.D. Department of Radiation Oncology, Koc University, Istanbul, Turkey

Department of Radiology, Hacettepe University, Ankara, Turkey

Ilker Tinay, M.D. Department of Urology, School of Medicine, Marmara University, Istanbul, Turkey

Funda Vakar-Lopez, M.D. Department of Pathology, University of Washington, Seattle, WA, USA

Gozde Yazici, M.D. Department of Radiation Oncology, Hacettepe University, Ankara, Turkey

Berna Akkus Yildirim, M.D. Department of Radiation Oncology, Başkent University, Adana, Turkey

Radiological Imaging in Urological Cancers

1

Mehmet Ruhi Onur and Muşturay Karçaaltıncaba

Abstract

The use of radiological imaging in urological cancers is increasing with improvements in imaging technologies and implementation of these techniques to clinical scenarios. Ultrasonography, computed tomography, and magnetic resonance imaging have enormous potentials in the diagnosis, staging, and surveillance of urological cancers. Emerging imaging techniques enable morphologic assessment of urological cancers with high spatial and contrast resolution. Functional imaging techniques reveal microstructure of tumors which can be used in the diagnosis, prediction of prognosis, and assessment of response to treatment and surveillance of tumors. Biopsyless diagnosis may be possible in the future particularly for renal and prostate tumors. In this chapter, current status of urooncologic imaging will be reviewed.

1.1 Introduction

Urological cancers constitute one of the most frequent encountered malignancies in urologic and oncologic practice. Imaging has a critical role in the diagnosis of urological tumors as well as staging and active surveillance. In addition to the morphologic and functional assessment of tumors, imaging techniques can be used to guide the interventional procedures including biopsy, preoperative embolization, or ablation providing palliative care or curative treatment. Optimal evaluation and treatment of urological cancers can be accomplished with appropriate use of imaging techniques for the diagnosis and staging of tumors, guidance for invasive procedures, and active surveillance of patients.

M.R. Onur, M.D. • M. Karçaaltıncaba, M.D. (✉)
Department of Radiology, Hacettepe University, Ankara, Turkey
e-mail: musturayk@yahoo.com

G. Ozyigit, U. Selek (eds.), *Principles and Practice of Urooncology*,
DOI 10.1007/978-3-319-56114-1_1

Ultrasonography (US) is usually the first preferred imaging technique in the diagnosis of urological cancers. As a noninvasive, inexpensive, easily accessible, and nonionizing radiation used imaging method, US can be used in patients as a first-step imaging technique in patients with suspected malignancy. US demonstrates solid and/or cystic content of the urological masses. Color-flow Doppler US (CDUS) can reveal blood flow within the mass. However grayscale US and CDUS have remarkable limitations in characterization of urological masses. Contrast-enhanced US (CEUS) can demonstrate the enhancement features of tumors which increase the likelihood of neoplastic nature of a mass and can be used in differentiation between benign and malignant urological masses. New emerging technologies promise increased capability for detection and characterization of urological cancers.

Computed tomography (CT) is the mainstay imaging technique utilized in radiologic assessment of renal, ureteral, and bladder cancers. With its multiplanar imaging capability acquired in a short scanning time, CT can demonstrate morphological imaging features, attenuation values, and contrast enhancement patterns of tumors. CT may be helpful to characterize urological cancers by comparison of density values of urological cancers represented by Hounsfield unit (HU) at unenhanced, early, and delayed phases after intravenous (IV) contrast administration.

Magnetic resonance imaging (MRI) is a problem-solving imaging technique in the radiologic assessment of urological cancers. Acquisition of multiple imaging sequences with high soft tissue contrast resolution assigns MRI as decision-making technique in difficult cases. Multiparametric MRI (mp-MRI) technique which consists of conventional MRI sequences such as T1-weighted (W), T2-W, dual-echo T1-W sequences combined with functional MRI sequences including diffusion-weighted imaging (DWI) and dynamic contrast-enhanced MRI (DCE-MRI) are being more increasingly used in detection and characterization of the urological cancers.

1.2 Renal Cancer

1.2.1 General Information

Renal cancers account for 3% of adult malignancies, occurring at a mean age of 65. Male predominance exists in renal cancers with a male to female ratio of 3:1 [1]. Renal cancers are more frequently detected at early stages due to frequent incidental presentation of renal tumors on cross-sectional imaging studies performed due to indications other than urological symptoms. The likelihood of malignancy is 80% in all solid renal lesions detected on imaging studies [2]. However 38% of renal lesions less than 1 cm are benign [3]. Detection of renal tumors on imaging studies necessitates differentiation between benign and malignant masses. In the setting of renal malignancy assessment of other kidney in terms of renal mass is mandatory since 5% of sporadic renal tumors present as bilateral multifocal renal masses [4, 5].

Best prognostic factors in renal cancers are grade and stage of the cancers determined with Fuhrman grading system and tumor-node-metastasis (TNM) staging system, respectively. Fuhrman grading system classifies renal carcinomas according to nuclear size and shape and the size of the nucleoli [1]. TNM staging system includes localization of renal cancers, extension of tumors to perirenal tissues, and metastatic involvement of lymph nodes and distant tissues and organs. Imaging techniques can determine the local and distant spread of renal cancers.

1.2.2 Imaging Techniques

1.2.2.1 Ultrasonography

Ultrasonography is helpful for initial screening of renal lesions as well as to discriminate cystic lesions from solid lesions and monitoring growth of previously determined lesion [6]. Renal cancers usually present as a focal, expansile mass with heterogeneous echogenicity different from adjacent hypoechoic renal parenchyma. Heterogeneous echogenicity and expansile nature of renal cancers are helpful in distinguishing renal cancers from pseudotumoral renal lesions such as column of Bertin and dromedary hump of the kidney. However detection of small renal cancers (<3 cm) confined in renal parenchyma without expansile appearance may be difficult with US especially if these cancers have isoechoic appearance similar to renal parenchyma. Renal cell carcinoma (RCC) as being most frequently encountered renal tumor usually manifests as hypo-, iso-, or hyperechoic expansile mass on US (Figs. 1.1 and 1.2).

Small renal masses (<3 cm) may more likely present with hyperechoic appearance than larger tumors [7]. Papillary RCCs usually appear as hypoechoic or isoechoic and rarely hyperechoic solid masses (Fig. 1.3) [8]. However it is nearly

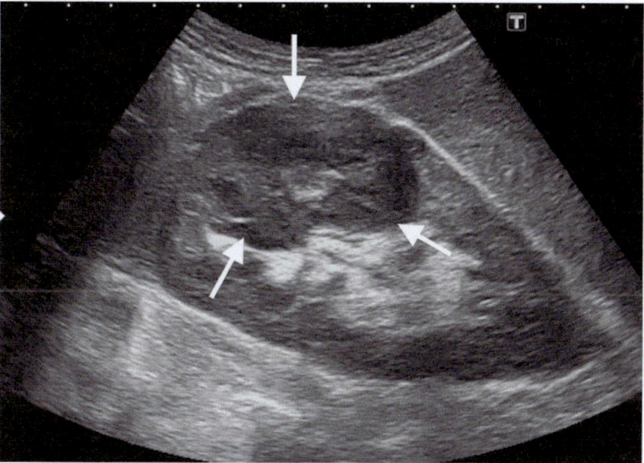

Fig. 1.1 Clear cell RCC. Grayscale US of a 78-year-old male demonstrates a hypoechoic expansile solid renal mass (*arrows*)

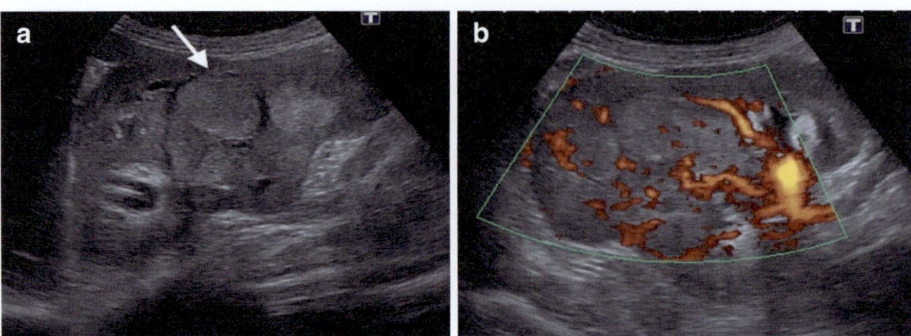

Fig. 1.2 Chromophobe RCC. (**a**) Grayscale US of a 56-year-old female with chromophobe RCC reveals multilobulated hyperechoic solid mass (*arrow*). (**b**) Power Doppler US demonstrates hypervascularity of the tumor

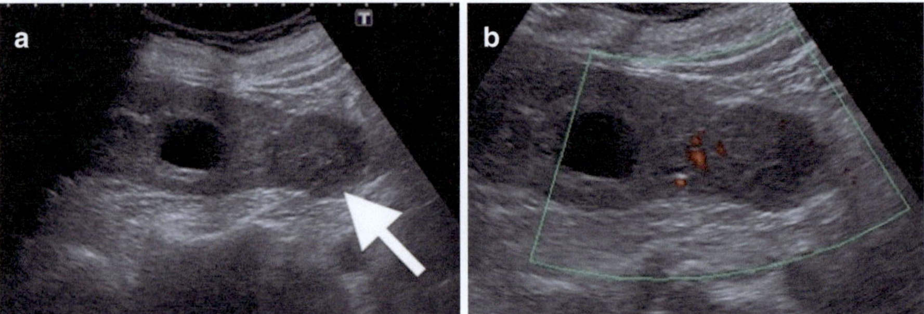

Fig. 1.3 Papillary cell RCC. (**a**) Grayscale US of a 66-year-old male with papillary RCC shows hypoechoic renal mass (*arrow*) arising from lower pole of the kidney and extending inferiorly. (**b**) Renal mass presents with low vascularity on power Doppler US

impossible to differentiate subtypes of RCCs such as clear cell RCC, papillary RCC, and chromophobe RCC by US due to similar sonographic features of these tumors on grayscale US and CDUS. Generally, papillary cell types of RCCs have less vascularity compared to other types of RCCs on CDUS (Fig. 1.3). Renal lymphomas and metastases may manifest as multifocal infiltrative masses (Fig. 1.4). Renal pelvis tumors, most frequently as transitional cell carcinomas (TCCs), present with a hypoechoic appearance within the hyperechoic renal sinus (Fig. 1.5). However TCCs or other tumors localized in renal pelvis are usually more susceptible to be missed on US compared to renal parenchymal tumors.

Cystic renal masses detected on US should be elaborated in terms of malignancy. Sonographic features that increase the likelihood of malignancy in complex renal cysts include thickened cyst wall, numerous or thickened or nodular septations within the cyst, presence of irregular or central calcifications, and the presence of blood flow in the septations or cyst wall (Fig. 1.6) [9]. US can be an important complementary method by revealing cystic nature of hyperdense,

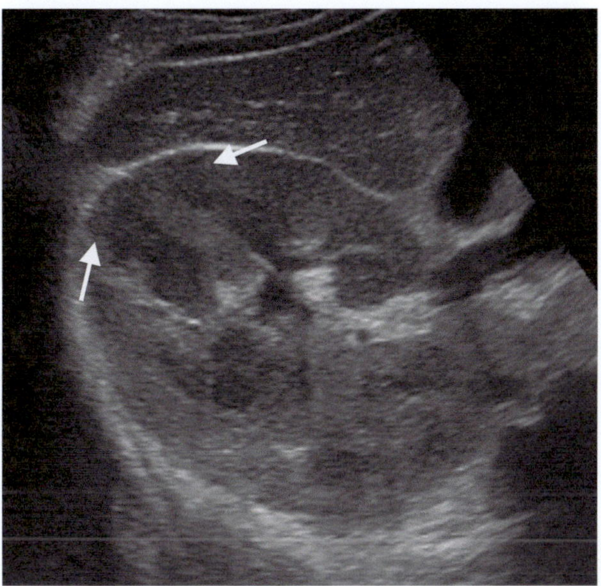

Fig. 1.4 Renal lymphoma. Grayscale US reveals multifocal hypoechoic infiltrative lesions (*arrows*) in the renal parenchyma representing lymphomatous involvement

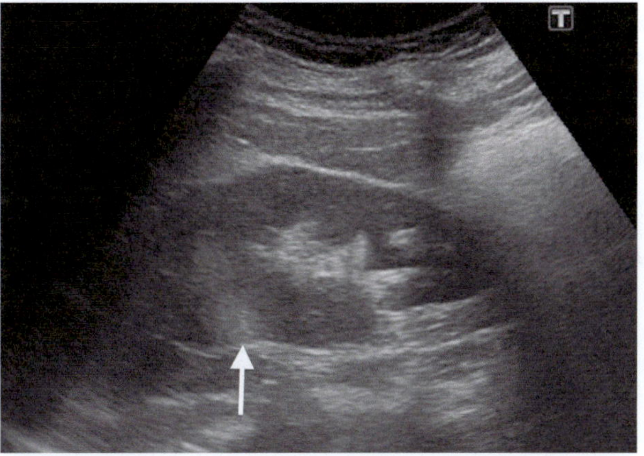

Fig. 1.5 Renal TCC. Grayscale US of a 72-year-old female with TCC demonstrates a hypoechoic solid mass (*arrow*) in the renal pelvis replacing hyperechoic renal sinus fat in the upper pole of the kidney

solid-appearing renal lesions on CT and solid nature of lesions which appear as cystic mass on CT [10].

Contrast-enhanced US seems to be a promising imaging technique for distinguishing benign and malignant renal tumors. A meta-analysis study including

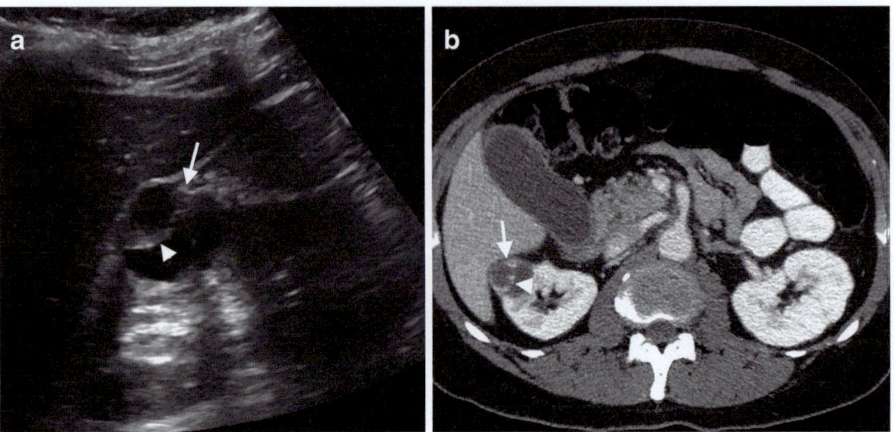

Fig. 1.6 Cystic RCC. (**a**) Grayscale US reveals cystic renal mass (*arrow*) containing thick septa (*arrowhead*). (**b**) Axial contrast-enhanced CT reveals cystic renal mass (*arrow*) in the right kidney with enhancing septa (*arrowhead*)

11 studies reported a pooled sensitivity of 88% and specificity of 80% in differentiation between benign and malignant renal tumors by CEUS [11].

Ultrasound elastography is an emerging technique based on measuring elasticity of biological tissues by calculating their response to manually applied force by US probe or propagating sound waves. Since malignant renal tumors are assumed to be stiffer than benign tumors, it has been suggested that US elastography can be used to differentiate benign and malignant renal tumors (Fig. 1.7). Although successful results imply the utility of US elastography in differentiation between benign and malignant renal tumors, determination of subtypes of renal tumors seems to be unpredictable by this technique [12].

Assessment of renal vein involvement is mandatory in case of renal cancers. Renal veins should be visualized from renal hilum to inferior vena cava (IVC) on CDUS to detect hypo- or hyperechoic filling defect with solid appearance in renal vein representing tumoral thrombus. CDUS is comparable to MRI for detecting tumoral extension to renal veins and inferior vena cava with a sensitivity of 86% and specificity of 94% [13–15].

Main limitation of US in assessment of renal tumors is difficulty to detect and characterize small renal masses. One study showed that 42% of renal lesions between 15 and 20 mm were not detected on US while CT detected 100% of lesions [16]. User dependency which may cause interobserver variability in follow-up of lesions is another limitation of US.

Intraoperative US yields high-resolution images in partial nephrectomies and enucleation of tumors. Intraoperative US can demonstrate new findings which were not detected on preoperative imaging in 10.6% of cases and alters the surgical management in 71.4% of patients with renal cancers [17].

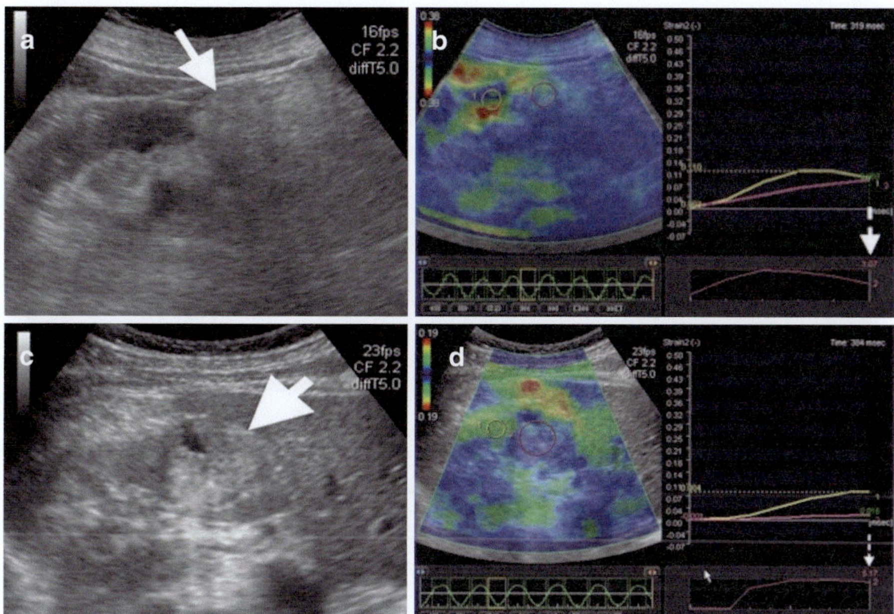

Fig. 1.7 Ultrasound elastography of renal masses. (**a**) Grayscale US image of a 48-year-old female demonstrates hyperechoic mass (*arrow*) representing angiomyolipoma. (**b**) Strain elastography of the mass depicts strain index value as 1.07 (*dashed arrow*) corresponding to benign renal mass. (**c**) Grayscale US image of a 55-year-old male with RCC reveals hyperechoic solid mass (*arrow*) in the kidney. (**d**) Strain elastography depicts strain index value of the mass as 5.17 (*dashed arrow*) representing increased stiffness and likelihood of malignancy of the mass

1.2.2.2 Computed Tomography

Computed tomography is the decision-making imaging technique in assessment of renal tumors. Awareness of sonographic imaging features of renal mass may be helpful for planning CT protocol since renal parenchymal or pelvis tumors should be scanned with different CT protocols. The use of intravenous (IV) iodinated contrast material and ionizing radiation in CT examination mandates appropriate planning of CT protocol. Multiphasic CT protocols used in the evaluation of renal mass include precontrast scanning and corticomedullary (scan delay 35–40 s after IV contrast injection), nephrographic (scan delay 70–90 s after IV contrast injection), and delayed excretory (scan delay 5–10 min after IV contrast injection) phases [18]. Precontrast images demonstrate calcifications in the renal masses and yield a baseline density measurement to compare enhancement degree and pattern of the tumors on contrast-enhanced images. Precontrast CT is also critical in depicting hypovascular hemorrhagic cysts which may be misdiagnosed on contrast-enhanced images as hypovascular papillary RCC [19]. In these cases, unenhanced CT demonstrates hyperdense appearance of hemorrhagic cysts secondary to high attenuation of the

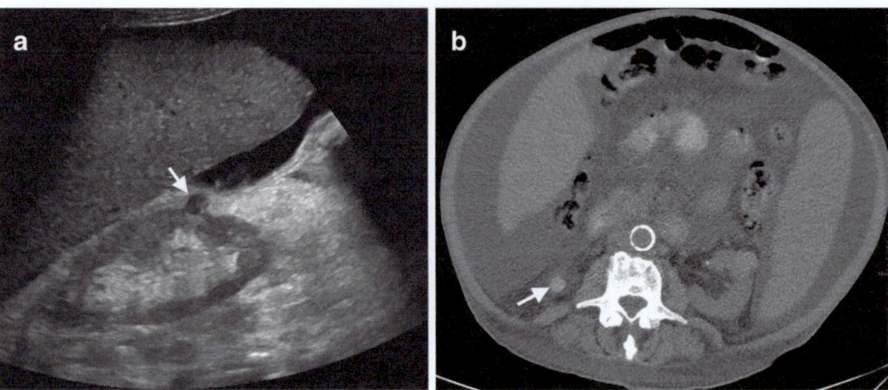

Fig. 1.8 Hemorrhagic cyst. (**a**) Grayscale US image of a 45-year-old female shows well-circumscribed hypoechoic cyst-like mass (*arrow*) located near the lower pole of the right kidney. The absence of posterior acoustic enhancement suggests probability of solid mass. (**b**) Precontrast axial CT image reveals hyperattenuation in the mass (*arrow*) representing hemorrhagic cyst

blood on CT and helps to realize pseudoenhancement of hemorrhagic cysts on contrast-enhanced CT images (Fig. 1.8). Corticomedullary images demonstrate lesion vascularity and renal vascular anatomy. Renal cortex enhances more than renal medulla in corticomedullary phase. Images acquired on this phase may help to distinguish hypervascular clear cell carcinoma from hypovascular papillary cell carcinoma [19]. However renal masses localized in renal medulla may be missed on corticomedullary phase images. In nephrographic phase renal parenchyma enhances homogeneously with similar enhancement in renal cortex and medulla. Renal tumors manifest as less enhancing solid or semisolid lesions compared to renal parenchyma (Fig. 1.9). This phase is the most helpful imaging phase for detection and characterization of renal masses [20]. Nephrographic phase images have superiority in detection especially small (<3 cm) renal masses in the renal parenchyma [18]. Excretory images are helpful to delineate renal collecting systems, ureters, and bladder with tumoral involvement of these structures (Fig. 1.9).

Malignant potential of a renal mass increases with presence of significant enhancement which is defined as an attenuation increase of at least 15–20 HU on postcontrast images with respect to the precontrast image [20]. Enhancement of a lesion up to 10 HU is defined as pseudoenhancement which may be encountered in some renal cysts. Enhancement of 10–20 HU in a renal mass on CT refers to indeterminate mass that necessitates assessment with MRI. Other scanning phases give additional valuable information for presurgical planning. Contrast enhancement characteristics of renal masses can be a distinguishing feature in prediction of subtypes of RCCs. Conventional type or clear cell type of RCC as being most frequently detected RCC subtype presents usually as well-circumscribed, heterogeneous mass containing usually two components as solid hypervascular portion and necrotic or hemorrhagic necrotic, avascular portion [21]. Typical clear cell RCC manifests with intense enhancement in the corticomedullary phase and less enhancement

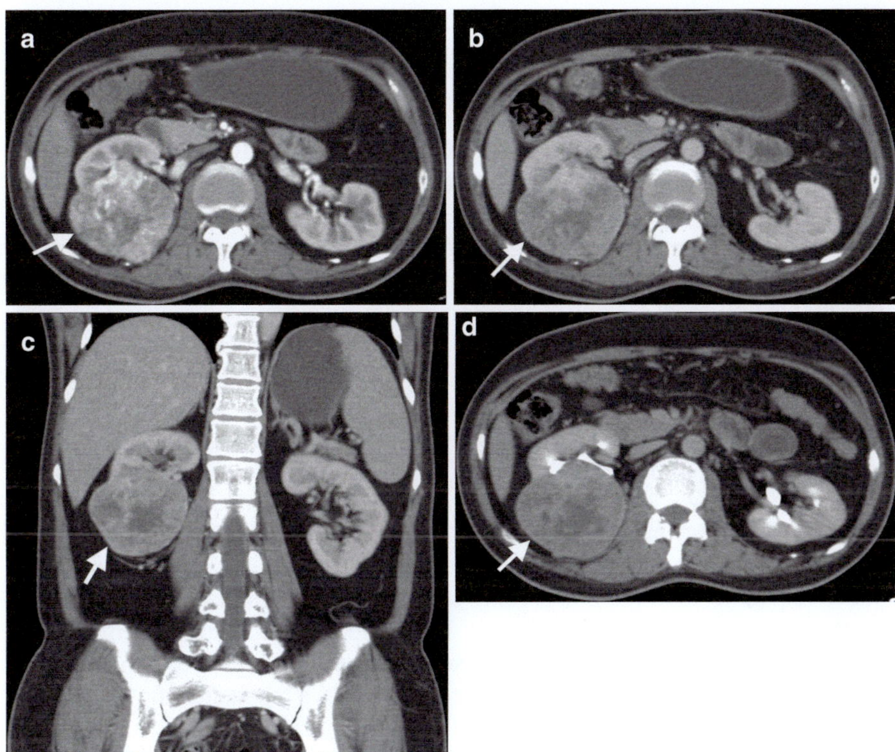

Fig. 1.9 Multiphasic CT of clear cell RCC. (**a**) Axial CT image obtained at corticomedullary phase reveals hypervascular solid mass (*arrow*) arising from the inferior pole of the right kidney. (**b**) Axial and (**c**) coronal CT images at nephrogram phase demonstrate solid mass (*arrows*) enhancing less than adjacent renal parenchyma. (**d**) Axial excretory phase CT image reveals splaying of inferior collecting system by the mass (*arrow*)

compared to renal parenchyma at nephrographic phase. Papillary RCCs were reported as homogeneously enhancing renal mass in comparison to renal parenchyma and other subtypes of RCC [22, 23]. A hypovascular solid renal mass without fat content usually suggests papillary RCC as 82% of the cases manifest with less than or equal to 40 HU enhancement [24].

Small renal lesions which are smaller than 10 mm constitute a challenge for both urooncologists and radiologists. Characterization of renal masses less than 1 centimeter is frequently difficult on CT [21]. If a renal parenchymal lesion appears hypodense compared with the renal cortex on precontrast CT images with the density values of <10 HU or <−20 HU regardless of density values after IV contrast administration, these lesions can be assumed to be a benign renal parenchymal lesion mostly renal cortical cyst and small angiomyolipoma, respectively [21]. When density measurement of small renal parenchymal lesions does not yield any informative value, these lesions can be defined as “indeterminate microlesion, with no suspect characteristics” and can be followed up with imaging [21].

Cystic renal masses detected on CT should be interrogated in terms of malignancy. Bosniak classification system is widely accepted as a reliable tool to define complicated cystic renal masses for likelihood of malignancy. Although Bosniak classification was firstly introduced as CT classification system, the classification scheme may also be applied to MRI [25]. According to Bosniak classification system, category I lesions refer to simple cysts. Category II lesions have smooth septa and minimal wall thickening. Category I and II lesions are benign lesions requiring no further workup. Category IIF lesions include well-marginated cysts with enhancing or nonenhancing multiple hairline-thin septa and nonenhancing high-attenuation renal lesions. These lesions are indeterminate moderately complicated cystic renal masses that require follow-up to demonstrate stability. Category III lesions have thickened wall or septa and include some imaging features suspicious of malignancy that may be managed surgically. The presence of solid component in cystic renal mass refers to Bosniak category IV lesion and indicates high suspicion for malignancy (Fig. 1.10). Category IV lesions are managed surgically. Pseudoenhancement which is characterized as increased density in the cyst wall or septa after IV contrast administration is a pitfall that can cause misdiagnosis of cystic renal malignancy. Pseudoenhancement of cystic renal masses results from volume averaging and beam-hardening effects on CT [22]. Smaller renal cysts tend to be more amenable to pseudoenhancement [26]. Hemorrhagic cysts can present with pseudoenhancement; however hyperdense appearance of hemorrhagic cysts on precontrast CT is characteristic for hemorrhagic cysts.

CT can easily identify macroscopic fat in renal masses. The diagnosis of angiomyolipoma can be established safely on CT when the density of a mass measured as <−20 HU with no content of calcification or necrosis [21]. However RCCs may rarely present with fat component. Fat content in a RCC mostly occurs in papillary cell type [27]. In the setting of fat-containing renal mass, the possibility of

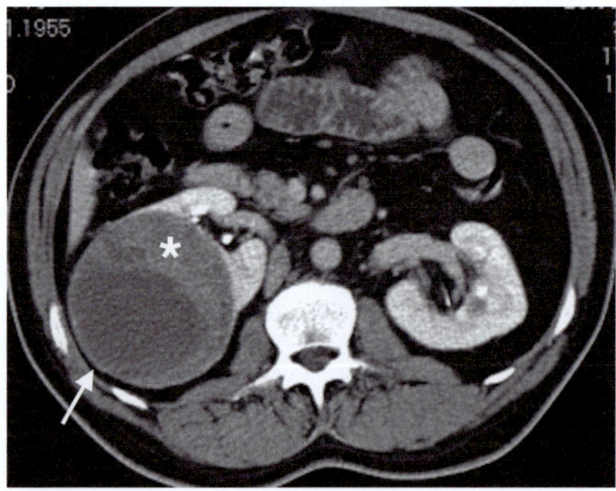

Fig. 1.10 Cystic RCC. Axial contrast-enhanced CT demonstrates cystic mass (*arrow*) with enhancing solid component (*asterisk*) classified as Bosniak category IV and surgically proved to be RCC

malignancy should be thought if a large, solid, infiltrating, and heterogeneous lesion is detected on CT. Calcifications may be encountered in 30% of RCCs which are typically central and irregular [21]. Invasion of the renal vein and inferior vena cava (IVC) occurs in 23% and 7% of RCCs, respectively [28] (Fig. 1.11).

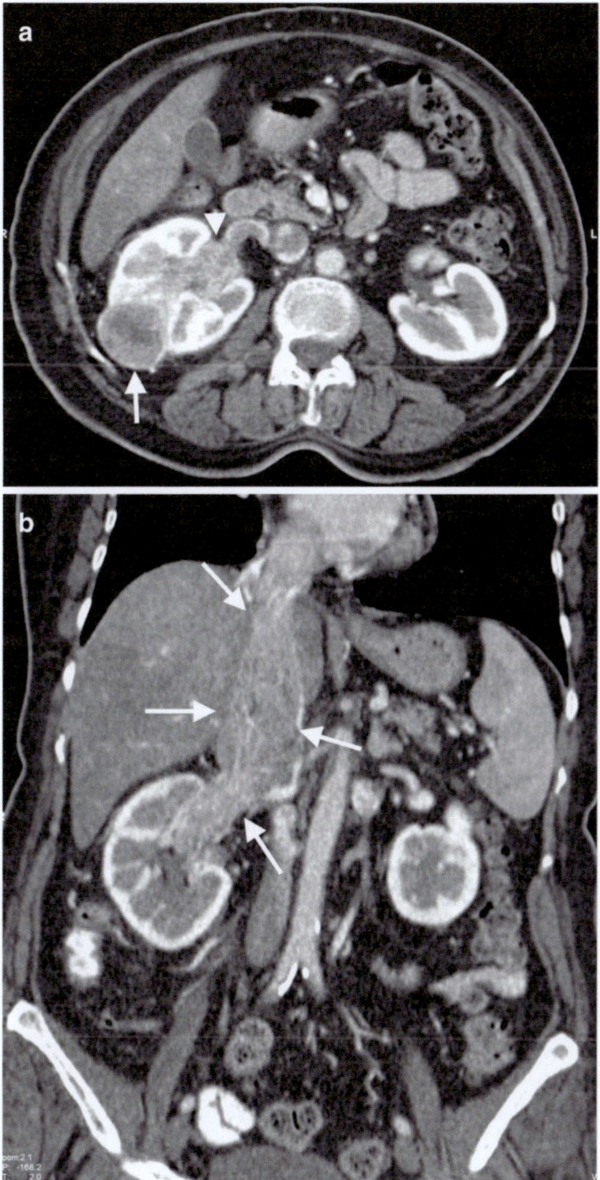

Fig. 1.11 RCC with venous invasion. (**a**) Axial contrast-enhanced CT of a 66-year-old female with RCC demonstrates a solid renal mass (*arrow*) in the interpolar region of the right kidney and invasion of the renal vein with tumor (*arrowhead*). (**b**) Coronal contrast-enhanced CT reveals tumoral invasion of the right renal vein and extension of the tumor thrombus to the right atrium through IVC (*arrows*)

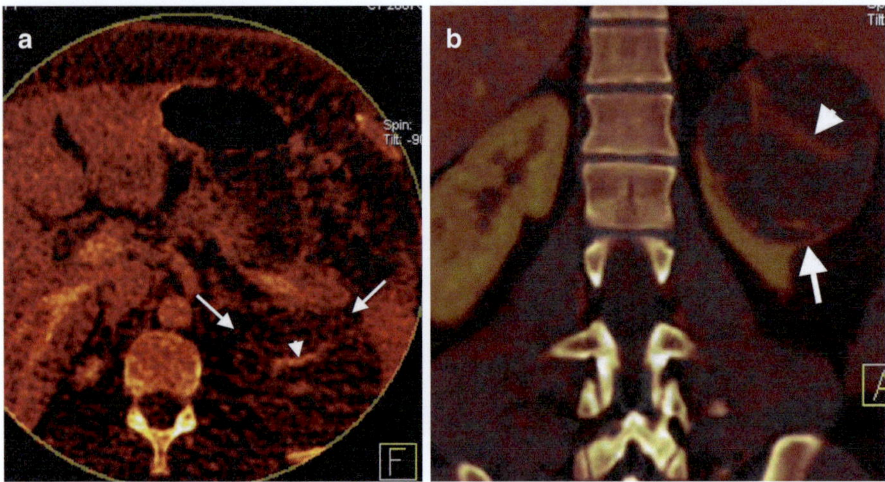

Fig. 1.12 Dual-energy CT of renal mass. Axial iodine overlay (**a**) and coronal mixed (**b**) images of DECT reveal a cystic mass (*arrows*) at the upper pole of the left kidney with a septum formation that uptakes iodine (*arrowhead*)

RENAL nephrometry scoring system is a numerical scoring system of imaging features of renal mass on CT or MRI including maximal tumor radius, exophytic versus endophytic nature of the tumor, relationship of the tumor to the collecting system or sinus, location relative to polar lines, and anterior or posterior tumor location [20]. It was reported that RENAL nephrometry scoring system can be used as a predictor of surgical outcomes of laparoscopic partial nephrectomy and histology and grade of RCCs [29].

Dual-energy CT (DECT) is an evolving CT technology, which is characterized by simultaneous acquisition of CT data with two different energies or peak tube voltages [30]. In this technology different tissues in the organs can be separated by attenuation difference behavior at two different tube voltage levels. Virtual unenhanced CT images can be acquired which contributes to decreasing ionizing radiation dose up to 47% compared to multiphasic CT examination [31]. Iodine content of the renal masses instead of attenuation values (HU) after IV contrast administration can be measured with this technique (Fig. 1.12). DECT can also be helpful to demonstrate pseudoenhancement of renal masses [32].

1.2.2.3 Magnetic Resonance Imaging

Magnetic resonance imaging (MRI) is a problem-solving tool in characterizing renal tumors with its high soft tissue contrast and multiplanar imaging capabilities [33]. MRI can depict water and fat content of renal tumors. Benign and malignant renal tumors may be more accurately differentiated by MRI due to capability of obtaining various sequences which enable to determine fat and water content of renal masses. MRI was shown to be better in evaluating renal lesions which were previously deemed indeterminate on CT [34].

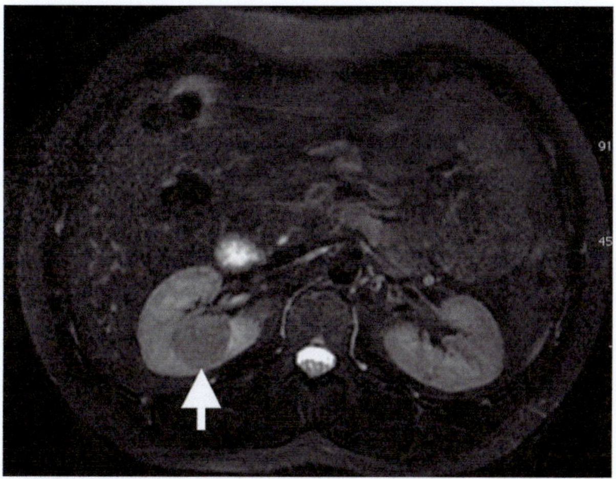

Fig. 1.13 Papillary RCC. Axial T2-W MRI of a 72-year-old male demonstrates a well-circumscribed hypointense mass (*arrow*) in the right kidney

Renal mass evaluation with MRI should include T1-W axial in- and out-of-phase gradient-echo sequence to identify macroscopic and microscopic fat, T2-W axial and coronal sequences to evaluate overall anatomy, renal collecting system, and complexity of cystic renal lesions and dynamic contrast-enhanced (DCE) T1-W fat-suppressed sequences consisting of corticomedullary, nephrographic, and excretory phases. Renal tumors usually appear hypointense on T1-W and hyperintense on T2-W images, while papillary cell RCCs manifest as hypointense lesions on T2-W images (Fig. 1.13). Cystic renal masses can be more easily and accurately characterized by MRI compared to CT. The presence and thickness of septa, wall thickness, and contrast enhancement patterns of renal cystic lesions can be depicted on DCE-MR images. Coronal T1-W images at excretory phase with administration of diuretics can delineate collecting system and ureters and may be helpful in the diagnosis of TCCs.

DWI technique is increasingly used in the assessment of renal tumors. Solid renal tumors demonstrate increased signal intensity on DW images and decreased signal intensity on ADC maps secondary to restricted diffusion of water molecules in renal tumors (Fig. 1.14). DWI has potential to discriminate malignant renal tumors from benign tumors with ADC measurements. It was shown that malignant renal masses have lower ADC values than benign renal masses (Fig. 1.15) [19]. The ADC values of clear cell RCC were shown to be significantly higher than chromophobe and papillary cell RCC which may be helpful to differentiate these subtypes of RCC [35, 36].

Superiority of MRI over other imaging techniques is most remarkable on renal cystic masses with high protein content and hemorrhage. Since these lesions demonstrate high density on precontrast images and may show pseudoenhancement on contrast-enhanced CT images, their diagnosis may be difficult on MDCT.

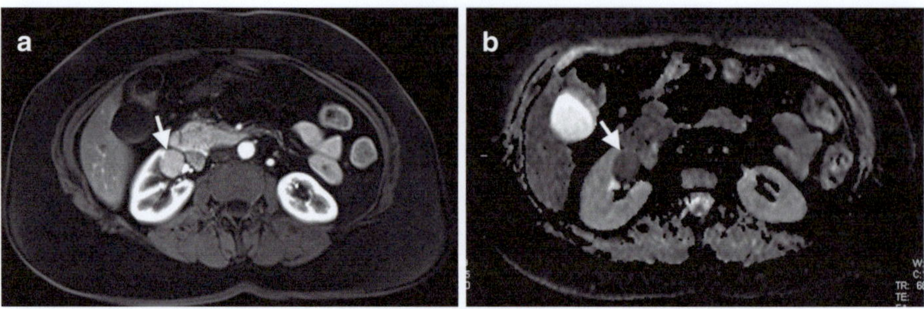

Fig. 1.14 DWI of renal cancer. (**a**) Contrast-enhanced T1-W MRI of a 62-year-old male with chromophobe RCC demonstrates enhancing solid mass (*arrow*) in the right kidney. (**b**) Renal mass presents with signal loss (*arrow*) secondary to restricted diffusion on ADC map

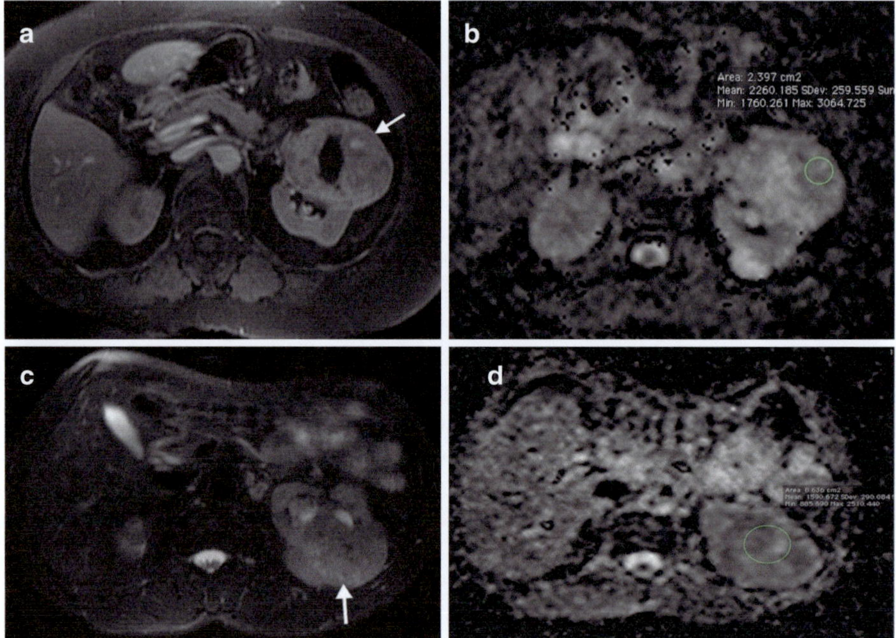

Fig. 1.15 ADC values of benign and malignant renal masses. (**a**) Axial contrast-enhanced fat-saturated T1-W image of a 44-year-old female with oncocytoma reveals enhancing solid mass (*arrow*) with nonenhancing central scar. (**b**) ADC value of the mass on ADC map image is measured as 2.26 mm^2/s. (**c**) Axial T2-W image of a 66-year-old male with chromophobe RCC reveals a hyperintense solid mass (*arrow*) arising from the left kidney. (**d**) ADC value of the mass on ADC map image is measured as 1.59 mm^2/s

MRI provides a solution for this problem with subtraction technique. With MRI subtraction technique, precontrast MR image of a T1-W hyperintense lesion can be subtracted from contrast-enhanced image of same lesion (Fig. 1.16). MRI was shown to be superior than CT on depicting additional septa, thickening of the wall

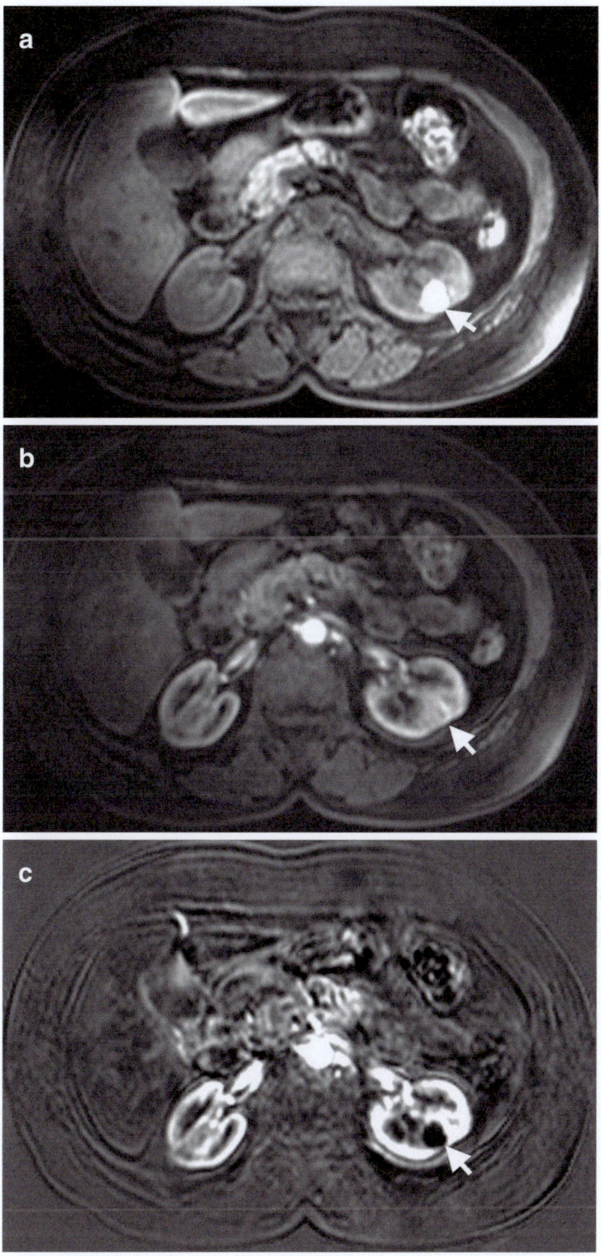

Fig. 1.16 Renal complex cyst on subtraction MRI. (**a**) Axial fat-suppressed T1-W image shows a hyperintense mass (*arrow*) in the left kidney. (**b**) Axial contrast-enhanced T1-W image demonstrates left kidney mass with hyperintense appearance (*arrow*) suggesting contrast enhancement. (**c**) Subtraction image reveals signal loss (*arrow*) in the mass confirming nonenhancement of the mass

or septa, or enhancement of the complex renal cysts [25]. Application of Bosniak criteria to cystic lesions on MRI may lead to upstaging of lesions in 10% of cases which were previously categorized on CT [25].

MRI is also a key imaging tool for differentiation between fat-poor angiomyolipomas (AMLs) from RCC. A study using combination of MR sequences reported sensitivity, specificity, and accuracy values of 73%, 99%, and 96%, respectively, in distinguishing AML from RCC [37].

Multiparametric MRI (mp-MRI) of the kidney refers to acquisition of DCE-MRI, DWI, and perfusion MRI for evaluation of renal tumors. Perfusion MRI techniques including arterial spin labeling (ASL) and blood-oxygen-level-dependent (BOLD) MRI were reported to be helpful in distinguishing between benign and malignant renal masses with the capability of obtaining high-temporal-resolution images compared to conventional dynamic MRI. ASL is characterized by using the endogenous contrast properties of arterial blood and noninvasively labeling inflowing spins without exogenous contrast material administration [38]. ASL was shown to be helpful in distinguishing between RCC and oncocytomas as well as between papillary RCCs from other subtypes of RCC [38, 39]. BOLD MRI may be helpful for distinguishing RCCs from AMLs at 3 T MRI and for differentiation between benign cystic lesions from RCCs [40].

Although gadolinium-based contrast agents that are used in MRI were thought as safe contrast agents before, it is well known that these patients especially ones with impaired kidney function are at the risk of nephrogenic systemic fibrosis. Therefore, the use of gadolinium contrast in patients with low glomerular filtration rate (<30 mL/min/1.73 m^2) is not recommended according to guidelines of American College of Radiology unless risk-benefit assessment favors the use of gadolinium contrast agent [20].

Malignant Tumors of Renal Pelvis

Transitional cell carcinomas and squamous cell carcinomas (SCC) represent 90% and 10% of pelvicalyceal malignant tumors (PMTs), respectively [41]. TCC may present as multifocal, synchronous, or metachronous lesions, which necessitate evaluation of all urinary tract with cross-sectional imaging studies. Computed tomography urography (CTU) enables evaluation of pelvicalyceal system of the kidneys, ureters, and bladder.

PMT manifest as focal mass or thickening of the wall of the urinary tract. US may not detect PMT presenting with thickening of the pelvis or ureteral wall. However focal mass forming PMT can be visualized on US as hypoechoic mass replacing hyperechoic renal sinus fat (Fig. 1.5).

CTU is essential for evaluating PMT especially for detection of synchronous lesions in the entire urinary tract. Mean attenuation value of these tumors (30 HU) is different from water (mean HU, 0), blood clot (mean HU, 50–75), and calculi (mean HU >100) [42]. PMTs enhance mildly or moderately on arterial phase images and manifest with washout on delayed phase images on CT [43]. Renal pelvis tumors most frequently manifest as filling defect in the renal pelvis at excretory

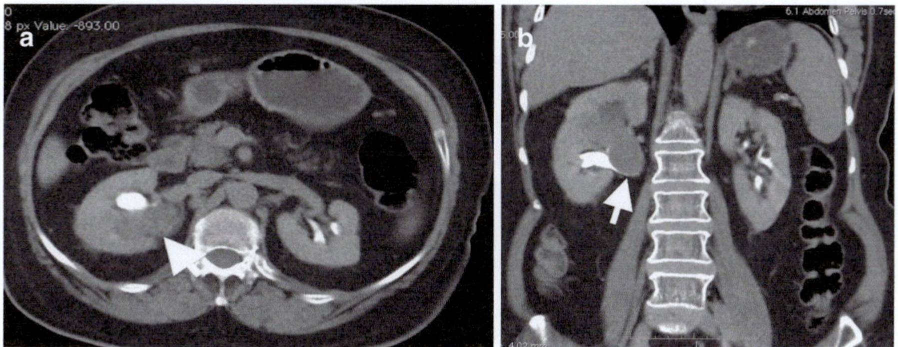

Fig. 1.17 Transitional cell carcinoma of renal pelvis. Axial (**a**) and coronal (**b**) CTU excretory phase images of a 74-year-old male reveal filling defect at the inferior portion of the renal pelvis and calyces caused by solid mass (*arrows*)

phase images (Fig. 1.17). Superficial TCCs can be diagnosed based on the CT features as focal or diffuse mural thickening, focally obstructed calyces, or sessile filling defects within the hyperdense pelvicalyceal system or ureters filled with iodinated contrast material. Renal collecting system may be expanded, and renal fat sinus may be compressed due to mass effect of the PMT. Renal parenchymal invasion may be observed on aggressive and advanced stage of TCC that represents 15% of these tumors and can mimic renal parenchymal malignancies invading renal collecting system [43]. Renal parenchymal invasion of PMT can be defined as obliterated renal sinus fat plane between the mass and renal parenchyma on CT. TCC is more likely to be located centrally and expand the kidney centrifugally with less likely causing contour irregularities compared to RCC invading renal collecting system [44]. CT may play an important role in staging of PMT; however it cannot distinguish T1 tumor (limited to uroepithelium and lamina propria) from T2 tumor (tumor invading the muscularis propria) [22]. Early-stage PMT (T1 and T2) can be distinguished from advanced-stage tumors such as T3 (invading peripelvic fat or renal parenchyma) and T4 (invading adjacent organs or abdominal wall or extending perinephric fat) [22].

Metastases

Renal metastases usually manifest as bilateral and multifocal masses. If a solid renal mass is detected in a patient with extrarenal malignancy and metastases in other organs, probability of the diagnosis of renal metastasis is more likely [45]. However in the absence of other organ metastasis, a solid renal mass is less likely to be a metastasis even in the setting of primary extrarenal malignancy [46]. Renal metastases frequently appear as more infiltrative and less vascular masses compared to clear cell RCCs in the renal parenchyma. Differentiation between primary renal malignancies and metastases is usually difficult according to imaging features on cross-sectional imaging which often necessitate biopsy of the mass in the setting of solitary solid renal mass in patients with extrarenal primary malignancy.

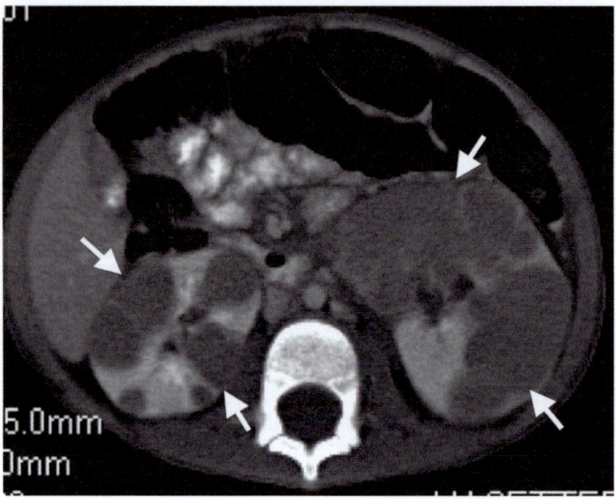

Fig. 1.18 Renal lymphoma. Axial contrast-enhanced CT demonstrates bilateral multiple focal renal parenchymal masses (*arrows*) suggesting lymphomatous involvement of the kidneys

Lymphoma

Lymphoma should be kept in mind in the differential diagnosis of extraprimary solid renal tumors since lymphoma is the third most common tumor involving the kidney after lung and breast cancer [47]. Primary renal lymphoma is a rare condition. Secondary renal lymphoma occurs due to invasion of the kidney by retroperitoneal lymphomatous tissue or hematogenous spread from distant sources. Renal lymphoma may present with diffuse infiltrating type or focal masses in the renal parenchyma.

US demonstrates hypoechoic, infiltrative focal masses in the renal parenchyma. CT is more helpful in the diagnosis of renal lymphoma than US. Diffuse infiltrating renal lymphoma may appear with nephromegaly and heterogeneously enhanced renal parenchyma on contrast-enhanced CT. Focal renal masses show homogeneous and a lower degree of enhancement than renal parenchyma with a relatively little mass effect (Fig. 1.18). Infiltrative renal lymphoma which arises from retroperitoneal lymphoid tissue presents with typical appearance that is characterized by infiltration of renal sinus without obstructing the renal collecting system and invasion of renal hilar vasculature. Renal contours are not usually deformed unless infiltrative lesion becomes enlarged and extended to perirenal fat tissue. Perirenal infiltration of lymphoma without parenchymal involvement is less common form of the disease.

Primary Renal Mesenchymal Tumors

Primary renal mesenchymal tumors are rare and include some imaging findings that can be helpful for diagnosis for these tumors. These tumors consist of leiomyosarcoma, liposarcoma, fibrosarcoma, malignant fibrous histiocytoma, rhabdomyosarcoma, osteosarcoma, chondrosarcoma, malignant peripheral nerve sheath tumor, synovial sarcoma, and angiosarcoma [41].

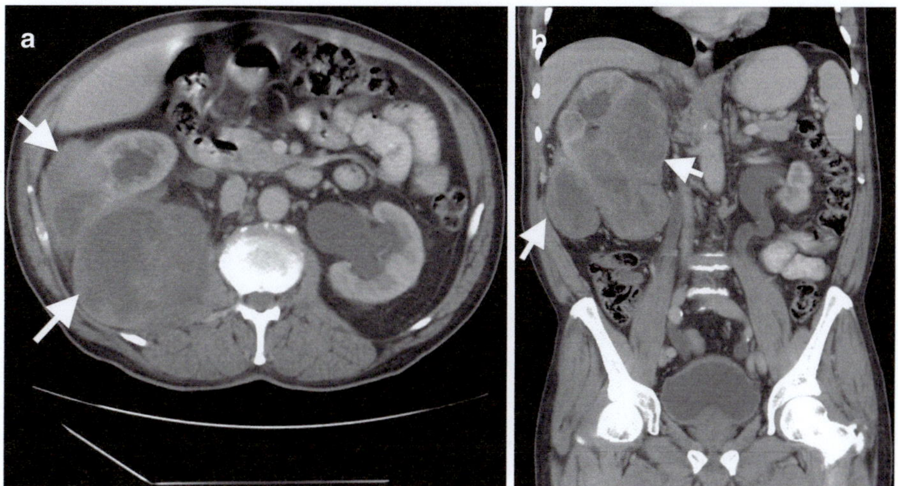

Fig. 1.19 Perirenal sarcoma. Axial (**a**) and coronal (**b**) contrast-enhanced CT images demonstrate large soft tissue mass (*arrows*) arising from renal capsule and extending to the perirenal area

Renal sarcomas arise from the peripheral part of the kidney, mostly renal capsule, and present as a peripherally extending, large, heterogeneous mass rather than parenchymal mass (Fig. 1.19). A smooth interface between sarcomas and renal parenchyma is usually visualized on CT or MRI. Necrosis with large area is more frequently encountered in sarcomas than RCC. Liposarcomas as one of the most frequently encountered mesenchymal tumors of the kidney should be differentiated from angiomyolipomas (AMLs) since both of these lesions contain large amount of fat tissue. Most characteristic differentiating imaging feature between these entities is the presence of renal parenchymal defect at the site of the AML's origin. It may be difficult to define the parenchymal defect in large AMLs. In this setting, the presence of intratumoral hemorrhage, the smaller oversize of the lesion, and the presence of other AMLs in the renal parenchyma may be helpful in distinguishing AML from liposarcoma.

1.2.3 Staging of Renal Tumors

Staging of renal tumors is conducted through TNM system. Preoperative planning and prognosis of renal cancers are associated with accurate staging. In renal cancer staging, it is important to determine perirenal tumor extension. Although perirenal tumor spread does not affect the treatment plan, it is a prognostic factor. Perirenal stranding which may be suggested as an indicator of perirenal tumoral spread on CT and MRI is not a reliable finding since 50% of renal tumors confined in the renal capsule was reported to present with perirenal stranding [48]. A pseudocapsule that is composed of compressed renal parenchyma and fibrosis envelopes renal tumors. An intact pseudocapsule which can be well demonstrated on T2-W MR images as

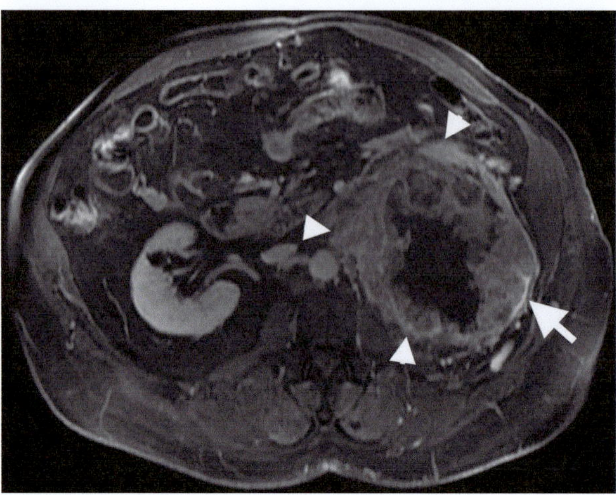

Fig. 1.20 Perirenal invasion of renal cancer. Axial fat-suppressed contrast-enhanced T1-W image shows tumoral mass (*arrows*) arising from the left kidney and invading perirenal fat tissue (*arrowheads*)

hypointense linear structure may represent absence of perirenal tumor spread [49]. Involvement of renal capsule or Gerota fascia can be better evaluated by MRI than CT due to superiority of MRI in depicting perirenal fat invasion and fat planes with its high contrast resolution (Fig. 1.20) [50].

Staging of renal tumors should include interrogation of venous extension of the tumors. Since patients with renal malignancy may be prone to venous thromboembolism, it is important to distinguish bland thrombus and tumoral thrombus in the setting of renal venous and/or IVC thrombosis. Bland thrombus of the venous system presents with nonenhanced filling defect confined to venous vessel, while tumoral thrombus usually appears as contrast enhanced, vessel expanding, and usually upward projected into the IVC on CT or MRI. MR imaging has been assumed as more capable than CT in evaluation of vascular extension, differentiation of perihilar lymph nodes from hilar vessels, and assessment of direct invasion of renal tumors to the adjacent tissues [21].

Renal cancers mostly metastasize to the lung, bone, brain, liver, and mediastinum [20]. Chest radiograph is the first step in the evaluation of lung metastases; however chest CT may be required in the presence of abnormal chest radiography findings.

Liver metastases can be detected on US examination. Solid or cystic lesions detected on US and suspected as metastatic lesions may be evaluated with CT or MRI. Renal cancer metastasis originated particularly from clear cell RCC manifest as hypervascular liver metastases.

1.2.4 Intervention in Renal Masses

The biopsy of renal masses is not usually required for management. Limited indications of renal mass biopsy include assessment of patients for percutaneous ablative treatment, high suspicion of renal metastasis from other tumors or lymphomatous involvement, suspected nephroblastoma in a young adult, and non-negligible probability of a benign histology with imaging features suggesting oncocytoma or low-fat angiomyolipoma [21].

Thermal ablation techniques including radio frequency ablation (RF), cryoablation, microwaves, laser, and focused ultrasound ablation have become generally well-known treatment alternatives for renal tumors in surgically at-risk patients. Since nearly 50% of renal tumors are detected incidentally and these tumors are usually at small size without advanced-stage treatment, strategy of these tumors may involve radiologically guided thermal ablation techniques [51]. Percutaneous ablation of renal tumors can be performed under the guidance of US, CT, or MRI. Percutaneous route has the advantages of less pain, immediate verification of ablation efficiency, shorter period of hospitalization, and reduced overall cost [52]. Thermal ablation techniques are usually used percutaneously; however laparoscopic thermal ablation may also be used in anteriorly positioned renal tumors. A meta-analysis study revealed overall complication rates of laparoscopic and percutaneous radio frequency techniques as 7.4% and 3.1%, respectively [52].

US guidance in renal tumor ablation enables fast and accurate positioning of the applicators. However formation of hyperechoic gas bubbles after RF ablation and ice crystals after cryotherapy may prevent visualization of posttreatment changes at the tumor site [53]. CT is the best guidance method for percutaneous ablation of renal tumors for localizing the tumor, controlling the procedure, and diagnosing immediate complications.

RF ablation is effective in renal tumors less than 4 cm, while cryoablation and microwave ablation techniques can be used in larger tumors. Local recurrence-free survival at 5 years after RF ablation was reported as 89–92% [54, 55]. Most recurrences after RF ablation occur during the first year [56]. Technical failure of this technique increases with size increase (>4 cm) and sinus extension of the tumor [57].

Cryotherapy is characterized by destruction of tumor cells using freeze/thaw cycles [53]. The freezing cycle produces ice crystals which cause denaturation of intracellular proteins, destruction of cell structures, and modification of cell membrane function. This cycle permits inflow of water into the intracellular compartment resulting in burst tumor cells. Cryoablation allows monitoring the ablation zone in real time which is important to visualize the tissue changes close to the adjacent sensitive organs. Central renal tumors are more available for cryotherapy as this technique does not damage the urothelium [53]. Cryotherapy has lower rates of reoperation (1.3%), tumor progression (5.2%), and frequency of metastases (1%) compared to RF with corresponding rates of 8.5%, 12.9%, and 2.5%, respectively [58].

In microwave ablation technique, larger tumors can be treated in less time with uniform cell death in the ablation zone since ablation is not limited by desiccation, carbonization, or thermal convection [59].

Complications of renal tumor ablation consist of bleeding (0–30%), pneumothorax (1–2%), pain (4.5%), thermal injuries of the digestive tract (0–1%) and urinary tract (less than 4%), infection (0–2%), and tumor dissemination [53].

Follow-up of patients with renal tumor ablation should be performed 2, 6, and 12 months after ablation with US, CT, or MRI in the first year, and annual follow-up is required in the following 5 years [53]. Necrotic and hemorrhagic changes in ablation zone may mimic recurrence with increased signal intensity on T1-W MR images. In the setting of this circumstance, subtraction MR images can reveal true unenhanced or enhanced area in the ablation zone.

1.3 Bladder Cancer

1.3.1 General Information

Bladder cancer is the sixth most commonly diagnosed malignancy in the United States [60]. Main purpose of imaging in bladder cancer is optimized pretreatment staging for guiding appropriate treatment. Staging of bladder cancer should include assessment of bladder wall involvement and local, regional, nodal, or distant visceral spread of the tumor. Bladder cancers most frequently manifest as non-muscle-invasive bladder cancer (NMIBC). As this form of bladder cancer has tendency to recur, close surveillance with imaging techniques is necessary. One quarter of patients with bladder cancer present as muscle-invasive bladder cancer (MIBC) [60]. Since radical cystectomy is required in the treatment of MIBC, local/regional extravesical tumor invasion and distant metastasis should be interrogated with CT or MRI.

Transitional cell carcinomas (TCCs) are the most frequently encountered bladder cancer. TCCs can be seen as papillary masses protruding to the bladder lumen or infiltrating mass causing focal or diffuse thickening of the bladder wall. Calcification rarely occurs in TCC. Squamous cell carcinomas are characterized by mass-like, aggressive, frequently calcified tumors often associated with chronic bladder wall inflammation or schistosomiasis. Adenocarcinomas mostly occur in patients with bladder exstrophy and urachal remnants usually localized in anterior and superior aspect of the bladder [61].

1.3.2 Imaging Features

1.3.2.1 Ultrasonography

Adequate distention of the bladder is essential for sonographic assessment of patients with suspicion of bladder cancer. Bladder cancers present as hypo- or isoechoic polypoid solid lesions protruding into the bladder lumen or sessile asymmetric thickening of bladder wall. CDUS usually demonstrates blood flow within the bladder cancer (Fig. 1.21). US has a sensitivity of 61–84% for polypoid bladder cancer larger than 5 mm [62]. Small polypoid tumors (<5 mm) can be easily missed on US. Hematomas can be differentiated from bladder tumors by visualizing mobility of hematomas with patient movement, absence of blood flow on CDUS, and fragmentation of solid-appearing mass by applying pressure by US transducer. US

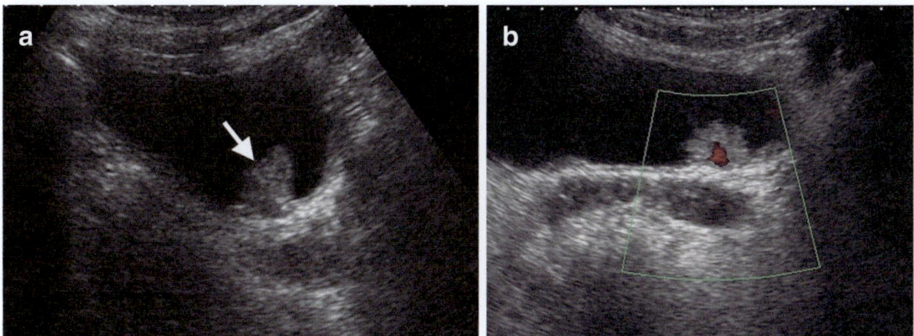

Fig. 1.21 Bladder cancer. (**a**) Grayscale US demonstrates solid papillary echogenic mass (*arrow*) arising from posterior wall of the bladder and protruding to the bladder lumen. (**b**) Power Doppler US reveals blood flow signal within the mass

can reveal the number, size, and appearance (sessile or pedicled) of bladder cancer and their topography relative to the prostatic urethra and to the ureteral meatus [63]. US can be more helpful in bladder cancer localized in a bladder diverticulum where cystoscopy may be insufficient for evaluation [64]. Three-dimensional (3D) virtual sonography combined with 2D sonography has a sensitivity of 96.4%, specificity of 88.8%, a positive predictive value (PPV) of 97.6%, and a negative predictive value (NPV) of 84.2% for detection of bladder cancer [65]. CEUS has higher sensitivity (88.5%) and specificity (88.9%) values for detection of bladder cancer compared to grayscale US [66].

1.3.2.2 Computed Tomography

CT is one of the most frequently used imaging techniques in detection, staging, and surveillance of the bladder cancer. American College of Radiology (ACR) appropriateness criteria refer CTU as the best initial imaging examination technique for the evaluation of hematuria [67]. CTU series generally include precontrast images and enhanced images at nephrographic phase and excretory phase. 3D reformatted images of the excretory phase of CTU demonstrate the entire urinary tract by delineating the tract with iodinated contrast agent. In order to reduce radiation dose during CTU, some institutions use split-bolus technique that refers to acquisition of nephrographic phase images and excretory phase images at same scanning time to demonstrate contrast-enhanced renal parenchyma and contrast agent-filled renal collecting system, ureters, and bladder in the same image series. This technique reduces the radiation dose of CTU; however contrast resolution of images may be diminished secondary to dilution of contrast agent in the urinary tract. Split-bolus technique reduces radiation dose and is comparable to that of intravenous urography (IVU) [65].

Stage T1 bladder cancers appear as pedunculated polypoid lesions or asymmetric thickening of the bladder wall on CT (Fig. 1.22). T2 tumors usually present as sessile lesions (Fig. 1.23). MDCT including excretory phase has 96% sensitivity and 99% specificity for detection of polypoid bladder cancers between 5 and 10 mm,

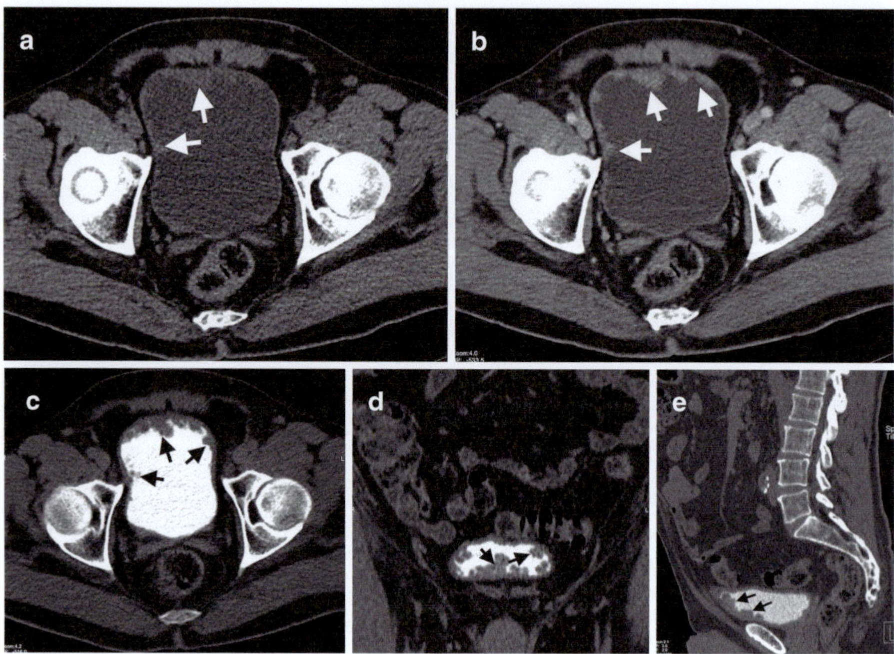

Fig. 1.22 Bladder cancer on CTU. (**a**) Axial precontrast CT image reveals thickening of anterior bladder wall with mild hyperdense appearance (*arrows*). (**b**) Axial contrast-enhanced CT image at venous phase demonstrates enhancement of the irregularly thickened anterior bladder wall (*arrows*). (**c**) Axial (**d**) coronal and (**e**) sagittal contrast-enhanced CT images at excretory phase reveal irregular filling defect in the anterior and inferior bladder wall (arrows) representing bladder cancer

89% sensitivity for polypoid lesions smaller than 5 mm, and 40% sensitivity for polypoid lesions smaller than 3 mm [68]. The specificity and NPV of CTU for detection of bladder cancer are higher in patients with hematuria than in patients without hematuria [69].

It should be kept in mind that the diagnostic efficiency of CT for detection of bladder cancer may be decreased when CT examination is performed shortly after bladder interventions such as biopsy or transurethral resection of the bladder (TURB). A study which compared the frequency of concordance between CT findings and histologic examinations showed that CT examinations performed 7 days after the bladder intervention were more in concordance with the histopathological results than CT examinations performed in the following 7 days after TURB [70].

CTU is frequently used in NMIBC patients to demonstrate involvement of upper urinary tract. CTU overweighs MRI in the evaluation of tumoral involvement in upper urinary tract owing to its higher spatial resolution [64]. Occult intramural or transmural extension of tumor and measurable pelvic lymphadenopathy suggestive of local spread of bladder cancer can be diagnosed with CT. Perivesical fat

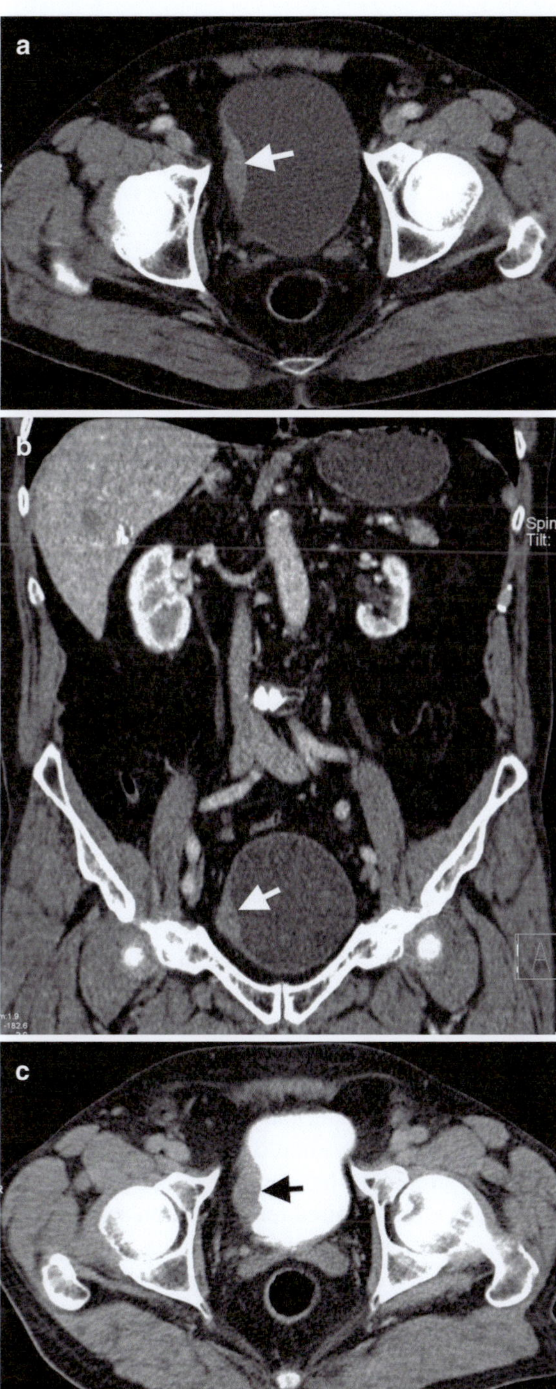

Fig. 1.23 Muscle-invasive bladder cancer on CTU. Axial (**a**) and coronal (**b**) contrast-enhanced CT images at venous phase reveal enhancing sessile mass (*arrow*) at the right bladder wall. (**c**) CTU image at excretory phase reveals filling defect (*arrow*) in the right bladder wall

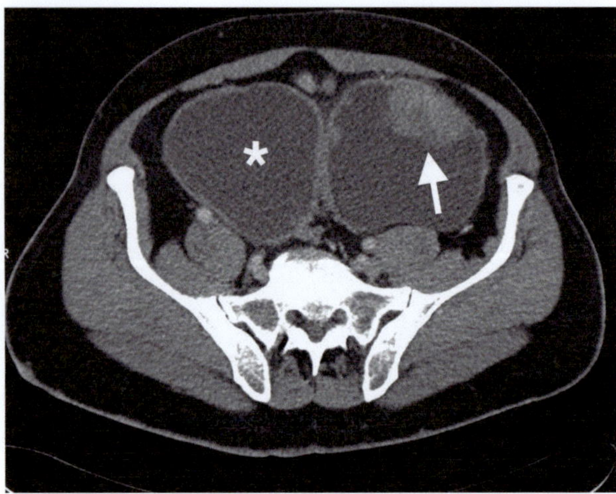

Fig. 1.24 Bladder cancer in diverticulum. Axial contrast-enhanced CT image demonstrates solid enhancing mass (*arrow*) arising from superior wall of the bladder diverticula (*asterisk*, bladder)

infiltration can be detected on CT with 89% sensitivity and 95% specificity values [68, 70]. Bladder tumors arising in the bladder diverticulum should be rigorously assessed in terms of perivesical fat invasion since muscularis mucosa layer is absent in the bladder diverticula (Fig. 1.24). Infiltration of prostate and seminal vesicles by bladder cancer can be detected on CT only when these organs were massively infiltrated. CT is helpful to assess possible invasion of digestive tract such as sigmoid colon or loops of the small intestine [68]. Distant metastasis including peritoneal carcinomatosis can also be detected with CT [71]. Multiplanar imaging capability of CT with thin slices provides 3D visualization of the entire urinary tract resembling IVU images. These 3D images may be easy to evaluate the urinary tract; however abnormalities visualized in 3D reconstructed images should be confirmed on axial images. In one study, 21 of 27 upper urinary tract neoplasms were missed using the 3D reconstructed images alone [72].

For monitoring NIMBC, CT urography is recommended every 2 years; however CT urography can be performed in the presence of positive cytology or any symptom indicating upper urinary tract involvement [68]. In monitoring patients with MIBC, CT urography should be performed every 6 months for 2 years after radical cystectomy followed by annual CT scanning [73].

Patients with impaired renal function are more susceptible to renal failure due to iodinated contrast agent nephrotoxicity which limits the use of CTU. Pelvic prostheses cause artifacts that prevent optimal assessment of bladder cancers especially localized at bladder base. Bladder cancers adjacent to prostate may be difficult to assess by CT since these lesions may be mistakenly defined as normal prostate or prostatic lesion protruding to the bladder lumen [74].

1.3.2.3 Magnetic Resonance Imaging

MRI technique in bladder cancer evaluation should include T2-weighted spin-echo sequences in at least three orthogonal and/or oblique planes, T1-weighted spin-echo axial sequence, fat-saturated T1-weighted axial sequence, and DWI and DCE-MRI sequences [63]. The use of endorectal coil may be more helpful to evaluate bladder cancers at the base, trigone, or posterior wall of the bladder [75]. Bladder cancers localized at the dome of the bladder can be interpreted better on sagittal and coronal planes. Lateral wall tumors are best evaluated on axial and coronal plane images. T2-W oblique sequences should be obtained perpendicular to the wall of the tumor to reduce partial volume effect that may cause false positivity in perivesical tumoral fat infiltration. Fat-saturated T1-weighted images are helpful to depict contours of the bladder [63].

Bladder cancers present with intermediate signal intensity similar to bladder wall muscle, hyperintense than urine and hypointense relative to perivesical fat on T1-W images. High signal intensity of perivesical fat on T1-W images diminishes in the presence of perivesical tumoral infiltration. On T2-weighted images, signal intensity of bladder cancers is lower than the signal from the urine and perivesical fat and higher than the wall (Fig. 1.25). A pedicle accompanies 75% of polypoid tumors [65]. This pedicle appears as a linear structure with poorly defined contours with lower signal intensity than that of the tumor on T2-W images. Contrast enhancement of tumor pedicle occurs later than tumor due to its fibrotic nature. Preservation of low signal intensity of the bladder wall indicates absence of muscle invasion by the tumor. MIBCs present with interruption of the hypointense bladder wall in tumor site on T2-W images (Fig. 1.26).

Contrast-enhanced T1-W images of MRI are helpful for detection and delineation contours of bladder cancers in order to determine perivesical infiltration. Bladder cancers are known as hypervascular tumors characterized by early enhancement compared to bladder wall. Contrast-enhanced images obtained at 15–25 s after IV gadolinium injection are more helpful in distinguishing bladder cancer from bladder wall. After that phase, uninvolved bladder wall becomes enhanced more than tumors. Missing early phase images of MRI due to technical reasons may result in underdiagnosis of especially small bladder cancers. Contrast-enhanced MRI may be misleading and cause false-positive results secondary to nodular or sessile contrast-enhanced lesions in the bladder wall mimicking bladder cancers in the following situations: inflammatory peritumoral neovascularization, post-biopsy, post-endovesical instillation, and post-radiotherapy fibrosis [65].

Contrast-enhanced dynamic MR images can differentiate T1 stage tumors from higher-stage tumors with 75–92% accuracy [76]. MRI examinations performed with endorectal coil can better delineate submucosal layer of the bladder wall, which may be helpful to differentiate T1 tumors from T2 tumors. The sensitivity and specificity values of MRI in distinguishing T2 stage or below from a T3 stage or higher were reported as 86% and 84%, respectively [77]. Invasion of bladder tumors to the adjacent organs such as the vagina, prostate, seminal vesicles, and

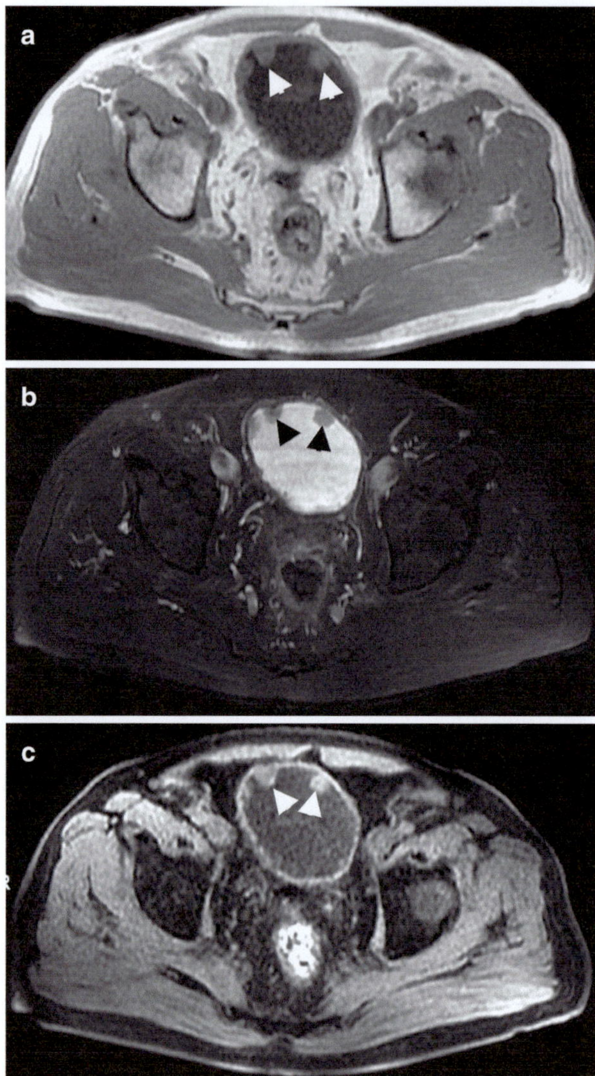

Fig. 1.25 Bladder cancer on MRI. (**a**) Axial fat-suppressed T1-W image reveals multifocal polypoid solid masses (*arrowheads*) arising from bladder wall with intermediate signal intensity. (**b**) Axial T2-W image reveals hypointense solid bladder wall masses (*arrowheads*) protruding to the hyperintense bladder lumen. (**c**) Axial fat-suppressed contrast-enhanced T1-W image reveals enhancement of tumors (*arrowheads*)

rectum can be best identified by MRI (Fig. 1.27). Axial and sagittal T2-W and contrast-enhanced MR images are more helpful to detect vaginal invasion.

DWI is used as a complementary imaging technique in evaluation of bladder cancers with MRI. This technique depicts molecular diffusion of water molecules in biological tissues. Restricted diffusion of water molecules causes increased signal

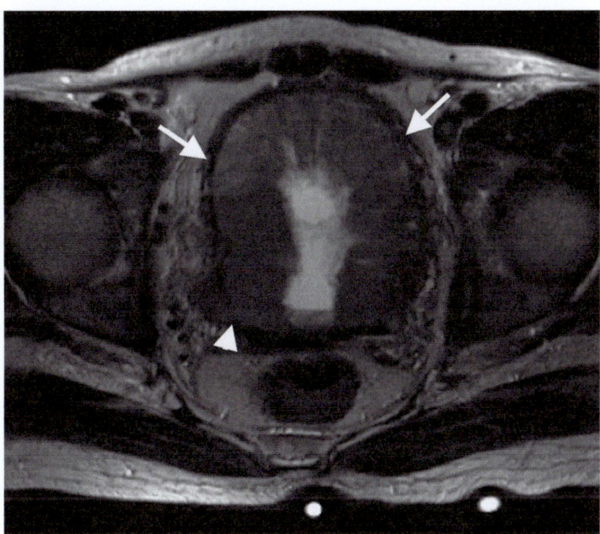

Fig. 1.26 Muscle-invasive bladder cancer on MRI. Axial T2-W image shows diffuse wall thickening (*arrows*) of the bladder wall representing bladder cancer. Interruption of the T2-W hypointense signal on the right posterolateral wall of the bladder (*arrowhead*) represents muscle invasion of the tumor

intensity on DW images and decreased ADC values on ADC maps. Bladder cancers have hyperintense appearance on DW images and low ADC values. The sensitivity, specificity, PPV, NPV, and accuracy values of DWI for detection of bladder cancer were reported as 98.1%, 92.3%, 100%, 92.3%, and 97%, respectively [78]. ADC value as a quantitative parameter representing water diffusivity is lower in bladder cancers compared to normal bladder wall and benign bladder lesions [79]. ADC values decrease with increasing stage and grade of the bladder cancers [79]. It has been shown that ADC values may be used to differentiate stage I or below tumors from stage II or higher tumors [80]. Grade 3 bladder cancers were shown to manifest with significantly lower ADC values than grade 1 or grade 2 bladder cancers [80].

Invasion of the bladder cancer to the pelvic walls and pelvic floor, seminal vesicles, and prostate is crucial for treatment planning. MRI is a more reliable technique than CT for detection of peritumoral spread of bladder cancers due to its high contrast resolution and its ability to obtain tumor-oriented oblique images which can be adapted to morphology and extension of the tumors. Bladder cancers localized in the dome or the base of the bladder can be assessed better with MRI than CT. Invasion of the pelvic wall is best evaluated by T2-W images and contrast-enhanced MR images. Seminal vesicle invasion by bladder cancer causes replacement of the hyperintense fat tissue with hypointense tumoral involvement on T1-W images. Tumoral invasion of the seminal vesicles causes disappearance of high signal intensity of seminal vesicles on T2-weighted images. It should be kept in mind that low T2 signal intensity in seminal vesicles may also be seen in elderly patients, severe alcoholism, a history of infection, local radiotherapy, or amyloidosis of the seminal vesicles. Invasion of the prostate by bladder cancer should be

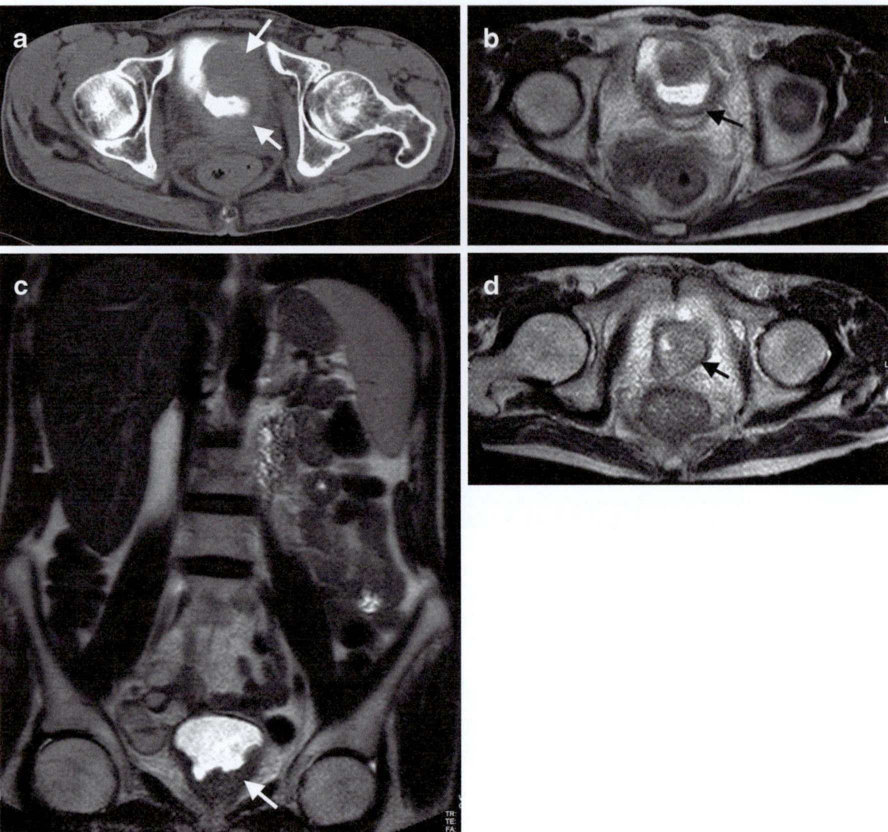

Fig. 1.27 Bladder cancer invasion into prostate. (**a**) CTU image demonstrates asymmetric tumoral wall thickening (*arrows*) of the left lateral and posteroinferior wall of the bladder. Axial (**b**) and coronal (**c**) T2-W images confirm the presence of bladder cancer with hypointense appearance (*arrows*) invading the inferior bladder wall. (**d**) Axial T2-W image at the prostate level reveals the invasion of the tumor to the left prostate gland resulting in hypointense appearance of left prostate gland (*arrow*) compared to the right gland

assessed on T2-W images. Interruption of the delineating contour between prostate and bladder and presence of a mass with similar signal intensity to the bladder cancer in the prostate parenchyma are signs of prostate invasion. Invasion of vaginal fornix, cervix, and uterine body should be interrogated with sagittal T2-W images. Pelvic muscles are thought to be involved in bladder cancer when signal intensity of the pelvic muscles resembles bladder cancer signal intensity on T1-W and T2-W images [63].

Imaging limited to the bladder is not sufficient in overall evaluation of bladder cancer. Upper urinary tract system evaluation is mandatory to demonstrate synchronous and metachronous urothelial tumors. MR urography (MRU) can be used with or without IV contrast injection to evaluate the upper urinary tract system. MRU is

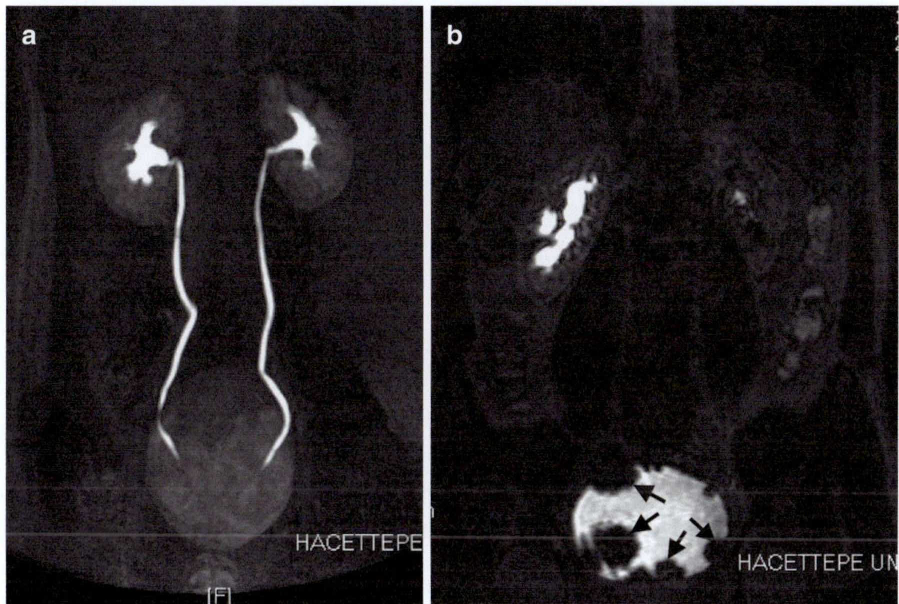

Fig. 1.28 MR urography. (**a**) MR urography of a patient without urinary tract malignancy shows entire urinary tract with high signal intensity. (**b**) MR urography of a patient with multifocal bladder cancer demonstrates multiple hypointense papillary-type bladder masses (*arrows*) protruding to the hyperintense bladder lumen

performed as a heavily T2-W image series on axial and coronal planes. Intravenous diuretic may be used to potentiate the dilatation of ureters and renal collecting system in order to demonstrate small and subtle synchronous and metachronous lesions (Fig. 1.28). MRU should be performed with 3D acquisition, and maximum intensity projection (MIP) images should be provided to assess the entire urinary tract.

1.3.3 Staging

T staging of bladder cancer refers to the depth of bladder wall invasion by the tumor which can be best depicted with MRI, since CT cannot demonstrate individual layers of the bladder wall. US is not a reliable technique in revealing the extent of invasion of the bladder wall and extravesical extension, but endoluminal or intravesical US introduced by a rigid cystoscope may demonstrate tumoral wall invasion although this technique is not widely used [61].

CT was reported to have an accuracy of 40–92% in staging of bladder cancer [81, 82]. In addition to the inaccuracy of T staging, microscopic or small volume of extravesical extension cannot be accurately depicted by CT [83]. Irregular interface between the bladder cancer and perivesical fat or tumoral overgrowth beyond the outer margin of the bladder wall indicates perivesical tumoral extension on CT [61].

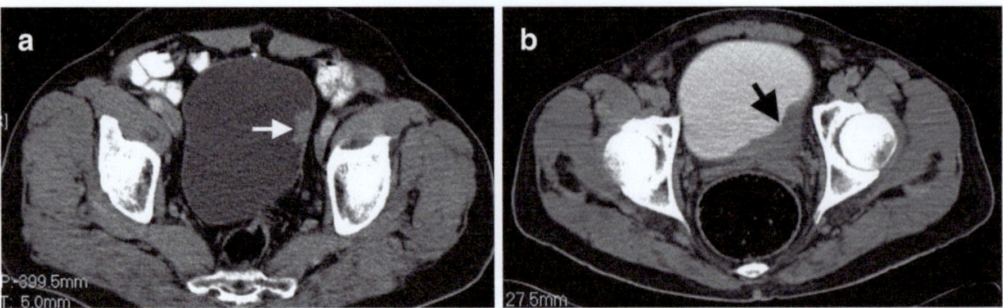

Fig. 1.29 CT in T staging of bladder cancer. (**a**) Axial contrast-enhanced CT image demonstrates an enhancing solid mass (*arrow*) arising from left bladder wall. There is no sign indicating perivesical tumor extension. (**b**) Axial CTU image shows bladder cancer at left posterolateral wall of the bladder with perivesical infiltration (*arrow*)

CT cannot distinguish T2a from T2b disease; however T3a tumors can be differentiated from T3b or higher-stage tumors [84] (Fig 1.29).

MRI is better than CT in detection of small tumors (<10 mm) and staging of superficial tumors [85]. Superficial (≤T1) and muscle-invasive (≥T2) bladder tumors can be differentiated with the accuracy values ranged from 75% to 92% with DCE-MRI [86, 87] (Fig. 1.30). DWI has accuracy values of 63.6%, 75.7%, 93.7%, and 87.5% for accurate staging of T1, T2, T3, and T4 bladder cancer, respectively [81].

1.3.3.1 Lymph Node Metastasis

Lymph node metastasis of bladder cancers can be evaluated with CT or MRI. Measurement of shortest axis of lymph node is commonly used for determining abnormality in the lymph nodes. A shortest diameter of 8 mm for pelvic lymph nodes and 1 cm for abdominal lymph nodes is assumed to be abnormal. However it is well known that lymph nodes may become enlarged in benign processes, mostly resulting from inflammatory causes. This mismatch necessitates assessment of morphological changes in the lymph nodes. Presence of necrosis in the lymph node which can be detected in lymph nodes larger than 2 cm, increased density around the involved lymph node secondary to tumoral infiltration and extracapsular spread are reliable imaging features to suggest malignant infiltration in the lymph nodes [63]. The accuracy values of CT and MRI for detection of lymph node metastasis are reported as 70–90% and 64–92%, respectively (Fig. 1.31) [88]. It is important to know that preoperative imaging by CT may result in false-negative rates of 25% [61]. DWI may also be used in detection of lymph nodes.

1.3.3.2 Metastasis Staging

Bladder cancers most frequently metastasize to the lungs, bone, liver, and brain [83]. Lung metastasis can be assessed by chest radiography in patients without high risk for metastasis. Chest CT is the choice of imaging for lung metastasis for high-risk patients.

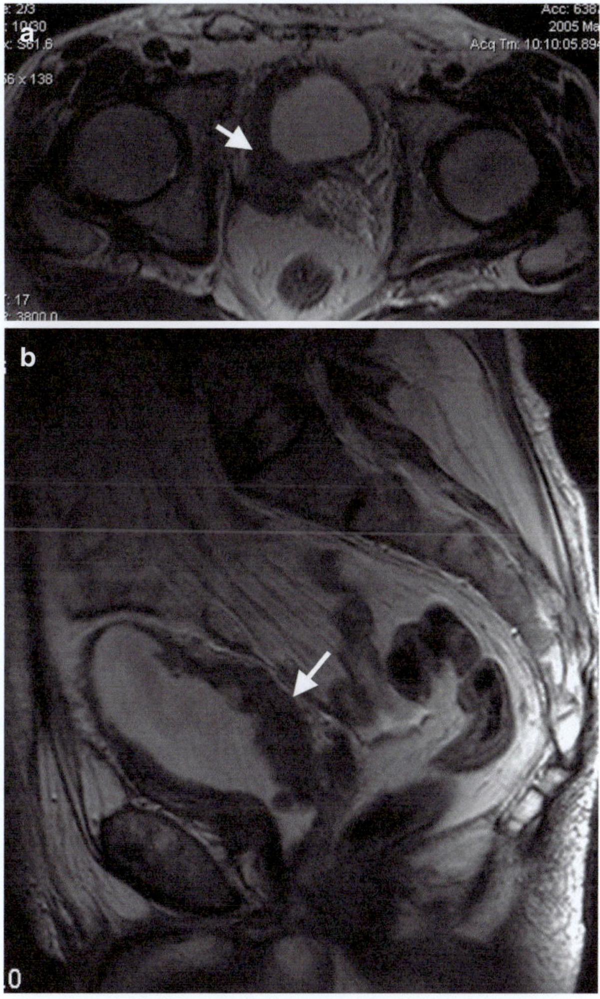

Fig. 1.30 Bladder cancer T staging with MRI. Axial (**a**) and sagittal (**b**) T2-W MR images show muscle-invasive hypointense bladder cancer in the right bladder wall (*arrows*) with perivesical invasion

MRI is more sensitive than bone scintigraphy for detection of bone metastasis. Routine evaluation of bone metastasis is not recommended in bladder cancer unless high suspicion exists.

1.3.4 Monitoring After Treatment

Follow-up imaging in bladder cancer is critical in management of patients, since up to 70% of patients with bladder cancer experience recurrence after treatment.

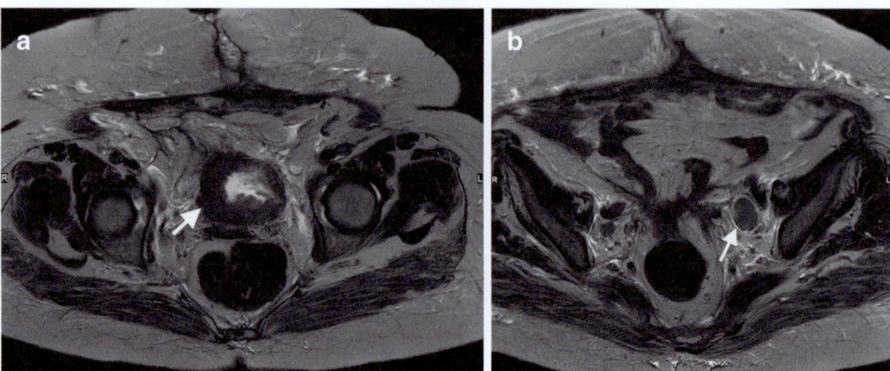

Fig. 1.31 Lymph node metastasis in bladder cancer. (**a**) Axial T2-W image demonstrates diffuse wall thickening (*arrow*) mostly prominent in right lateral wall secondary to bladder cancer. (**b**) Axial T2-W image at iliac vessel level shows left iliac lymphadenopathy (*arrow*) with intermediate signal intensity suggesting lymph node metastasis

Follow-up imaging of bladder cancers to detect recurrence should be performed with MRI. Contrast-enhanced T1-W and DW images are most helpful to depict tumoral masses which may present as a pelvic mass after radical cystectomy or lymph node involvement [63].

NMIBC do not necessitate periodic imaging surveillance of upper urinary tract except for those with a high risk of recurrence [89, 90]. Follow-up imaging of patients who underwent radical cystectomy depends on the pathologic stage of the tumor after cystectomy. Patients with advanced disease undergo routine CTU or MRI within the first 2 to 3 years to depict local or distant recurrence [91]. Routine surveillance of upper urinary tract with CTU is recommended in patients with muscle-invasive cancer [91, 92].

1.4 Prostate Cancer

1.4.1 General Information

Prostate cancer imaging improved tremendously with the advances in US and MRI. Imaging techniques aim to demonstrate size, location, and extension of the primary prostate cancer [93]. Implementation of new techniques enabled radiologists to detect prostate cancer foci in the prostate gland as well as to provide a precise map of the position of the tumor foci and post-therapeutic recurrences, which may decrease the need for random prostate biopsies in the evaluation of prostate cancer. US evaluation of prostate cancer has been increasingly used with implementation of elastography technique. Importance of MRI in prostate cancer has been increasing after the implementation of multiparametric MRI that include dynamic sequences, DWI, and T2-W images. Main standpoints in imaging of prostate cancer are standardization of MRI technique, interpretation, and reporting, which is the goal of recently introduced PI-RADS version 2 [94].

1.4.2 Imaging Features

1.4.2.1 Ultrasonography

Main role of US in prostate cancer imaging is to detect malignancy in prostate parenchyma and to guide prostate cancer biopsy. The use of wide-angle transrectal probe enables physicians to visualize normal prostate gland and abnormal areas and to define suspicious areas for malignancy. Prostate cancer usually presents as a hypoechoic mass in the peripheral zone of the prostate gland on grayscale transrectal US (TRUS) (Fig. 1.32). Color-flow Doppler US can demonstrate increased vascularity in tumor region. US can detect 60% of prostate cancers. Specificity of US for detection of prostate cancer is low since only 50% of hypoechoic lesions in prostate gland represent prostate cancer and inflammatory and infectious processes cause increased vascularity in prostate gland mimicking prostate cancer [95, 96].

Ultrasonography in prostate cancer is mainly used for guiding interventional procedures. Main concerns of TRUS-guided 12-core systematic biopsy technique include poor lesion visualization secondary to low spatial resolution, undersampling of small volume, difficulty of sampling from transitional zone and anteriorly located tumors, and high detection rates of small clinically insignificant prostate cancer that may result in overtreatment [97, 98]. These pitfalls lead to decreased true positive result as 25–30% of TRUS-guided biopsy in detecting prostate cancer [99]. New US techniques adapted to US-guided prostate biopsy including elastography, contrast-enhanced US (CEUS), and mp-MRI TRUS fusion biopsy improved diagnostic performance of TRUS-guided biopsy [100].

Elastography is an emerging US technology that measures stiffness of tissues. US elastography can be performed with two methods as strain elastography (SE) and shear wave elastography (SWE). Strain elastography is a semiquantitative US elastography technique that depicts compression and decompression of tissues in response to mechanical force applied by US probe. Stiffer lesions displace less than

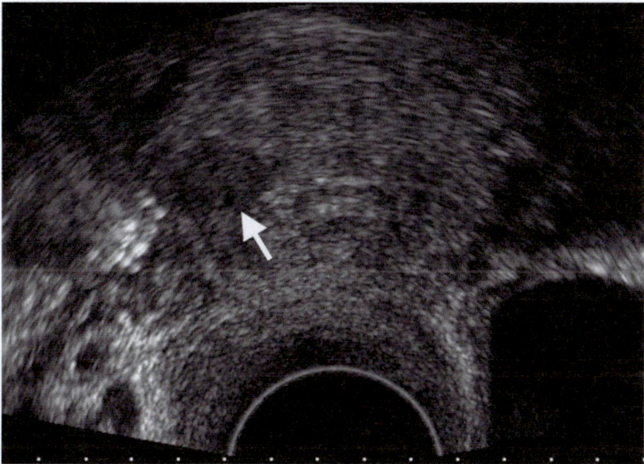

Fig. 1.32 Prostate cancer. TRUS image of a 66-year-old male demonstrates a hypoechoic area (*arrow*) in the peripheral prostate gland which was proved to be prostate cancer after biopsy

soft tissues, and this difference can be displayed on US monitor as color-coded images. Ratio of displacements of different areas pointed out by region of interest (ROI) can be automatically calculated on US elastography, and these ratios which are called as strain index values can be used to detect prostate cancer and differentiate prostate cancer from prostate gland and benign prostate lesions. The PPV and NPV of SE for detection of prostate cancer range between 57% and 87% and 72% and 87%, respectively [101].

SWE differs from SE with capability of providing shear wave velocity values of biological tissues. SWE measures the velocity of shear waves propagated from tissues that are exposed to acoustic waves by US probe. Stiffer tissues produce faster shear waves than soft tissues which may be used to differentiate benign and malignant lesions. SWE using TRUS biopsy was reported to have a sensitivity of 96% and NPV of 99% for detection of prostate cancer lesions 0.3 cm or larger [102]. SWE using TRUS-guided biopsy can decrease the biopsy rate by 53% [101].

Contrast-enhanced US can be performed with injection of microbubbles as an intravascular contrast agent. CEUS enables real-time visualization of microvessel density of prostate lesions and determine the most vascularized lesions in the setting of multinodular prostate gland resulting in improved PPV of TRUS biopsy. Since microvessel density of prostate lesions correlates with Gleason score of prostate carcinoma, CEUS can be used to detect lesions more accurately than color-flow Doppler or power Doppler US [103]. Sensitivity, specificity, and NPV of CEUS in prostate cancer were reported as 70%, 74%, and 72%, respectively. These values are higher than grayscale and CDUS which have sensitivity values as 39% and 41%, respectively [103]. A suspicious lesion in the prostate gland is 3.5 times and is more likely to be malignant when identified by CEUS [104].

Mp-MRI-fused TRUS biopsy is a novel technique that is characterized by combining Mp-MRI images and TRUS images to perform TRUS-guided biopsies. In this technique TRUS and mp-MR images can be fused cognitively or by software. Cognitive fusion refers to fusion of mp-MRI images and TRUS images cognitively by TRUS operator. After assessment of mp-MRI images and determination of suspicious area on MRI, TRUS operator mentally fuses suspicious areas on MRI with real-time US images during biopsy. Performing biopsy with mp-MRI has been shown to increase the accuracy of TRUS-guided prostate biopsy [99]. Second fusion technique is software-based fusion of mp-MRI images obtained before biopsy with real-time TRUS images obtained during biopsy.

Suspicious areas on mp-MRI can be superimposed to real-time TRUS images to guide biopsy [105]. Misregistration of images on the same level can occur due to patient motion and deformation of prostate tissue during transrectal probe scanning [99]. Thirty percent of high-risk cancers missed on standard extended sextant biopsy were detected by following mp-MRI TRUS fusion biopsy [106]. This procedure reduces sampling errors and detects 30% more high-risk prostate cancer (GS $\geq 4 + 3$ and up) and 17% fewer lower risk (GS $\leq 3 + 4$ and up) [106].

Mp-MRI TRUS fusion biopsies are especially helpful in the diagnosis of prostate cancers which are missed on standard TRUS-guided biopsies (Fig. 1.33). These prostate cancers are usually localized in the anterior zone of the prostate [107].

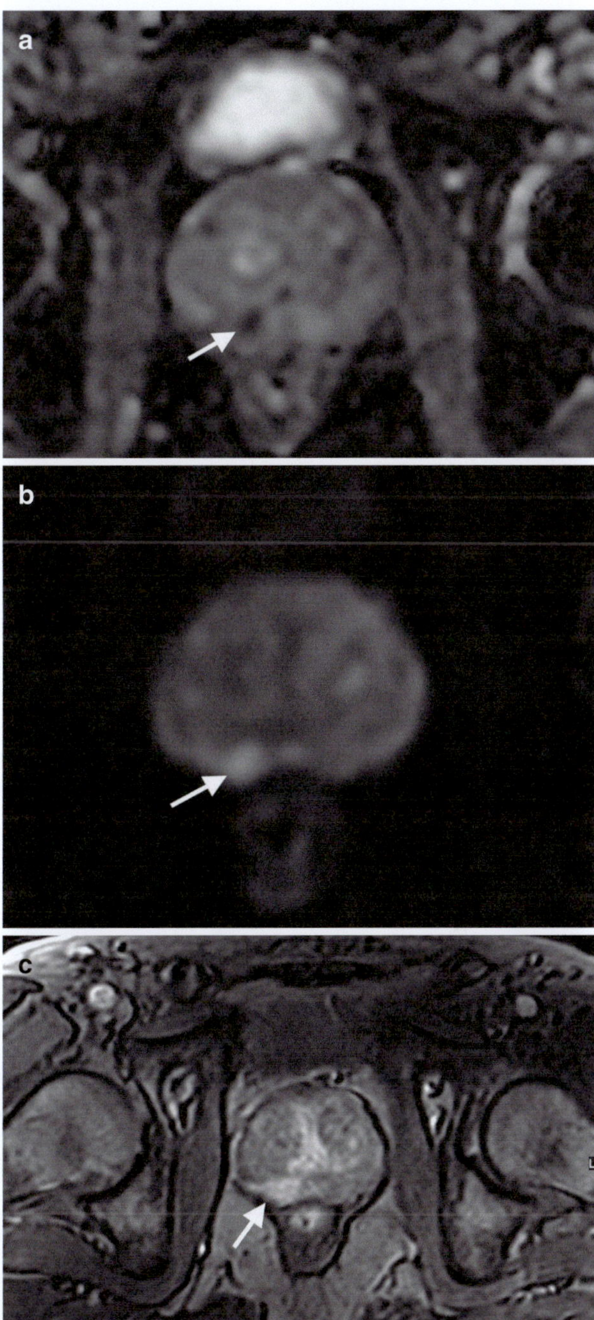

Fig. 1.33 A 57-year-old man presented with rising PSA with negative 12-core TRUS-guided biopsy 2 years ago. Mp-MRI including ADC map (**a**), DWI (**b**), and axial contrast-enhanced T1-W image at arterial phase (**c**) images showed 5 mm PI-RADS lesion (*arrows*) in right posteromedial mid-peripheral gland. Cognitive MRI fusion and TRUS-guided biopsy result was Gleason 3 + 4 tumor

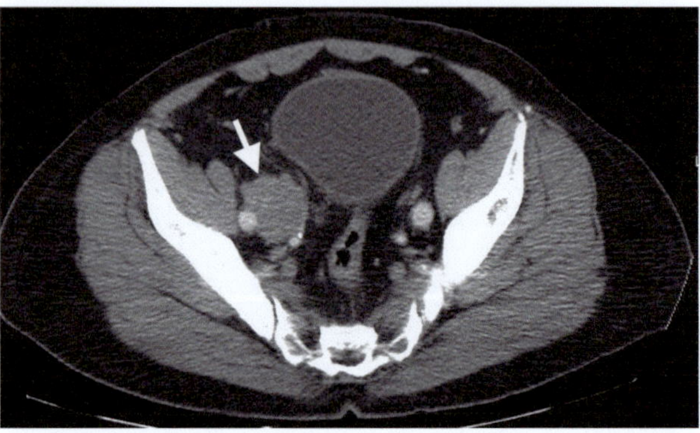

Fig. 1.34 Lymph node metastasis from prostate cancer. Axial contrast-enhanced CT image of a 67-year-old male with prostate cancer demonstrates enlarged right parailiac lymph nodes (*arrow*) secondary to metastasis

1.4.2.2 Computed Tomography

CT cannot be used in evaluation of tumoral lesions confined to the prostatic capsule due to its low contrast resolution. Involvement of lymph nodes and distant metastasis can be assessed with CT in prostate cancer (Fig. 1.34). CT evaluation of patients with suspected prostate cancer should include the prostate dimensions, presence of intravesical prostatic protrusion and the length of protrusion, any asymmetry in prostate contour, and presence of pelvic and para-aortic lymphadenopathy with size measurements [93]. Sensitivity and specificity of CT for detection of lymph node metastasis are 42% and 82%, respectively [108]. Recurrence after prostatectomy cannot be reliably detected with CT due to low sensitivity (36%) of technique [109]. CT can detect recurrent tumors larger than 2 cm [109].

1.4.2.3 Magnetic Resonance Imaging

MRI is a safe and well-tolerated imaging technique, which is being increasingly used in the detection of prostate cancer. Diagnosis, preoperative evaluation, and planning of treatment can be conducted with MRI. MRI of prostate cancer includes anatomic and functional imaging sequences. Cancer foci in the gland can be identified, and aggressive tumor foci can be distinguished from less significant foci to guide diagnosis and targeted treatment of cancer. MRI can overcome shortcomings of blinded transrectal biopsies that has low sensitivity in special areas of prostate such as base and the extreme apex, the anterior compartment, and periurethral area [110]. Mp-MRI has a sensitivity of 86%, specificity of 94%, and NPV of 95% for detection of significant size prostate cancer (>0.5 cm^3) (Fig. 1.35) [111–114]. Mp-MRI not only detects and characterizes the cancerous lesions but also depicts recurrences of prostate cancer.

MRI can diagnose prostate cancer foci that are invisible on US and allow optimal biopsy sites. After biopsy MRI can confirm the presence or absence of a significant lesion in the setting of detected microfoci in TRUS-guided biopsy which can alter the management of the patient ranging between active surveillance and surgery.

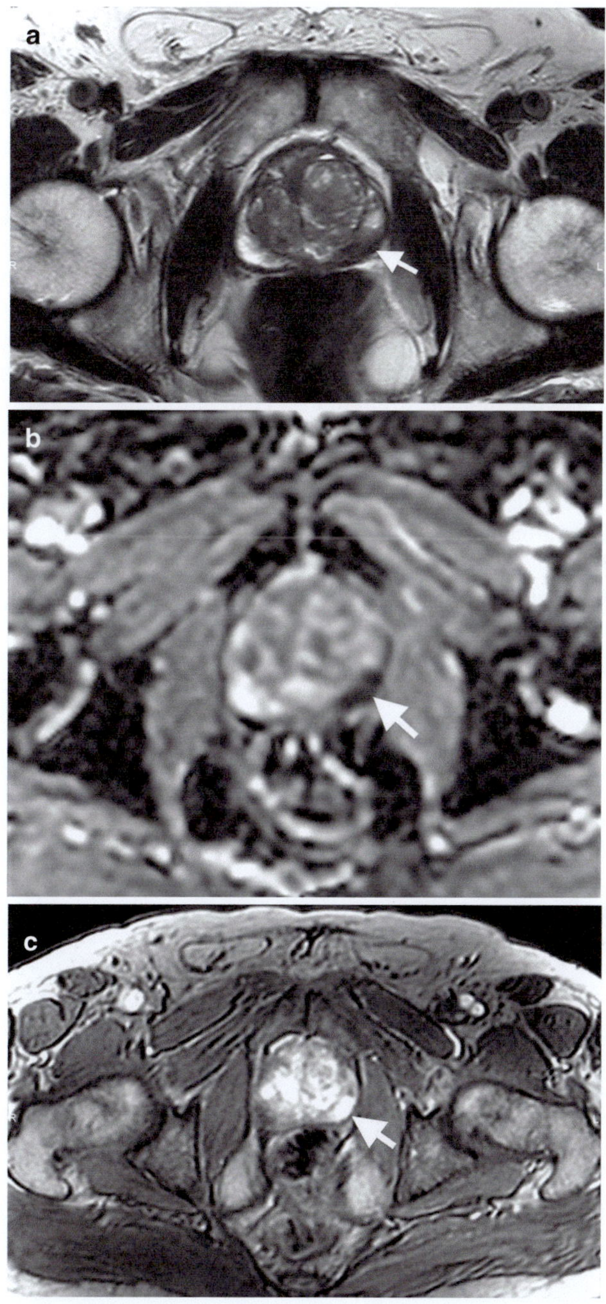

Fig. 1.35 Prostate cancer on MRI. (**a**) Axial T2-W image of a 74-year-old male demonstrates hypointense cancer area (*arrow*) in the left posterior peripheral zone. (**b**) ADC map shows signal loss (*arrow*) in the cancer region. (**c**) DCE-MRI at early phase reveals avid enhancement (*arrow*) of the lesion

Intraprostatic extension of the tumor can be depicted by MRI which is important for the planning of surgery or focused treatment. Staging of prostate cancer can be accurately performed by revealing extension of tumor to seminal vesicles and other extracapsular areas. MRI should be performed at least 6 weeks after biopsy to reduce artifacts from hemorrhage after biopsy [107]. However it was reported that the detection of clinically significant cancers is not likely to be compromised by post-biopsy hemorrhage which makes unnecessary to delay the MRI [115].

Prostate cancer MRI can be performed with 1.5 Tesla (T) MRI using endorectal coil or 3 T with or without endorectal coil. Endorectal coil along with a pelvic phased-array coil is recommended in 1.5 T MR scanners due to high sensitivity of endorectal coil for detecting prostate cancer and to improve staging by precise visualization of surrounding pelvic tissue, extraprostatic extension, and seminal vesicle invasion [116]. Higher magnet strength (3 T) can eliminate the need for endorectal coil with sufficient resolution and increased signal-to-noise ratio [117].

Anatomic imaging sequences of MRI in prostate cancer include multiplanar images of T1-W and T2-W sequences. Mp-MRI sequences consist of dynamic contrast-enhanced images, DWI, and T2-weighted images. T1-W images are helpful to recognize post-biopsy hemorrhage and metastases to the lymph nodes and pelvic bones. Prostate cancers manifest on T2-W images as low signal focal or diffuse lesions mostly in the peripheral zone of prostate gland. However specificity of low signal appearance of prostate cancer is low, since prostatic intraepithelial neoplasia, prostatitis, biopsy-related hemorrhage, changes from hormone therapy, and postradiation fibrosis may also present as low attenuated lesions (Fig. 1.36) [108]. Transitional zone tumors present with the appearance of non-circumscribed, moderately hypointense lesions resembling erased charcoal or smudgy fingerprint appearance on T2-W images (Fig. 1.37) [115]. T2-W images can also demonstrate prostatic capsule invasion and extraprostatic extension of tumor on axial images

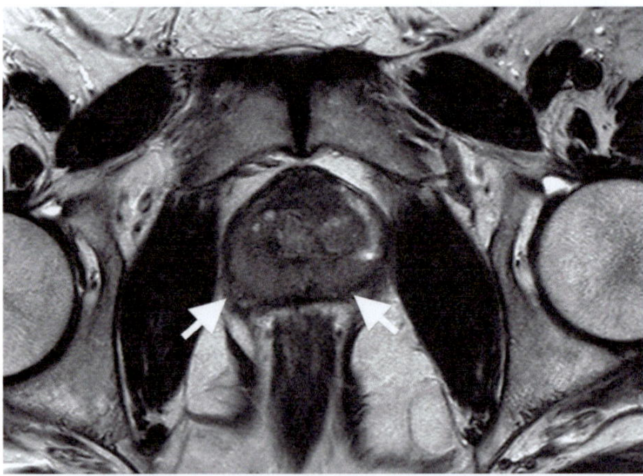

Fig. 1.36 Prostatitis mimicking prostate cancer. Axial T2-W MR image reveals diffuse hypointense appearance of peripheral prostate gland (*arrows*) mimicking malignancy

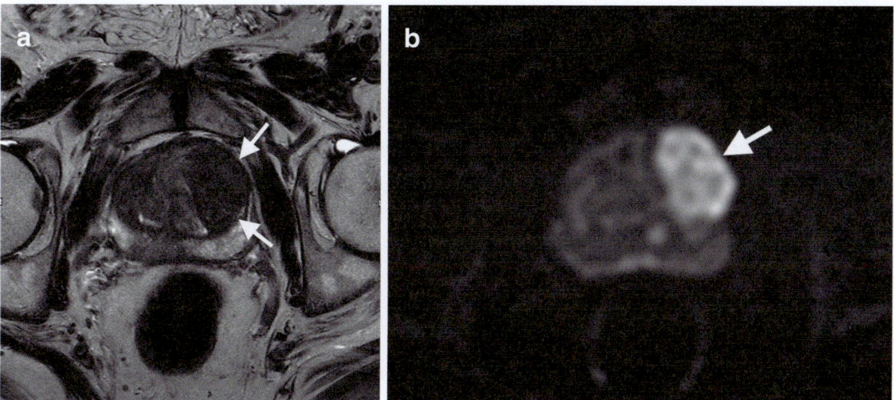

Fig. 1.37 Prostate cancer in transitional zone. (**a**) T2-W image reveals a hypointense mass (*arrows*) in mid-transitional zone of prostate. (**b**) DWI of prostate shows increased signal intensity of the mass (*arrow*) suggesting malignancy

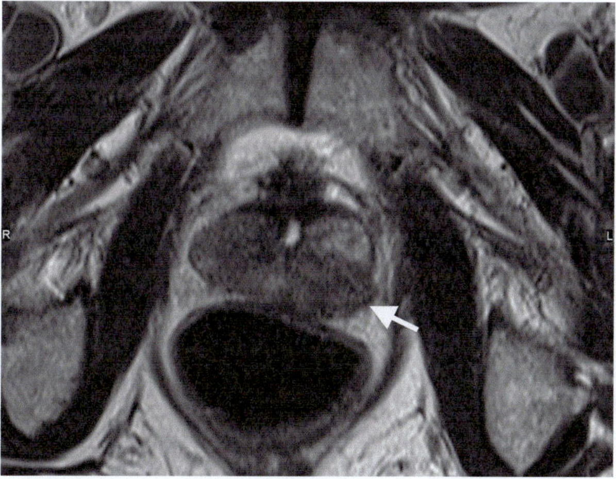

Fig. 1.38 Prostate cancer with capsule invasion. Axial T2-W image demonstrates hypointense mass in left posterolateral peripheral prostate gland. Interruption of prostate capsule in tumoral region suggests capsule invasion (*arrow*). Histopathology confirmed invasion of capsule by the tumor

(Fig. 1.38). Seminal vesicle invasion manifests with loss of high signal intensity of the seminal vesicles with contour abnormalities on T2-W images. Recurrent prostate cancers present as a soft tissue mass with intermediate signal intensity in the low signal fibrotic prostatectomy area.

DWI is one of the main imaging sequences of mp-MRI of the prostate. It is important to obtain DWI at high diffusion gradients represented by high *b* values (*b*, 1500) since DWI at low *b* values has limited accuracy for detection of prostate cancer. Prostate cancer presents with increased signal intensity on DW images and low signal intensity on ADC maps. Prostate cancer can also be assessed quantitatively by ADC map which yields lower ADC values in prostate cancer compared to normal parenchyma. There is also inverse correlation between ADC values and Gleason scores [118]. The sensitivity and specificity values of DWI in detection of prostate cancer in a meta-analysis were 76% and 86%, respectively [119]. The sensitivity of MRI increases from 67–74% to 78–88%, and specificity increases from 77–79% to 88–89% when the DWI is added to T2-W imaging alone [120]. Main limitations of DWI are reduced anatomic detail compared to T2W images, spatial distortion, and signal loss due to magnetic susceptibility effects.

Dynamic contrast-enhanced imaging (DCE) is a functional sequence with a fast temporal resolution (less than 10 s) obtained by T1-W gradient-echo sequence [99]. DCE-MRI is based on tumor angiogenesis that is characterized by vessel formation and increased permeability [121]. Tumors comprise greater interstitial space compared to normal tissues which make tumors more susceptible to contrast accumulation. Contrast enhancement parameters including mean transit time (MTT), blood flow, permeability of the surface area, and interstitial volume are greater in tumors than normal parenchymal organs. Dynamic series of contrast-enhanced images of the prostate can reveal hypervascular prostate cancers more precisely than static contrast-enhanced images [122]. Prostate cancers manifest with early enhanced lesions on DCE-MRI. Relative peak enhancement and wash-in rate were shown to be most useful parameters in detection of prostate cancer in the peripheral zone [123]. The presence of postcontrast early arterial enhancement can upgrade PI-RADS 3 lesion to PI-RADS 4 category [124]. Transitional zone is more susceptible to overlap between normal and cancerous tissues of perfusion parameters [124]. DCE-MRI is especially useful in detecting tumors located in anterior fibromuscular stroma and apex and recurrent prostate cancer, which may be difficult to detect on T2-W images (Fig. 1.39). Improvement in the detection of extracapsular extension and seminal vesicle invasion can be done with DCE-MRI [125].

MR spectroscopic imaging is a three-dimensional chemical shift imaging technique which assesses the relative concentration of different chemical compounds in tissues. The healthy prostate gland includes a high level of citrate and polyamines [124]. Prostate cancer manifests with decreased citrate and polyamine and increased choline levels [126]. High choline plus creatine to citrate (CC/C) ratio indicates prostate cancer [127]. MRS can be useful for determining the presence of cancer, determining lesion aggressiveness, and detecting recurrence [128]. MRS scoring system which is based on the choline plus creatinine (Ch + Cr) to citrate (Ci) ratio, choline-to-creatinine ratios, and polyamine levels assigns spectral voxels a score between 1 and 5. A score of 4 or 5 indicates high likelihood of malignancy with the sensitivity values of 64–93% and specificity values of 84.6% and 89.3%, respectively [124]. Detection, localization, and estimation of aggressiveness of prostate cancer have been reported to be improved with the use of MRS in addition to prostate MRI [126]. However due to problems in standardization, acquisition, and interpretation of MR spectroscopy, it is not used by PI-RADS version 2 classification.

Report of prostate MRI should include prostate dimensions, any asymmetry in the prostate contour, any abnormal signal or contrast enhancement in the peripheral

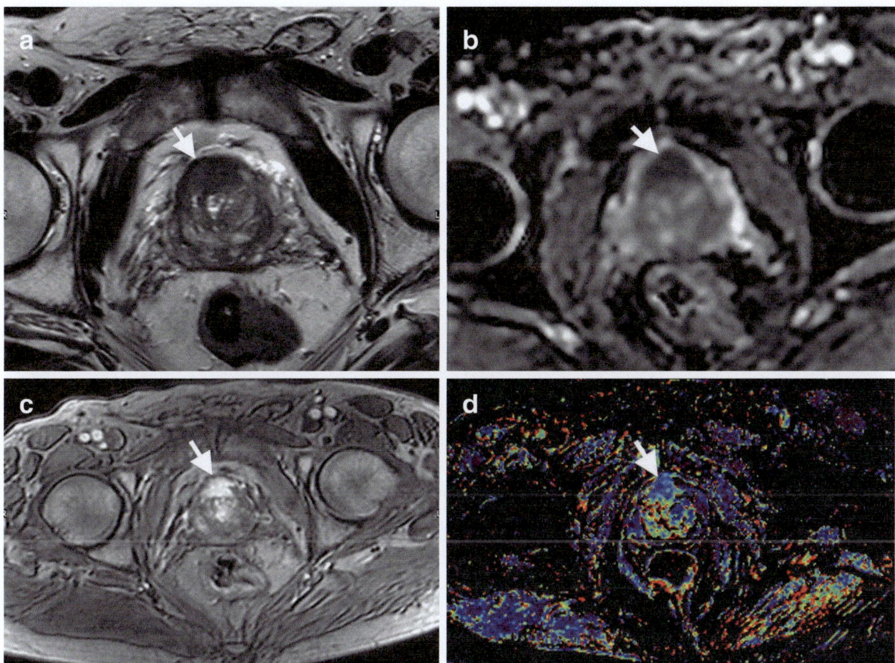

Fig. 1.39 DCE-MRI of prostate cancer in anterior fibromuscular stroma. Prostate cancer localized in anterior part of prostate appears hypointense on T2-W (**a**) and ADC (**b**) images. (**c**) Prostate cancer enhances after IV gadolinium administration (*arrow*). (**d**) Perfusion MRI shows increased perfusion of the tumor (*arrow*, *blue-coded area*) compared to nonneoplastic prostate

or transitional zone, presence of intravesical protrusion and the length of protrusion, loss of periprostatic fat plane, seminal vesicle signal intensity and asymmetry, and presence of pelvic and para-aortic lymphadenopathy [93].

Prostate MRI findings in prostate cancer have been standardized as Prostate Imaging Reporting and Data System (PI-RADS). The aim of PI-RADS is to promote standardization in acquisition, interpretation, and reporting of mp-MRI of prostate cancer by establishing minimum acceptable technical parameters for prostate mp-MRI, standardize the terminology and content of reports, and categorize the lesions according to levels of suspicion or risk for malignancy [115]. Updated PI-RADS by European Society of Urogenital Radiology (ESUR) is called PI-RADS version 2 [129]. Prostate is divided into 39 regions (36 for the prostate, 2 for the seminal vesicles, and 1 for the external urethral sphincter) in PI-RADS. Mapping of prostate gland aids to localize the findings detected on MRI which is helpful for discussion of management and treatment plan between physicians and guiding targeted prostate biopsy. After localization of lesions in the prostate gland, likelihood of malignancy is scored in a five-point scale according to findings on T2-W, DWI, and DCE images (Table 1.1) [130]. In PI-RADS volume of the prostate should be reported. DWI is the primary determining sequence for peripheral zone (Fig. 1.40). Minimum requirement of measurement is largest dimension on axial image [115].

Table 1.1 PI-RADS™ v3 assessment categories [115]

PI-RADS 1	Very low (clinically significant cancer is highly unlikely to be present)
PI- RADS 2	Low (clinically significant cancer is unlikely to be present)
PI-RADS 3	Intermediate (the presence of clinically significant cancer is equivocal)
PI-RADS 4	High (clinically significant cancer is likely to be present)
PI-RADS 5	Very high (clinically significant cancer is highly likely to be present)

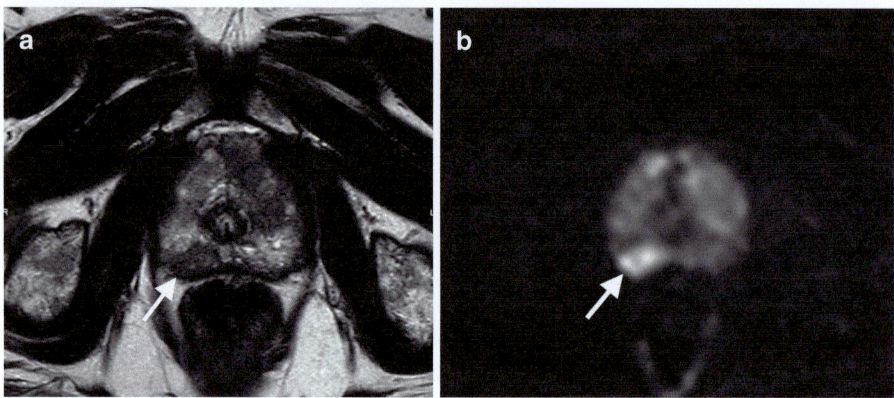

Fig. 1.40 PI-RADS 5 prostate cancer. (**a**) Axial T2-W image demonstrates hypointense area (*arrow*) in right posterior peripheral gland consistent with prostate cancer. (**b**) DWI reveals increased signal intensity (*arrow*) secondary to diffusion restriction

The diameter of lesions in peripheral zone should be measured on ADC images, while transition zone lesions should be measured on T2-W images [115].

PI-RADS necessitate mapping of the prostate lesions. For the mapping, sector map including 36 regions should be used, and "index (dominant) lesion" should be identified. Index lesion refers to lesion that yields highest PI-RADS assessment category. In the setting of multifocal lesions, the largest lesion usually has highest Gleason score and extracapsular extension is usually encountered in this lesion.

With the use of mp-MRI, the sensitivity for the detection of prostate cancer ranges between 74% and 82%, specificity ranges between 68% and 88%, and NPV ranges between 65% and 94% [131, 132]. Prostatic lesions which was scored as (PI-RADS ≥4) on mp-MRI were shown to be correlated with higher risk of cancer on fusion biopsy and final pathology [133] (Fig. 1.41). High NPV of mp-MRI may avoid standard 12-core prostate biopsy. Combination of negative TRUS biopsy and negative mp-MRI may obviate the need for repeat biopsy [99].

It should be kept in mind that PI-RADS does not include recommendations for the management. Management of patients should be based on laboratory and clinical history, physical examination findings, and standards of care besides mp-MRI findings.

The MRI features of extraprostatic disease are summarized in Table 1.2.

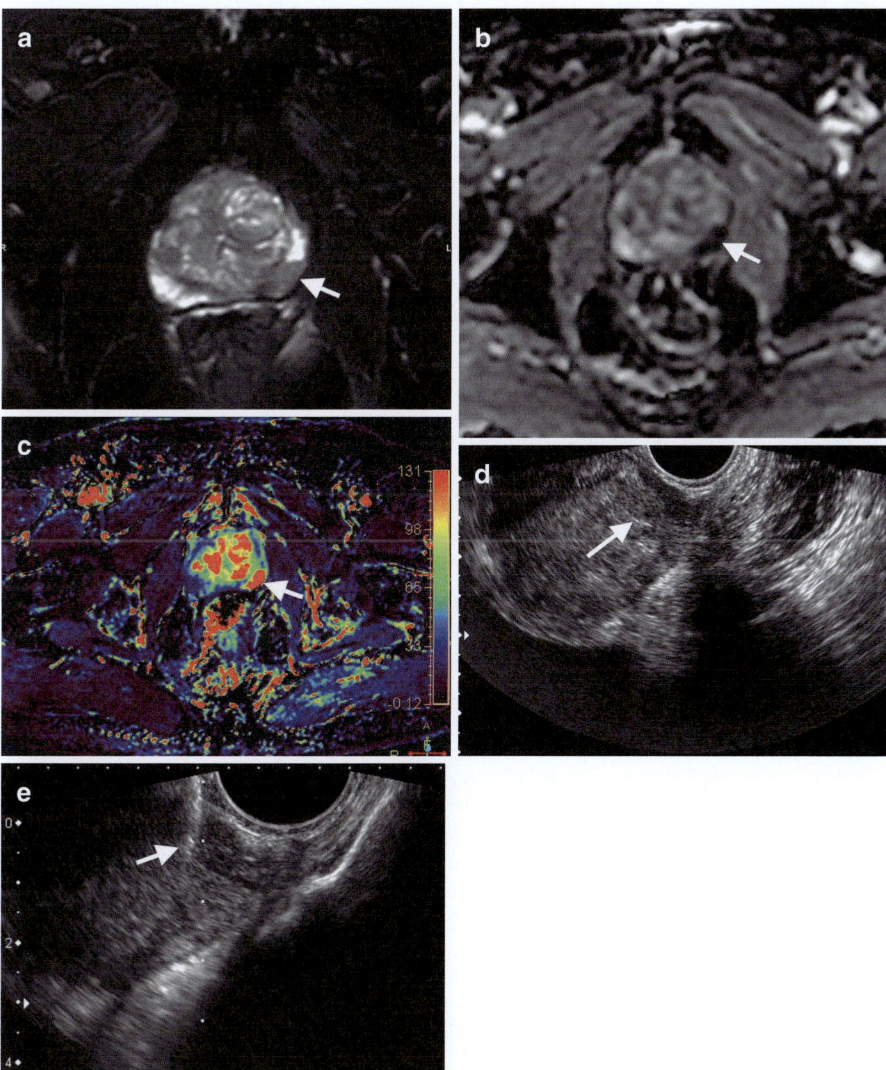

Fig. 1.41 PI-RADS 5 prostate cancer. (**a**) Axial T2-W image reveals left peripheral tumor with hypointense appearance (*arrow*). (**b**) Tumor presents with diminished signal (*arrow*) on ADC map secondary to depleted diffusion. (**c**) Perfusion MRI reveals increased perfusion (*arrow*) of tumor. (**d**) Tumor manifests as hypoechoic mass (*arrow*) on TRUS. (**e**) TRUS-guided biopsy of the mass (*arrow*) depicted prostate cancer with Gleason score of 9

Table 1.2 Signs of extraprostatic extension [115]

Signs of extraprostatic extension
Asymmetry or invasion of the neurovascular bundles
Bulging prostatic contour
Irregular or spiculated margin
Obliteration of the rectoprostatic angle
Tumor-capsule interface of greater than 1.0 cm
Breach of the capsule with evidence of tumor extension

1.4.3 Local Staging of Patients with Biopsy-Proven Prostate Cancer

Mp-MRI improves sensitivity and the PPV of detecting organ-confined prostate carcinoma [134]. Local or metastatic spread of prostate cancer should be detected after the diagnosis of prostate cancer. Local spread of prostate cancer includes extracapsular spread, neurovascular bundle invasion, seminal vesicle invasion, and adjacent organ spread. T1 tumors refer to clinically unapparent (neither palpable nor visible at imaging) tumors. T2 tumors are confined within the prostate gland. T3a tumors extend beyond the prostatic capsule; T3b tumors invade the seminal vesicle. T4 tumors are characterized as fixed or invade adjacent structures other than seminal vesicles (e.g., bladder, rectum, pelvic wall) [135]. The role of mp-MRI in detecting extracapsular extension is controversial. Poor sensitivity (47%) was obtained with mp-MRI in detecting extraprostatic extension [136]. Mp-MRI has a sensitivity ranging between 13% and 95% and specificity ranging between 49% and 97%, respectively [137]. Invasion of seminal vesicles can be determined with a sensitivity of 23–80% and specificity of 81–99% [137].

The apex of prostate should be carefully assessed in local staging of prostate cancer since involvement of external urethral sphincter may result in surgical- or radiotherapy-induced injury and impaired urinary continence [115].

Invasion of neurovascular bundle and seminal vesicles should be inspected on high-resolution T2-W images and DCE T1-W images (Table 1.3) (Figs. 1.42 and 1.43).

Table 1.3 Signs of seminal vesicle invasion [115]

Signs
Focal or diffuse low T2 signal intensity
Abnormal contrast enhancement within and/or along the seminal vesicles
Restricted diffusion
Obliteration of the angle between base of the prostate and the seminal vesicle

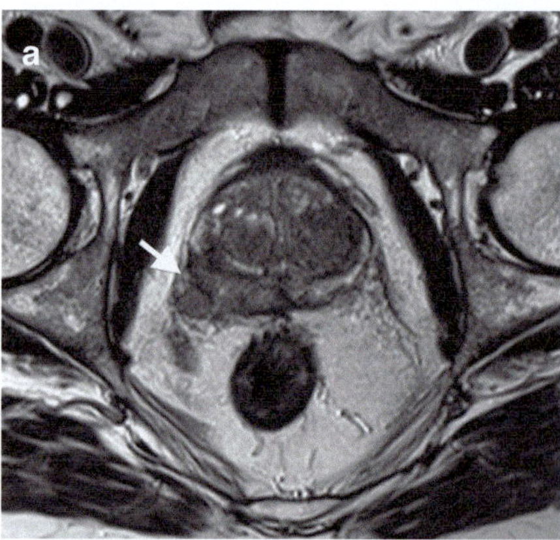

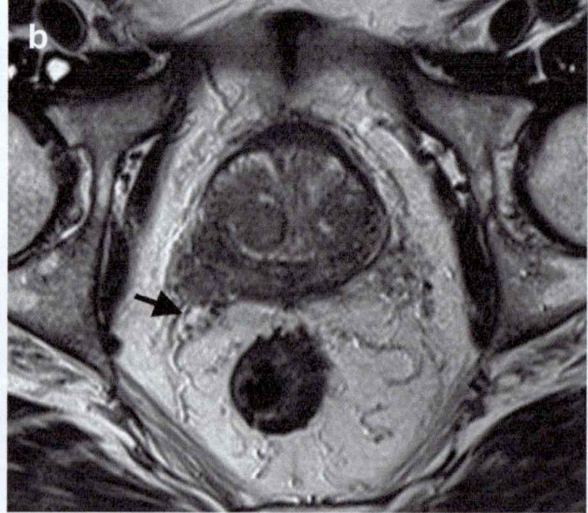

Fig. 1.42 Prostate capsule and neurovascular invasion in prostate cancer. T2-W images performed for local staging of prostate cancer show tumor in the right peripheral gland with (**a**) extracapsular extension (arrow) and (**b**) neurovascular bundle invasion (*arrow*)

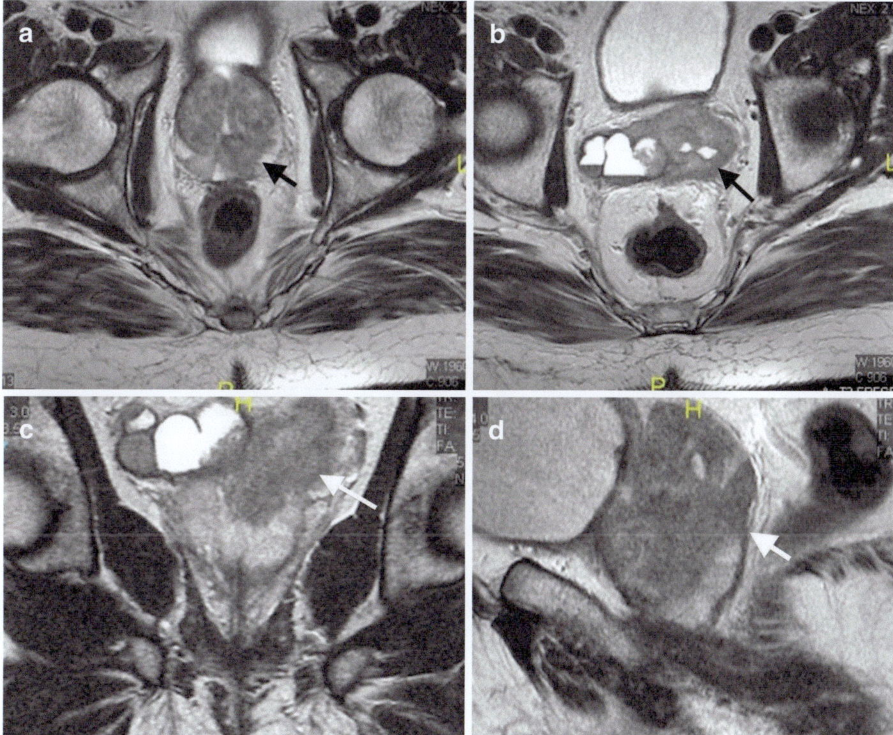

Fig. 1.43 Prostate cancer with seminal vesical invasion. T2-W images performed for local staging of prostate cancer (*arrow*) (**a**) show left seminal vesical invasion (arrows) on axial (**b**), coronal (**c**), and sagittal (**d**) images

1.4.3.1 Lymph Node Metastasis

Metastasis to the lymph nodes represents poor prognosis in prostate cancer [93]. In lymph node assessment, common femoral, obturator, external iliac, internal iliac, common iliac, pararectal, presacral, paracaval, and para-aortic lymph nodes should be inspected. Lymph node metastasis can be detected on mp-MRI including T2-W and postcontrast T1 sequences with 39% sensitivity and 82% specificity [108]. Benign and malignant lymph nodes can be distinguished with 86% sensitivity, 85% specificity, and 86% accuracy [138]. Imaging of lymph nodes on mp-MRI after intravenous administration of lymphotropic superparamagnetic nanoparticles can differentiate malignant lymph nodes from benign lymph nodes with a sensitivity of 100% on a per-patient basis analysis [139]. It has been shown that mp-MRI has higher sensitivity (91%) than conventional MRI (35%) on node-by-node analysis [139]. Accuracy of MRI is increased with IV administration of lymphotrophic superparamagnetic nanoparticles in especially lymph nodes less than 1 cm [137].

1.4.3.2 Distant Metastasis

Prostate cancer most commonly metastasizes to the bone, particularly the axial skeleton following the distribution of the skull, thorax, pelvis, spine, and proximal long bones [93]. MRI detects bone metastasis with a sensitivity of 100% and specificity

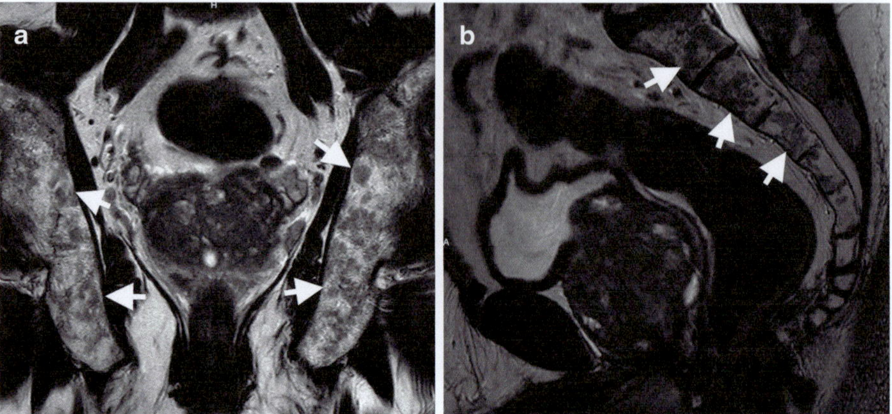

Fig. 1.44 Bone metastasis. Coronal (**a**) and sagittal (**b**) T2-W MR images of a 74-year-old man reveal multiple hypointense bone metastasis (*arrows*) of prostate cancer replacing hyperintense bone marrow

of 88%, while bone scintigraphy detects the metastasis with 46% sensitivity and 32% specificity [140]. Bone lesions that were detected on bone scans can be characterized on MRI. Bone metastases present with diminished signal intensity within the high-signal bone marrow fat (Fig. 1.44).

1.4.3.3 Preprocedural Assessment

The use of mp-MRI in prostate cancer is not limited only for detection, characterization, and staging of the lesions, but also it can be used in preprocedural assessment of patients including nerve-sparing surgery, radiation therapy, and focal therapy [99]. It was shown that appropriate assessment with mp-MRI can alter treatment in 30% of cases [141]. Areas with extracapsular extension are widely excised, and selective excision is preferred for areas without extracapsular extension which result in sparing the neurovascular bundles [134]. Mp-MRI can also be helpful with identifying lesions to guide focal laser ablation and HIFU therapies.

Planning of radiation therapy for prostate cancer necessitates accurate delineation of prostate cancer, cancer volume, and tumor extent in order to increase the therapeutic radiation dose to malignant lesions and decrease the radiation dose to the urethra and periprostatic regions free of tumoral invasion [142]. Determining volume and extent of tumors to the periprostatic regions can also be used to increase utility and efficacy and safety of local therapies such as brachytherapy, cryosurgical ablation, and high-frequency focused ultrasound.

High NPV of mp-MRI (98%) for clinically significant prostate cancer raised a question as mp-MRI can be used as a screening tool for clinically significant prostate cancer and prevent unnecessary biopsy procedures. Swedish study reported that if PSA ≥1.8 and positive MRI findings were used, biopsy rates may be reduced by 26% [143]. Although mp-MRI is not generally accepted as a screening tool for prostate cancer, a biparametric MRI including T2-W and DWI sequences may be performed in patients for screening as a fast imaging technique before biopsy since majority of information yielded from mp-MRI gleaned from these sequences [144].

1.4.3.4 Metabolic Imaging

Although ^{1}H spectroscopy and FDG-PET were used to depict metabolic properties of prostate cancer, utility of these techniques was not generally accepted due to low spatial resolution, long acquisition time, and limited additional benefit. Hyperpolarized ^{13}C MR imaging as a new metabolic imaging technique depicts conversion of pyruvate to lactate, despite oxygen-rich environment in prostate cancer [145]. This technique was recently shown to demonstrate elevated lactate/pyruvate ratios in biopsy-proven prostate cancer [146].

1.4.3.5 Evaluation of Recurrence

Recurrence of prostate cancer is almost always evaluated by mp-MRI; however efficacy of T2W sequence, DWI, and MRS is limited due to postsurgical or post-radiotherapy or local therapy changes resulting in fibrosis (Figs. 1.45, 1.46). DCE-MRI is helpful in these situations since recurrent cancer tissue presents with early enhancement while posttreatment changes manifest as delayed enhancing regions (Fig. 1.47) [147]. The sensitivity and specificity of DCE-MRI for detection of

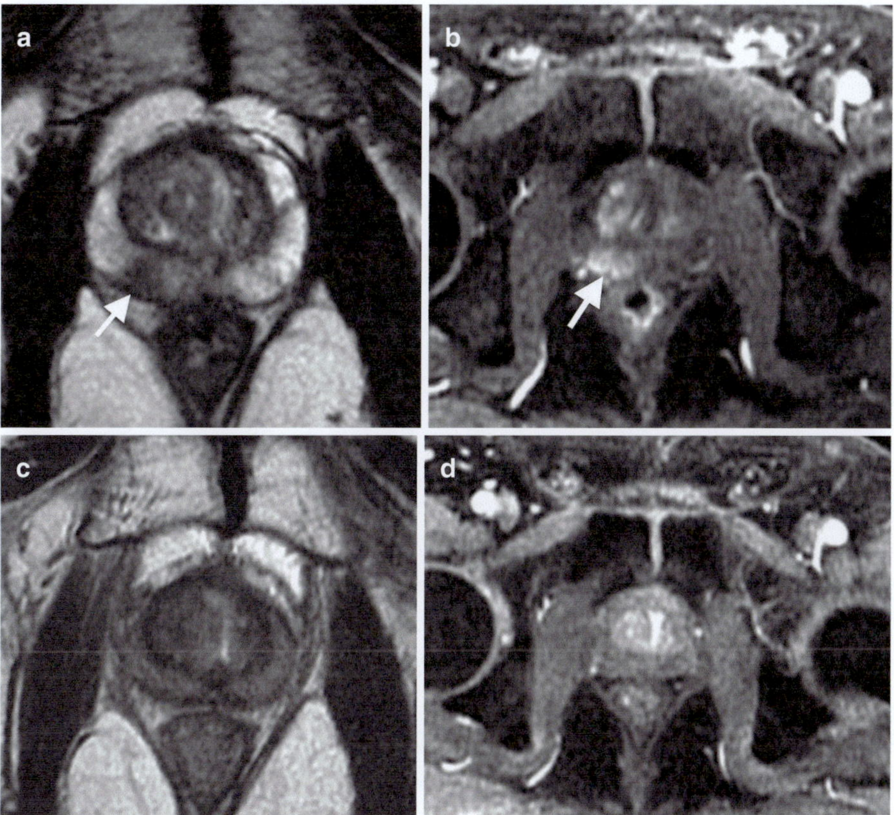

Fig. 1.45 Prostate cancer in the right peripheral gland (arrows) seen as low signal on T2-W image (**a**) and hypervascular (**b**) on postcontrast T1-W image disappeared after radiation treatment at corresponding images (**c** and **d**)

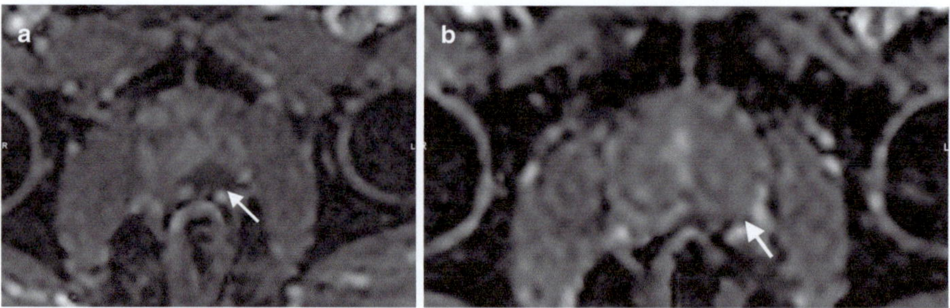

Fig. 1.46 Prostate cancer in the left peripheral gland seen as low signal (*arrow*) on ADC map (**a**) disappeared (*arrow*) after radiation treatment (**b**)

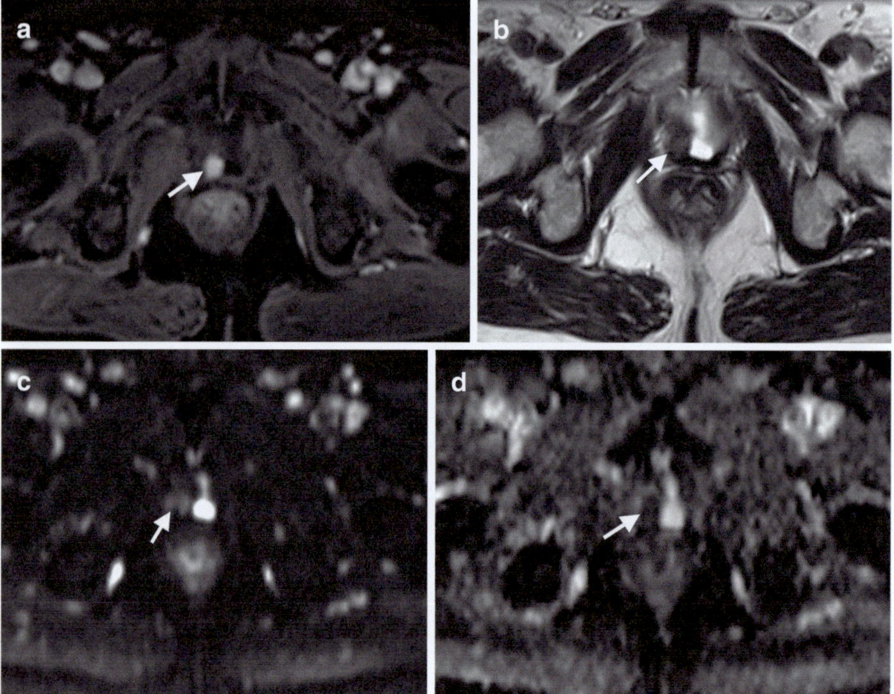

Fig. 1.47 A 65-year-old man presented with rising PSA after radical prostatectomy. Axial post-contrast (**a**), T2-W (**b**), and DWI images (**c**) and ADC map (**d**) show local recurrent tumor (*arrows*) measuring 12 mm

recurrent prostate cancer after radical prostatectomy were reported as 85% and 95%, respectively [148].

Conclusion

Advanced MRI techniques may be helpful in assessment aggressiveness of the renal tumors. Detection, staging, and follow-up of bladder tumors can be conducted with imaging techniques mostly with CT or MRI. Suspected or proven bladder tumors are most commonly initially evaluated by CT. MRI provides additional necessary information about the local invasion of bladder wall layers and extension to perivesical area. Multiparametric MRI is a promising tool to detect, localize, and accurately biopsy clinically significant prostate cancer. Advanced MRI techniques such as DWI are promising for differentiation between benign and malignant tumors, prediction aggressiveness, and treatment response of bladder tumors. US, CT, and MRI can be used to assess prostate cancer, lymph node status, and bone metastasis. Accurate reporting in prostate cancer in accordance with updated guidelines has gained importance to appropriate management of patients. Selection of patients with prostate cancer to local therapy or systemic treatment relies on appropriate assessment and accurate reporting.

References

1. Compérat E, Camparo P. Histological classification of malignant renal tumours at a time of major diagnostic and therapeutic changes. Diagn Interv Imaging. 2012;93:221–31.
2. Patard JJ, Leray E, Rioux-Leclercq N, et al. Prognostic value of histologic subtypes in renal cell carcinoma: a multicenter experience. J Clin Oncol. 2005;23:2763–71.
3. Thompson RH, Kurta JM, Kaag M, et al. Tumor size is associated with malignant potential in renal cell carcinoma. J Urol. 2009;181:2033–6.
4. Patel MI, Simmons R, Kattan MW, et al. Long-term follow-up of bilateral sporadic renal tumors. Urology. 2003;61:921–5.
5. Richstone L, Scherr DS, Reuter VR, et al. Multifocal renal cortical tumors: frequency, associated clinicopathological features and impact on survival. J Urol. 2004;171:615–20.
6. Zirinsky K, Auh YH, Rubenstein WA, et al. CT of the hyperdense renal cyst: sonographic correlation. AJR Am J Roentgenol. 1984;143:151–6.
7. Forman HP, Middleton WD, Melson GL, et al. Hyperechoic renal cell carcinomas: increase in detection at US. Radiology. 1993;188:431–4.
8. Press GA, McClennan BL, Melson GL, et al. Papillary renal cell carcinoma: CT and sonographic evaluation. AJR Am J Roentgenol. 1984;143:1005–9.
9. Hartman DS, David CJ Jr, Goldman SM, et al. Renal lymphoma: radiologic-pathologic correlation of 21 cases. Radiology. 1982;144:759–66.
10. Markic D, Krpina K, Ahel J, Spanjol J, Grskovic A, Stifter S, et al. Different presentations of renal cell cancer on ultrasound and computerized tomography. Urologia. 2014;81:228–32.
11. Wang C, Yu C, Yang F, Yang G. Diagnostic accuracy of contrast- enhanced ultrasound for renal cell carcinoma: a meta-analysis. Tumour Biol. 2014;35:6343–50.
12. Onur MR, Poyraz AK, Bozgeyik Z, Onur AR, Orhan I. Utility of semiquantitative strain elastography for differentiation between benign and malignant solid renal masses. J Ultrasound Med. 2015;34:639–47.

13. Habboub HK, Abu-Yousef MM, Williams RD, See WA, Schweiger GD. Accuracy of color Doppler sonography in assessing venous thrombus extension in renal cell carcinoma. Am J Roentgenol. 1997;168:267–71.
14. Hricak H, Thoeni RF, Carroll PR, Demas BE, Marotti M, Tanagho EA. Detection and staging of renal neoplasms: a reassessment of MR imaging. Radiology. 1988;166:643–9.
15. Roubidoux MA, Dunnick NR, Sostman HD, Leder RA. Renal carcinoma: detection of venous extension with gradient-echo MR imaging. Radiology. 1992;182:269–72.
16. Jamis-Dow CA, Choyke PL, Jennings SB, et al. Small (< or 5 3-cm) renal masses: detection with CT versus US and pathologic correlation. Radiology. 1996;198:785–8.
17. Bhosale PR, Wei W, Ernst RD, Bathala TK, Reading RM, Wood CG, et al. Intraoperative sonography during open partial nephrectomy for renal cell cancer: does it alter surgical management. Am J Roentgenol. 2014;203:822–7.
18. Zhang J, Lefkowitz RA, Bach A. Imaging of kidney cancer. Radiol Clin North Am. 2007;45:119–47.
19. Sankineni S, Brown A, Cieciera M, Choyke PL, Turkbey B. Imaging of renal cell carcinoma. Urol Oncol. 2016;34:147–55.
20. Kang SK, Kim D, Chandarana H. Contemporary imaging of the renal mass. Curr Urol Rep. 2011;12:11–7.
21. Hélénon O, Eiss D, Debrito P, Merran S, Correas JM. How to characterise a solid renal mass: a new classification proposal for a simplified approach. Diagn Interv Imaging. 2012;93:232–45.
22. Zhang J, Lefkowitz RA, Ishill NM, et al. Solid renal cortical tumors: differentiation with CT. Radiology. 2007;244:494–504.
23. Herts BR, Coll DM, Novick AC, et al. Enhancement characteristics of papillary renal neoplasms revealed on triphasic helical CT of the kidneys. AJR Am J Roentgenol. 2002;178:367–72.
24. Couvidat C, Eiss D, Merran S, Vieillefond A, Correas JM, Hélénon O. Papillary renal cell carcinoma: spectrum of imaging findings with pathologic correlation. Chicago, United States, RSNA annual meeting; 2008 30th November–5th December.
25. Israel GM, Hindman N, Bosniak MA. Evaluation of cystic renal masses: comparison of CT and MR imaging by using the Bosniak classification system. Radiology. 2004;231:365–71.
26. Abdulla C, Kalra MK, Saini S, et al. Pseudoenhancement of simulated renal cysts in a phantom using different multidetector CT scanners. AJR Am J Roentgenol. 2002;179:1473–6.
27. Lesavre A, Correas JM, Merran S, Grenier N, Vieillefond A, Hélénon O. CT of papillary renal cell carcinoma with cholesterol necrosis mimicking angiomyolipomas. AJR Am J Roentgenol. 2003;181:143–5.
28. Kallman DA, King BF, Hattery RR, Charboneau JW, Ehman RL, Guthman DA, et al. Renal vein and inferior vena cava tumor thrombus in renal cell carcinoma: CT, US, MRI and venacavography. J Comput Assist Tomogr. 1992;16:240–7.
29. Kutikov A, Smaldone MC, Egleston BL, et al. Anatomic features of enhancing renal masses predict malignant and high-grade pathology: a preoperative nomogram using the RENAL nephrometry score. Eur Urol. 2011;60:241–8.
30. Karçaaltıncaba M, Aktaş A. Dual-energy CT revisited with multidetector CT: review of principles and clinical applications. Diagn Interv Radiol. 2011;17:181–94.
31. Graser A, Becker CR, Staehler M, et al. Single phase dual-energy CT allows for characterization of renal masses as benign or malignant. Invest Radiol. 2010;45:399–405.
32. Mileto A, Nelson RC, Paulson EK, Marin D. Dual-Energy MDCT for Imaging the Renal Mass. AJR Am J Roentgenol. 2015;204:W640–7.
33. Pretorius ES, Wickstrom ML, Siegelman ES. MR imaging of renal neoplasms. Magn Reson Imaging Clin N Am. 2000;8:813–36.
34. Willatt JM, Hussain HK, Chong S, Kappil M, Azar SF, Liu PS, et al. MR imaging in the characterization of small renal masses. Abdom Imaging. 2014;39:761–9.
35. Taouli B, Thakur RK, Mannelli L, Babb JS, Kim S, Hecht EM, et al. Renal lesions: characterization with diffusion-weighted imaging versus contrast-enhanced MR imaging. Radiology. 2009;251:398–407.

36. Wang H, Cheng L, Zhang X, Wang D, Guo A, Gao Y, et al. Renal cell carcinoma: diffusion-weighted MR imaging for subtype differentiation at 3.0 T. Radiology. 2010;257:135–43.
37. Sasiwimonphan K, Takahashi N, Leibovich BC, Carter RE, Atwell TD, Kawashima A. Small (< 4 cm) renal mass: differentiation of angiomyolipoma without visible fat from renal cell carcinoma utilizing MR imaging. Radiology. 2012;263:160–8.
38. Lanzman RS, Robson PM, Sun MR, Patel AD, Mentore K, Wagner AA, et al. Arterial spin-labeling MR imaging of renal masses: correlation with histopathologic findings. Radiology. 2012;265:799–808.
39. Wagstaff PG, Zondervan PJ, de la Rosette JJ, Laguna MP. The role of imaging in the active surveillance of small renal masses. Curr Urol Rep. 2014;15:386.
40. Min JH, Kim CK, Park BK, Kim E, Kim B. Assessment of renal lesions with blood oxygenation level-dependent MRI at 3T:preliminary experience. Am J Roentgenol. 2011;197:W489–94.
41. Rha SE, Byun JY, Jung SE, et al. The renal sinus: pathologic spectrum and multimodality imaging approach. Radiographics. 2004;24:S117–31.
42. Urban BA, Buckley J, Soyer P, et al. CT appearance of transitional cell carcinoma of the renal pelvis: Part 1. early-stage disease. AJR Am J Roentgenol. 1997;169:157–61.
43. Browne RF, Meehan CP, Colville J, et al. Transitional cell carcinoma of the upper urinary tract: spectrum of imaging findings. Radiographics. 2005;25:1609–27.
44. Urban BA, Buckley J, Soyer P, et al. CT appearance of transitional cell carcinoma of the renal pelvis: Part 2. advanced-stage disease. AJR Am J Roentgenol. 1997;169:163–8.
45. Curry NS. Small renal masses (lesions smaller than 3 cm): imaging evaluation and management. AJR Am J Roentgenol. 1995;164:355–62.
46. Israel GM, Krinsky GA. MR imaging of the kidneys and adrenal glands. Radiol Clin North Am. 2003;41:145–59.
47. Cohan RH, Dunnick NR, Leder RA, et al. Computed tomography of renal lymphoma. J Comput Assist Tomogr. 1990;14:933–8.
48. Johnson CD, Dunnick NR, Cohan RH, et al. Renal adenocarcinoma: CT staging of 100 tumors. AJR Am J Roentgenol. 1987;148:59–63.
49. Roy C Sr, El Ghali S, Buy X, et al. Significance of the pseudocapsule on MRI of renal neoplasms and its potential application for local staging: a retrospective study. AJR Am J Roentgenol. 2005;184:113–20.
50. Narumi Y, Miyazaki T, Hatanaka Y, et al. MR imaging evaluation of renal carcinoma. Abdom Imaging. 1997;22:216–25.
51. Jayson M, Sanders H. Increased incidence of serendipitously discovered renal cell carcinoma. Urology. 1998;51:203–5.
52. Hui GC, Tuncali K, Tatli S, Morrison PR, Silverman SG. Comparison of percutaneous and surgical approaches to renal tumor ablation: metaanalysis of effectiveness and complication rates. J Vasc Interv Radiol. 2008;19:1311–20.
53. Cornelis F, Balageas P, Le Bras Y, Rigou G, Boutault JR, Bouzgarrou M, Grenier N. Radiologically-guided thermal ablation of renal tumours. Diagn Interv Imaging. 2012;93:246–61.
54. Gervais DA, Arellano RS, McGovern FJ, McDougal WS, Mueller PR. Radiofrequency ablation of renal cell carcinoma: part 2. Lessons learned with ablation of 100 tumors. AJR. 2005;185:72–80.
55. Mylona S, Kokkinaki A, Pomoni M, Galani P, Ntai S, Thanos L. Percutaneous radiofrequency ablation of renal cell carcinomas in patients with solitary kidney: 6 years experience. Eur J Radiol. 2009;69:351–6.
56. Zagoria RJ, Traver MA, Werle DM, Perini M, Hayasaka S, Clark PE. Oncologic efficacy of CT-guided percutaneous radiofrequency ablation of renal cell carcinomas. AJR. 2007;189:429–36.
57. Veltri A, Grosso M, Castagneri F, Garetto I, Sacchetto P, Tosetti I, et al. Radiofrequency thermal ablation of small tumors in transplanted kidneys: an evolving nephron-sparing option. J Vasc Interv Radiol. 2009;20:674–9.

58. Kunkle DA, Uzzo RG. Cryoablation or radiofrequency ablation of the small renal mass: a meta-analysis. Cancer. 2008;113:2671–80.
59. Wright AS, Sampson LA, Warner TF, Mahvi DM, Lee FT. Radiofrequency versus microwave ablation in a hepatic porcine model. Radiology. 2005;236:132–9.
60. Rais-Bahrami S, Pietryga JA, Nix JW. Contemporary role of advanced imaging for bladder cancer staging. Urol Oncol. 2016;34:124–33.
61. Purysko AS, Leão Filho HM, Herts BR. Radiologic imaging of patients with bladder cancer. Semin Oncol. 2012;39:543–58.
62. Datta SN, Allen GM, Evans R, Vaughton KC, Lucas MG. Urinary tract ultrasonography in the evaluation of haematuria – a report of over 1,000 cases. Ann R Coll Surg Engl. 2002;84:203–5.
63. Roy C. Tumour pathology of the bladder: the role of MRI. Diagn Interv Imaging. 2012;93:297–309.
64. Totaro A, Pinto F, Brescia A, Racioppi M, Cappa E, D'Agostino D, Volpe A, Sacco E, Palermo G, Valentini A, Bassi P. Imaging in bladder cancer: present role and future perspectives. Urol Int. 2010;85:373–80.
65. Kocakoc E, Kiris A, Orhan I, Poyraz AK, Artas H, Firdolas F. Detection of bladder tumors with 3-dimensional sonography and virtual sonographic cystoscopy. J Ultrasound Med. 2008;27:45–53.
66. Nicolau C, Bunesch L, Sebastia C, Salvador R. Diagnosis of bladder cancer: contrast-enhanced ultrasound. Abdom Imaging. 2010;35:494–503.
67. ACR Appropriateness Criteria. Hematuria. American College of Radiology. 2008. Accessed www.acr.org
68. M R. Tumours of the bladder: what does the urologist expect from imaging? Diagn Interv Imaging. 2012;93:291–6.
69. Sadow CA, Silverman SG, O'Leary MP, JE S. Bladder cancer detection with CT urography in an Academic Medical Center. Radiology. 2008;249:195–202.
70. Kim JK, Park SY, Ahn HJ, Kim CS, KS C. Bladder cancer: analysis of multi-detector row helical CT enhancement pattern and accuracy in tumor detection and perivesical staging. Radiology. 2004;231:725–31.
71. Turkbey B, Basaran C, Karcaaltincaba M, Akpinar E, Oguz B, Akata D, Ozmen MN, O A. Peritoneal carcinomatosis in urinary bladder cancer. Clin Imaging. 2008;32:192–5.
72. Caoili EM, Cohan RH, Inampudi P, Ellis JH, Shah RB, Faerber GJ, Montie JE. MDCT urography of upper tract urothelial neoplasms. AJR Am J Roentgenol. 2005;184:1873–81.
73. Pfister C, Roupret M, Wallerand H, Davin JL, Quintens H, Guy L, et al. Recommandations en onco-urologie 2010: tumeurs urothéliales. Prog Urol. 2010;20:S255–74.
74. Turney BW, Willatt JM, Nixon D, Crew JP, Cowan NC. Computed tomography urography for diagnosing bladder cancer. BJU Int. 2006;98:345–8.
75. Zhang J, Gerst S, Lefkowitz RA, Bach A. Imaging of bladder cancer. Radiol Clin North Am. 2007;45:183–205.
76. Tuncbilek N, Kaplan M, Altaner S, Atakan IH, Süt N, Inci O, et al. Value of dynamic contrast enhanced MRI and correlation with tumor angiogenesis in bladder cancer. AJR. 2009;192:949–55.
77. Scattoni V, Da Pozzo LF, Colombo R. Dynamic gadolinium enhanced magnetic resonance imaging in staging of superficial bladder cancer. J Urol. 1996;155:1594–5.
78. Abou-El-Ghar ME, El-Assmy A, Refaie HF, El-Diasty T. Bladder cancer: diagnosis with diffusion-weighted MR imaging in patients with gross hematuria. Radiology. 2009;251:415–21.
79. Dağgülli M, Onur MR, Fırdolaş F, Onur R, Kocakoç E, Orhan İ. Role of diffusion MRI and apparent diffusion coefficient measurement in the diagnosis, staging and pathological classification of bladder tumors. Urol Int. 2011;87:346–52.
80. Takeuchi M, Sasaki S, Ito M, Okada S, Takahashi S, Tatsuya K, et al. Diffusion weighted MR imaging – accuracy for diagnosing t stage and estimating histologic grade. Radiology. 2009;251:112–21.
81. El-Assmy A, Abou-El-Ghar ME, Mosbah A, et al. Bladder tumour staging: comparison of diffusion- and T2-weighted MR imaging. Eur Radiol. 2009;19:1575–81.

82. Barentsz JO, Ruijs SH, Strijk SP. The role of MR imaging in carcinoma of the urinary bladder. AJR Am J Roentgenol. 1993;160:937–47.
83. ACR Appropriateness Criteria. Pretreatment staging of invasive bladder cancer. American College of Radiology. 2009. Accessed www.acr.org
84. Bindu NS, Nagaraj SH, Dushyant VS. State of the art cross-sectional imaging in bladder cancer. Curr Probl Diagn Radiol. 2007;36:83–96.
85. Tachibana M, Baba S, Deguchi N, et al. Efficacy of gadolinium-diethylenetriaminepentaacetic acid-enhanced magnetic resonance imaging for differentiation between superficial and muscle-invasive tumor of the bladder: a comparative study with computerized tomography and transurethral ultrasonography. J Urol. 1991;145:1169–73.
86. Kim B, Semelka RC, Ascher SM, Chalpin DB, Carroll PR, Hricak H. Bladder tumor staging: comparison of contrast enhanced CT, T1- and T2-weighted MR imaging, dynamic gadolinium-enhanced imaging, and late gadolinium-enhanced imaging. Radiology. 1994;193:239–45.
87. Tanimoto A, Yuasa Y, Imai Y, et al. Bladder tumor staging: comparison of conventional and gadolinium-enhanced dynamic MR imaging and CT. Radiology. 1992;185:741–7.
88. Swinnen G, Maes A, Pottel H, et al. FDG-PET/CT for the preoperative lymph node staging of invasive bladder cancer. Eur Urol. 2010;57:641–7.
89. American Urological Association. Bladder Cancer Clinical Guideline Update Panel. The management of bladder cancer: diagnosis and treatment recommendations. American Urological Association Education and Research, Inc; 2007 (reviewed and validity confirmed 2010). Accessed www.auanet.org
90. Brausi M, Witjes JA, Lamm D, et al. A review of current guidelines and best practice recommendations for the management of nonmuscle invasive bladder cancer by the International Bladder Cancer Group. J Urol. 2011;186:2158–67.
91. Beyersdorff D, Zhang J, Schöder H, Bochner B, Hricak H. Bladder cancer: can imaging change patient management? Curr Opin Urol. 2008;18:98–104.
92. Yoshida S, Koga F, Kawakami S, et al. Initial experience of diffusion-weighted magnetic resonance imaging to assess therapeutic response to induction chemoradiotherapy against muscle-invasive bladder cancer. Urology. 2010;75:387–91.
93. Tabatabaei S, Saylor PJ, Coen J, Dahl DM. Prostate cancer imaging: what surgeons, radiation oncologists, and medical oncologists want to know. AJR Am J Roentgenol. 2011;196:1263–6.
94. Mertan FV, Greer MD, Shih JH, George AK, Kongnyuy M, Muthigi A, Merino MJ, Wood BJ, Pinto PA, Choyke PL, Turkbey B. Prospective Evaluation of the Prostate Imaging Reporting and Data System Version 2 for Prostate Cancer Detection. J Urol. 2016;196:690–6.
95. Dyke CH, Toi A, Sweet JM. Value of random ultrasound-guided transrectal prostate biopsy. Radiology. 1990;176:345–9.
96. Ghai STA. Role of transrectal ultrasonography in prostate cancer. Radiol Clin North Am. 2012;50:1061–73.
97. Volkin D, Turkbey B, Hoang AN, et al. Multiparametric magnetic resonance imaging (MRI) and subsequent MRI/ultrasonography fusion guided biopsy increase the detection of anteriorly located prostate cancers. BJU Int. 2014;114:E43–9.
98. Nevoux P, Ouzzane A, Ahmed HU, et al. Quantitative tissue analyses of prostate cancer foci in an unselected cystoprostatectomy series. BJU Int. 2012;110:517–23.
99. Marko J, Gould CF, Bonavia GH, Wolfman DJ. State-of-the-art imaging of prostate cancer. Urol Oncol. 2016;34:134–46.
100. Brown AM, Elbuluk O, Mertan F, Sankineni S, Margolis DJ, Wood BJ, Pinto PA, Choyke PL, Turkbey B. Recent advances in image-guided targeted prostate biopsy. Abdom Imaging. 2015;40:1788–99.
101. Barr RG. Elastography in clinical practice. Radiol Clin North Am. 2014;52:1145.
102. Correas J, Tissier A, Khairoune A, et al. Prostate cancer: diagnostic performance of real-time shear-wave elastography. Radiology. 2015;275:280–9.
103. Pallwein L, Mitterberger M, Pelzer A, Bartsch G, Strasser H, Pinggera GM, Aigner F, Gradl J, Zur Nedden D, Frauscher F. Ultrasound of prostate cancer: recent advances. Eur Radiol. 2008;18:707–15.

104. Halpern EJ, Frauscher F, Rosenberg M, Gomella LG. Directed biopsy during contrast-enhanced sonography of the prostate. AJR Am J Roentgenol. 2002;178:915–9.
105. Pinto PA, Chung PH, Rastinehad Ardeshir R, et al. Magnetic resonance imaging/ultrasound fusion guided prostate biopsy improves cancer detection following transrectal ultrasound biopsy and correlates with multiparametric magnetic resonance imaging. J Urol. 2011;186:1281–5.
106. Siddiqui MM, Rais-Bahrami S, Turkbey B, et al. Comparison of MR/ultrasound fusion-guided biopsy with ultrasound-guided biopsy for the diagnosis of prostate cancer. JAMA. 2015;313:390–7.
107. Vourganti S, Rastinehad A, Yerram NK, et al. Multiparametric magnetic resonance imaging and ultrasound fusion biopsy detect prostate cancer in patients with prior negative transrectal ultrasound biopsies. J Urol. 2012;188:2152–7.
108. Barchetti F, Panebianco V. Multiparametric MRI for recurrent prostate cancer post radical prostatectomy and postradiation therapy. Biomed Res Int. 2014:316272.
109. Turkbey B, Shah VP, Pang Y, et al. Is apparent diffusion coefficient associated with clinical risk scores for prostate cancers that are visible on 3-T MR images? Radiology. 2011;258:488–95.
110. Berman RM, Brown AM, Chang SD, Sankineni S, Kadakia M, Wood BJ, Pinto PA, Choyke PL, Turkbey B. DCE MRI of prostate cancer. Abdom Radiol (NY). 2016;41:844–53.
111. Villers A, Puech P, Mouton D, Leroy X, Ballereau C, Lemaitre L. Dynamic contrast enhanced, pelvic phased array magnetic resonance imaging of localized prostate cancer for predicting tumor volume: correlation with radical prostatectomy findings. J Urol. 2006;176:2432–7.
112. Lemaitre L, Puech P, Poncelet E, Bouye S, Leroy X, Biserte J, et al. Dynamic contrast-enhanced MRI of anterior prostate cancer: morphometric assessment and correlation with radical prostatectomy findings. Eur Radiol. 2009;19:470–80.
113. Puech P, Potiron E, Lemaitre L, Leroy X, Haber GP, Crouzet S, et al. Dynamic contrast-enhanced-magnetic resonance imaging evaluation of intraprostatic prostate cancer: correlation with radical prostatectomy specimens. Urology. 2009;74:1094–9.
114. Delongchamps NB, Rouanne M, Flam T, Beuvon F, Liberatore M, Zerbib M, et al. Multiparametric magnetic resonance imaging for the detection and localization of prostate cancer: combination of T2-weighted, dynamic contrast-enhanced and diffusion-weighted imaging. BJU Int. 2011;107:1411–8.
115. Weinreb JC, Barentsz JO, Choyke PL, Cornud F, Haider MA, Macura KJ, Margolis D, Schnall MD, Shtern F, Tempany CM, Thoeny HC, Verma S. PI-RADS prostate imaging – reporting and data system: 2015, version 2. Eur Urol. 2016;69:16–40.
116. Torricelli P, Barberini A, Cinquantini F, Sighinolfi M, Cesinaro AM. 3-T MRI with phased-array coil in local staging of prostatic cancer. Acad Radiol. 2008;15:1118–25.
117. Lourenco AP, Donegan L, Khalil H, Mainiero MB. Improving outcomes of screening breast MRI with practice evolution: initial clinical experience with 3T compared to 1.5T. J Magn Reson Imaging. 2014;39:535–9.
118. Coakley FV, Qayyum A, Kurhanewicz J. Magnetic resonance imaging and spectroscopic imaging of prostate cancer. J Urol. 2003;170:S69–75.
119. Testa C, Schiavina R, Lodi R, et al. Prostate cancer: sextant localization with MR imaging, MR spectroscopy, and 11C-choline PET/CT. Radiology. 2007;244:797–806.
120. Lim HK, Kim JK, Kim KA, Cho KS. Prostate cancer: apparent diffusion coefficient map with T2-weighted images for detection – a multireader study. Radiology. 2009;250:145–51.
121. Brawer MK, Deering RE, Brown M, Preston SD, Bigler SA. Predictors of pathologic stage in prostatic carcinoma: the role of neovascularity. Cancer. 1994;73:678–87.
122. Verma S, Turkbey B, Muradyan N, Rajesh A, Cornud F, Haider MA, Choyke PL, Harisinghani M. Overview of dynamic contrast-enhanced MRI in prostate cancer diagnosis and management. AJR Am J Roentgenol. 2012;198:1277–88.
123. Kim JK, Hong SS, Choi YJ, et al. Wash-in rate on the basis of dynamic contrast- enhanced MRI: usefulness for prostate cancer detection and localization. J Magn Reson Imaging. 2005;22:639–46.

124. Verma S, Rajesh A. A clinically relevant approach to imaging prostate cancer: review. AJR Am J Roentgenol. 2011;196(3 Suppl):S1–10; Quiz S11–4.
125. Bloch BN, Furman-Haran E, Helbich TH, Lenkinski RE, Degani H, Kratzik C, et al. Prostate cancer: accurate determination of extracapsular extension with high-spatial-resolution dynamic contrast-enhanced and T2-weighted MR imaging – initial results. Radiology. 2007;245:176–85.
126. Kurhanewicz J, Vigneron DB, Hricak H, Narayan P, Carroll P, Nelson SJ. Three-dimensional H-1 MR spectroscopic imaging of the in situ human prostate with high (0.24-0.7-cm3) spatial resolution. Radiology. 1996;198:795–805.
127. Junker D, Quentin M, Nagele U, et al. Evaluation of the PI-RADS scoring system for mpMRI of the prostate: a whole-mount step- section analysis. World J Urol. 2015;33:1023–30.
128. Itou Y, Nakanishi K, Narumi Y, Nishizawa Y, Tsukuma H. Clinical utility of apparent diffusion coefficient (ADC) values in patients with prostate cancer: can ADC values contribute to assess the aggressiveness of prostate cancer? J Magn Reson Imaging. 2011;33:167–72.
129. de Rooij M, Hamoen EH, Futterer JJ, Barentsz JO, Rovers MM. Accuracy of multiparametric MRI for prostate cancer detection: a meta-analysis. Am J Roentgenol. 2014;202:343–51.
130. Ouzzane A, Puech P, Lemaitre L, et al. Combined multiparametric MRI and targeted biopsies improve anterior prostate cancer detection, staging, and grading. Urology. 2011;78:1356–62.
131. Villeirs GM, De Meerleer GO, DeVisschere PJ, Fonteyne VH, Verbaeys AC, Oosterlinck W. Combined magnetic resonance imaging and spectroscopy in the assessment of high grade prostate carcinoma in patients with elevated PSA: a single-institution experience of 356 patients. Eur J Radiol. 2011;77:340–5.
132. Akin O, Hricak H. Imaging of prostate cancer. Radiol Clin North Am. 2007;45:207–22.
133. George AK, Pinto PA, Rais-Bahrami S. Multiparametric MRI in the PSA screening era. Biomed Res Int. 2014;2014:465816.
134. George AK, Turkbey B, Valayil SG, Muthigi A, Mertan F, Kongnyuy M, Pinto PA. A urologist's perspective on prostate cancer imaging: past, present, and future. Abdom Radiol (NY). 2016;41:805–16.
135. Boonsirikamchai P, Choi S, Frank SJ, Ma J, Elsayes KM, Kaur H, Choi H. MR imaging of prostate cancer in radiation oncology: what radiologists need to know. Radiographics. 2013;33:741–61.
136. Raskolnikov D, George AK, Rais-Bahrami S, et al. The role of magnetic resonance image guided prostate biopsy in stratifying men for risk of extracapsular extension at radical prostatectomy. J Urol. 2015;194:105–11.
137. Harisinghani MG, Barentsz J, Hahn PF, et al. Noninvasive detection of clinically occult lymph-node metastases in prostate cancer. N Engl J Med. 2003;348:2491–9.
138. Zhang J, Hricak H, Shukla-Dave A, et al. Clinical stage T1c prostate cancer: evaluation with endorectal MR imaging and MR spectroscopic imaging. Radiology. 2009;253:425–34.
139. Augustin H, Fritz GA, Ehammer T, Auprich M, Pummer K. Accuracy of 3-tesla magnetic resonance imaging for the staging of prostate cancer in comparison to the part in tables. Acta Radiol. 2009;50:562–9.
140. Lecouvet FE, Geukens D, Stainier A, Jamar F, Jamart J, d'Othée BJ, Therasse P, Vande Berg B, Tombal B. Magnetic resonance imaging of the axial skeleton for detecting bone metastases in patients with high-risk prostate cancer: diagnostic and cost-effectiveness and comparison with current detection strategies. J Clin Oncol. 2007;25:3281–7.
141. Park BH, Jeon HG, Jeong BC, Seo SI, Lee HM, Choi HY, Jeon SS. Influence of magnetic resonance imaging in the decision to preserve or resect neurovascular bundles at robotic assisted laparoscopic radical prostatectomy. J Urol. 2014;192:82–8.
142. Sciarra A, Barentsz J, Bjartell A, et al. Advances in magnetic resonance imaging: how they are changing the management of prostate cancer. Eur Urol. 2011;59:962–77.
143. Grenabo Bergdahl A, Wilderäng U, Aus G, et al. Role of magnetic resonance imaging in prostate cancer screening: a pilot study within the Goteborg randomised screening trial. Eur Urol. 2016;70:566–73.

144. Fascelli M, Rais-Bahrami S, Sankineni S, et al. Combined biparametric prostate MRI and prostate specific antigen in the detection of prostate cancer: a validation study in a biopsy naive patient population. Urology. 2016;88:125–34.
145. Ciccarese C, Santoni M, Massari F, et al. Metabolic alterations in renal and prostate cancer. Curr Drug Metab. 2016;17:150–5.
146. Nelson SJ, Kurhanewicz J, Vigneron DB, et al. Metabolic imaging of patients with prostate cancer using hyperpolarized [1-^{13}C]pyruvate. Sci Transl Med. 2013;14:198ra108.
147. Kara T, Akata D, Akyol F, Karçaaltıncaba M, Özmen M. The value of dynamic contrast-enhanced MRI in the detection of recurrent prostate cancer after external beam radiotherapy: correlation with transrectal ultrasound and pathological findings. Diagn Interv Radiol. 2011;17:38–43.
148. Coakley FV, Hricak H, Wefer AE, Speight JL, Kurhanewicz J, Roach M. Brachytherapy for prostate cancer: endorectal MR imaging of local treatment-related changes. Radiology. 2001;219:817–21.

Management of Non-muscle-Invasive and Muscle-Invasive Bladder Cancers

2

Ilker Tinay and N. Aydin Mungan

Abstract

Bladder cancer (BC) is the 7th most commonly diagnosed cancer in men worldwide, while it declines to 11th when both sexes are considered. The worldwide age-standardized incidence rate (per 100,000 person/years) is 9.0 for men and 2.2 for women. Europe has among the highest incidence rates of BC in the world, where the age-standardized incidence rate is 19.1 for men and 4.0 for women. The overall burden was greater in men; however varying incidence trends by gender were reported recently in some countries, with rates drop in male and increase in female population. The management of BC should be tailored according to the disease stage, grade, and patient-related factors at the presentation. In this chapter, we will discuss the management of non-muscle-invasive disease and the surgical management of muscle-invasive disease.

2.1 Introduction

Bladder cancer (BC) is the 7th most commonly diagnosed cancer in men worldwide, while it declines to 11th when both sexes are considered [1]. The worldwide age-standardized incidence rate (per 100,000 person/years) is 9.0 for men and 2.2 for women. An estimated 76,960 new cases of BC will be diagnosed in the United States (USA) in 2016 [2]. Bladder cancer, the fourth most common

I. Tinay, M.D.
Department of Urology, School of Medicine, Marmara University, Istanbul, Turkey

N.A. Mungan, M.D. (✉)
Department of Urology, Bulent Ecevit University, Zonguldak, Turkey
e-mail: anmungan@yahoo.com

G. Ozyigit, U. Selek (eds.), *Principles and Practice of Urooncology*,
DOI 10.1007/978-3-319-56114-1_2

cancer in males, is 3.3 times more prevalent in men than in women in the USA. Europe has among the highest incidence rates of BC in the world, where the age-standardized incidence rate is 19.1 for men and 4.0 for women [1]. The overall burden was greater in men; however varying incidence trends by gender were reported recently in some countries, with rates drop in male and increase in female population [1]. Worldwide, age-standardized mortality rate (per 100,000 person/years) was 3.2 for men vs. 0.9 for women in 2012 [1]. Although mortality declines were generally observed in Europe, mortality rates in European men were by far the highest recorded worldwide [1]. In 2016, approximately 16,390 deaths (11,820 men and 4570 women) will result from BC, which is the eighth most common in male population and the fourth most common in patients >80 years of age in the USA [2]. Regarding the mortality, again the affliction was greater in men; however as with the incidence trends by sex in some countries, mortality rates decline in men and increase in women [1]. Disparities in terms of healthcare systems, management protocols, or access to facilities, particularly between countries at different levels of development, could explain the differences reported in BC incidence, survival, and mortality rates between countries [1].

At presentation, approximately 75% of patients with BC present with non-muscle-invasive disease confined to the mucosa (pathological stage Ta and/or carcinoma in situ) or submucosa (pathological stage T1), and almost 50% of these patients have low-grade disease [3, 4] (Fig. 2.1). The remaining 25% of BC patients present with muscle-invasive or metastatic disease and most of these tumors are high-grade lesions [3, 5]. In non-muscle-invasive BC, the most important prognostic factor is grade [5], and the latest grading system was introduced in 2004 by the World Health Organization (WHO) and updated in 2016 [6, 7]. This grading system categorizes urothelial carcinoma as "low grade" or "high grade" and includes another category, "papillary urothelial neoplasm of low malignant potential (PUNLMP)." For invasive BC, the most important prognostic factor is clinical and pathological stage, which is based on the depth of tumor invasion and metastasis status [5].

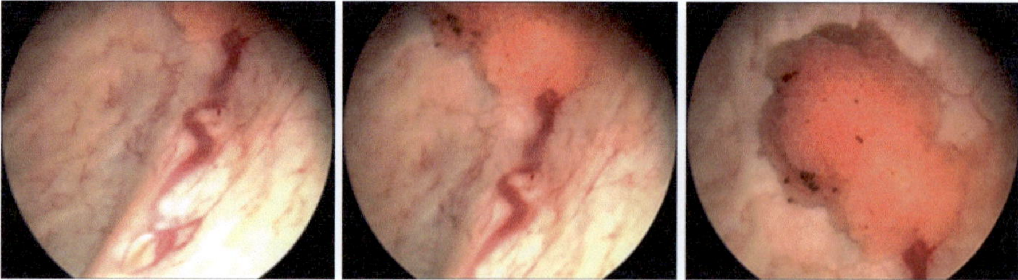

Fig. 2.1 Cystoscopic appearance of a bladder tumor with a feeding vessel and papillary nature (Courtesy of Marmara University Department of Urology)

The management of BC should be tailored according to the disease stage, grade, and patient-related factors at the presentation. In this chapter, we will discuss the management of non-muscle-invasive disease and the surgical management of muscle-invasive disease. Target volume delineation radiotherapy guidelines, bladder preservation approaches, systemic chemotherapies, targeted therapies, and immunotherapy in BC will be discussed in the following chapters.

2.2 Management of Non-muscle-Invasive Bladder Cancer

The initial step for the diagnosis of bladder tumors is transurethral resection (TUR) to remove all visible tumors with sufficient surgical margins and depth (Fig. 2.2), which also represents the initial approach in the management of non-muscle-invasive bladder cancer (NMIBC). However, the diagnosis of NMIBC requires close follow-up with potentially additional treatments since reported 5-year rates of NMIBC recurrence range from 50% to 70% and progression to muscle-invasive disease range from 10% to 30% [5].

The management of NMIBC is based on the pathological findings of the TUR specimen: histology, tumor grade, pathological T stage, presence or absence of the muscularis propria, and carcinoma in situ. Using these pathological findings together with tumor size, tumor quantity, and number of previous recurrences, NMIBC has been categorized as low-, intermediate-, or high-risk groups for recurrence and progression by European Association of Urology (EAU) and National Institute for Health and Care Excellence (NICE) [4, 8] (Table 2.1). It should be noted that the major difference between EAU and NICE risk groups is that EAU categorizes patients with multiple or recurrent >3 cm pTa low-grade tumors as high-risk disease, while it has been defined as intermediate-risk disease by NICE [9]. Based on these risk groups, national and international societies developed practical recommendations for the management of NMIBC [4, 8, 10, 11].

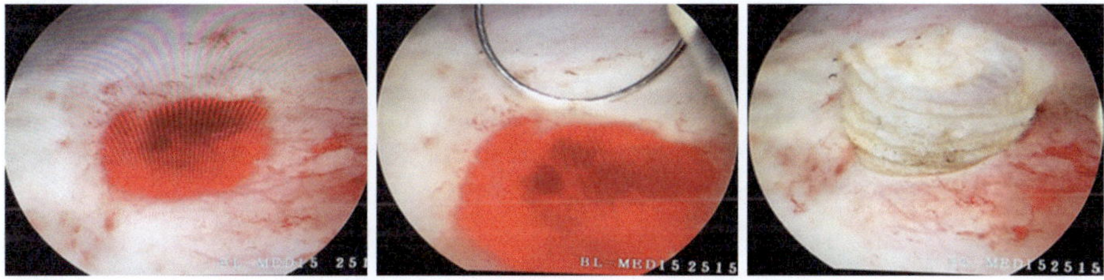

Fig. 2.2 Cystoscopic appearance of a suspicious bladder lesion and transurethral resection of this lesion with sufficient surgical margins and depth (Courtesy of Marmara University Department of Urology)

Table 2.1 NMIBC risk groups according to the EAU and NICE guidelines

NMIBC risk groups	EAU guidelines [4]	NICE guidelines [8]
Low	New solitary pTa low grade (G1/2) <3 cm	Solitary pT1 low grade (G1/2) <3 cm Papillary urothelial neoplasm of low malignant potential
Intermediate	All others	Solitary pTa low grade (G1/2) >3 cm Multifocal pTa low grade (G1/2) pTa high grade (G2) Any pTaG2 (unspecified) Any low risk with recurrence <12 months
High	Any pT1 pTa high-grade (G3) pCIS Multiple/recurrent AND >3 cm Ta low grade (G1/2)	Any pT1 pTa high-grade (G3) pCIS Aggressive variants—nested/micropapillary
Highest	T1G3/HG associated with concurrent bladder CIS, multiple and/or large T1G3/HG and/or recurrent T1G3/HG T1G3/HG with CIS in the prostatic urethra, unusual histology of urothelial carcinoma, lymphovascular invasion	Not exists

2.3 Repeat/Restaging Transurethral Resection

To more correctly evaluate stage and improve response to adjuvant intravesical treatments, the value of a repeat or restaging transurethral resection after the initial transurethral resection has been proven [12–14]. A second transurethral resection corrects clinical staging errors in 9–49% of cases and detects residual tumor in 26–83% of cases [15]. Major guidelines support the role of repeat resection within 2–6 weeks after primary resection in cases of incomplete resection and in cases of high-grade pTa where detrusor was not present. In addition, EAU, International Consultation on Urological Diseases (ICUD), and National Comprehensive Cancer Network (NCCN) recommend a repeat resection in all pT1 tumors. ICUD and NICE suggest a second resection in all high-risk tumors even in cases with detrusor present in primary resection. EAU mentions two select circumstances regarding carcinoma in situ (CIS): incomplete resection, if no muscle is present in the initial resection except CIS, and all high-grade lesions except primary CIS [4].

A second resection is particularly warranted for T1 tumors since 2–28% of them prove to be muscle invasive, thus requiring a change in management [15]. Our group recently showed that the interval between first and second TUR should be ≤42 days in order to attain lower recurrence and progression rates in patients with high-risk NMIBC treated with maintenance intravesical Bacillus Calmette-Guérin (BCG) therapy [16].

2.4 Intravesical Chemotherapy

For patients with NMIBC, a single immediate instillation of intravesical chemotherapy (IVC) (e.g., mitomycin, epirubicin, or doxorubicin) after transurethral resection is recommended by all guidelines. The optimum timing is within 6 h after transurethral resection, and delaying instillation for more than 24 h was found to increase recurrence rates by nearly twofold [17]. A meta-analysis of randomized trials supported that IVC prolongs recurrence-free interval (hazard ratio [HR], 0.62; 95% confidence interval [CI], 0.50–0.77) and early recurrences of NMIBC were 12% less likely in the intervention population when administered immediately after TUR [18]. Another meta-analysis of randomized trials reported benefit from IVC in patients with low-risk and intermediate-risk disease (HR, 0.65; 95%CI, 0.58–0.74) but not in patients with high-risk disease [19]. Although a single immediate instillation of IVC for recurrent tumors has been considered as a non-useful treatment option, in the recent EAU guidelines, it has been recommended in patients with previous low recurrence rate (less than or equal to one recurrence per year) and expected EORTC recurrence score <5 [4].

Although low-risk BC patients would only require a single instillation of IVC, this is subtherapeutic for intermediate-risk disease and an induction course 3–4 weeks after TURBT is recommended by all guidelines. A randomized trial comparing three different regimes of IVC failed to show any difference between a 6-month and a 1-year regime in a predominantly intermediate-risk cohort [20]. For patients with intermediate-risk NMIBC, a meta-analysis of randomized trials showed benefit from the addition of 1 year of maintenance IVC after transurethral resection (1-year recurrence HR 0.56) [21]. However, the exact induction regime and the need for maintenance instillation are uncertain, and yet no studies have shown decreased progression rates with IVC [21].

2.5 Intravesical Immunotherapy

All guidelines advocate the use of intravesical BCG immunotherapy after TURBT in high-risk NMIBC. Several randomized studies have compared BCG with various IVCs [22]. In these studies, not only was BCG superior in terms of reducing recurrences, but also it was the only intravesical treatment that delayed disease progression [23]. Data from these studies are further supported by five meta-analyses confirming the superiority of intravesical BCG over intravesical MMC in both high-risk papillary and CIS tumors [22, 24]. It should be noted that a reduction of 32–59% in tumor recurrence only achieved when maintenance BCG was used. Two meta-analyses compared intravesical BCG vs. MMC and reported 27–34% reduction in progression rates for patients treated with induction and maintenance BCG [25, 26]. In order to augment the effect of intravesical therapies, a randomized trial comparing BCG followed by electromotive mitomycin with BCG alone reported promising results with lower rates of disease progression (9.3% vs. 21.9%) and mortality (21.5% vs. 32.4%) in combination group [27].

Intravesical BCG treatment is also a valuable option for patients with intermediate-risk disease. A recent randomized trial showed that in high-risk disease, recurrence-free survival was greatest when maintenance BCG was delivered at full dose for 3 years; however, for intermediate-risk NMIBC, 1 year of maintenance treatment was adequate [28]. Another recent randomized trial compared BCG with hyperthermic administration of mitomycin in intermediate- and high-risk patients and reported a higher 24-month relapse-free survival rate with mitomycin (78.1% vs. 64.8%) but no difference in progression [29]. However these recent findings require further validation.

All guidelines recommend the BCG induction regime of once a week for 6 weeks, which was first described by Morales 40 years ago [30]. However, different maintenance protocols exist ranging from 6 once weekly instillations every 6 months for 2 years to monthly instillations for 2 years [31, 32]. The most commonly used protocol is based on the Southwest Oncology Group study, where the maintenance group received 3 once weekly BCG at 3 and 6 months followed by 3 once weekly BCG every 6 months for up to 3 years [33].

2.6 Treatment Alternatives During the Global Shortage of BCG

Bacillus Calmette-Guérin is a live vaccine and historically the Connaught strain has been dominantly used for the intravesical treatment. Sanofi, who produces this strain, had major production problems in 2012, and their supply had to be withdrawn from the market for security reasons. This put added pressure on the other strains, such as Tice, Tokyo, RIVM, etc., and an increased demand for intravesical treatment alternatives [34, 35]. As we mentioned above, the term NMIBC represents a heterogeneous group of patients, and subclassification is helpful to manage these patients. It is also possible to subgroup patients, who ideally should be managed with intravesical BCG treatment, and make treatment recommendations:

2.6.1 Alternative BCG Schedules

- **Patients already on treatment:** BCG maintenance can be stopped after the first year in patients without CIS and continued for up to 3 years in patients with CIS at a reduced 1/3 dose [35]. In the EORTC-GU trial, this approach did not seem to lead to more tumor progression; however a higher risk of recurrence has been noticed in the very high-risk group [36].
- **New patients:** A reduced dose of 1/3 BCG for both induction and maintenance for 1 year has been investigated by the same EORTC-GU trial, and this treatment regimen was also not associated with an increased progressing rate as compared to full dose regimen [36].

2.6.2 Alternative Intravesical Chemotherapy Applications

- **Mitomycin C with maintenance:** Although intravesical BCG treatment was associated with superior treatment results in the RCTs, a significant response in terms of recurrence rates should be noticed with the use of maintenance mitomycin C even in high-risk patients [22]. Based on these results, an alternative treatment schedule with induction and maintenance mitomycin C seems to be a sensible alternative, especially for high-risk NMIBC patients without highest-risk features [35].
- **Delivery of chemotherapy with thermal energy:** Thermal energy appears to optimize the absorption of several intravesical agents, and several devices are available to deliver thermo-chemotherapy for the treatment of NMIBC [34, 35]. A recent systemic review and meta-analysis reported a 59% reduction in recurrence rate for this approach compared to traditional chemotherapy instillations [37].
- **Electromotive drug administration:** This approach uses an electric current to augment transepithelial drug penetration. Data of two RCTs from the same group suggest that this administration appears to increase bladder uptake of MMC, resulting in an improved response rate in high-risk group [27, 38]. Although short-term results appear equivalent to BCG, long- term efficacy data are lacking by the time of this review.
- **Intravesical gemcitabine:** A recent review reported similar results with gemcitabine in intermediate-risk group compared to intravesical BCG therapy; however inferior results were reported for high-risk group. Today this treatment mainly reserved for BCG-refractory patients [39].

2.7 Future Perspectives

Intravesical drug delivery is challenged by the difficulty of establishment of a suitable and effective drug concentration because of periodical discharge of the bladder. In this context, bio-adhesive colloidal drug delivery systems have emerged as promising delivery systems for intravesical chemotherapeutic agents. Recently, we have reported on different cationic nanoparticles for the effective delivery of mitomycin C for NMIBC [40–42]. Similarly we also showed that cationic nanoparticles provide a significantly improved perspective in intravesical immunotherapy of bladder tumors [43]. Further studies and especially in human trials with biocompatible cationic nanoparticles are required for more effective intravesical therapies in NMIBC.

2.8 Treatment of Disease Unresponsive to or Relapsing After BCG Vaccination

Treatment failures of BCG can be stratified into the three categories: no response to BCG (BCG-refractory disease), relapse after BCG, and BCG intolerance [44, 45]. The EAU panel categorized these instances under the title "unsuccessful treatment with intravesical BCG" (Table 2.2) [4].

Table 2.2 EAU categories for unsuccessful intravesical BCG treatments

BCG failure	Whenever a MIBC is detected during follow-up. BCG-refractory tumor: 1. If HG non-muscle-invasive papillary tumor is present at 3 month 2. If CIS (without concomitant papillary tumor) is present at both 3 and 6 months 3. If HG tumor appears during BCG therapy (patients with low-grade recurrence during or after BCG treatment are not considered a BCG failure) HG recurrence after BCG: Recurrence of HG/grade 3 (WHO 2004/1973) tumor after completion of BCG maintenance, despite an initial response
BCG intolerance	Severe side effects that prevent further BCG instillation before completing induction.

Recently, the US Food and Drug Administration, the International Bladder Cancer Group, and the American Society of Clinical Oncology GU Cancers Group introduced another subcategory called "BCG unresponsive," basically to assist patient selection for clinical trial enrolment after the worldwide shortage of BCG [46, 47]. This category includes BCG-refractory disease and a subset of the patients with relapsing BCG who have recurrence within 6 months of last exposure to BCG during maintenance treatment. These patients are at highest risk of recurrence and progression, do not benefit from continued BCG, and are strongly recommended to undergo radical cystectomy. However, patients with late BCG relapse (more than 1–2 years after last BCG exposure) and who are unwilling to undergo RC can try another course of salvage intravesical treatment with repeat intravesical induction BCG, BCG with interferon α2a, gemcitabine, or valrubicin [5].

In EAU guidelines, for BCG-refractory category, the recommendation is either RC or bladder-preserving strategies in patients unsuitable for cystectomy [4]. For high-grade recurrence, RC, repeat BCG, or bladder-preserving strategies are recommended. For non-high-grade recurrences after BCG in primary intermediate tumors, repeat intravesical BCG/chemotherapy or RC is recommended. The NICE guideline recommends all patients who fail induction course BCG to be considered for RC [8]. If the patient's clinical situation is unsuitable for RC, further intravesical therapy may be considered, but there was considerable uncertainty regarding the optimal next steps. At the present time, treatments other than RC must be considered oncologically inadequate in patients with BCG failure.

2.9 Upfront Cystectomy for Very High-Risk NMIBC

High-risk NMIBC is a heterogeneous disease and recently the definition of "very high-risk disease" has been introduced with the recommendation of upfront radical cystectomy as the initial management to improve survival [4]. The evidence is solid that high-grade pT1 BC with coexisting CIS is associated with an increased risk of recurrence and progression [48]. EORTC nomograms also suggest that in patients treated with intravesical BCG (with a maintenance protocol), previous recurrence rate and presence of multifocal disease were associated with progression and death [49].

In addition, the diagnosis of "micropapillary" variant histology has been reported to be refractory to BCG with 67% risk of disease progression [50].

Based on these data, patients with very high-risk NMIBC include those with multiple and/or large high-grade T1 tumors, micropapillary variant histology, coexistent CIS in the bladder or prostatic urethra, or presence of lymphovascular invasion in TUR pathology [51–53]. EAU, NICE, NCCN, and ICUD suggest early cystectomy as an alternative to intravesical BCG in these very high-risk tumors. ICUD specifically identify young patients with pT1 disease with at least one adverse prognostic factor listed above, where EAU suggest that patients with large tumors (>3 cm) are also candidates of early cystectomy [4, 44].

2.10 Surgical Management of Muscle-Invasive Bladder Cancer

Standard radical cystectomy (RC) techniques include removal of the distal ureters together with the urethra, adjacent vagina, and uterus in women or prostate and seminal vesicles in men [54]. Radical cystectomy with bilateral pelvic lymphadenectomy and often preceded by neo-adjuvant cisplatin-based chemotherapy is the gold standard surgical treatment for muscle-invasive BC [5, 54]. Minimally invasive radical cystectomy (MIRC) techniques, namely, laparoscopic- and robot-assisted RC, are being increasingly applied for the treatment of muscle-invasive BC, and short- to medium-term results are promising for both techniques in terms of postoperative morbidity and oncologic outcomes [55]. For the optimization of erectile function and urinary continence after RC, nerve-sparing and pelvic organ-sparing techniques have been reported [56]. Nerve-sparing RC is applicable for both women and men, except there is doubt for the local tumor control such as patients with clinical T3–T4 tumors [5, 56]. However, the long-term oncological safety for prostate and/or seminal vesicle sparing RC in men remains in question since whole-mount processing of the prostate demonstrates urothelial cancer in 20–40% and prostate adenocarcinoma in 40–50 % of patients in the final pathology [57, 58].

The extent of pelvic lymph node dissection (PLND) during RC is a subject of debate. An extended PLND includes all lymph nodes (LNs) between the aortic bifurcation and common iliac vessels (proximally), the genitofemoral nerve (laterally), the circumflex iliac vein and LNs of Cloquet (distally), and the internal iliac vessels (posteriorly), including the obturator fossa and the presacral LNs anterior to the sacral promontory (Fig. 2.3). A recent meta-analysis showed that an extended pelvic lymph node dissection should be done as it results in more accurate staging, better regional control, and improved survival than the more restricted dissection and less than complete lymphadenectomy [59]. The number of removed LNs for a sufficient determination of LN staging in each patient is currently not standardized [60]. Studies reported that higher numbers of examined LNs are related to increased CSS and overall survival (OS) rates. Herr reported 5-year OS rates of 33% in patients with 0–5 examined LNs compared to 79% with >14 nodes [61]. A multi-institutional cooperative bladder cancer group study reported a recommendation of

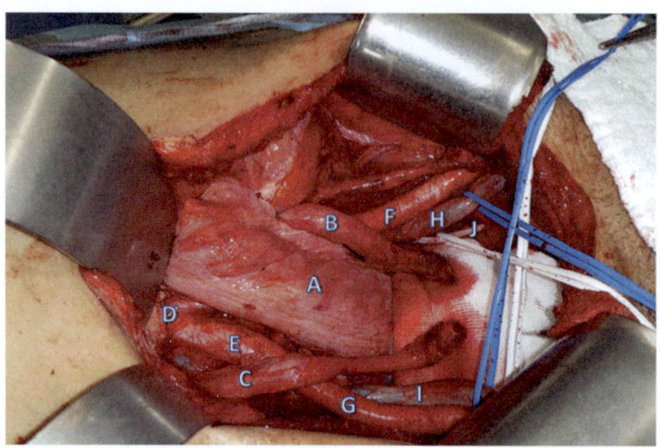

Fig. 2.3 Appearance of the pelvic area after radical cystectomy and extended lymphadenectomy. (**A**) Sigmoid colon, (**B**) left ureter, (**C**) right ureter, (**D**) aortic bifurcation, (**E**) right common iliac artery, (**F**) left external iliac artery, (**G**) right external iliac artery, (**H**) left external iliac vein, (**I**) right external iliac vein, (**J**) left obturator nerve (Courtesy of Marmara University Department of Urology)

a minimum removal of 10 to 14 LNs [62]. Two ongoing prospective randomized trials, AB 25/02-LEA by German Association of Urogenital Oncology and SWOG-S1011 by Southwest Oncology Group, are testing whether extended pelvic lymphadenectomy results in better survival or locoregional control than standard bilateral pelvic lymphadenectomy [63, 64].

Radical cystectomy is associated with significant postoperative mortality, where 30-day mortality rates were reported between 1.2% and 3.2% and 90-day mortality rates varies between 2.3% and 8% [54, 65, 66]. Early complication rates within 30 days after the surgery were reported between 20% and 60% in studies using multi-institutional cystectomy databases and large single center cohorts [67]. Enhanced recovery protocols, avoiding bowel preparation and nasogastric tube, starting with early feeding, using nonnarcotic pain management, cholinergic and μ-opioid antagonists, after radical cystectomy, aim to reduce perioperative morbidity [68, 69]. However the experience with these recovery protocols is limited. In general, lower morbidity and (perioperative) mortality are seen with high-volume surgeons and hospitals [70, 71].

A randomized trial [72] of robotic-assisted laparoscopic versus open radical cystectomy showed no difference in morbidity or length of hospital stay but longer operative time and increased cost in the robotic group, similar to results from the CORAL study from the UK [73]. A propensity-matched comparison study of morbidity and costs of open and robot-assisted radical cystectomies reported similar major complication rates (Clavien grade ≥3) between open- and robot-assisted RC. However robot-assisted RC had 46% decreased odds of minor complications (Clavien grade <3) [74]. Two prospective randomized clinical trials comparing open and robotic radical cystectomy are in progress, but final results have not been reported yet [5, 75].

Late morbidity after radical cystectomy is usually linked to the type of urinary diversion. Generally, ileal conduits represent least complication-prone and most commonly performed urinary diversion, where neobladders represent more complex diversions with high patient commitment during rehabilitation period. The largest single site experience with neobladders reported at least 1 complication within 90 days of surgery in 58% of patients, where 36% had minor (grades 1 to 2) and 22% had major (grades 3 to 5) complications [76]. However, studies comparing different types of diversions showed no significant differences in early and late morbidities after neobladder, ileal conduit, and Indiana pouch [77–79].

The results of a large and multi-institutional series show that in patients with localized invasive transitional cell carcinoma, radical cystectomy and pelvic lymphadenectomy are associated with mean recurrence-free and bladder cancer-specific survival of 58% and 66% at 5 years [80]. The largest single site study with more than 1000 patients reported recurrence-free survival and overall survival of 68% and 66% at 5 years and 60% and 43% at 10 years, respectively [81]. When divided by pathological T stage, 5-year recurrence-free survival was 76% in patients with pT1 tumors, 74% for pT2, 52% for pT3, and 36% for pT4 [81]. A recent analysis using Surveillance, Epidemiology and End Results database revealed an increased stage-specific 5-year survival rate for all stages, except for metastatic disease between 1973 and 2009 [82].

Conclusion

The initial step for the diagnosis of bladder tumors is transurethral resection (TUR) to remove all visible tumors with sufficient surgical margins and depth, which also represents the initial approach in the management of non-muscle-invasive bladder cancer (NMIBC). For patients with NMIBC, a single immediate instillation of intravesical chemotherapy (IVC) (e.g., mitomycin, epirubicin, or doxorubicin) after transurethral resection is recommended by all guidelines. Intravesical BCG treatment is also a valuable option for patients with intermediate-risk disease. All guidelines recommend the BCG induction regime of once a week for 6 weeks. Radical cystectomy with bilateral pelvic lymphadenectomy often preceded by neo-adjuvant cisplatin-based chemotherapy is the gold standard surgical treatment for muscle-invasive BC. The extent of pelvic lymph node dissection (PLND) during RC is a subject of debate.

References

1. Antoni S, Ferlay J, Soerjomataram I, Znaor A, Jemal A, Bray F. Bladder cancer incidence and mortality: a global overview and recent trends. Eur Urol. 2016;71:96–108.
2. Siegel RL, Miller KD, Jemal A. Cancer statistics, 2016. CA Cancer J Clin. 2016;66(1):7–30.
3. Miller KD, Siegel RL, Lin CC, Mariotto AB, Kramer JL, Rowland JH, et al. Cancer treatment and survivorship statistics, 2016. CA Cancer J Clin. 2016;66(4):271–89.
4. Babjuk M, Bohle A, Burger M, Capoun O, Cohen D, Comperat EM, et al. EAU guidelines on non-muscle-invasive urothelial carcinoma of the bladder: update 2016. Eur Urol. 2017;71:447–61.

5. Kamat AM, Hahn NM, Efstathiou JA, Lerner SP, Malmstrom PU, Choi W, et al. Bladder cancer. Lancet. 2016;338:2796–810.
6. Epstein JI. The new World Health Organization/International Society of Urological Pathology (WHO/ISUP) classification for TA, T1 bladder tumors: is it an improvement? Crit Rev Oncol Hematol. 2003;47(2):83–9.
7. Humphrey PA, Moch H, Cubilla AL, Ulbright TM, Reuter VE. The 2016 WHO classification of tumours of the urinary system and male genital organs-part B: prostate and bladder tumours. Eur Urol. 2016;70(1):106–19.
8. Bladder cancer: diagnosis and management. London: National Institute for Health and Clinical Excellence Guidance; 2015.
9. Tan WS, Rodney S, Lamb B, Feneley M, Kelly J. Management of non-muscle invasive bladder cancer: a comprehensive analysis of guidelines from the United States, Europe and Asia. Cancer Treat Rev. 2016;47:22–31.
10. Brausi M, Witjes JA, Lamm D, Persad R, Palou J, Colombel M, et al. A review of current guidelines and best practice recommendations for the management of nonmuscle invasive bladder cancer by the International Bladder Cancer Group. J Urol. 2011;186(6):2158–67.
11. Hall MC, Chang SS, Dalbagni G, Pruthi RS, Seigne JD, Skinner EC, et al. Guideline for the management of nonmuscle invasive bladder cancer (stages Ta, T1, and Tis): 2007 update. J Urol. 2007;178(6):2314–30.
12. Guevara A, Salomon L, Allory Y, Ploussard G, de la Taille A, Paul A, et al. The role of tumor-free status in repeat resection before intravesical bacillus Calmette-Guerin for high grade Ta, T1 and CIS bladder cancer. J Urol. 2010;183(6):2161–4.
13. Sfakianos JP, Kim PH, Hakimi AA, Herr HW. The effect of restaging transurethral resection on recurrence and progression rates in patients with nonmuscle invasive bladder cancer treated with intravesical bacillus Calmette-Guerin. J Urol. 2014;191(2):341–5.
14. Divrik RT, Yildirim U, Zorlu F, Ozen H. The effect of repeat transurethral resection on recurrence and progression rates in patients with T1 tumors of the bladder who received intravesical mitomycin: a prospective, randomized clinical trial. J Urol. 2006;175(5):1641–4.
15. Miladi M, Peyromaure M, Zerbib M, Saighi D, Debre B. The value of a second transurethral resection in evaluating patients with bladder tumours. Eur Urol. 2003;43(3):241–5.
16. Baltaci S, Bozlu M, Yildirim A, Gokce MI, Tinay I, Aslan G, et al. Significance of the interval between first and second transurethral resection on recurrence and progression rates in patients with high-risk non-muscle-invasive bladder cancer treated with maintenance intravesical Bacillus Calmette-Guerin. BJU Int. 2015;116(5):721–6.
17. Kaasinen E, Rintala E, Hellstrom P, Viitanen J, Juusela H, Rajala P, et al. Factors explaining recurrence in patients undergoing chemoimmunotherapy regimens for frequently recurring superficial bladder carcinoma. Eur Urol. 2002;42(2):167–74.
18. Perlis N, Zlotta AR, Beyene J, Finelli A, Fleshner NE, Kulkarni GS. Immediate post-transurethral resection of bladder tumor intravesical chemotherapy prevents non-muscle-invasive bladder cancer recurrences: an updated meta-analysis on 2548 patients and quality-of-evidence review. Eur Urol. 2013;64(3):421–30.
19. Sylvester RJ, Oosterlinck W, Holmang S, Sydes MR, Birtle A, Gudjonsson S, et al. Systematic review and individual patient data meta-analysis of randomized trials comparing a single immediate instillation of chemotherapy after transurethral resection with transurethral resection alone in patients with stage pTa-pT1 urothelial carcinoma of the bladder: which patients benefit from the instillation? Eur Urol. 2016;69(2):231–44.
20. Hendricksen K, Witjes WP, Idema JG, Kums JJ, van Vierssen Trip OB, de Bruin MJ, et al. Comparison of three schedules of intravesical epirubicin in patients with non-muscle-invasive bladder cancer. Eur Urol. 2008;53(5):984–91.
21. Huncharek M, Geschwind JF, Witherspoon B, McGarry R, Adcock D. Intravesical chemotherapy prophylaxis in primary superficial bladder cancer: a meta-analysis of 3703 patients from 11 randomized trials. J Clin Epidemiol. 2000;53(7):676–80.
22. Malmstrom PU, Sylvester RJ, Crawford DE, Friedrich M, Krege S, Rintala E, et al. An individual patient data meta-analysis of the long-term outcome of randomised studies comparing

intravesical mitomycin C versus bacillus Calmette-Guerin for non-muscle-invasive bladder cancer. Eur Urol. 2009;56(2):247–56.
23. Kamat AM, Porten S. Myths and mysteries surrounding bacillus Calmette-Guerin therapy for bladder cancer. Eur Urol. 2014;65(2):267–9.
24. Sylvester RJ, van der Meijden AP, Witjes JA, Kurth K. Bacillus calmette-guerin versus chemotherapy for the intravesical treatment of patients with carcinoma in situ of the bladder: a meta-analysis of the published results of randomized clinical trials. J Urol. 2005;174(1):86–91. discussion-2
25. Sylvester RJ, van der MA, Lamm DL. Intravesical bacillus Calmette-Guerin reduces the risk of progression in patients with superficial bladder cancer: a meta-analysis of the published results of randomized clinical trials. J Urol. 2002;168(5):1964–70.
26. Bohle A, Bock PR. Intravesical bacille Calmette-Guerin versus mitomycin C in superficial bladder cancer: formal meta-analysis of comparative studies on tumor progression. Urology. 2004;63(4):682–6. discussion 6–7
27. Di Stasi SM, Giannantoni A, Giurioli A, Valenti M, Zampa G, Storti L, et al. Sequential BCG and electromotive mitomycin versus BCG alone for high-risk superficial bladder cancer: a randomised controlled trial. Lancet Oncol. 2006;7(1):43–51.
28. Brausi M, Oddens J, Sylvester R, Bono A, van de Beek C, van Andel G, et al. Side effects of Bacillus Calmette-Guerin (BCG) in the treatment of intermediate- and high-risk Ta, T1 papillary carcinoma of the bladder: results of the EORTC genito-urinary cancers group randomised phase 3 study comparing one-third dose with full dose and 1 year with 3 years of maintenance BCG. Eur Urol. 2014;65(1):69–76.
29. Arends TJ, Nativ O, Maffezzini M, de Cobelli O, Canepa G, Verweij F, et al. Results of a randomised controlled trial comparing intravesical chemohyperthermia with mitomycin C versus Bacillus Calmette-Guerin for adjuvant treatment of patients with intermediate- and high-risk non-muscle-invasive bladder cancer. Eur Urol. 2016;69(6):1046–52.
30. Morales A, Eidinger D, Bruce AW. Intracavitary Bacillus Calmette-Guerin in the treatment of superficial bladder tumors. 1976. J Urol. 2002;167(2 Pt 2):891–3. discussion 3–5
31. Palou J, Laguna P, Millan-Rodriguez F, Hall RR, Salvador-Bayarri J, Vicente-Rodriguez J. Control group and maintenance treatment with bacillus Calmette-Guerin for carcinoma in situ and/or high grade bladder tumors. J Urol. 2001;165(5):1488–91.
32. Badalament RA, Herr HW, Wong GY, Gnecco C, Pinsky CM, Whitmore WF Jr, et al. A prospective randomized trial of maintenance versus nonmaintenance intravesical bacillus Calmette-Guerin therapy of superficial bladder cancer. J Clin Oncol. 1987;5(3):441–9.
33. Lamm DL, Blumenstein BA, Crissman JD, Montie JE, Gottesman JE, Lowe BA, et al. Maintenance bacillus Calmette-Guerin immunotherapy for recurrent TA, T1 and carcinoma in situ transitional cell carcinoma of the bladder: a randomized Southwest Oncology Group Study. J Urol. 2000;163(4):1124–9.
34. Mostafid AH, Palou Redorta J, Sylvester R, Witjes JA. Therapeutic options in high-risk non-muscle-invasive bladder cancer during the current worldwide shortage of bacille Calmette-Guerin. Eur Urol. 2015;67(3):359–60.
35. Veeratterapillay R, Heer R, Johnson MI, Persad R, Bach C. High-risk non-muscle-invasive bladder cancer-therapy options during intravesical BCG shortage. Curr Urol Rep. 2016; 17(9):68.
36. Oddens J, Brausi M, Sylvester R, Bono A, van de Beek C, van Andel G, et al. Final results of an EORTC-GU cancers group randomized study of maintenance bacillus Calmette-Guerin in intermediate- and high-risk Ta, T1 papillary carcinoma of the urinary bladder: one-third dose versus full dose and 1 year versus 3 years of maintenance. Eur Urol. 2013;63(3):462–72.
37. Lammers RJ, Witjes JA, Inman BA, Leibovitch I, Laufer M, Nativ O, et al. The role of a combined regimen with intravesical chemotherapy and hyperthermia in the management of non-muscle-invasive bladder cancer: a systematic review. Eur Urol. 2011;60(1):81–93.
38. Di Stasi SM, Giannantoni A, Stephen RL, Capelli G, Navarra P, Massoud R, et al. Intravesical electromotive mitomycin C versus passive transport mitomycin C for high risk superficial bladder cancer: a prospective randomized study. J Urol. 2003;170(3):777–82.

39. Shelley MD, Jones G, Cleves A, Wilt TJ, Mason MD, Kynaston HG. Intravesical gemcitabine therapy for non-muscle invasive bladder cancer (NMIBC): a systematic review. BJU Int. 2012;109(4):496–505.
40. Bilensoy E, Sarisozen C, Esendagli G, Dogan AL, Aktas Y, Sen M, et al. Intravesical cationic nanoparticles of chitosan and polycaprolactone for the delivery of Mitomycin C to bladder tumors. Int J Pharm. 2009;371(1–2):170–6.
41. Erdogar N, Iskit AB, Mungan NA, Bilensoy E. Prolonged retention and in vivo evaluation of cationic nanoparticles loaded with Mitomycin C designed for intravesical chemotherapy of bladder tumours. J Microencapsul. 2012;29(6):576–82.
42. Erdogar N, Iskit AB, Eroglu H, Sargon MF, Mungan NA, Bilensoy E. Cationic core-shell nanoparticles for intravesical chemotherapy in tumor-induced rat model: safety and efficacy. Int J Pharm. 2014;471(1–2):1–9.
43. Erdogar N, Iskit AB, Eroglu H, Sargon MF, Mungan NA, Bilensoy E. Antitumor efficacy of Bacillus Calmette-Guerin loaded cationic nanoparticles for intravesical immunotherapy of bladder tumor induced rat model. J Nanosci Nanotechnol. 2015;15(12):10156–64.
44. Kamat AM, Sylvester RJ, Bohle A, Palou J, Lamm DL, Brausi M, et al. Definitions, end points, and clinical trial designs for non-muscle-invasive bladder cancer: recommendations from the international bladder cancer group. J Clin Oncol. 2016;34(16):1935–44.
45. Lamm D, Persad R, Brausi M, Buckley R, Witjes JA, Palou J, et al. Defining progression in nonmuscle invasive bladder cancer: it is time for a new, standard definition. J Urol. 2014;191(1):20–7.
46. Jarow J, Maher VE, Tang S, Ibrahim A, Kim G, Sridhara R, et al. Development of systemic and topical drugs to treat non-muscle invasive bladder cancer. Bladder Cancer. 2015;1(2): 133–6.
47. Lerner SP, Dinney C, Kamat A, Bivalacqua TJ, Nielsen M, O'Donnell M, et al. Clarification of bladder cancer disease states following treatment of patients with intravesical BCG. Bladder Cancer. 2015;1(1):29–30.
48. Sylvester RJ, van der Meijden AP, Oosterlinck W, Witjes JA, Bouffioux C, Denis L, et al. Predicting recurrence and progression in individual patients with stage Ta T1 bladder cancer using EORTC risk tables: a combined analysis of 2596 patients from seven EORTC trials. Eur Urol. 2006;49(3):466–5. discussion 75–7
49. Cambier S, Sylvester RJ, Collette L, Gontero P, Brausi MA, van Andel G, et al. EORTC nomograms and risk groups for predicting recurrence, progression, and disease-specific and overall survival in non-muscle-invasive stage Ta-T1 urothelial bladder cancer patients treated with 1–3 years of maintenance Bacillus Calmette-Guerin. Eur Urol. 2016;69(1):60–9.
50. Kamat AM, Gee JR, Dinney CP, Grossman HB, Swanson DA, Millikan RE, et al. The case for early cystectomy in the treatment of nonmuscle invasive micropapillary bladder carcinoma. J Urol. 2006;175(3 Pt 1):881–5.
51. Segal R, Yafi FA, Brimo F, Tanguay S, Aprikian A, Kassouf W. Prognostic factors and outcome in patients with T1 high-grade bladder cancer: can we identify patients for early cystectomy? BJU Int. 2012;109(7):1026–30.
52. Martin-Doyle W, Leow JJ, Orsola A, Chang SL, Bellmunt J. Improving selection criteria for early cystectomy in high-grade t1 bladder cancer: a meta-analysis of 15,215 patients. J Clin Oncol. 2015;33(6):643–50.
53. Willis DL, Fernandez MI, Dickstein RJ, Parikh S, Shah JB, Pisters LL, et al. Clinical outcomes of cT1 micropapillary bladder cancer. J Urol. 2015;193(4):1129–34.
54. Alfred Witjes J, Lebret T, Comperat EM, Cowan NC, De Santis M, Bruins HM, et al. Updated 2016 EAU guidelines on muscle-invasive and metastatic bladder cancer. Eur Urol. 2017;71:462–75.
55. Challacombe BJ, Bochner BH, Dasgupta P, Gill I, Guru K, Herr H, et al. The role of laparoscopic and robotic cystectomy in the management of muscle-invasive bladder cancer with special emphasis on cancer control and complications. Eur Urol. 2011;60(4):767–75.
56. Kessler TM, Burkhard FC, Studer UE. Clinical indications and outcomes with nerve-sparing cystectomy in patients with bladder cancer. Urol Clin North Am. 2005;32(2):165–75.

57. Patel SG, Cookson MS, Barocas DA, Clark PE, Smith JA Jr, Chang SS. Risk factors for urothelial carcinoma of the prostate in patients undergoing radical cystoprostatectomy for bladder cancer. BJU Int. 2009;104(7):934–7.
58. Bruins HM, Djaladat H, Ahmadi H, Sherrod A, Cai J, Miranda G, et al. Incidental prostate cancer in patients with bladder urothelial carcinoma: comprehensive analysis of 1476 radical cystoprostatectomy specimens. J Urol. 2013;190(5):1704–9.
59. Bi L, Huang H, Fan X, Li K, Xu K, Jiang C, et al. Extended vs non-extended pelvic lymph node dissection and their influence on recurrence-free survival in patients undergoing radical cystectomy for bladder cancer: a systematic review and meta-analysis of comparative studies. BJU Int. 2014;113(5b):E39–48.
60. May M, Herrmann E, Bolenz C, Brookman-May S, Tiemann A, Moritz R, et al. Association between the number of dissected lymph nodes during pelvic lymphadenectomy and cancer-specific survival in patients with lymph node-negative urothelial carcinoma of the bladder undergoing radical cystectomy. Ann Surg Oncol. 2011;18(7):2018–25.
61. Herr HW. Extent of surgery and pathology evaluation has an impact on bladder cancer outcomes after radical cystectomy. Urology. 2003;61(1):105–8.
62. Herr H, Lee C, Chang S, Lerner S. Bladder Cancer Collaborative G. Standardization of radical cystectomy and pelvic lymph node dissection for bladder cancer: a collaborative group report. J Urol. 2004;171(5):1823–8. discussion 7–8.
63. Juergen E, Gschwend MMH, Lehmann J, Ruebben H, Albers P, Heidenreich A, de Geeter P, Wolff JM, Frohneberg D, Schnoeller T, Kälble T, Stoeckle M, Stenzl A, Mueller M. Limited versus extended pelvic lymphadenectomy in patients with bladder cancer undergoing radical cystectomy: Survival results from a prospective, randomized trial (LEA AUO AB 25/02). J Clin Oncol. 2016;34(Suppl):4503.
64. Lerner SP, Tangen CM, Svatek RS, Koppie TM, Alva A, La Rosa FG, Pal SK, Daneshmand S, Dinney CPN, Kibel AS, Pohar K, Canter DJ, Kassouf W, Bangs R, Thompson IM. A phase iii surgical trial to evaluate the benefit of a standard versus an extended pelvic lymphadenectomy performed at time of radical cystectomy for muscle invasive urothelial cancer: SWOG S1011 (NCT #01224665). J Urol. 2015;193(4):e807.
65. Aziz A, May M, Burger M, Palisaar RJ, Trinh QD, Fritsche HM, et al. Prediction of 90-day mortality after radical cystectomy for bladder cancer in a prospective European multicenter cohort. Eur Urol. 2014;66(1):156–63.
66. Isbarn H, Jeldres C, Zini L, Perrotte P, Baillargeon-Gagne S, Capitanio U, et al. A population based assessment of perioperative mortality after cystectomy for bladder cancer. J Urol. 2009;182(1):70–7.
67. Lavallee LT, Schramm D, Witiuk K, Mallick R, Fergusson D, Morash C, et al. Peri-operative morbidity associated with radical cystectomy in a multicenter database of community and academic hospitals. PLoS One. 2014;9(10):e111281.
68. Daneshmand S, Ahmadi H, Schuckman AK, Mitra AP, Cai J, Miranda G, et al. Enhanced recovery protocol after radical cystectomy for bladder cancer. J Urol. 2014;192(1):50–5.
69. Persson B, Carringer M, Andren O, Andersson SO, Carlsson J, Ljungqvist O. Initial experiences with the enhanced recovery after surgery (ERAS) protocol in open radical cystectomy. Scand J Urol. 2015;49(4):302–7.
70. Morgan TM, Barocas DA, Keegan KA, Cookson MS, Chang SS, Ni S, et al. Volume outcomes of cystectomy – is it the surgeon or the setting? J Urol. 2012;188(6):2139–44.
71. Ravi P, Bianchi M, Hansen J, Trinh QD, Tian Z, Meskawi M, et al. Benefit in regionalisation of care for patients treated with radical cystectomy: a nationwide inpatient sample analysis. BJU Int. 2014;113(5):733–40.
72. Bochner BH, Dalbagni G, Sjoberg DD, Silberstein J, Keren Paz GE, Donat SM, et al. Comparing open radical cystectomy and robot-assisted laparoscopic radical cystectomy: a randomized clinical trial. Eur Urol. 2015;67(6):1042–50.
73. Khan MS, Gan C, Ahmed K, Ismail AF, Watkins J, Summers JA, et al. A single-centre early phase randomised controlled three-arm trial of open, robotic, and laparoscopic radical cystectomy (CORAL). Eur Urol. 2016;69(4):613–21.

74. Leow JJ, Reese SW, Jiang W, Lipsitz SR, Bellmunt J, Trinh QD, et al. Propensity-matched comparison of morbidity and costs of open and robot-assisted radical cystectomies: a contemporary population-based analysis in the United States. Eur Urol. 2014;66(3):569–76.
75. Smith ND, Castle EP, Gonzalgo ML, Svatek RS, Weizer AZ, Montgomery JS, et al. The RAZOR (randomized open vs robotic cystectomy) trial: study design and trial update. BJU Int. 2015;115(2):198–205.
76. Hautmann RE, de Petriconi RC, Volkmer BG. Lessons learned from 1000 neobladders: the 90-day complication rate. J Urol. 2010;184(3):990–4. quiz 1235
77. Monn MF, Kaimakliotis HZ, Cary KC, Pedrosa JA, Flack CK, Koch MO, et al. Short-term morbidity and mortality of Indiana pouch, ileal conduit, and neobladder urinary diversion following radical cystectomy. Urol Oncol. 2014;32(8):1151–7.
78. Kim SH, Yu A, Jung JH, Lee YJ, Lee ES. Incidence and risk factors of 30-day early and 90-day late morbidity and mortality of radical cystectomy during a 13-year follow-up: a comparative propensity-score matched analysis of complications between neobladder and ileal conduit. Jpn J Clin Oncol. 2014;44(7):677–85.
79. Lee RK, Abol-Enein H, Artibani W, Bochner B, Dalbagni G, Daneshmand S, et al. Urinary diversion after radical cystectomy for bladder cancer: options, patient selection, and outcomes. BJU Int. 2014;113(1):11–23.
80. Shariat SF, Karakiewicz PI, Palapattu GS, Lotan Y, Rogers CG, Amiel GE, et al. Outcomes of radical cystectomy for transitional cell carcinoma of the bladder: a contemporary series from the Bladder Cancer Research Consortium. J Urol. 2006;176(6 Pt 1):2414–22; discussion 22.
81. Stein JP, Lieskovsky G, Cote R, Groshen S, Feng AC, Boyd S, et al. Radical cystectomy in the treatment of invasive bladder cancer: long-term results in 1054 patients. J Clin Oncol. 2001;19(3):666–75.
82. Abdollah F, Gandaglia G, Thuret R, Schmitges J, Tian Z, Jeldres C, et al. Incidence, survival and mortality rates of stage-specific bladder cancer in United States: a trend analysis. Cancer Epidemiol. 2013;37(3):219–25.

Target Volume Delineation Guidelines in Bladder Cancer

3

Melis Gultekin, Sezin Yuce Sari, Pervin Hurmuz, Gozde Yazici, Fadil Akyol, and Gokhan Ozyigit

Abstract

The use of radiotherapy (RT) in the treatment of bladder cancer has been decreasing through the years. There is no role of RT in carcinoma in situ and Ta and Tl tumors. However, irradiation may have a role in high-grade or recurrent T1 lesions. There is no prospective randomized trial comparing surgery with RT in muscle-invasive bladder cancer. In T2–T4a disease without lymph node (LN) involvement, RT can be combined with concurrent chemotherapy in medically fit patients. However, there is no rationale of RT in patients with LN or distant metastasis except for palliative reasons. The gross tumor volume (GTV), clinical target volume (CTV), planning target volume (PTV), and organs at risk (OAR) should be delineated separately in each slice based on the recommendations in the International Commission on Radiation Units and Measurements (ICRU) reports 50 and 62. The only delineation guideline for the RT in bladder cancer has been reported by the Australian and New Zealand Faculty of Radiation Oncology Genito-Urinary Group.

3.1 Anatomy

The urinary bladder is a muscular organ located in the pelvis, inferior to the pubic bone when empty, but may extend up into the abdomen to the umbilicus when full. The bladder has an apex, a base (posterior surface), a superior surface, two inferolateral surfaces, a trigone, and a neck. The apex ends as a fibrous cord above the pubic bone which connects the bladder to the allantois. This part is the remnant of the fetal urachus from which many tumors can arise. The base is separated from the

M. Gultekin, M.D. • S. Yuce Sari, M.D. (✉) • P. Hurmuz, M.D. • G. Yazici, M.D.
F. Akyol, M.D. • G. Ozyigit, M.D.
Department of Radiation Oncology, Hacettepe University, Ankara, Turkey
e-mail: sezin_yuce@hotmail.com

G. Ozyigit, U. Selek (eds.), *Principles and Practice of Urooncology*,
DOI 10.1007/978-3-319-56114-1_3

rectum by the ureters, vas deferens, and seminal vesicles in men and the uterus and vagina in women. A V-shaped structure is formed by the seminal vesicles at the base, and the vas deferens enters the middle of this structure. Both ureters enter the bladder slightly superior and lateral to the seminal vesicles. The superior surface is the only surface covered with peritoneum and is in close proximity to the uterus, ileum, and sigmoid colon. The inferolateral surfaces are surrounded by loose connective tissue and in close proximity to the pubic bone, levator ani, and obturator internus muscles. The neck of the bladder is the most inferior part which is adjacent to the prostate and urethra. The retropubic space separates the bladder from the pubic bone anteriorly.

3.2 Role of Radiotherapy for Locoregional Disease

The use of radiotherapy (RT) in the treatment of bladder cancer has been decreasing through the years. There is no role of RT in carcinoma in situ, Ta, and Tl tumors. However, irradiation may have a role in high-grade or recurrent T1 lesions [1–4]. There is no prospective randomized trial comparing surgery with RT in muscle-invasive bladder cancer. In T2–T4a disease without lymph node (LN) involvement, RT can be combined with concurrent chemotherapy in medically fit patients [5, 6]. However, there is no rationale of RT in patients with LN or distant metastasis except for palliative reasons.

In North America, split schedules of RT have been used. An interval cystoscopy is followed by 39–40 Gy RT in 1.8–2 Gy fraction doses, and after an interim cystoscopy for the detection of response, RT proceeds to a total dose of 64–66 Gy with long-term survival rates [7, 8]. However, only 65% of patients retain a functioning bladder, whereas others undergo salvage cystectomy [9]. On the other hand, in the United Kingdom a single radical course of RT is administered to the whole bladder to a total dose of 64 Gy in 32 fractions or a hypofractionated schedule of 55 Gy in 20 fractions, following the transurethral resection for bladder tumor (TURBT) [10, 11].

3.3 Target Volume Delineation

In the conventional era, the superior border was at the L5-S1 vertebrae interspace, and the inferior border was inferior to the obturator foramina (1.5 cm inferior to the bladder neck and/or prostatic urethra). On the anterior-posterior fields, the lateral borders were 1.5–2 cm lateral to the bony pelvis. On the lateral fields, the anterior border was 1 cm posterior to the anterior of the symphysis pubis, and the posterior border was 1–3 cm posterior to the tumor detected on imaging techniques. The boost dose was prescribed to the whole bladder with 1.5–2 cm margins.

For modern conformal RT techniques, the patient is first immobilized with a kneefix and feetfix in supine position for the planning computed tomography

(CT). The arms should be on the chest in order to keep them away from the treatment area. The rectum should be empty, and daily enema can be used. The bladder is recommended to be empty by most authors in order to minimize the risk of geographic miss and also to decrease the irradiated volumes. However, a full bladder moves the intestines and rectum out of the field and decreases the toxicity rate. For this reason, we prefer a full bladder for the extended field RT in our clinic. However, the boost dose should be administered with an empty bladder, and a second planning CT should be taken if the extended field was administered with a full bladder. At the Mass General Hospital, a Foley catheter is inserted into the bladder after the patient has voided [12]. They measure the postvoiding urine residual and replace it by an equal volume of bladder contrast with an additional 25 mL of contrast in order to define the inner walls of the bladder and 15 mL of air in order to visualize the anterior portion of the bladder on the lateral simulation film.

To define the isocenter, three radiopaque pellet markers are placed: one at the anterior midline and two at the right and left lateral point, respectively, on the skin. Intravenous contrast injection is not routinely recommended. The CT scan is acquired in 3–5 mm slices from 3 cm superior to the base of the bladder or bottom of L5, whichever is more superior, to the inferior of ischial tuberosities. The gross tumor volume (GTV), clinical target volume (CTV), planning target volume (PTV), and organs at risk (OAR) should be delineated separately in each slice based on the recommendations in the International Commission on Radiation Units and Measurements (ICRU) reports 50 and 62 [13, 14].

The only delineation guideline for the RT of bladder cancer has been reported by the Australian and New Zealand Faculty of Radiation Oncology Genito-Urinary Group [15].

3.4 Definitive Radiotherapy for the Intact Bladder

3.4.1 Gross Tumor Volume

The GTV can be difficult to define on CT only, and magnetic resonance imaging (MRI) can help the delineation process. It is defined as any gross residual disease seen at cystoscopy or by imaging techniques including the disease seen or palpated outside the bladder wall. Following a complete TURBT for a tumor that does not extend outside the bladder wall, there is no definable GTV.

3.4.2 Clinical Target Volume

CTV1 is the whole bladder, tumor bed (after TUR), proximal urethra, bladder neck and/or prostatic urethra (in case of prostatic fossa involvement), and, if existent, extravesical extension with a 0.5-cm margin. This field is irradiated with 45–50 Gy in 1.8–2 Gy fraction doses. The reason for delineating the whole bladder is that bladder cancer is generally multifocal and recurs in a multifocal manner [16]. Besides, delineating the microscopic extent of the tumor on a planning CT is difficult. If elective nodal irradiation is to be administered, pelvic LNs are also delineated in CTV1 and receive the same dose. CTV2 for the boost dose is formed with a 0.5-cm margin to the GTV2 and irradiated to a total dose of 60–65 Gy. Another boost technique is to irradiate the whole bladder with an additional 8 Gy and then give a boost dose of 12 Gy to the tumor alone. However, if the site of the tumor is not clear, then the whole bladder is recommended to be treated to the total dose [15].

All anatomical variations such as cystocele and diverticulum should be included in the CTV. If there is involvement of ureteric orifice, distal urethra should be encompassed in the CTV with a 1-cm margin [17]. The prostate is involved in up to 43% of patients with bladder cancer [18, 19]. The risk of urethral involvement, and therefore prostatic involvement, is increased with the existence of carcinoma in situ in the bladder, multifocal tumors, and involvement of the trigone/bladder neck. If any one of these risk factors is present, the whole prostate gland can be included in the CTV1. If there is macroscopic involvement of the prostate and/or urethra, the prostate should be included in both CTV1 and CTV2 [15].

In female patients, the rate of urethral involvement was found 7–46% in cystectomy series [20]. Urethral involvement was shown to be associated with the involvement of bladder neck [20]. Another potential site for microscopic invasion is the anterior vaginal wall in patients with urethral involvement [20]. However, it is difficult to determine microscopic vaginal involvement without cystectomy, and delineating the vagina is not routinely recommended. If there is anterior vaginal wall involvement on imaging or clinical examination, then the vagina should be included in CTV1 together with the proximal urethra.

CTV delineation including pelvic LNs in a muscle-invasive bladder cancer patient treated with bladder-preserving multimodal approach image-guided RT (IGRT) is depicted in Fig. 3.1. Boost volume for the same patient is shown in Fig. 3.2.

3.4.3 Role of Elective Nodal Irradiation

There are conflicting data on elective nodal irradiation in the treatment of bladder cancer. The rate of LN involvement is approximately 25% according to radical cystectomy series, and this finding helps to indicate the need for extensive LN dissection (LND) and adjuvant chemotherapy [10, 21, 22]. The number of dissected LNs is directly correlated with the outcome of patients, independent of the N stage [23, 24]. Based on these findings, elective nodal irradiation may provide a survival benefit in patients that did not undergo LND whether they are involved or not, with the expense of additional toxicity. However, pelvic control and survival rates are not decreased with irradiation of the bladder alone when used together with chemotherapy [25].

The BC20001 study reported a low rate of nodal relapse both in patients that received RT alone (7%) and in patients that received chemoradiotherapy (5%) [26]. In a randomized trial which compares 45 Gy of whole pelvic RT including elective nodal irradiation and 20 Gy boost dose with bladder-only irradiation of 65 Gy, no difference was found in the rates of pelvic nodal relapse and overall survival in patients with complete response [27]. Therefore, it may be reasonable to electively irradiate the pelvic lymphatic regions in patients that cannot receive concurrent chemotherapy.

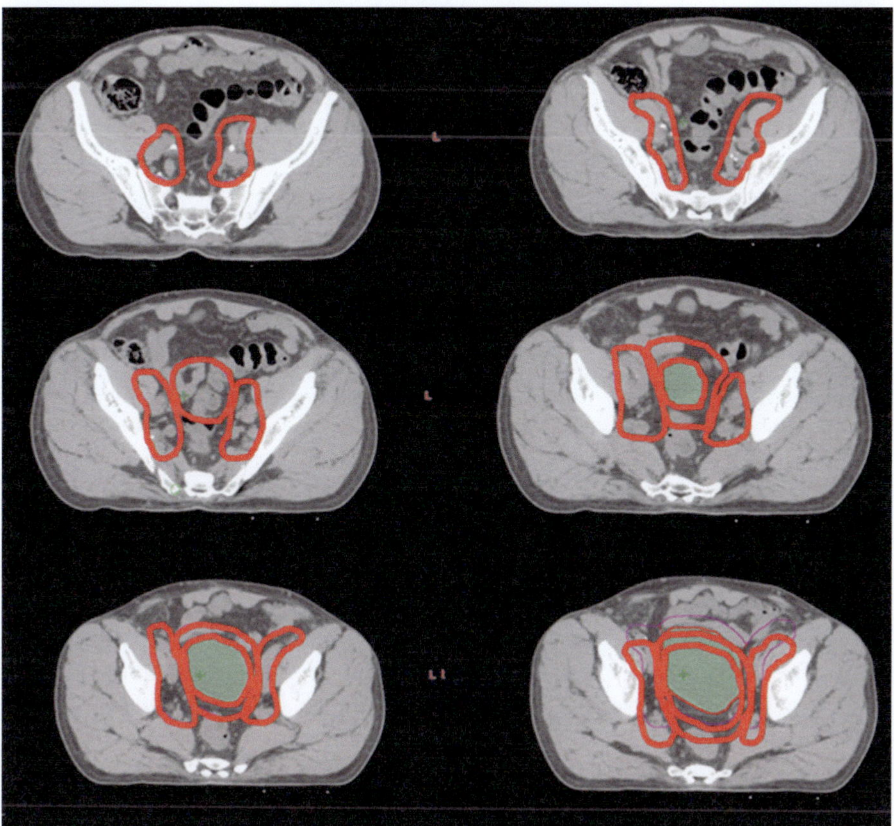

Fig. 3.1 CTV delineation for a muscle-invasive bladder cancer patient treated with definitive IGRT

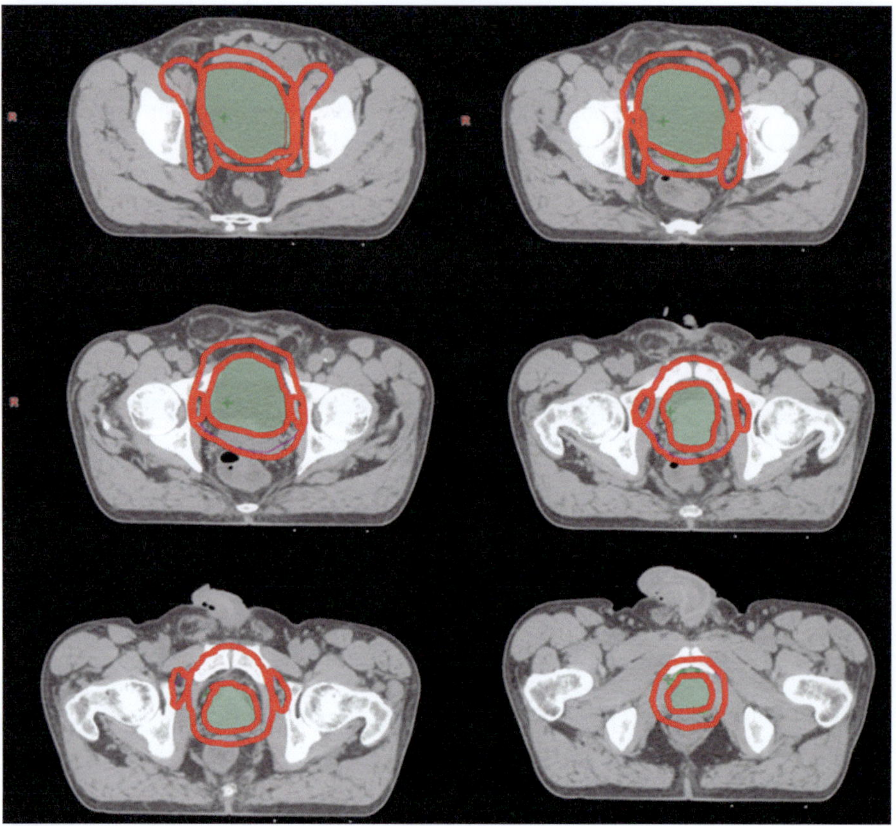

Fig. 3.1 (continued)

3.4.4 Planning Target Volume

Some authors define the whole bladder as PTV with a 1.5-cm margin to the uninvolved outer bladder wall and the extravesical extent of the tumor with a 2-cm margin. In other instances, the PTV is formed with a 2-cm margin to the CTV in order to adequately cover all errors based on setup and organ motion. It was shown that the bladder wall can move beyond 1.5 cm at least once during a course of treatment in over 60% of patients and the GTV can move outside the PTV on at least one course of treatment in over 20% of patients [28–30]. Graham et al. [31] recommend adding margins of 1.6 cm anteriorly and posteriorly, 1.4 cm laterally, 3 cm superiorly, and 1.4 cm inferiorly; however, this will certainly cause increased rate of radiation-related toxicity. Meijer et al. [32], on the other hand, recommend margins of 1 cm anteriorly and laterally, 1.2 cm inferiorly, 1.4 cm posteriorly, and 2 cm superiorly. To overcome this issue, daily image-guided therapy can be administered, or insertion of fiducial markers in the

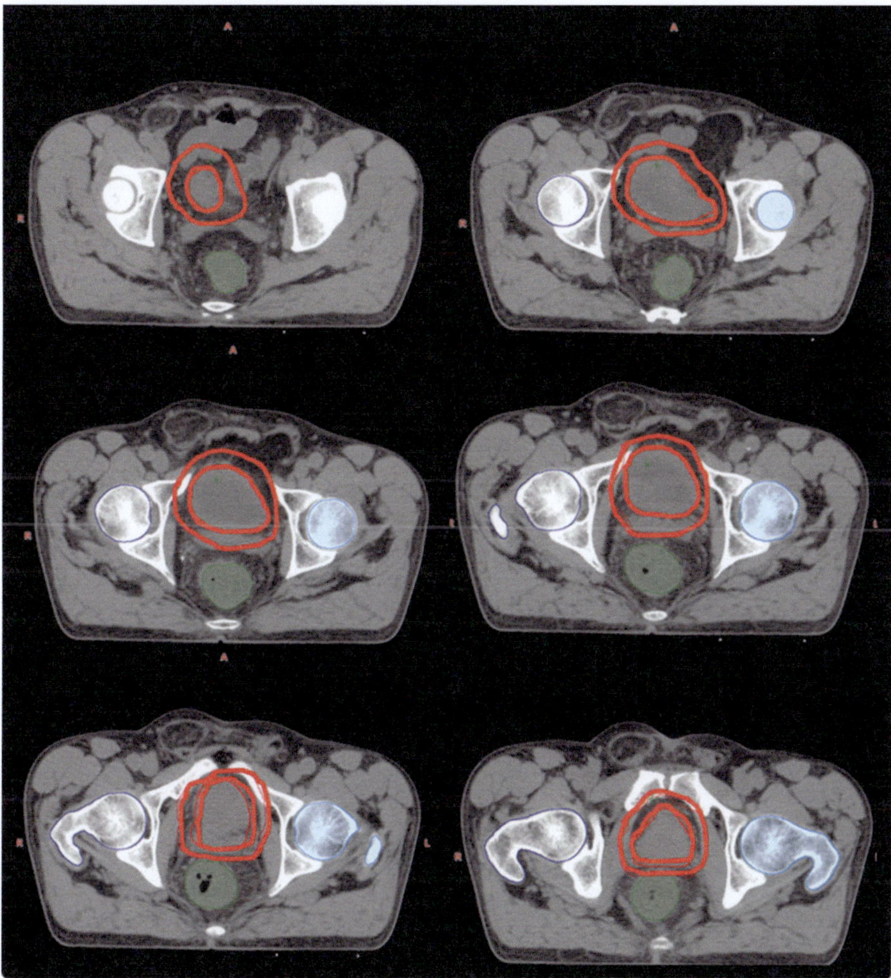

Fig. 3.2 Boost volume delineation for a muscle-invasive bladder cancer patient treated with definitive IGRT

bladder wall around the tumor bed can be another solution. The use of these techniques can decrease the margins <1.5 cm [33]. However, besides the movement of the bladder, the change of its shape is also challenging. Therefore, margins for the PTV do not seem to be reduced at any time soon. The recommended margins for the PTV are 1–1.5 cm in all directions and 2–2.5 cm in the superior direction when using conventional RT [15]. The inferior margin can be reduced to 1 cm if the prostate or urethra has been included. One should also consider which walls of the bladder are involved by the cancer and the relative mobility of this particular portion of the bladder.

3.5 Adjuvant Setting

If surgery is planned to a patient with bladder cancer, RT may have a role in the pre- or postoperative setting. Preoperative RT has been questioned because of the fact that it delays the time to definitive surgery and increases its morbidity, as well as it may compromise the surgeon's ability to perform continent urinary diversions. On the other hand, the survival benefit of preoperative RT was only shown for clinical T3 and T4 tumors [34, 35]. The only prospective randomized trial of postoperative RT which includes patients with transitional cell and squamous cell bladder cancer revealed increased local control and disease-free survival rates compared to observation after surgery [36]. However, the morbidity of postoperative RT is higher than preoperative RT because of the large volumes occupied by the small bowel after cystectomy. It was reported that the incidence of small bowel obstruction was >30% with 50 Gy in conventional fractionation [37]. Therefore, preoperative RT is a safer option; however, if postoperative RT is to be administered, dose reduction is recommended with a small RT field in order to minimize radiation-induced toxicity.

Conclusion

Patient-based treatment planning is the standard approach in bladder cancer RT. Recommended simulation and delineation techniques are summarized in this chapter. If these recommendations are applied in clinical practice, the variations in treatment techniques between institutions can be minimized.

References

1. van der Werf-Messing B, Hop WC. Carcinoma of the urinary bladder (category T1NxM0) treated either by radium implant or by transurethral resection only. Int J Radiat Oncol Biol Phys. 1981;7(3):299–303.
2. Van der Steen-Banasik EM, Visser AG, Reinders JG, Heijbroek RP, Idema JG, Janssen TG, et al. Saving bladders with brachytherapy: implantation technique and results. Int J Radiat Oncol Biol Phys. 2002;53(3):622–9.
3. Rodel C, Grabenbauer GG, Kuhn R, Dunst J, Papadopoulos T, Schrott KM, et al. Invasive bladder cancer: organ preservation by radiochemotherapy. Front Radiat Ther Oncol. 2002;36:118–30.
4. Weiss C, Wolze C, Engehausen DG, Ott OJ, Krause FS, Schrott KM, et al. Radiochemotherapy after transurethral resection for high-risk T1 bladder cancer: an alternative to intravesical therapy or early cystectomy? J Clin Oncol. 2006;24(15):2318–24.
5. Coppin CM, Gospodarowicz MK, James K, Tannock IF, Zee B, Carson J, et al. Improved local control of invasive bladder cancer by concurrent cisplatin and preoperative or definitive radiation. The National Cancer Institute of Canada Clinical Trials Group. J Clin Oncol. 1996;14(11):2901–7.
6. Hoskin PJ, Rojas AM, Bentzen SM, Saunders MI. Radiotherapy with concurrent carbogen and nicotinamide in bladder carcinoma. J Clin Oncol. 2010;28(33):4912–8.
7. Kaufman DS, Winter KA, Shipley WU, Heney NM, Wallace HJ 3rd, Toonkel LM, et al. Phase I-II RTOG study (99-06) of patients with muscle-invasive bladder cancer undergoing transurethral surgery, paclitaxel, cisplatin, and twice-daily radiotherapy followed by selective bladder preservation or radical cystectomy and adjuvant chemotherapy. Urology. 2009;73(4):833–7.

8. Mak RH, Zietman AL, Heney NM, Kaufman DS, Shipley WU. Bladder preservation: optimizing radiotherapy and integrated treatment strategies. BJU Int. 2008;102(9 Pt B):1345–53.
9. Kaufman DS, Winter KA, Shipley WU, Heney NM, Chetner MP, Souhami L, et al. The initial results in muscle-invading bladder cancer of RTOG 95-06: phase I/II trial of transurethral surgery plus radiation therapy with concurrent cisplatin and 5-fluorouracil followed by selective bladder preservation or cystectomy depending on the initial response. Oncologist. 2000;5(6):471–6.
10. Stein JP, Lieskovsky G, Cote R, Groshen S, Feng AC, Boyd S, et al. Radical cystectomy in the treatment of invasive bladder cancer: long-term results in 1054 patients. J Clin Oncol. 2001;19(3):666–75.
11. Dalbagni G, Genega E, Hashibe M, Zhang ZF, Russo P, Herr H, et al. Cystectomy for bladder cancer: a contemporary series. J Urol. 2001;165(4):1111–6.
12. Efstathiou JA, Zietman A Coen JJ, Shipley WU. Bladder cancer. In: Gunderson LL, Tepper JE Clinical radiation oncology. 3rd ed. China: Elsevier Saunders; 2012. 1099–1123.
13. Measurements. ICoRUa. ICRU Report 50: prescribing, recording and reporting photon beam therapy. Bethesda, Maryland, USA; 1993.
14. Measurements. ICoRUa. ICRU Report 62: prescribing, recording and reporting photon beam therapy (supplement to ICRU report 50). Bethesda, Maryland, USA; 1999.
15. Hindson BR, Turner SL, Millar JL, Foroudi F, Gogna NK, Skala M, et al. Australian & New Zealand Faculty of Radiation Oncology Genito-Urinary Group: 2011 consensus guidelines for curative radiotherapy for urothelial carcinoma of the bladder. J Med Imaging Radiat Oncol. 2012;56(1):18–30.
16. Brausi M, Collette L, Kurth K, van der Meijden AP, Oosterlinck W, Witjes JA, et al. Variability in the recurrence rate at first follow-up cystoscopy after TUR in stage Ta T1 transitional cell carcinoma of the bladder: a combined analysis of seven EORTC studies. Eur Urol. 2002;41(5):523–31.
17. Foroudi F, Wong J, Haworth A, Baille A, McAlpine J, Rolfo A, et al. Offline adaptive radiotherapy for bladder cancer using cone beam computed tomography. J Med Imaging Radiat Oncol. 2009;53(2):226–33.
18. Richards KA, Parks GE, Badlani GH, Kader AK, Hemal AK, Pettus JA. Developing selection criteria for prostate-sparing cystectomy: a review of cystoprostatectomy specimens. Urology. 2010;75(5):1116–20.
19. Shen SS, Lerner SP, Muezzinoglu B, Truong LD, Amiel G, Wheeler TM. Prostatic involvement by transitional cell carcinoma in patients with bladder cancer and its prognostic significance. Hum Pathol. 2006;37(6):726–34.
20. Stein JP, Penson DF, SD W, Skinner DG. Pathological guidelines for orthotopic urinary diversion in women with bladder cancer: a review of the literature. J Urol. 2007;178(3 Pt 1):756–60.
21. Kassouf W, Agarwal PK, Herr HW, Munsell MF, Spiess PE, Brown GA, et al. Lymph node density is superior to TNM nodal status in predicting disease-specific survival after radical cystectomy for bladder cancer: analysis of pooled data from MDACC and MSKCC. J Clin Oncol. 2008;26(1):121–6.
22. Buscarini M, Josephson DY, Stein JP. Lymphadenectomy in bladder cancer: a review. Urol Int. 2007;79(3):191–9.
23. Herr HW, Faulkner JR, Grossman HB, Natale RB, deVere White R, Sarosdy MF, et al. Surgical factors influence bladder cancer outcomes: a cooperative group report. J Clin Oncol. 2004;22(14):2781–9.
24. Koppie TM, Vickers AJ, Vora K, Dalbagni G, Bochner BH. Standardization of pelvic lymphadenectomy performed at radical cystectomy: can we establish a minimum number of lymph nodes that should be removed? Cancer. 2006;107(10):2368–74.
25. Sengelov L, von der Maase H. Radiotherapy in bladder cancer. Radiother Oncol. 1999;52(1):1–14.
26. James ND, Hussain SA, Hall E, Jenkins P, Tremlett J, Rawlings C, et al. Radiotherapy with or without chemotherapy in muscle-invasive bladder cancer. N Engl J Med. 2012; 366(16):1477–88.

27. Tunio MA, Hashmi A, Qayyum A, Mohsin R, Zaeem A. Whole-pelvis or bladder-only chemoradiation for lymph node-negative invasive bladder cancer: single-institution experience. Int J Radiat Oncol Biol Phys. 2012;82(3):e457–62.
28. Turner SL, Swindell R, Bowl N, Marrs J, Brookes B, Read G, et al. Bladder movement during radiation therapy for bladder cancer: implications for treatment planning. Int J Radiat Oncol Biol Phys. 1997;39(2):355–60.
29. Harris SJ, Buchanan RB. An audit and evaluation of bladder movements during radical radiotherapy. Clin Oncol (R Coll Radiol). 1998;10(4):262–4.
30. Sur RK, Clinkard J, Jones WG, Taylor RE, Close HJ, Chaturvedi A, et al. Changes in target volume during radiotherapy treatment of invasive bladder carcinoma. Clin Oncol (R Coll Radiol). 1993;5(1):30–3.
31. Graham J, Gee A, Hilton S, et al. Geometric uncertainties in radiotherapy of the prostate and bladder. In: Geometric uncertainties in radiotherapy. London: British Institute of Radiology; 2003.
32. Meijer GJ, Rasch C, Remeijer P, Lebesque JV. Three-dimensional analysis of delineation errors, setup errors, and organ motion during radiotherapy of bladder cancer. Int J Radiat Oncol Biol Phys. 2003;55(5):1277–87.
33. Roof KS, Mazal A, Sarkar S, et al. A three-dimensional CT based analysis of inter-fraction bladder motion during radiotherapeutic treatment of bladder cancer. Int J Radiat Oncol Biol Phys. 2004;60:S430.
34. Parsons JT, Million RR. Planned preoperative irradiation in the management of clinical stage B2-C (T3) bladder carcinoma. Int J Radiat Oncol Biol Phys. 1988;14(4):797–810.
35. Cole CJ, Pollack A, Zagars GK, Dinney CP, Swanson DA, von Eschenbach AC. Local control of muscle-invasive bladder cancer: preoperative radiotherapy and cystectomy versus cystectomy alone. Int J Radiat Oncol Biol Phys. 1995;32(2):331–40.
36. Zaghloul MS, Awwad HK, Akoush HH, Omar S, Soliman O, el Attar I. Postoperative radiotherapy of carcinoma in bilharzial bladder: improved disease free survival through improving local control. Int J Radiat Oncol Biol Phys. 1992;23(3):511–7.
37. Reisinger SA, Mohiuddin M, Mulholland SG. Combined pre- and postoperative adjuvant radiation therapy for bladder cancer – a ten year experience. Int J Radiat Oncol Biol Phys. 1992;24(3):463–8.

Bladder Preservation Therapies in Bladder Cancer

4

Ozan Cem Guler and Cem Onal

Abstract

Intravesical therapies with close monitoring are adequate for superficial disease, and chemotherapy and palliative radiotherapy are the main treatment options in metastatic stages. For muscle-invasive disease, treatment strategies are basically divided into two groups: surgery vs. trimodality treatment (TMT) that involves transurethral resection (TUR) of tumor tissues and concurrent radiochemotherapy (RCT); radiotherapy (RT) monotherapy is not recommended as primary curative option, and multimodality treatment is currently regarded only as an alternative in selected, well-informed, and compliant patients in whom cystectomy is not considered for clinical or personal reasons.

4.1 Introduction

Bladder cancer is the fifth most common malignancy in men, accounting for 5% of all cancer in males, and the ninth most common cancer in men and women combined [1]. Even though histological types may vary from countries, vast majority of the patients had urothelial (transitional cell) carcinoma histology. However, squamous cell carcinoma increases with schistosomal infection [2]. Mainly, urinary bladder cancer has three stages: superficial, muscle-invasive, and metastatic disease. Localized bladder cancer is divided into non-muscle-invasive (Ta, T1, Tis) and muscle-invasive (T2a–T4b) disease.

O.C. Guler, M.D. (✉)
Department of Radiation Oncology, Karadeniz Technical University, Trabzon, Turkey
e-mail: hcemonal@hotmail.com

C. Onal, M.D.
Department of Radiation Oncology, Başkent University, Adana, Turkey

G. Ozyigit, U. Selek (eds.), *Principles and Practice of Urooncology*,
DOI 10.1007/978-3-319-56114-1_4

Intravesical therapies with close monitoring are adequate for superficial disease, and chemotherapy and palliative radiotherapy are the main treatment options in metastatic stages. For muscle-invasive disease, treatment strategies are basically divided into two groups: surgery vs. trimodality treatment (TMT) that involves transurethral resection (TUR) of tumor tissues and concurrent radiochemotherapy (RCT). In many regions of Europe, radical radiotherapy is the treatment and cystectomy is reserved for nonresponding or recurring patients, while in the USA, treatment of muscle-invasive bladder cancer almost always entails a radical cystectomy. Although the current "European Association of Urology" [3] guidelines suggest radical cystectomy as the standard treatment for localized muscle-invasive bladder cancer, radiotherapy (RT) monotherapy is not recommended as primary curative option, and multimodality treatment is currently regarded only as an alternative in selected, well-informed, and compliant patients in whom cystectomy is not considered for clinical or personal reasons [4].

Radiotherapy plays an important role in organ-sparing oncological treatment regimens in most cancers. Although RT has been used in the management of bladder cancer for decades, it has not been widely accepted as a sole treatment to achieve bladder preservation; however, it has been largely ignored in the quest for the cure of locally advanced bladder cancer. Innovation in technology lets the radiation oncologists to make more comprehensive approaches. It is feasible to protect the normal tissues while delivering higher doses to tumor within new modalities. As a consequence of higher doses, improvement in local control may be acquired. In this chapter, we mainly assess the current role of RT and novel approaches in the treatment of urinary bladder cancer, focusing on TMT in muscle-invasive bladder cancer (MIBC).

4.2 Management of Non-muscle-Invasive Bladder Cancer

The majority of the patients with bladder cancer are diagnosed in the early stages. Non-muscle-invasive bladder cancer (NMIBC) consists of Ta, Tis, or T1 lesions. Although T1 bladder cancer is accepted as superficial tumor, lamina propria invasion is observed, that is rich in blood vessels and lymphatics causing hematogenous and lymphatic metastasis. The main treatment of such disease includes TUR of bladder tumor (TUR-BT) with or without intravesical chemotherapy and/or immunotherapy since it has a high risk of recurrence and progression to muscle-invasive disease [5, 6]. This choice is based on risk factors such as stage (whether the lamina propria is involved or not), tumor grade, tumor size, multifocality, whether the tumor is recurrent or not, and patient's tolerance. The immunotherapy with bacillus Calmette-Guérin (BCG) is the treatment of choice for superficial bladder cancer, whereas intravesical chemotherapy usually consists of mitomycin-C (MMC) [7, 8]. Also, intravesical gemcitabine may be used as a chemotherapeutic agent in the treatment of NMIBC [9]. Immunotherapy or chemotherapy can be used alone or in combination. Maintenance therapy after TUR-BT is generally needed in patients with NMIBC.

In comparison to intravesical therapy, RT/radiochemotherapy (RCT) can provide advantage by treating the micrometastases in the deeper muscle layer and pelvic lymph nodes which are seen in 5–10% of pT1 lesions [10].

Disease that is refractory to immunotherapy and/or chemotherapy, progression to muscle-invasive disease, and recurrent diseases that cannot be managed endoscopically are candidates for surgery. Duncan et al. [11] reported a local control rate of 28% and 5-year overall survival rate of 61% in 190 patients treated with bladder-only RT. In a study by Gospodarowicz et al. [12], the local control and disease-specific survival rates were 20% and 32%, respectively, for multiple tumors. All of these studies are based on RT-only regimen. However, there are a few data assessing the role of RCT for NMIBC. Weiss et al. [13] reported treatment outcomes from 141 patients with high-risk T1 bladder cancer treated with initial TUR-BT followed by RT alone or RCT. The RT dose was 55.8 Gy administered 4–6 weeks after TUR-BT with pelvic nodes receiving a median dose of 50.4 Gy. Although complete response rates at the first cystoscopy were similar in RT and RCT groups (82% vs. 87%), 5-year failure rate was higher in RT group compared to RCT arm (64% vs. 46%). With a median follow-up of 62 months, 10-year OS and DSS rates were 51% and 7%, respectively, and 50% of overall patients had their bladder preserved. In a randomized trial of 210 patients, the study by Harland et al. [14] examined the efficacy of RT for pT1G3 disease. Thirty-seven centers compared radical radiotherapy with standard conservative therapy in patients with unifocal disease with no carcinoma in situ (CIS) and radical radiotherapy alone vs. intravesical therapy in patients with multifocal disease or CIS. After a median follow-up of 44 months, no survival benefit was observed with RT.

4.3 Treatment of Muscle-Invasive Disease

4.3.1 Monotherapy

Radical cystectomy is still accepted as the gold standard treatment for MIBC [15]. This surgical procedure includes removal of whole bladder and dissection of regional lymph nodes. Additionally, the prostate and seminal vesicles are removed in men, and the uterus, cervix, ovaries, and anterior vagina are removed in women. This operation is usually performed using an open technique. Since high perioperative complication rates of open RC, minimally invasive surgical techniques such as laparoscopic or robotic surgery have been explored. Despite all these techniques, it is not possible to avoid potential morbidity or mortality of RC. Also bladder preservation therapies have a remarkable quality-of-life (QOL) advantage with similar oncological outcomes.

Urothelial bladder cancer is sensitive to cisplatin-based chemotherapeutics, with survival benefit demonstrated in patients with MIBC. Neoadjuvant chemotherapy-only regimen is widely used in perioperative settings in locally advanced patients [16]. However, the benefit of adjuvant RT is still controversial. Although cisplatin-based chemotherapy regimens are widely used in patients with MIBC with high-risk features after RC, there are no randomized clinical data that have been shown to date.

Bladder preservation therapies are basically divided into two groups: single modality and TMT. Single modality treatment consists of TUR alone, partial cystectomy, RT, or chemotherapy alone. The results of such treatments have inferior outcomes compared to RC or TMT. Two recently published results of comparative studies have reported similar 5-year and 10-year survival rates between radical cystectomy and RT alone [17–19]. In a 10-year retrospective study with 458 patients undergoing RT or cystectomy, no significant difference in 10-year overall survival was observed between RT and radical cystectomy (22% vs. 24%) [19]. In a systematic review, the reported 5-year local control rate ranged between 35 and 45% with a 5-year OS of 25–40% with RT monotherapy [20]. Consequently, RT monotherapy is often reserved for patients deemed unsuitable for cystectomy because of advanced age or comorbidity. There are few studies demonstrating the effectiveness of RT as a treatment option in terms of local control and survival in elderly patients with locally advanced bladder cancer not suitable for cystectomy [21]. Langsenlehner et al. [21] reported complete response rates of 65% and local control rate of 53% after 3 years in 75 bladder cancer patients treated with 50–50.4 Gy course of conformal RT. However, 35% of patients died from bladder cancer.

4.3.2 Multimodal Approach

Optimal bladder preservation therapy is TMT and comprises TUR-BT followed by concurrent RCT. Preliminary studies demonstrated complete response rate to endoscopic resection followed by chemotherapy was nearly twice that achieved by chemotherapy alone and addition of RT further improved disease-free survival with intact bladder [22–24]. The use of bladder-preserving strategies, such as combining RT and chemotherapy after maximal TUR is an effective alternative to radical cystectomy [11, 13, 25–28]. The extension of TUR-BT is very important in this treatment, and it should be as complete as possible in maximally safe procedure.

Since the late 1980s several centers have investigated the bladder preservation strategy as an alternative to radical cystectomy. This strategy is multidisciplinary, entailing maximal TUR-BT, followed by combined RCT [13, 26, 29–38] (Table 4.1). Three centers (the University of Erlangen, Germany; the Massachusetts General Hospital [MGH], MA, USA; and the University of Paris V, France) together with the Radiation Therapy Oncology Group (RTOG) in a multi-institutional setting have the largest experience. All reached the conclusion that patients who completely respond to TMT (61–87% in different series) are those who shall reap the benefits of long-term survival, while for those who cannot attain CR, cystectomy is the appropriate option. Cystoscopy is performed after a few weeks of RCT to assess the treatment response. If any residual disease (macro- or microscopic) remains, bladder preservation is aborted by cystectomy. On the other hand, if CR is achieved, a consolidation phase of RCT is carried out. The Massachusetts General Hospital reported the results of 348 patients with MIBC who were treated with combined

Table 4.1 Bladder preservation trials

Author (year)	*n*	RT course	RT dose (Gy)	OS	CSS	CR (%)	Salvage RC (%)
[a]Housset et al. (1993)	54	Split course	44 (bid)	3y, 59%	3y, 62%	74	–
[a]Shipley et al. (1998)	62	Split course	64.8	5y, 49%	–	60	25.8
[a]James et al. (2012)	182	Continuous	55–64	5y, 48%	–	–	11.4
[a]Tunio et al. (2012)	200	Continuous	65	5y, 52%	–	93	–
Kaufman et al. (2000)	34	Split course	44 (bid)	–	3y, 83%	67	29.4
Hussain et al. (2004)	41	Continuous	55 Gy in 20	2y, 50%	2y, 68%	71	19.5
Peyromaure et al. (2004)	43	Split course	24 Gy in 8 (bid)	–	3y, 75%	74.4	25.6
Kragelj et al. (2005)	84	Continuous	64	9y, 25%	9y, 51%	78	8.3
Cogna et al. (2006)	113	Continuous	64	–	5y, 50%	70	15
Weiss et al. (2007)	112	Continuous	55.8–59.4	5y, 74%	5y, 82%	88	17
Aboziada et al. (2009)	50	Split course	66	1.5y, 100%	1.5y, 84%	60	28
Choudhury et al. (2011)	50	Continuous	52.5 Gy in 20	5y, 65%	5y, 78%	82	14
Lagrange et al. (2011)	51	Split course	63	8y, 36%	–	–	33.3
Zapatero et al. (2011)	39	Split course	64.8	5y, 73%	5y, 82%	80	33

[a]Prospective studies

Abbreviations: *RT* radiotherapy, *OS* overall survival, *CSS* cause-specific survival, *CR* complete response, *RC* radical cystectomy

RCT [39]. The authors reported complete response (CR) rate of 72%, with 5- and 10-year OS rates of 52% and 35%, respectively. The 5- and 10-year DSS rates were 64% and 59%, respectively. Patients were excluded if they had pathologically proven positive nodes or hydronephrosis. All MGH protocols had in common the use of TUR-BT, concomitant cisplatin-based RT, and cystectomy if complete response was not achieved.

At the University of Erlangen, the authors retrospectively analyzed 415 patients with MIBC. The treatment included TUR-BT followed 4 weeks later by RCT up to a dose of 45–54 Gy to the bladder and pelvic nodes, and then whole bladder dose is boosted to 55.8–59.4 Gy total dose, depending upon the completeness of TUR-BT. Six to eight weeks after completion of therapy, response is assessed by cystoscopy. If the response is incomplete, cystectomy is indicated. The complete response rates for all patients and radiotherapy alone were 72% and 61%, respectively. The 5- and 10-year OS rates were 51% and 31%, while salvage cystectomy rates were 20% [40].

The Bladder Cancer 2001 (BC2001) study was the first randomized study investigating the role of chemotherapy to TUR-BT followed by radiotherapy in MIBC [31]. The chemotherapy regimen consisted of 5-FU and MMC. The 2-year DFS was significantly improved in the combined treatment arm compared to RT alone (67% vs. 54%, $p = 0.03$). Also there was a trend favoring RCT arm in 5-year OS rates (48% vs. 35%; $p = 0.16$). The National Cancer Institute of Canada (NCIC) investigated the addition of cisplatin chemotherapy to RT for organ-sparing treatment modality [25]. There was a statistically significant reduction in pelvic recurrences in patients treated with concurrent RCT compared to RT alone (29% vs. 52%); however, no statistically significant difference in OS was observed.

Several investigative protocols were carried out by the "Radiation Therapy Oncology Group" (RTOG). The first one, RTOG 85-12, consisted of induction RT with cisplatin; thereafter patients with complete response received additional RT and a third dose of cisplatin [41]. In RTOG 88-02 study, the toxicity of adding neoadjuvant, cisplatin, methotrexate, and vinblastine (CMV) to the combined treatment was evaluated [42]. The good tolerability of the regimen in this study led to RTOG 89-03, a randomized phase III trial assessing the efficacy of neoadjuvant CMV [27]. However, this study was stopped early due to unacceptably high toxicity rates in the CMV arm. Moreover, the addition of neoadjuvant CMV did not show any benefit in terms of complete response and overall survival or bladder preservation rates. RTOG 95-06 evaluated the accelerated hypofractionated scheme [30]. Although overall survival and bladder preservation rates were encouraging, grade 3 or more genitourinary toxicity rates were a concern. RTOG 97-06 also evaluated the efficacy of hypofractionated RT scheme [43]. In RTOG 99-06, paclitaxel was added to the concomitant cisplatin and gemcitabine in the adjuvant setting leading to an excellent complete rate of 87% [44].

Radiation dose and schedule vary within countries, but the most acceptable fractionation is 40–46 Gy to the pelvic lymph nodes and bladder with a boost to tumor a total dose of 60–66 Gy. Cisplatin is the most common concurrent chemotherapy agent. The main goal of this chemotherapy is being a radiosensitizer. After performing TUR-BT, the bladder preservation protocols usually belong to one of the three categories (Fig. 4.1). In the first scheme RT is delivered to patients who attain pathological complete remission after a full dose of chemotherapy. The second scheme includes induction chemotherapy with two to three cycles of CMV and then RCT for the responders. The third scheme entails concomitant RCT either with moderate dose followed by cystoscopy and consolidation RCT or to give high-dose RCT and to perform cystoscopy after completion of the dose. For all schemes, cystectomy is indicated for those who attained non-complete response. A cystoscopy with re-biopsy should be performed for assessment of therapy response. This evaluation could be done at the end of TMT (continuous course) or before planning to the boost volumes after 40–46 Gy (split course). In the latter, patients responding to the treatment were treated for boost to the tumor, while nonresponders were offered for salvage RC. Five-year overall survival (OS) and cancer-specific survival rates range from 36% to 74% and 50% to 82%, respectively. Salvage cystectomy rates were 25–30% [45].

Advanced age is not a contraindication for TMT. As older patients are more likely to have significant comorbidities, treatment should be interpreted carefully. Especially kidney function test (BUN and creatinine), electrolytes, and fluid intake should be taken into consideration with attention. RTOG pooled analysis of patients aged 75 or more showed no significant differences in CR or DSS.

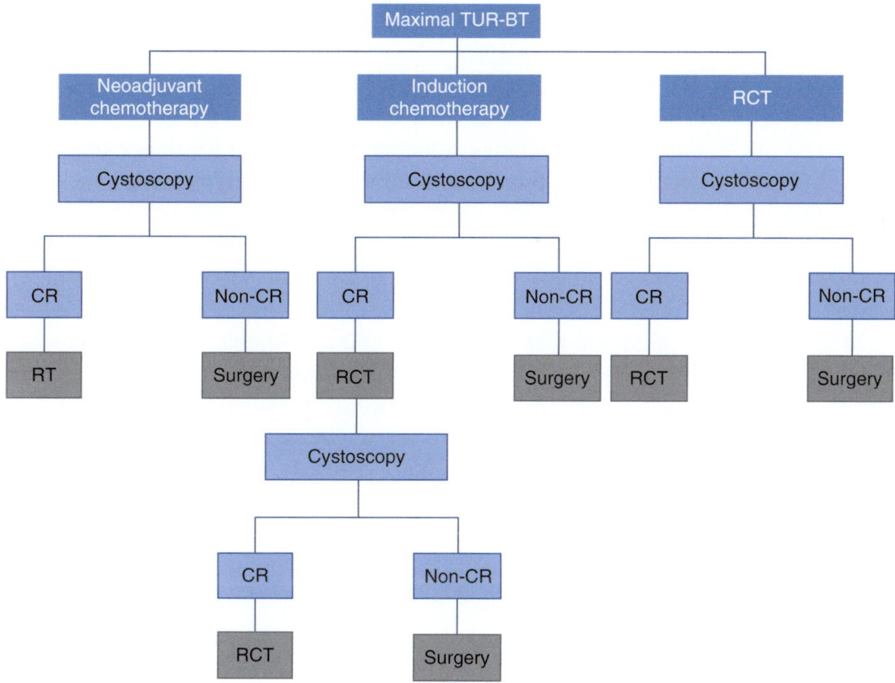

Fig. 4.1 Bladder preservation protocols usually belong to one of the three categories

4.4 Metastatic Disease and Recurrences

Distant metastasis is much more frequent compared to local control in bladder cancer. In patients with RC, 5-year locoregional control rates are up to 80%, but 5-year OS was ranging from 40 to 60% [16, 46]. Cisplatin and gemcitabine are the treatment of choice in most patients with metastatic bladder carcinoma. Response rates to the first-line treatment are satisfactory, but eventually most of the patients develop progression and need second-line treatment. It is hard to mention cure in metastatic disease, but patients with node-only metastatic disease or lung carcinoma may be cured by chemotherapy. Radiotherapy is always an integral part of treatment in patients with metastatic disease. As in other cancer types, it may be used for palliative intent for local disease such as the bone or brain. Hematuria is the most common cause to refer to radiotherapy in patients with metastatic bladder cancer. Also stereotactic radiosurgery (SRS) has a potential in patients with a small number of metastasis in bladder cancer.

If TMT approach fails, management of the local recurrences may be challenging due to local side effects of such treatment. Salvage cystectomy is indicated for patients who develop invasive recurrences. In modern prospective series, salvage cystectomy rates were ranging from 11 to 26% [27, 31].

4.5 Irradiation Techniques

Historically, most of the published data about bladder cancer RT is about two-dimensional conventional RT. Nowadays, 3D-conformal RT is the current standard in most of the clinical trials. IMRT has emerged as an option for image guidance. Advances in RT planning, verification, positioning, and delivery provide a means to optimize RT for bladder cancer and overcome difficulties, which have previously limited the success of this treatment, and also offer the opportunity to reduce the irradiated normal tissue volumes while delivering more intensive and increased RT dose.

Intensity modulated radiotherapy (IMRT) is a new technique which allows more accurate delivery of required doses or beyond to the tumor while protecting adjacent organs or structures. This technique is widely used in radiotherapy and replaced the three-dimensional radiotherapy (3D-RT) in the treatment of MIBC. Fractionation schedules and treatment fields vary from centers. There is no randomized trial comparing the conventional fractionation and BID. The most accepted approach is 40–45 Gy to the entire bladder, prostatic/proximal urethra, and the lymph nodes in the pelvis following by boost 20 Gy to the tumor a total dose of 65–66 Gy. Treating only bladder for a total dose of 64 Gy in 2 Gy fractions is performed by some groups (i.e., the UK).

4.5.1 Simulation, Target Volume, and Fields

All simulations are performed with empty bladder in supine position. This makes more reproducible and predictable positioning of bladder. 3D-CT simulation is essential for treatment. Patients underwent 3-mm-slice-thickness CT from mid-L4 to the lower edge of lesser trochanters. Intravenous contrast could be used in suspicious cases, not as clinical routine.

Treatment of urinary bladder cancer involves two phases of RT. The pelvic lymph nodes, prostate, and bladder are target volumes in the first phase. The second phase boosts the bladder alone. The pelvic lymph nodes consist of obturator and internal and external iliac lymphatics. As there might be occult stromal invasion, prostatic urethra and the first 2 cm of proximal urethra need to be covered in men and women, respectively. The top border of the field starts at the level of the bifurcation of the common iliac vessels and does not include the entire pelvis (Figs. 4.2 and 4.3).

4.5.2 Tumor Localization

Tumor location is essential for determining the target volume. For this purpose, operative notes during cystoscopy and histology reports should be available, and cross-sectional imaging is mandatory. Standard supine position is the treatment position of choice. Computed tomography simulation is the gold standard for treatment planning, for adequate coverage of the whole bladder [47]. Intravesical

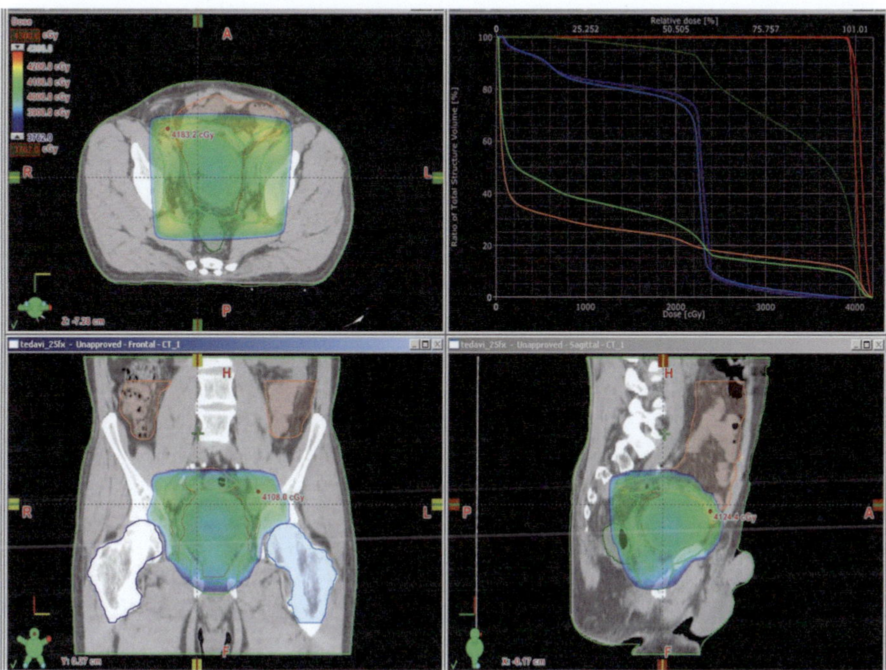

Fig. 4.2 Treatment of urinary bladder cancer involves two phases of RT. The pelvic lymph nodes, prostate, and bladder are target volumes in the first phase

contrast (30–70 mL) may also be administered via a catheter, with or without additional air (15–30 mL). It is necessary to make sure that the use of contrast does not result in considerable difference of the bladder volume in planning and during daily treatment delivery [48].

Although there is no randomized trial favoring the inclusion of the pelvic nodes in the radiation volume, elective nodal irradiation aims at eradication of micrometastatic disease in the pelvis. However, this approach results in irradiation of a large target volume, encompassing significant amounts of the small bowel and rectum. This can lead to greater gastrointestinal toxicity and potentially limit treatment intensification [49]. The question of whether to include lymph nodes or not in CTV has never been the issue of any randomized trial. Centers that irradiate the bladder alone do not report either increased pelvic failure rates or reduced survival, although direct comparisons are difficult [50]. Retrospective studies comparing patients receiving irradiation to the locoregional lymph nodes with patients treated with small fields to the bladder only showed a significantly worse treatment outcome on irradiation of the nodes [51].

However, the bias of treating the more advanced cases with locoregional nodes may be the reason for these inferior results [52]. However, reviewing the extended pelvic lymphadenectomy data in bladder cancer showed that several prospective and retrospective studies proved that the extent of lymphadenectomy and the

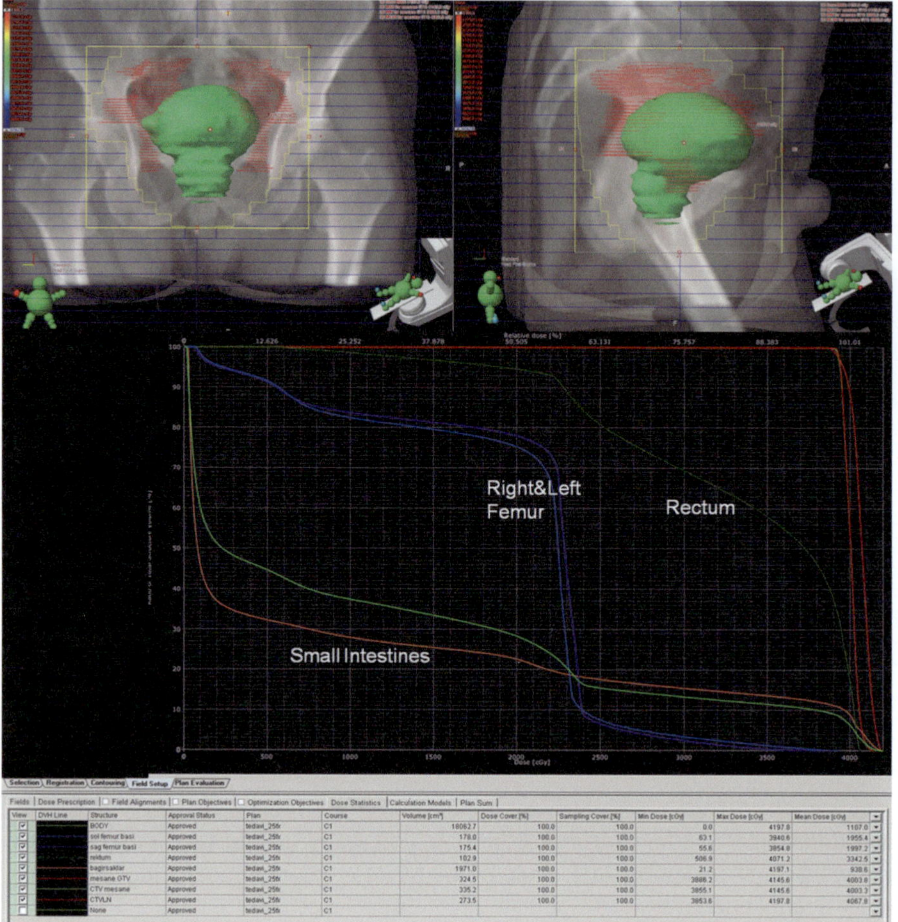

Fig. 4.3 Beam eye views and dose volume histogram for the first phase of radiotherapy

number of dissected nodes determine the survival rates, even in node-negative patients [53]. This may reflect the importance of eradication of the disease in the lymph nodes, even in its microscopic form, and in bladder cancer end results. With the advancement in radiotherapeutic techniques, it is expected that radiation can improve the tumor control probability and reduce normal tissue complication probability in such patients.

4.5.3 Target Delineation

The CTV for irradiating the bladder should encompass the entire outer circumference of the bladder, any extravesical disease spread, and any region deemed to be at risk of microscopic disease spread whenever whole bladder irradiation is the plan. For 3D planning, gross tumor volume (GTV) is determined including the bladder with any extravesical extension. Upon irradiation of bladder tumor, the determination of the tumor is mostly guided by MRI-fused images and/or other diagnostic modalities, including cystoscopic bladder maps and fiducial markers placed transurethrally.

Macroscopic visible tumor on CT/MRI or cystoscopy is delineated as gross tumor volume (GTV), if possible. The entire bladder, pelvic lymph nodes (obturator, external and internal iliacs), and prostate and prostatic urethra in men and the 2 cm of the proximal urethra in women are included in the first phase of clinical tumor volume (CTV1). In the second phase of the treatment, pelvic lymph nodes were excluded from clinical tumor volume (CTV2). Small bowel and rectum are delineated at organs at risks (OARs). Individualized planning tumor volume (PTV) margins are used for each center. 1.5–2 cm is the most commonly used isotropic margins for CTV to PTV, and it may be reduced with IGRT. It is shown that bladder wall movement of more than 1.5 cm occurs at least once during a course of treatment in more than 60% of patients (Figs. 4.4 and 4.5) [54].

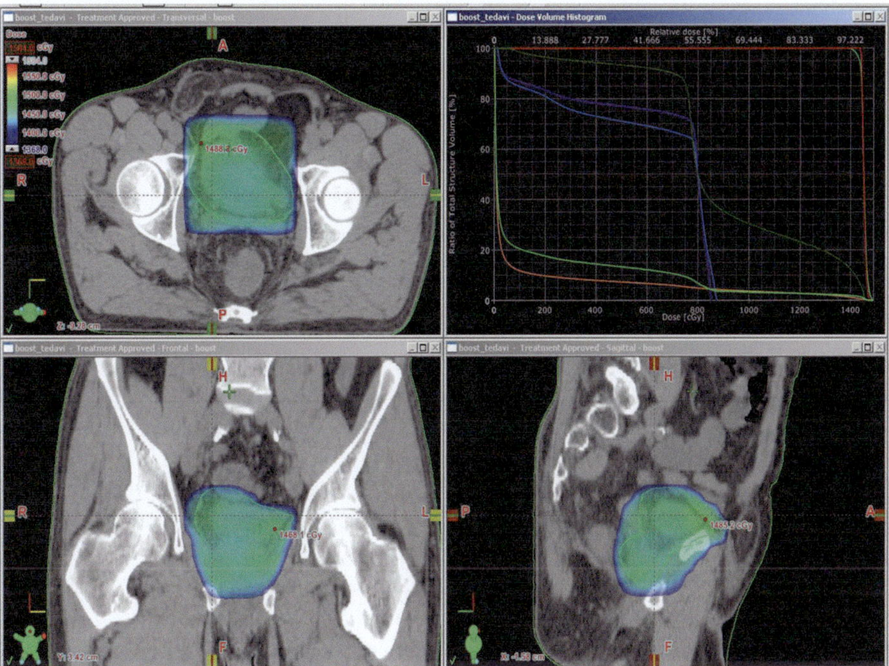

Fig. 4.4 In the second phase of the treatment, pelvic lymph nodes were excluded from clinical tumor volume. Small bowel and rectum are delineated at organs at risks (OARs). Individualized planning tumor volume (PTV) margins are used for each center

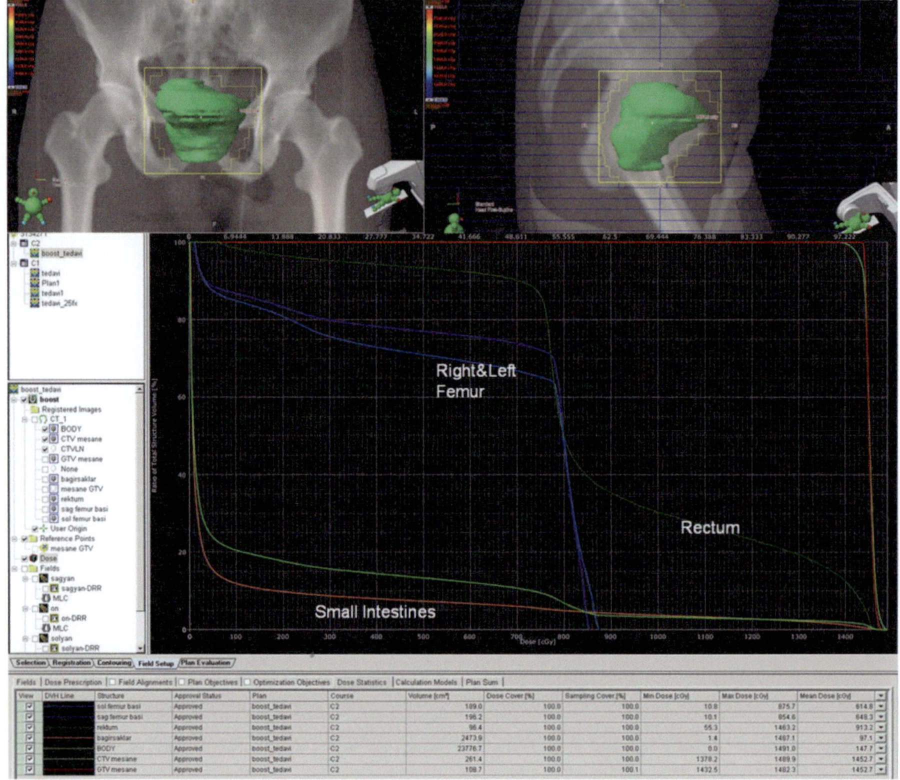

Fig. 4.5 Beam eye views and dose volume histogram for the second phase of radiotherapy (boost plan)

4.5.4 Doses and RT Schedules

There are two main RT schedules in the treatment of urinary bladder cancer. In the first one, CTV1 is treated up to 46 Gy and a boost of 65–66 Gy delivered to CTV2 in once-daily 1.8–2 Gy fractions, 5 days per week [25, 40]. In the second one, twice-daily concomitant boost is used, and CTV1 is treated up to 45 Gy in 1.8 Gy fractions and CTV2 is boosted to 67.5 Gy in 1.5 Gy fractions. Typically, 40–45 Gy is delivered to the pelvic lymph nodes and entire bladder, while the whole bladder boosts additional 20–24 Gy.

The major difference between these schedules is that the first regimen allows the physician to assess the early treatment response following the delivery of the first phase. Repeat cystoscopy/biopsy after 3 weeks of treatment break may distinguish the nonresponder patients and lead them to immediate radical cystectomy.

4.5.5 IMRT and IGRT

Day-to-day variations in bladder size, shape, and position are the major technical difficulties in urinary bladder cancer RT. These variations may result in inadequate dose homogeneity while increasing the dose to surrounding normal tissues. Also, the need of larger treatment margins might result in the irradiation of significant volumes of small bowel and rectum. The use of fiducial markers may allow a decrease in PTV expansion. Daily image-guided therapy is the only way to reduce the margins significantly. Also, if the daily treatment is centered on the bladder rather than referenced to bony anatomy, smaller margins could be feasible.

Estimated bladder tolerance in partial bladder irradiation is 80 Gy if one third of the bladder is spared. Partial bladder irradiation does allow for the delivery of a higher dose to the tumor than whole bladder radiation without increase in morbidity [49].

4.5.6 Brachytherapy

Brachytherapy is combined with EBRT to provide a radiation boost to the primary tumor. Although there are no randomized trials comparing the radical cystectomy vs. EBRT + brachytherapy, in selected population, outcomes appear to be similar [55, 56]. Because of lacking clinical data, the use of brachytherapy is not recommended in clinical routine.

Conclusion

All the oncological approaches have the same primary goal: to cure the cancer. In this case, bladder preservation is a secondary consideration. TMT regimen has equivalent oncological outcomes to radical surgery with improved QOL not only for medically unfit patients for RC but also patients who desire to keep their native bladder. Radiotherapy plays an important role in nearly all stages of bladder carcinoma.

References

1. Torre LA, Siegel RL, Ward EM, Jemal A. Global cancer incidence and mortality rates and trends – an update. Cancer Epidemiol Biomarkers Prev. 2016;25(1):16–27. doi:10.1158/1055-9965.EPI-15-0578.
2. Zaghloul MS, Mousa AG. Trimodality treatment for bladder cancer: does modern radiotherapy improve the end results? Expert Rev Anticancer Ther. 2010;10(12):1933–44. doi:10.1586/era.10.156.
3. Secin FP, Karanikolas N, Gopalan A, Bianco FJ, Shayegan B, Touijer K, et al. The anterior layer of Denonvilliers' fascia: a common misconception in the laparoscopic prostatectomy literature. J Urol. 2007;177(2):521–5. doi:10.1016/j.juro.2006.09.028.

4. Stenzl A, Cowan NC, De Santis M, Jakse G, Kuczyk MA, Merseburger AS, et al. The updated EAU guidelines on muscle-invasive and metastatic bladder cancer. Eur Urol. 2009;55(4):815–25. doi:10.1016/j.eururo.2009.01.002.
5. Babjuk M, Oosterlinck W, Sylvester R, Kaasinen E, Bohle A, Palou-Redorta J, et al. EAU guidelines on non-muscle-invasive urothelial carcinoma of the bladder, the 2011 update. Actas Urol Esp. 2012;36(7):389–402. doi:10.1016/j.acuro.2011.12.001.
6. Burger M, Oosterlinck W, Konety B, Chang S, Gudjonsson S, Pruthi R, et al. ICUD-EAU international consultation on bladder cancer 2012: non-muscle-invasive urothelial carcinoma of the bladder. Eur Urol. 2013;63(1):36–44. doi:10.1016/j.eururo.2012.08.061.
7. Babjuk M, Oosterlinck W, Sylvester R, Kaasinen E, Bohle A, Palou-Redorta J, et al. EAU guidelines on non-muscle-invasive urothelial carcinoma of the bladder. Eur Urol. 2008;54(2):303–14. doi:10.1016/j.eururo.2008.04.051.
8. Hall MC, Chang SS, Dalbagni G, Pruthi RS, Seigne JD, Skinner EC, et al. Guideline for the management of nonmuscle invasive bladder cancer (stages Ta, T1, and Tis): 2007 update. J Urol. 2007;178(6):2314–30. doi:10.1016/j.juro.2007.09.003.
9. Shelley MD, Jones G, Cleves A, Wilt TJ, Mason MD, Kynaston HG. Intravesical gemcitabine therapy for non-muscle invasive bladder cancer (NMIBC): a systematic review. BJU Int. 2012;109(4):496–505. doi:10.1111/j.1464-410X.2011.10880.x.
10. Stein JP, Lieskovsky G, Cote R, Groshen S, Feng AC, Boyd S, et al. Radical cystectomy in the treatment of invasive bladder cancer: long-term results in 1,054 patients. J Clin Oncol. 2001;19(3):666–75. doi:10.1200/jco.2001.19.3.666.
11. Duncan W, Quilty PM. The results of a series of 963 patients with transitional cell carcinoma of the urinary bladder primarily treated by radical megavoltage X-ray therapy. Radiother Oncol. 1986;7(4):299–310.
12. Gospodarowicz MK, Rider WD, Keen CW, Connolly JG, Jewett MA, Cummings BJ, et al. Bladder cancer: long-term follow-up results of patients treated with radical radiation. Clin Oncol (R Coll Radiol). 1991;3(3):155–61.
13. Weiss C, Wolze C, Engehausen DG, Ott OJ, Krause FS, Schrott KM, et al. Radiochemotherapy after transurethral resection for high-risk T1 bladder cancer: an alternative to intravesical therapy or early cystectomy? J Clin Oncol. 2006;24(15):2318–24. doi:10.1200/JCO.2006.05.8149.
14. Harland SJ, Kynaston H, Grigor K, Wallace DM, Beacock C, Kockelbergh R, et al. A randomized trial of radical radiotherapy for the management of pT1G3 NXM0 transitional cell carcinoma of the bladder. J Urol. 2007;178(3 Pt 1):807–13; discussion, 13. doi:10.1016/j.juro.2007.05.024.
15. Gakis G, Efstathiou J, Lerner SP, Cookson MS, Keegan KA, Guru KA, et al. ICUD-EAU International Consultation on Bladder Cancer 2012: radical cystectomy and bladder preservation for muscle-invasive urothelial carcinoma of the bladder. Eur Urol. 2013;63(1):45–57. doi:10.1016/j.eururo.2012.08.009.
16. Grossman HB, Natale RB, Tangen CM, Speights VO, Vogelzang NJ, Trump DL, et al. Neoadjuvant chemotherapy plus cystectomy compared with cystectomy alone for locally advanced bladder cancer. N Engl J Med. 2003;349(9):859–66. doi:10.1056/NEJMoa022148.
17. Chahal R, Sundaram SK, Iddenden R, Forman DF, Weston PM, Harrison SC. A study of the morbidity, mortality and long-term survival following radical cystectomy and radical radiotherapy in the treatment of invasive bladder cancer in Yorkshire. Eur Urol. 2003;43(3):246–57.
18. Kotwal S, Choudhury A, Johnston C, Paul AB, Whelan P, Kiltie AE. Similar treatment outcomes for radical cystectomy and radical radiotherapy in invasive bladder cancer treated at a United Kingdom specialist treatment center. Int J Radiat Oncol Biol Phys. 2008;70(2):456–63. doi:10.1016/j.ijrobp.2007.06.030.
19. Munro NP, Sundaram SK, Weston PM, Fairley L, Harrison SC, Forman D, et al. A 10-year retrospective review of a nonrandomized cohort of 458 patients undergoing radical radiotherapy or cystectomy in Yorkshire, UK. Int J Radiat Oncol Biol Phys. 2010;77(1):119–24. doi:10.1016/j.ijrobp.2009.04.050.
20. Rene NJ, Cury FB, Souhami L. Conservative treatment of invasive bladder cancer. Curr Oncol. 2009;16(4):36–47.

21. Langsenlehner T, Doller C, Quehenberger F, Stranzl-Lawatsch H, Langsenlehner U, Pummer K, et al. Treatment results of radiation therapy for muscle-invasive bladder cancer. Strahlenther Onkol. 2010;186(4):203–9. doi:10.1007/s00066-010-2053-1.
22. Hall RR, Newling DW, Ramsden PD, Richards B, Robinson MR, Smith PH. Treatment of invasive bladder cancer by local resection and high dose methotrexate. Br J Urol. 1984;56(6):668–72.
23. Herr HW, Bajorin DF, Scher HI. Neoadjuvant chemotherapy and bladder-sparing surgery for invasive bladder cancer: ten-year outcome. J Clin Oncol. 1998;16(4):1298–301. doi:10.1200/jco.1998.16.4.1298.
24. Prout GR Jr, Shipley WU, Kaufman DS, Heney NM, Griffin PP, Althausen AF, et al. Preliminary results in invasive bladder cancer with transurethral resection, neoadjuvant chemotherapy and combined pelvic irradiation plus cisplatin chemotherapy. J Urol. 1990;144(5):1128–34. discussion 34–6
25. Coppin CM, Gospodarowicz MK, James K, Tannock IF, Zee B, Carson J, et al. Improved local control of invasive bladder cancer by concurrent cisplatin and preoperative or definitive radiation. The National Cancer Institute of Canada Clinical Trials Group. J Clin Oncol. 1996;14(11):2901–7. doi:10.1200/jco.1996.14.11.2901.
26. Chung PW, Bristow RG, Milosevic MF, Yi QL, Jewett MA, Warde PR, et al. Long-term outcome of radiation-based conservation therapy for invasive bladder cancer. Urol Oncol. 2007;25(4):303–9. doi:10.1016/j.urolonc.2006.09.015.
27. Shipley WU, Winter KA, Kaufman DS, Lee WR, Heney NM, Tester WR, et al. Phase III trial of neoadjuvant chemotherapy in patients with invasive bladder cancer treated with selective bladder preservation by combined radiation therapy and chemotherapy: initial results of Radiation Therapy Oncology Group 89-03. J Clin Oncol. 1998;16(11):3576–83. doi:10.1200/jco.1998.16.11.3576.
28. Rodel C, Weiss C, Sauer R. Trimodality treatment and selective organ preservation for bladder cancer. J Clin Oncol. 2006;24(35):5536–44. doi:10.1200/JCO.2006.07.6729.
29. Sangar VK, McBain CA, Lyons J, Ramani VA, Logue JP, Wylie JP, et al. Phase I study of conformal radiotherapy with concurrent gemcitabine in locally advanced bladder cancer. Int J Radiat Oncol Biol Phys. 2005;61(2):420–5. doi:10.1016/j.ijrobp.2004.05.074.
30. Housset M, Maulard C, Chretien Y, Dufour B, Delanian S, Huart J, et al. Combined radiation and chemotherapy for invasive transitional-cell carcinoma of the bladder: a prospective study. J Clin Oncol. 1993;11(11):2150–7. doi:10.1200/jco.1993.11.11.2150.
31. James ND, Hussain SA, Hall E, Jenkins P, Tremlett J, Rawlings C, et al. Radiotherapy with or without chemotherapy in muscle-invasive bladder cancer. N Engl J Med. 2012;366(16):1477–88. doi:10.1056/NEJMoa1106106.
32. Tunio MA, Hashmi A, Qayyum A, Mohsin R, Zaeem A. Whole-pelvis or bladder-only chemoradiation for lymph node-negative invasive bladder cancer: single-institution experience. Int J Radiat Oncol Biol Phys. 2012;82(3):e457–62. doi:10.1016/j.ijrobp.2011.05.051.
33. Hussain SA, Stocken DD, Peake DR, Glaholm JG, Zarkar A, Wallace DM, et al. Long-term results of a phase II study of synchronous chemoradiotherapy in advanced muscle invasive bladder cancer. Br J Cancer. 2004;90(11):2106–11. doi:10.1038/sj.bjc.6601852.
34. Peyromaure M, Slama J, Beuzeboc P, Ponvert D, Debre B, Zerbib M. Concurrent chemoradiotherapy for clinical stage T2 bladder cancer: report of a single institution. Urology. 2004;63(1):73–7.
35. Kragelj B, Zaletel-Kragelj L, Sedmak B, Cufer T, Cervek J. Phase II study of radiochemotherapy with vinblastine in invasive bladder cancer. Radiother Oncol. 2005;75(1):44–7. doi:10.1016/j.radonc.2005.01.007.
36. Aboziada MA, Hamza HM, Abdlrahem AM. Initial results of bladder preserving approach by chemo-radiotherapy in patients with muscle invading transitional cell carcinoma. J Egypt Natl Canc Inst. 2009;21(2):167–74.
37. Choudhury A, Cowan R. Bladder preservation multimodality therapy as an alternative to radical cystectomy for treatment of muscle invasive bladder cancer. BJU Int. 2011;108(9):E313. doi:10.1111/j.1464-410X.2011.10672_3.x.

38. Choudhury A, Swindell R, Logue JP, Elliott PA, Livsey JE, Wise M, et al. Phase II study of conformal hypofractionated radiotherapy with concurrent gemcitabine in muscle-invasive bladder cancer. J Clin Oncol. 2011;29(6):733–8. doi:10.1200/JCO.2010.31.5721.
39. Efstathiou JA, Spiegel DY, Shipley WU, Heney NM, Kaufman DS, Niemierko A, et al. Long-term outcomes of selective bladder preservation by combined-modality therapy for invasive bladder cancer: the MGH experience. Eur Urol. 2012;61(4):705–11. doi:10.1016/j.eururo.2011.11.010.
40. Rodel C, Grabenbauer GG, Kuhn R, Papadopoulos T, Dunst J, Meyer M, et al. Combined-modality treatment and selective organ preservation in invasive bladder cancer: long-term results. J Clin Oncol. 2002;20(14):3061–71.
41. Tester W, Porter A, Asbell S, Coughlin C, Heaney J, Krall J, et al. Combined modality program with possible organ preservation for invasive bladder carcinoma: results of RTOG protocol 85-12. Int J Radiat Oncol Biol Phys. 1993;25(5):783–90.
42. Tester W, Caplan R, Heaney J, Venner P, Whittington R, Byhardt R, et al. Neoadjuvant combined modality program with selective organ preservation for invasive bladder cancer: results of Radiation Therapy Oncology Group phase II trial 8802. J Clin Oncol. 1996;14(1):119–26. doi:10.1200/jco.1996.14.1.119.
43. Kaufman D, Raghavan D, Carducci M, Levine EG, Murphy B, Aisner J, et al. Phase II trial of gemcitabine plus cisplatin in patients with metastatic urothelial cancer. J Clin Oncol. 2000;18(9):1921–7. doi:10.1200/jco.2000.18.9.1921.
44. Kaufman DS, Winter KA, Shipley WU, Heney NM, Wallace HJ 3rd, Toonkel LM, et al. Phase I-II RTOG study (99-06) of patients with muscle-invasive bladder cancer undergoing transurethral surgery, paclitaxel, cisplatin, and twice-daily radiotherapy followed by selective bladder preservation or radical cystectomy and adjuvant chemotherapy. Urology. 2009;73(4):833–7. doi:10.1016/j.urology.2008.09.036.
45. Ploussard G, Daneshmand S, Efstathiou JA, Herr HW, James ND, Rodel CM, et al. Critical analysis of bladder sparing with trimodal therapy in muscle-invasive bladder cancer: a systematic review. Eur Urol. 2014;66(1):120–37. doi:10.1016/j.eururo.2014.02.038.
46. Zehnder P, Studer UE, Skinner EC, Dorin RP, Cai J, Roth B, et al. Super extended versus extended pelvic lymph node dissection in patients undergoing radical cystectomy for bladder cancer: a comparative study. J Urol. 2011;186(4):1261–8. doi:10.1016/j.juro.2011.06.004.
47. Rothwell RI, Ash DV, Jones WG. Radiation treatment planning for bladder cancer: a comparison of cystogram localisation with computed tomography. Clin Radiol. 1983;34(1):103–11.
48. Muren LP, Smaaland R, Dahl O. Organ motion, set-up variation and treatment margins in radical radiotherapy of urinary bladder cancer. Radiother Oncol. 2003;69(3):291–304.
49. Cowan RA, McBain CA, Ryder WD, Wylie JP, Logue JP, Turner SL, et al. Radiotherapy for muscle-invasive carcinoma of the bladder: results of a randomized trial comparing conventional whole bladder with dose-escalated partial bladder radiotherapy. Int J Radiat Oncol Biol Phys. 2004;59(1):197–207. doi:10.1016/j.ijrobp.2003.10.018.
50. Fokdal L, Hoyer M, von der Maase H. Treatment outcome and prognostic variables for local control and survival in patients receiving radical radiotherapy for urinary bladder cancer. Acta Oncol. 2004;43(8):749–57. doi:10.1080/02841860410018629.
51. Davidson SE, Symonds RP, Snee MP, Upadhyay S, Habeshaw T, Robertson AG. Assessment of factors influencing the outcome of radiotherapy for bladder cancer. Br J Urol. 1990;66(3):288–93.
52. Fokdal L, Hoyer M, von der Maase H. Radical radiotherapy for urinary bladder cancer: treatment outcomes. Expert Rev Anticancer Ther. 2006;6(2):269–79. doi:10.1586/14737140.6.2.269.
53. Leissner J, Ghoneim MA, Abol-Enein H, Thuroff JW, Franzaring L, Fisch M, et al. Extended radical lymphadenectomy in patients with urothelial bladder cancer: results of a prospective multicenter study. J Urol. 2004;171(1):139–44. doi:10.1097/01.ju.0000102302.26806.fb.

54. Turner SL, Swindell R, Bowl N, Marrs J, Brookes B, Read G, et al. Bladder movement during radiation therapy for bladder cancer: implications for treatment planning. Int J Radiat Oncol Biol Phys. 1997;39(2):355–60.
55. Blank LE, Koedooder K, van Os R, van de Kar M, van der Veen JH, Koning CC. Results of bladder-conserving treatment, consisting of brachytherapy combined with limited surgery and external beam radiotherapy, for patients with solitary T1-T3 bladder tumors less than 5 cm in diameter. Int J Radiat Oncol Biol Phys. 2007;69(2):454–8. doi:10.1016/j.ijrobp.2007.03.014.
56. van der Steen-Banasik E, Ploeg M, Witjes JA, van Rey FS, Idema JG, Heijbroek RP, et al. Brachytherapy versus cystectomy in solitary bladder cancer: a case control, multicentre, East-Netherlands study. Radiother Oncol. 2009;93(2):352–7. doi:10.1016/j.radonc.2009.04.020.

Systemic Therapy for Bladder Cancer

5

Nil Molinas Mandel and Selen Mandel

Abstract

The gold standard of muscle-invasive bladder cancer is radical cystectomy. Before surgery three cycles of neoadjuvant chemotherapy can improve the overall survival and decrease the risk of recurrence. For operated high-risk without neoadjuvant therapy patients, adjuvant chemotherapy can be a good option. The primary treatment of metastatic bladder cancer is cisplatin-based chemotherapy. However, even though it is considered sensitive to chemotherapy, the average survival is 15 months and even less if there is an organ metastasis. For these patients 5-year survival rate is 5–20%. Several studies have shown different mutations in muscle-invasive bladder cancer. These mutations are being studied as a targeted therapy option for cases where chemotherapy is not sufficient. Although there is not a specifically approved treatment model for metastatic bladder cancer, targeted therapy is becoming a significant choice. According to the mutation analysis of the Cancer Genome Atlas (TCGA) project, there are three major pathway abnormalities in metastatic bladder cancer: regulation of cell cycle, RTK/RAS/PIK3, and chromatin abnormalities. The studies about the treatment of bladder cancers with cell cycle regulators, mTOR inhibitors, and EGFR inhibitors will be highly important in the future. Immunotherapy with the checkpoint inhibitors (an anti-PD1 therapy with atezolizumab, durvalumab) improves survival.

N.M. Mandel, M.D. (✉)
Department of Medical Oncology, VKF Amerikan Hospital, Istanbul, Turkey
e-mail: nmmandel@gmail.com

S. Mandel
Bezmialem School of Medicine, Istanbul, Turkey

G. Ozyigit, U. Selek (eds.), *Principles and Practice of Urooncology*,
DOI 10.1007/978-3-319-56114-1_5

5.1 Introduction

Sixty percent of early stage bladder cancers turn into muscle-invasive cancer [1]. Among other cancer types, high-grade invasive bladder cancer and urothelial cancers are considered as chemotherapy-sensitive tumors. DNA-damaging agent "cisplatin" is stated as the most effective drug for this particular cancer [2, 3].

5.2 Systemic Therapies in Muscle-Invasive Bladder Cancer

Even with the developments in surgical techniques, in muscle-invasive bladder cancers, 5-year survival rates for surgery alone are 48–66% [1–5]. For patients considered undergoing a radical cystectomy for invasive bladder cancers, it is suggested to give systemic chemotherapy prior to definitive surgery. Neoadjuvant chemotherapy decreases the risk of recurrence and prolongs the overall survival compared to surgery alone [1, 4].

In 60–70% of patients with invasive bladder cancer, the cancer is limited to the bladder and does not spread to the lymph nodes [6]. The recurrence rate of those patients is 15–25% [7]. In 20–30% of the patients, the tumor is outside the bladder or invades the fatty tissue surrounding the bladder. The recurrence rate of the patients in this group is 45–55%. In 20–30% of the invasive bladder cancers, lymph node metastasis can be discovered during surgery [8]. These patients have poor prognosis, and the chance of disease-free survival is 25–35% [1, 7].

The prognosis is poor for patients with recurrence following a radical surgery. Neoadjuvant chemotherapy lowers the risk of recurrence [9]. However, the physician may decide to direct the patient to surgery first without neoadjuvant chemotherapy. This decision is based on the patient's conditions as well as a physician's experience with prior cases [4, 10]. Following the surgery, the patients are evaluated for prognosis based on the invasion level of the tumor and lymph node metastasis. High-risk patients of this group are candidates for adjuvant chemotherapy [7].

There are some disadvantages of neoadjuvant chemotherapy besides the advantages which is listed as early treatment of microscopic disease, determination of in vivo chemotherapy sensitivity, and early treatment response to chemotherapy which could provide a sight of prognosis [10, 11]. Despite these listed advantages, the surgical stage of the current disease will not be known and unnecessary chemotherapy administrations could be possible, and thus the main disadvantage was the overtreatment with chemotherapy [11]. Also, chemoresistant patient's subgroup could miss the cystectomy options as a treatment. The toxicity caused by chemotherapy would postpone the timing of effective surgery [12, 13].

Depending on the results of meta-analysis, cisplatin-based chemotherapy schemas before definitive surgery provide 5–8% increase in overall survival [1]. Based on these results, neoadjuvant chemotherapy has to be discussed with patients diagnosed with muscle-invasive N0M0 [1, 9, 11, 13].

For adjuvant chemotherapy, an updated meta-analysis of nine randomized trials including 945 patients demonstrated an OS benefit [hazard ratio (HR) 0.77,

$p = 0.049$] and DFS benefit (HR 0.66, $p = 0.014$) among those who received cisplatin-based adjuvant chemotherapy [6]. The DFS benefit was increased among patients with lymph node involvement [6].

Radical cystectomy and extended lymphadenectomy are usually accepted to be the gold standard in treatment of muscle-invasive bladder cancer [14–20]. Bladder-sparing treatment approaches could be a reasonable approach for patients refusing radical cystectomy or patients with suitable tumor characteristics [14]. Concomitant radiochemotherapy (radiotherapy with cisplatin) is the most suitable and common way of treatment [15, 18, 19]. The initial prospective, randomized trial of radiotherapy alone versus concomitant chemoradiotherapy in muscle-invasive bladder cancer demonstrated an improved local control rate when cisplatin was added to radiation therapy [5].

A cystoscopy with bladder biopsy is mandatory for response evaluation, either midway through treatment or 2–3 months thereafter. If persistent or recurrent disease is observed at response evaluation or during follow-up (cystoscopy and urinary cytology every 3 months during the first 2 years and every 6 months thereafter), prompt salvage cystectomy is recommended when possible [7]. Clinical criteria helpful in determining whether patients are ideal for bladder preservation include an early tumor stage (including high-risk T1 disease, T2 <5 cm), a visibly complete TURBT, an absence of associated CIS, and a ureteral obstruction and adequate bladder capacity and function [8, 15].

5.3 Treatment of Advanced and Metastatic Disease

5.3.1 DNA-Targeted Chemotherapy

First trials of chemotherapy in advanced high-grade bladder or urothelial cancers demonstrated that a DNA-damaging cisplatin is an active drug [21]. Another active drug for metastatic bladder cancer is methotrexate. Combining cisplatin with an S-phase-specific antifolate drug methotrexate demonstrated higher response rates [22]. Methotrexate irreversibly blocks thymidylate synthase and dihydrofolate reductase enzymes, making the cell be blocked at the S phase [23]. In the following studies, it is showed that adding vinblastine and doxorubicine to this two-drug combined therapy achieved higher response rates. In addition to partial response, it was seen that complete responses could also be achieved [24]. Known as MVAC, this four-drug (methotrexate, vinblastine, Adriamycin (doxorubicin), and cisplatin) regimen is accepted as standard of care and used in different doses as well as dosage ranges [23]. It is seen that the addition of granulocyte colony-stimulating factor (G-CSF) in high-dose treatments achieved higher response rate; however, the toxicity is noted to increase accordingly. Following the 1990s, MVAC regimen is accepted as the first-line chemotherapy [25].

The search for an alternative to the highly toxic MVAC treatment has started. By the end of the 1990s, a synthetic pyrimidine antimetabolite gemcitabine was discovered. Gemcitabine inhibits the DNA synthesis at the S phase, by inhibiting DNA polymerase and ribonucleotide reductase, thus halting cell cycle progression [22].

The studies showed that gemcitabine, either alone or combined with cisplatin, is an effective agent in the treatment of advanced urothelial cancers. At a randomized phase 3 trial, with 505 metastatic bladder cancer patients, MVAC regimen was compared to gemcitabine and cisplatin combination (GC) [22, 23]. Following this trial, GC was accepted as the first-line chemotherapy, since it had a better safety profile. Response rates were above 50%, and the overall survivals were 15 and 12 months, respectively [22, 23].

Poor performance score (Karnofsky PS of <80%) and the evidence of visceral dissemination are important poor prognostic factors for overall survival [21].

5.3.2 Targeted Therapies

In 2014, the comprehensive molecular characterization of muscle-invasive bladder cancer (MIBC) by the Cancer Genome Atlas (TCGA) Research Network produced many new insights into the genetic makeup of MIBC3 [26]. Integrated analysis of mRNA, microRNA, and protein expression in 129 muscle-invasive tumors yielded four distinct clusters resembling the intrinsic subtypes identified in breast cancer [27]. Clusters I and II were similar to luminal A breast cancer and had high mRNA and protein expression of differentiation markers, including GATA3 and FOXA1. Cluster III and IV tumors were similar to basal breast cancer and had high expression of stem/progenitor cytokeratins [27].

Genetic alterations in the mTOR, FGFR, EGFR, and HER2 pathways have long been recognized in subsets of bladder cancer. TCGA and other studies have identified actionable drug targets in over 60% of the tumors interrogated [26, 28]. Disappointingly, no trial to date has proven efficacy for any rationally designed targeted agent in advanced UC.

Several phase II studies were evaluating the role of angiogenesis inhibitors such as bevacizumab, sunitinib, pazopanib, sorafenib, aflibercept, mTOR inhibitors as everolimus, EGFR inhibitors as cetuximab, erlotinib, gefitinib, and HER2 inhibitors as trastuzumab [29].

5.3.3 Immunotherapy

Patients with metastatic urothelial carcinoma have few treatment options after failure of platinum-based chemotherapy [27, 30, 31].

The recent introduction of anti-PD-L1 (programmed death ligand 1) treatment for metastatic UC was met with great enthusiasm [30, 31]. PD-L1 negatively regulates T-cell function by binding to its receptor programmed death 1 (PD-1 or B7-1) on activated T lymphocytes and other immune cells [30, 31]. The overexpression of PD-L1 in the tumor microenvironment is thought to be the mechanism by which tumor evasion of the host immune system occurs. Blockade of the PD-L1 pathway with a high-affinity engineered human anti-PD-L1 monoclonal immunoglobulin-G1 antibody (atezolizumab) was shown to improve objective response rate in a heavily pretreated population with poor prognostic features [31, 32]. Extended median overall survival ranging from 7.9 to 11.4 months was observed. One-year overall survival ranged between 36% and 48% compared with the historic rate of 20% from a pooled analysis [33].

Objective response rate, progression-free survival, and overall survival were found to be directly related to PD-L1 expression status on the infiltrating immune cells (ICs). In addition, treatment response correlated with mutation load and was found to be the highest in the luminal tumors subtyped within cluster II of the TCGA scheme [32]. The finding that PD-L1 was more efficacious in tumors with higher mutation load was consistent with patterns recognized in other malignancies [34]. Non-synonymous somatic mutations are thought to increase tumor neoantigen burden, leading to increased T-cell recognition and more potent tumoricidal activities unleashed by PD-L1 treatment.

The primary analysis (data cutoff May 5, 2015) showed that compared with a historical control overall response rate of 10%, treatment with atezolizumab resulted in a significantly improved RECIST v1.1 objective response rate for each prespecified immune cell group (IC2/IC3: 27% [95% CI 19–37], $p < 0.0001$; IC1/IC2/IC3: 18% [11–22], $p = 0.0004$) and in all patients (15% [10–18], $p = 0.0058$) [31]. With longer follow-up (data cutoff Sept 14, 2015), by independent review, objective response rates were 26% (95% CI 18–36) in the IC2/IC3 group, 18% [11–22] in the IC1/IC2/IC3 group, and 15% [10–17] overall in all 310 patients. With a median follow-up of 11.7 months (95% CI 11.4–12.2), ongoing responses were recorded in 38 (84%) of 45 responders [31]. Exploratory analyses showed the Cancer Genome Atlas (TCGA) subtypes and mutation load to be independently predictive for response to atezolizumab. Grade 3–4 treatment-related adverse events, of which fatigue was the most common (5 patients [2%]), occurred in 50 (16%) of 310 treated patients. Grade 3–4 immune-mediated adverse events occurred in 15 (5%) of 310 treated patients, with pneumonitis, increased aspartate aminotransferase, increased alanine aminotransferase, rash, and dyspnea being the most common. No treatment-related deaths occurred during the study [31].

Atezolizumab showed durable activity and good tolerability in this patient population. Increased levels of PD-L1 expression on immune cells were associated with increased response. This report is the first to show the association of TCGA subtypes with response to immune checkpoint inhibition and to show the importance of mutation load as a biomarker of response to this class of agents in advanced urothelial carcinoma [31].

Conclusion

Among other cancer types, high-grade invasive bladder cancer and urothelial cancers are considered as chemotherapy-sensitive tumors. DNA-damaging agent "cisplatin" is stated as the most effective drug for this particular cancer. The primary treatment of metastatic bladder cancer is cisplatin-based chemotherapy. Three cycles of neoadjuvant chemotherapy can improve overall survival and decrease the risk of recurrence. However, even though it is considered sensitive to chemotherapy, the average survival is 15 months and even less if there is an organ metastasis. For these patients 5-year survival rate is still poor.

References

1. Vale C. Advanced bladder cancer meta-analysis collaboration. Neoadjuvant chemotherapy in invasive bladder cancer: a systematic review and meta-analysis. Lancet. 2003;361(9373):1927–34.
2. Witjes JA, et al. Muscle-invasive and metastatic bladder cancer. EAU guidelines. 2013.
3. Gakis G, Efstathiou J, Lerner SP, et al. ICUD-EAU international consultation on bladder cancer 2012: radical cystectomy and bladder preservation for muscle- invasive urothelial carcinoma of the bladder. Eur Urol. 2013;63:45–57.
4. Stein S, John P, et al. Radical cystectomy in the treatment of invasive bladder cancer: long-term results in 1,054 patients. J Clin Oncol. 2001;19(3):666–75.
5. Coppin CM, et al. Improved local control of invasive bladder cancer by concurrent cisplatin and preoperative or definitive radiation. The National Cancer Institute of Canada Clinical Trials Group. J Clin Oncol. 1996;14(11):2901–7.
6. Leow JJ, Martin-Doyle W, Rajagopal PS, et al. Adjuvant chemotherapy for invasive bladder cancer: a 2013 updated systematic review and meta-analysis of randomized trials. Eur Urol. 2014;66:42–54.
7. Bellmunt J, Orsola A, Leow JJ, Wiegel T, De Santis M, Horwich A. On behalf of the ESMO Guidelines Working Group. 2014
8. Milosevic M, Gospodarowicz M, Zietman A, et al. Radiotherapy for bladder cancer. Urology. 2007;69:80–92.
9. Schultz PK, et al. Neoadjuvant chemotherapy for invasive bladder cancer: prognostic factors for survival of patients treated with M-VAC with 5-year follow-up. J Clin Oncol. 1994;12(7):1394–401.
10. Madersbacher S, et al. Radical cystectomy for bladder cancer today—a homogeneous series without neoadjuvant therapy. J Clin Oncol. 2003;21(4):690–6.
11. Chedgy EC, et al. Using the neoadjuvant chemotherapy paradigm to develop precision therapy for muscle-invasive bladder cancer. Urol Oncol Semin Orig Invest. 2016;34(10):469–76.
12. Sonpavde G, et al. Chemotherapy for muscle-invasive bladder cancer: better late than never? J Clin Oncol. 2016:JCO654442.
13. Zargar H, Espiritu PN, Fairey AS, Mertens LS, Dinney CP, Mir MC, et al. Multicenter assessment of neoadjuvant chemotherapy for muscle-invasive bladder cancer. Eur Urol. 2015;67:241–9.
14. Shipley WU, et al. An update of combined modality therapy for patients with muscle invading bladder cancer using selective bladder preservation or cystectomy. J Urol. 1999;162(2):445–50.
15. Shipley WU, Winter KA, Kaufman DS, Lee WR, Heney NM, Tester WR, Doggett RS. Phase III trial of neoadjuvant chemotherapy in patients with invasive bladder cancer treated with selective bladder preservation by combined radiation therapy and chemotherapy: initial results of Radiation Therapy Oncology Group 89-03. J Clin Oncol. 1998;16(11):3576–83.
16. William T, et al. Combined modality program with possible organ preservation for invasive bladder carcinoma: results of RTOG protocol 85-12. Int J Radiat Oncol Biol Phys. 1993;25(5):783–90.
17. Herr HW, Dotan Z, Donat SM, Bajorin DF. Defining optimal therapy for muscle invasive bladder cancer. J Urol. 2007;177(2):437–43.
18. Kachnic LA, et al. Bladder preservation by combined modality therapy for invasive bladder cancer. J Clin Oncol. 1997;15(3):1022–9.
19. Balar A, Bajorin DF, Milowsky MI. Management of invasive bladder cancer in patients who are not candidates for or decline cystectomy. Ther Adv Urol. 2011;3(3):107–17.
20. James ND, et al. Radiotherapy with or without chemotherapy in muscle-invasive bladder cancer. N Engl J Med. 2012;366(16):1477–88.
21. Witjes JA, Compérat E, Cowan NC, et al. EAU guidelines on muscle-invasive and metastatic bladder cancer: summary of the 2013 Guidelines. Eur Urol. 2014;65:778–92.

22. Von der Maase H, et al. Gemcitabine and cisplatin versus methotrexate, vinblastine, doxorubicin, and cisplatin in advanced or metastatic bladder cancer: results of a large, randomized, multinational, multicenter, phase III study. J Clin Oncol. 2000;18(17):3068–77.
23. Von der Maase H, et al. Long-term survival results of a randomized trial comparing gemcitabine plus cisplatin, with methotrexate, vinblastine, doxorubicin, plus cisplatin in patients with bladder cancer. J Clin Oncol. 2005;23(21):4602–8.
24. Bellmunt J, et al. Randomized phase III study comparing paclitaxel/cisplatin/gemcitabine and gemcitabine/cisplatin in patients with locally advanced or metastatic urothelial cancer without prior systemic therapy: EORTC Intergroup Study 30987. J Clin Oncol. 2012;30(10):1107–13.
25. Garcia JA, Dreicer R. Systemic chemotherapy for advanced bladder cancer: update and controversies. J Clin Oncol. 2006;24(35):5545–51.
26. The Cancer Genome Atlas Research Network. Comprehensive molecular characterization of urothelial bladder carcinoma. Nature. 2014;507:315–22.
27. Lerner SP. Targeted therapies for metastatic bladder cancer. J Urol. 2015;193:8–9.
28. Iyer G, Al-Ahmadie H, Schultz N, et al. Prevalence and co-occurrence of actionable genomic alterations in high-grade bladder cancer. J Clin Oncol. 2013;31(25):3133–40.
29. Zho Z, Shen Z, Xu C. Targeted therapy for advanced urothelial cancer of the bladder: where do we stand? Anticancer Agents Med Chem. 2012;12(9):1081–7.
30. McDermott DF, et al. Atezolizumab, an anti–programmed death-ligand 1 antibody, in metastatic renal cell carcinoma: long-term safety, clinical activity, and immune correlates from a phase Ia study. J Clin Oncol. 2016;34(8):833–42.
31. Rosenberg JE, Hoffman-Censits J, Powles T, et al. Atezolizumab in patients with locally advanced and metastatic urothelial carcinoma who have progressed following treatment with platinum-based chemotherapy: a single-arm, multicentre, phase 2 trial. Lancet. 2016;387(10030):1909–20.
32. Powles T, Eder JP, Fine GD, et al. MPDL3280A (anti-PD-L1) treatment leads to clinical activity in metastatic bladder cancer. Nature. 2014;515(7528):558–62.
33. Agarwal N, Bellmunt J, Maughan BL, et al. Six-month progression-free survival as the primary endpoint to evaluate the activity of new agents as second-line therapy for advanced urothelial carcinoma. Clin Genitourin Cancer. 2014;12(2):130–7.
34. Yadav M, Jhunjhunwala S, Phung QT, et al. Predicting immunogenic tumour mutations by combining mass spectrometry and exome sequencing. Nature. 2014;515(7528):572–6.

Targeted Therapies and Immunotherapy in Bladder Cancer

6

Mehmet Ali Nahit Şendur and Sercan Aksoy

Abstract

Cisplatin-based combination chemotherapy is still the standard first-line regimen for the treatment of metastatic urothelial carcinoma. Although the efficacy of targeted therapies was shown in most of the solid tumors, no targeted agent was approved until now in bladder cancer. Due to the preliminary phase II results of gemcitabine, cisplatin plus bevacizumab demonstrated promising objective response rate, overall survival, and progression-free survival in the first-line treatment of metastatic bladder cancer; a phase III is ongoing. The major advances in understanding the genetic background of urothelial tumors open up a new therapeutic area. Although the application of checkpoint inhibitors in bladder cancer is in its starting phase, the available results suggest that patients with metastatic disease and positive programmed death-ligand-1 (PD-L1) expression will derive the highest clinical benefit. Atezolizumab, an anti-PD-L1 monoclonal antibody, was approved by the Food and Drug Administration for the treatment of patients with locally advanced or metastatic urothelial carcinoma whose disease progressed after previous platinum-based chemotherapy. Both pembrolizumab and nivolumab, anti-PD-1 monoclonal antibodies, demonstrated antitumor activity with tolerable safety in patients with recurrent or metastatic urothelial cancer patients. Combination therapies to treat bladder cancer, involving cytotoxic chemotherapy, antiangiogenic agents, and immune checkpoint inhibitors, are currently ongoing.

M.A.N. Şendur, M.D.
Department of Medical Oncology, Ankara Yıldırım Beyazıt University, Ankara, Turkey

S. Aksoy, M.D. (✉)
Department of Medical Oncology, Hacettepe University Cancer Institute, Ankara, Turkey
e-mail: saksoy07@yahoo.com

G. Ozyigit, U. Selek (eds.), *Principles and Practice of Urooncology*,
DOI 10.1007/978-3-319-56114-1_6

6.1 Introduction

An estimated 76,960 new cases (58,950 men, 18,010 women) of urinary bladder will be diagnosed in the United States in 2016. Bladder cancer is the fourth most common diagnosed cancer in men and is more than three times prevalent than women [1]. Transitional cell carcinoma is the most predominant histologic type, and it accounts for 90% of all bladder cancers. Although most of the patients present with noninvasive bladder cancer, approximately 25% of the patients develop distant metastases either at the time of diagnosis or later [2].

Systemic chemotherapy is the cornerstone of treatment for unresectable or metastatic urothelial carcinomas. The first-line standard of care in metastatic bladder cancer is platinum-based combination chemotherapy. Gemcitabine plus cisplatin (GC) combination or methotrexate, vinblastine, adriamycin, and cisplatin (MVAC) regimens are standard regimens in unresectable or metastatic urothelial carcinomas, if patients fit enough to tolerate cisplatin [2, 3]. MVAC is one of the standard first-line options based on the results of two randomized clinical trials [4, 5]. In a prospective randomized trial, 110 patients with metastatic urothelial tumor were randomly assigned to MVAC or cisplatin, cyclophosphamide, plus adriamycin combination chemotherapy regimens [4]. In this study, the objective response rate (ORR) (65 vs 46%; $P < 0.05$) and overall survival (OS) (median, 48.3 weeks vs 36.1 weeks) were significantly higher in patients treated with MVAC regimen. In another randomized trial of 269 patients with advanced urothelial carcinoma who were randomly assigned to treatment with either MVAC or single-agent cisplatin, MVAC regimen is associated with significantly higher ORR (39 vs 12%; $P < 0.0001$), higher median progression-free survival (PFS) (10.0 vs 4.3 months), and higher median OS (12.5 vs 8.2 months; $P = 0.0002$) compared to the single-agent cisplatin arm [5]. In MVAC regimen, grade 3 or 4 leukopenia, mucositis, granulocytopenic fever, and drug-related mortality were more common compared to cisplatin single-agent arm.

In a randomized phase III trial in which 405 patients were randomly assigned to either GC or MVAC, similar ORR (GC, 49%; MVAC, 46%), similar PFS (7.7 months in GC and 8.3 months in MVAC), and similar OS (14.0 months in GC, 15.2 months in MVAC, HR, 1.09; 95% confidence interval (CI), 0.88 to 1.34, $P = 0.66$) results were reported [2, 6]. In MVAC group, compared to GC group, patients had more grade 3/4 neutropenia (82 vs 71%), neutropenic fever (14 vs 2%), neutropenic sepsis (12 vs 1%), mucositis (22 vs 1%), and alopecia (55 vs 11%). Until now, no significant OS benefit was achieved with triplet regimens or sequential combination regimens in the first-line treatment of patients with metastatic urothelial carcinoma [7, 8]. Due to high tolerability and less toxicity compared to MVAC, these results strengthen the role of GC as a standard first-line regimen in patients with locally advanced and metastatic bladder cancer.

Cisplatin-based combinations are the standard first-line regimens, but carboplatin-based chemotherapy is frequently substituted due to ineligible for cisplatin or to improve tolerability. Although direct comparative effectiveness of cisplatin and carboplatin is lacking in randomized trials, a total of 286 patients with metastatic urothelial carcinoma from four randomized trials were analyzed in a meta-analysis [9]. Although PFS and OS results were inadequate to compare cisplatin- and carboplatin-based regimens, cisplatin-based chemotherapy was significantly associated with higher rates of complete response (RR = 3.54; 95% CI 1.48–8.49; $P = 0.005$) and ORR (RR = 1.34; 95% CI 1.04–1.71; $P = 0.02$). Thus cisplatin-based combinations are associated with higher response rates.

In the randomized phase II/III EORTC 30986 trial, 238 chemotherapy-naïve patients unfit for cisplatin-based chemotherapy (glomerular filtration rate <60 but >30 mL/min) and/or a poor performance status (ECOG ≥2) were randomly assigned to treatment with carboplatin and gemcitabine or methotrexate, carboplatin, and vinblastine regimens [10]. There were no significant differences in OS (9.3 vs 8.1 months, respectively, $P = 0.64$), PFS (6 vs 4 months, respectively), and ORR (41 vs 30%, respectively) between the two treatment groups, but the incidence of severe acute toxicities was higher for patients treated with methotrexate, carboplatin, and vinblastine regimen. Thus gemcitabine plus carboplatin can be the first-line standard regimen for patients with advanced urothelial carcinoma unfit for cisplatin-based chemotherapy.

A number of chemotherapy drugs have single-agent activity in patients with metastatic urothelial carcinoma in previously treated patients such as platinum compounds, gemcitabine, vinblastine, doxorubicin, epirubicin, methotrexate, paclitaxel, docetaxel, and ifosfamide mostly dependent phase II trials [11]. Unfortunately, responses to single-agent chemotherapy are generally of short duration with no consistent improvement in survival. Vinflunine, a novel third-generation microtubule-inhibitor vinca alkaloid, is the only drug that tested in a valid randomized phase III trial in patients progressing after first-line treatment with platinum-containing combination chemotherapy [12, 13]. In this study, a total of 370 patients with advanced transitional cell carcinoma of urothelial tract who progressed after first-line platinum-containing regimen were randomly assigned to vinflunine plus best supportive care or best supportive care. Overall response rate, disease control, and PFS were all statistically significant favoring vinflunine plus best supportive care ($P = 0.006$, $P = 0.002$, and $P = 0.001$, respectively). Although, in the intent-to-treat population, no significant OS difference (6.9 vs 4.6 months, $P = 0.287$) was achieved, after adjusting for prognostic factors (HR = 0.77; 95% CI, 0.61–0.98, $P = 0.036$) and in the eligible population ($n = 357$), the median OS was significantly longer in vinflunine plus best supportive care than best supportive care group alone (6.9 vs 4.3 months, respectively, $P = 0.040$). This trial reached the highest level of evidence ever reported for second-line treatment. In Europe, vinflunine is the only approved chemotherapy drug in this setting, but there is no standard accepted second-line regimen all over the world.

Despite ORR, PFS, and OS rates were improved with cisplatin-based combinations in patients with metastatic urothelial carcinoma, most of the patients progressed within 6–8 months, and median survival was not more than 15 months according to the previous randomized trials. The aim of this chapter is to review the results of new targeted therapies and immunotherapy in unresectable or metastatic bladder cancer.

6.2 Targeted Agents

Molecular analysis identified genetic and epigenetic alterations in high-grade urothelial carcinomas, and about 60% of these alterations can be targeted by drugs already approved for use in other indications or in clinical trials [14]. Previous studies showed the amplification of FGFR1, CCND1, and MDM2. Alterations in regulators of G1-S cell cycle progression, such as TP53 and RB, FGFR3 mutations and translocations, and PTEN deletions can also occur. In addition to recurrent mutations in the receptor tyrosine kinases, RAS/RAF, PI3K, AKT, and mammalian target of rapamycin (mTOR) pathways were identified [15, 16]. The RAS signaling pathway appears to have a major role in the development of low-grade, noninvasive lesions; 30–40% are characterized by activating mutations in the HRAS gene. Molecular analyses identified kinase-activating fibroblast growth factor receptors-3 (FGFR3) gene fusions in up to 70% of urothelial cancers, an upstream tyrosine kinase receptor involved in cellular proliferation and angiogenesis [17].

In the Cancer Genome Atlas project, an integrated analysis of 131 urothelial carcinomas was investigated to provide a comprehensive landscape of molecular alterations [14]. In this comprehensive analysis, potential therapeutic targets were identified in 69% of the tumors, 42% of urothelial carcinomas had genomic alterations targets phosphatidylinositol-3-OH kinase/AKT/mTOR pathway, and 45% had genomic alterations targets including ERBB2 RTK/MAPK pathway.

Although FGFR3 mutations are associated with cellular proliferation, differentiation, migration, and angiogenesis, FGFR mutations are a common feature of low-grade noninvasive papillary urothelial bladder cancer; it rarely occurs in high-grade invasive bladder cancer. FGFR3 mutations are a common feature in noninvasive urothelial bladder cancer and occur at a lower frequency (12–15%) in high-grade metastatic urothelial carcinomas [14]. In contrary to FGFR3 mutations, FGFR1 overexpression was observed in all stages of bladder carcinomas [18]. Tyrosine kinase inhibitors, monoclonal anti-FGFR antibodies, and FGF-trapping molecules that targeted FGFR are currently under development. In a phase II trial in patients with progressive advanced urothelial carcinoma, dovitinib, a FGFR3 included broad tyrosine kinase inhibitor, had very limited activity in both FGFR3-mutated and FGFR3 wild-type groups [19]. Phase I and II trials of BGJ398, a pan-inhibitor of FGFR, are still currently ongoing.

In the Cancer Genome Atlas project, 42% of urothelial carcinomas had genomic alterations targets phosphatidylinositol-3-OH kinase/AKT/mTOR pathway [14]. This pathway is an essential pathway involved in cell growth, cell survival, and cell metabolism. The role of buparlisib (BKM120), an oral PI3K inhibitor, is currently investigated in a phase II clinical trial in the second-line setting for patients with metastatic urothelial carcinoma. In a phase II study, 37 patients with advanced urothelial carcinoma who progressed after platinum-based therapy were treated with everolimus, an mTOR inhibitor, 10 mg/day until progressive disease or unacceptable toxicity [20]. The primary endpoint disease control rate was 27% at 8 weeks. In a whole-genome sequencing analysis of 109 patients with metastatic bladder cancer treated with everolimus, tuberous sclerosis complex 1 (TSC1) mutations was found in 8% of tumors and correlated with everolimus sensitivity [21].

The human epidermal growth factor receptor-2 (HER2) status is important for the management of early and metastatic breast cancer and for the metastatic gastric cancer, for both prognosis and prediction of the response to targeted therapies [22, 23]. Approximately 15–25% of all breast cancers and 20% of all metastatic gastric cancers are HER2 positive and display gene amplification or HER2 overexpression [23–26]. Accurate determination of HER2 status may be of prognostic and predictive value for the targeted therapies. In invasive urothelial bladder carcinomas, the true incidence of HER2 overexpression and/or amplification remains uncertain ranging from 23 to 80% for overexpression and from 0 to 32% for amplification [27]. Lae and colleagues investigated 1005 primary invasive urothelial bladder carcinomas for HER2 evaluation and reported that HER2 overexpression was found in 9.2% of tumor samples and 5.1% of invasive bladder carcinomas had a HER2 gene amplification by FISH confirmation [27]. HER2-positive patients with metastatic urothelial carcinomas had more metastatic sites and visceral metastasis than did HER2-negative patients [28, 29]. Several clinical trials are currently ongoing to identify potential candidates for targeted therapy in locally advanced or metastatic bladder cancer patients with HER2 overexpression. A single-arm phase II study evaluating trastuzumab in combination with paclitaxel, gemcitabine, and carboplatin in 44 patients with HER2-positive urothelial carcinoma showed a 70%, 9.3, and 14.1 months response rate, median time to progression, and survival, respectively [28]. In another phase II trial, patients with advanced or metastatic urothelial carcinoma overexpressing HER2 were randomly assigned to gemcitabine + platinum combination with or without trastuzumab [30]. In this trial, among 563 screened patients, 75 (13.3%) were HER2 positive (IHC 2+/3+ and FISH+). In both arms, no significant difference was found in terms of PFS, ORR, and OS. In a single-arm, prospective phase II study, 59 patients with locally advanced or metastatic transitional cell carcinoma were treated with second-line lapatinib, an EGFR and a HER2 inhibitor, and the primary endpoint ORR >10% was observed only in one (1.7%) patient [31]. The median OS was significantly prolonged in patients with tumors that overexpressed EGFR and/or HER2 ($P = 0.0001$). In a phase II/III, double-blind, randomized trial, 348 patients with HER1-/HER2-positive metastatic bladder cancer were randomly assigned to maintenance lapatinib versus placebo after first-line chemotherapy, and it shows that lapatinib maintenance did not improve the primary outcome PFS (4.6 months in lapatinib arm, 5.3 months in placebo, HR: 1.04, $P = 0.77$) [32]. Similarly, OS and ORR did not significantly differ with maintenance lapatinib in HER1-/HER2-positive metastatic bladder cancer. Despite promising therapeutic targets, EGFR inhibitors have not reached their goal in the clinic with disappointing activity in the treatment of urothelial carcinoma. Although previous trials targeting HER2 were inconclusive in metastatic urothelial carcinoma, new agents targeting HER2 may be more effective. Trastuzumab emtansine (T-DM1) has promising antitumor effects in preclinical models of HER2-positive bladder cancer models [33].

In a phase II randomized trial to determine the efficacy of EGFR inhibition in urothelial cancers, 39 patients with chemotherapy-refractory metastatic urothelial cancer who have progressed after one previous treatment were randomly assigned to cetuximab with and without paclitaxel [34]. Although the single-agent cetuximab arm closed early due to 82% of first 11 patients progressed by 8 weeks, the combination arm showed 25% ORR with median 10.5 months OS. Cetuximab plus paclitaxel combination showed promising activity in the second-line treatment of patients with metastatic urothelial carcinoma.

Several antiangiogenic drugs have been approved in a different tumor types, but most of the majority of such agents failed to demonstrate clinical activity in advanced-stage urothelial carcinoma, either in monotherapy or in combination with cytotoxic chemotherapy [35, 36]. In a single-arm phase II study, chemotherapy-naïve patients with metastatic or unresectable urothelial carcinoma were treated with gemcitabine, cisplatin, plus bevacizumab combination as first line [37]. A total 43 patients were treated with combination, and the ORR was 72%, PFS was 8.2 months, and OS was 19.1 months. Due to gemcitabine, cisplatin plus bevacizumab demonstrated promising OS and PFS; a phase III is ongoing.

6.3 Immunotherapy

Based on the immunogenic properties of some solid tumors, immunotherapy was launched as one of the treatment modalities in cancer therapy many decades ago. Bladder cancer is a highly immunogenic cancer type due to high mutational load which is associated with triggering the immune response as tumor antigens. Intravesical bacillus Calmette-Guérin (BCG) is the first Food and Drug Administration (FDA)-approved immunotherapy that significantly reduced the risk of recurrence in patients with noninvasive urothelial bladder cancer by stimulating immune response and thus is a standard treatment for non-muscle invasive bladder cancer [38, 39]. A systematic literature review of 13 randomized controlled trials (RCTs) with 2548 patients examined the role of receiving intravesical chemotherapy immediately in patients with non-muscle invasive bladder cancer [40]. In this systematic review, recurrence-free interval prolonged by 38% (HR: 0.62; 95% CI, 0.50–0.77; $p < 0.001$), and early recurrences were 12% less compared to control group population.

Immune system is well balanced between co-activator and co-inhibitor signals. Immune checkpoints are very important step for regulating host immune system by blocking immune response, preventing normal tissue damage, and autoimmunity. Programmed cell death protein 1 (PD-1), programmed cell death protein ligand 1 (PD-L1), and cytotoxic T-lymphocyte-associated protein 4 (CTLA-4) are the main components of immune checkpoints [41]. Checkpoint inhibitors that targeted to CTLA-4 and PD-1 have been studied more extensively in solid tumors and demonstrated significant response with these agents.

Cancer cell, which have abnormal antigen expression due to many genetics and epigenetic abnormalities, can be detected and eradicated by host immune system.

T cells are chief elements of the host immunity. Immune response is initiated by the recognition of tumor-specific antigen presented by the major histocompatibility complex (MHC) on the surface of antigen-presenting cells (dendritic cells, macrophage, etc.). After interaction between MHC and T-cell receptor (TCR), several co-stimulators are secreted for enhancing to immune response. Consequently, innate and adaptive immune systems are activated, and active immune systems detect and eradicate cancer cells before tumors become clinically apparent, also called immune surveillance. However, immune system is tightly regulated by co-stimulatory and inhibitory molecules; therefore, balance between stimulatory and inhibitory molecules are crucial to maintain immune response. In the physiologic condition, co-inhibitor molecules can avoid excessive immune response and, consequently, prevent normal tissue damaged and autoimmunity.

PD-1, PD-L1, and CTLA-4 receptors located on the surface of the T-cell lymphocytes are demonstrated as a clinical target. PD-1 inhibits T-cell activation by interaction with PD-L1 (B7-H1) and PD-L2 (B7-DC) receptor expressed by tumor, stroma, and immune cells [42]. PD-1 is mainly expressed on activated T cell (CD4+–CD8+) and also natural killer and B cells and tumor-infiltrating lymphocytes (TILs) [43]. PD-L2 is also upregulated in dendritic cells, macrophage, and lymphoid tissue with response to microenvironmental stimuli [44]. Unlike PD-L1, PD-L2 is not usually overexpressed on the surface of tumor cells. Therefore, data about relationship with PD-L2 receptor overexpression and immune response was not known exactly yet.

In 2012, for the first time, the safety and activity of anti-PD-1 nivolumab was investigated in phase I trial, and it was reported that objective responses were seen in patients with advanced malignant melanoma or renal cell cancer or non-small cell lung cancer (NSCLC) [45]. In recent years, the significant activity of nivolumab was shown in different lines of patients with advanced malignant melanoma, renal cell cancer, and NSCLC, and the significant activity of pembrolizumab was shown in different lines of patients with advanced malignant melanoma and NSCLC according to the randomized phase III trials [46–51]. After the efficacy and marked improvement of the treatment response with anti-PD-1 inhibitors were shown in advanced malignant melanoma, NSCLC, and renal cell carcinoma, many trials are still ongoing in patients with other type of cancers. Recently, bladder cancers are also one of the fields where data evolve about the use of immune checkpoint inhibitors.

The role of PD-L1 was evaluated as a mechanism for local stage progression in urothelial carcinoma (UC) of the bladder. PD-L1 expression is associated with high-grade tumors and with advanced stage. In an immunohistochemical evaluation of high-grade urothelial carcinomas, PD-L1 expression was observed in 7% of pTa, 16% of pT1, 23% of pT2, 30% of pT3/pT4, and 45% of carcinoma in situ (CIS) tumors [52]. In a pooled analysis of 61 studies in the literature, PD-L1 expression was reported in 44.9% of urothelial carcinomas [53].

Recent advances showed that anti-PD-1 and anti-PD-L1 agents as named checkpoint inhibitors have demonstrated promising activity in bladder cancer [54, 55]. Atezolizumab (MPDL3280A) is a IgG1 monoclonal anti-PD-L1 antibody designed to interfere with the binding of PD-L1 ligand to its two receptors, PD-1 and B7.1, thus restoring anticancer T-cell activity. In a single-arm, two-cohort, phase II, Imvigor210 trial, patients with inoperable locally advanced or metastatic urothelial carcinoma whose disease had progressed after previous platinum-based chemotherapy received treatment with intravenous atezolizumab (1200 mg, every 3 weeks) [56]. PD-L1 expression on tumor-infiltrating immune cells was assessed prospectively by immunohistochemistry: IC0 (<1%), IC1 (≥1% but <5%), and IC2/IC3 (≥5%). Compared to historical cohort, ORR of 10%, treatment with atezolizumab resulted in a significantly improved primary endpoint ORR for each defined immune cell group (IC2/IC3, 26%; $P < 0.0001$; IC1/IC2/IC3, 18%, $P = 0.0004$) and overall in 310 patients (15%, $P = 0.0058$). The median PFS was 2.1 months in all patients and was similar in all immune cell groups. The median OS was 11.4 months in patients in the IC2/IC3 group, whereas it was 8.8 months in the IC1/IC2/IC3 group and 7.9 months in all immune cell groups. Atezolizumab showed good tolerability, no treatment-related deaths occurred during the study, and most treatment-related adverse events were mild to moderate in nature. Grade 3–4 adverse events occurred in 50 (16%) of 310 treated patients, and fatigue (2%) is the most common. These data moved atezolizumab for approval by the US Food and Drug Administration (FDA) in May 2016 in the treatment of patients with locally advanced or metastatic urothelial carcinoma whose disease has worsened during or following platinum-containing chemotherapy or within 12 months of receiving platinum-containing chemotherapy, either before (neoadjuvant) or after (adjuvant) surgical treatment.

In a recent single-arm, phase II study, previously untreated 123 patients with locally advanced or metastatic urothelial cancer who were cisplatin ineligible were treated with atezolizumab 1200 mg every 3 weeks [57]. The primary endpoint ORR was 23%; the complete response rate was 9% ($n = 11$). Median PFS was 2.7 months in all patients and 4.1 months in IC2/IC3 patients. Median overall survival was 15.9 months with a 17.2 months follow-up. In conclusion, atezolizumab showed promising activity in untreated metastatic urothelial cancer who were cisplatin ineligible with good safety profile.

In the phase Ib KEYNOTE-012 study, patients with recurrent, metastatic, or persistent urothelial cancer of the bladder, renal pelvis, ureter, or urethra were treated with pembrolizumab, an anti-PD-1 antibody [58]. Median follow-up was 13 months; ORR was 25%. Patients with ≥1% PD-L1 staining on tumor cells had a 33% ORR, whereas only 9% in <1% PD-L1 staining patients treated with pembrolizumab. PFS at 12 months was 19%, and median duration of response had not been achieved at the interim analysis. In phase I/II, CHECKMATE-032, open-label study, patients with urothelial carcinoma of the renal pelvis, ureter, bladder, or urethra whose disease progressed after previous platinum-based chemotherapy were treated with nivolumab, an anti-PD1 monoclonal antibody, 3 mg/kg intravenously every 2 weeks [59]. A total of 86 patients were enrolled, and ORR was 24.4% of 78 patients treated with nivolumab, and ORR did not demonstrate significant difference in ORR (24.0 vs 26.2%) according to the PD-L1(+) and PD-L1(−) patients with metastatic urothelial cancer, respectively. Median overall survival was 9.7 months with 46% 1-year OS rate. Median overall survival was 16.2 months in patients with

PD-L1 ≥ 1%, whereas 9.9 months in patients with PD-L1 < 1%. Median PFS was 5.5 months in patients with PD-L1 ≥ 1% and 2.8 months in patients with PD-L1 < 1%. Grade 3–4 treatment-related adverse events occurred 22% of patients. Both pembrolizumab and nivolumab demonstrated antitumor activity with tolerable safety in patients with recurrent or metastatic urothelial cancer patients.

Intravesical BCG immunotherapy is still the gold standard treatment of non-muscle invasive bladder cancer more than three decades. An alternative regulatory pathway that limits immune response in diseases including cancer has been recently elucidated. Immune checkpoint inhibitors have been found to play a major role in maintaining peripheral T-cell tolerance. In limited clinical trials, PD-1/PD-L1 blockade has shown promise as salvage therapy for metastatic chemotherapy-refractory urothelial carcinoma. Atezolizumab, an anti-PD-L1 monoclonal antibody, was approved by FDA for the treatment of patients with locally advanced or metastatic urothelial carcinoma whose disease progressed after previous platinum-based chemotherapy. Understanding of PD-1 and PD-L1 as checkpoints in metastatic disease suggests that its blockade may be useful in the treatment of patients with earlier-stage disease. Phase III trials of atezolizumab, nivolumab, and pembrolizumab are still ongoing in both early and advanced stages.

Conclusion

Gemcitabine plus cisplatin is still a standard first-line regimen in patients with locally advanced and metastatic bladder cancer. A promising new immunotherapeutic agent has arrived in the form of checkpoint inhibition.

References

1. Siegel RL, Miller KD, Jemal A. Cancer statistics, 2016. CA Cancer J Clin. 2016;66(1):7–30.
2. von der Maase H, Hansen SW, Roberts JT, et al. Gemcitabine and cisplatin versus methotrexate, vinblastine, doxorubicin, and cisplatin in advanced or metastatic bladder cancer: results of a large, randomized, multinational, multicenter, phase III study. J Clin Oncol. 2000;18(17):3068–77.
3. von der Maase H, Sengelov L, Roberts JT, et al. Long-term survival results of a randomized trial comparing gemcitabine plus cisplatin, with methotrexate, vinblastine, doxorubicin, plus cisplatin in patients with bladder cancer. J Clin Oncol. 2005;23(21):4602–8.
4. Logothetis CJ, Dexeus FH, Finn L, et al. A prospective randomized trial comparing MVAC and CISCA chemotherapy for patients with metastatic urothelial tumors. J Clin Oncol. 1990;8(6):1050–5.
5. Loehrer PJ Sr, Einhorn LH, Elson PJ, et al. A randomized comparison of cisplatin alone or in combination with methotrexate, vinblastine, and doxorubicin in patients with metastatic urothelial carcinoma: a cooperative group study. J Clin Oncol. 1992;10(7):1066–73.
6. Roberts JT, von der Maase H, Sengelov L, et al. Long-term survival results of a randomized trial comparing gemcitabine/cisplatin and methotrexate/vinblastine/doxorubicin/cisplatin in patients with locally advanced and metastatic bladder cancer. Ann Oncol. 2006;17(Suppl 5):v118–22.
7. Bellmunt J, von der Maase H, Mead GM, et al. Randomized phase III study comparing paclitaxel/cisplatin/gemcitabine and gemcitabine/cisplatin in patients with locally advanced or metastatic urothelial cancer without prior systemic therapy: EORTC intergroup study 30987. J Clin Oncol. 2012;30(10):1107–13.

8. Milowsky MI, Nanus DM, Maluf FC, et al. Final results of sequential doxorubicin plus gemcitabine and ifosfamide, paclitaxel, and cisplatin chemotherapy in patients with metastatic or locally advanced transitional cell carcinoma of the urothelium. J Clin Oncol. 2009;27(25):4062–7.
9. Galsky MD, Chen GJ, Oh WK, et al. Comparative effectiveness of cisplatin-based and carboplatin-based chemotherapy for treatment of advanced urothelial carcinoma. Ann Oncol. 2012;23(2):406–10.
10. De Santis M, Bellmunt J, Mead G, et al. Randomized phase II/III trial assessing gemcitabine/carboplatin and methotrexate/carboplatin/vinblastine in patients with advanced urothelial cancer who are unfit for cisplatin-based chemotherapy: EORTC study 30986. J Clin Oncol. 2012;30(2):191–9.
11. Bellmunt J, Orsola A, Leow JJ, et al. Bladder cancer: ESMO practice guidelines for diagnosis, treatment and follow-up. Ann Oncol. 2014;25(Suppl 3):iii40–8.
12. Bellmunt J, Fougeray R, Rosenberg JE, et al. Long-term survival results of a randomized phase III trial of vinflunine plus best supportive care versus best supportive care alone in advanced urothelial carcinoma patients after failure of platinum-based chemotherapy. Ann Oncol. 2013;24(6):1466–72.
13. Bellmunt J, Theodore C, Demkov T, et al. Phase III trial of vinflunine plus best supportive care compared with best supportive care alone after a platinum-containing regimen in patients with advanced transitional cell carcinoma of the urothelial tract. J Clin Oncol. 2009;27(27):4454–61.
14. Cancer Genome Atlas Research Network. Comprehensive molecular characterization of urothelial bladder carcinoma. Nature. 2014;507(7492):315–22.
15. Forbes SA, Bindal N, Bamford S, et al. COSMIC: mining complete cancer genomes in the catalogue of somatic mutations in cancer. Nucleic Acids Res. 2011;39(Database issue):D945–50.
16. Goebell PJ, Knowles MA. Bladder cancer or bladder cancers? Genetically distinct malignant conditions of the urothelium. Urol Oncol. 2010;28(4):409–28.
17. Hurst CD, Platt FM, Taylor CF, et al. Novel tumor subgroups of urothelial carcinoma of the bladder defined by integrated genomic analysis. Clin Cancer Res. 2012;18(21):5865–77.
18. Tomlinson DC, Lamont FR, Shnyder SD, et al. Fibroblast growth factor receptor 1 promotes proliferation and survival via activation of the mitogen-activated protein kinase pathway in bladder cancer. Cancer Res. 2009;69(11):4613–20.
19. Milowsky MI, Dittrich C, Duran I, et al. Phase 2 trial of dovitinib in patients with progressive FGFR3-mutated or FGFR3 wild-type advanced urothelial carcinoma. Eur J Cancer. 2014;50(18):3145–52.
20. Seront E, Rottey S, Sautois B, et al. Phase II study of everolimus in patients with locally advanced or metastatic transitional cell carcinoma of the urothelial tract: clinical activity, molecular response, and biomarkers. Ann Oncol. 2012;23(10):2663–70.
21. Iyer G, Hanrahan AJ, Milowsky MI, et al. Genome sequencing identifies a basis for everolimus sensitivity. Science. 2012;338(6104):221.
22. Slamon DJ, Leyland-Jones B, Shak S, et al. Use of chemotherapy plus a monoclonal antibody against HER2 for metastatic breast cancer that overexpresses HER2. N Engl J Med. 2001;344(11):783–92.
23. Bang YJ, Van Cutsem E, Feyereislova A, et al. Trastuzumab in combination with chemotherapy versus chemotherapy alone for treatment of HER2-positive advanced gastric or gastro-oesophageal junction cancer (ToGA): a phase 3, open-label, randomised controlled trial. Lancet. 2010;376(9742):687–97.
24. Slamon DJ, Clark GM, Wong SG, et al. Human breast cancer: correlation of relapse and survival with amplification of the HER-2/neu oncogene. Science. 1987;235(4785):177–82.
25. Wolff AC, Hammond ME, Schwartz JN, et al. American Society of Clinical Oncology/College of American Pathologists guideline recommendations for human epidermal growth factor receptor 2 testing in breast cancer. Arch Pathol Lab Med. 2007;131(1):18–43.
26. Dawood S, Broglio K, Buzdar AU, et al. Prognosis of women with metastatic breast cancer by HER2 status and trastuzumab treatment: an institutional-based review. J Clin Oncol. 2010;28(1):92–8.

27. Lae M, Couturier J, Oudard S, et al. Assessing HER2 gene amplification as a potential target for therapy in invasive urothelial bladder cancer with a standardized methodology: results in 1005 patients. Ann Oncol. 2010;21(4):815–9.
28. Hussain MH, MacVicar GR, Petrylak DP, et al. Trastuzumab, paclitaxel, carboplatin, and gemcitabine in advanced human epidermal growth factor receptor-2/neu-positive urothelial carcinoma: results of a multicenter phase II National Cancer Institute trial. J Clin Oncol. 2007;25(16):2218–24.
29. Lonn U, Lonn S, Friberg S, et al. Prognostic value of amplification of c-erb-B2 in bladder carcinoma. Clin Cancer Res. 1995;1(10):1189–94.
30. Oudard S, Culine S, Vano Y, et al. Multicentre randomised phase II trial of gemcitabine+platinum, with or without trastuzumab, in advanced or metastatic urothelial carcinoma overexpressing Her2. Eur J Cancer. 2015;51(1):45–54.
31. Wulfing C, Machiels JP, Richel DJ, et al. A single-arm, multicenter, open-label phase 2 study of lapatinib as the second-line treatment of patients with locally advanced or metastatic transitional cell carcinoma. Cancer. 2009;115(13):2881–90.
32. Powles T, Huddart RA, Elliott T, et al. A phase II/III, double-blind, randomized trial comparing maintenance lapatinib versus placebo after first line chemotherapy in HER1/2 positive metastatic bladder cancer patients. J Clin Oncol. 2015;33(suppl):abstr 4505.
33. Hayashi T, Seiler R, Oo HZ, et al. Targeting HER2 with T-DM1, an antibody cytotoxic drug conjugate, is effective in HER2 over expressing bladder cancer. J Urol. 2015;194(4): 1120–31.
34. Wong YN, Litwin S, Vaughn D, et al. Phase II trial of cetuximab with or without paclitaxel in patients with advanced urothelial tract carcinoma. J Clin Oncol. 2012;30(28):3545–51.
35. Garcia J, Santome L, Anido U, et al. Metastatic bladder cancer: second-line treatment and recommendations of the genitourinary tumor division of the Galician oncologic society (SOG-GU). Curr Oncol Rep. 2016;18(12):72.
36. Rose TL, Milowsky MI. Improving systemic chemotherapy for bladder cancer. Curr Oncol Rep. 2016;18(5):27.
37. Hahn NM, Stadler WM, Zon RT, et al. Phase II trial of cisplatin, gemcitabine, and bevacizumab as first-line therapy for metastatic urothelial carcinoma: Hoosier Oncology group GU 04-75. J Clin Oncol. 2011;29(12):1525–30.
38. Redelman-Sidi G, Glickman MS, Bochner BH. The mechanism of action of BCG therapy for bladder cancer—a current perspective. Nat Rev Urol. 2014;11(3):153–62.
39. Gandhi NM, Morales A, Lamm DL. Bacillus Calmette-Guerin immunotherapy for genitourinary cancer. BJU Int. 2013;112(3):288–97.
40. Perlis N, Zlotta AR, Beyene J, et al. Immediate post-transurethral resection of bladder tumor intravesical chemotherapy prevents non-muscle-invasive bladder cancer recurrences: an updated meta-analysis on 2548 patients and quality-of-evidence review. Eur Urol. 2013;64(3):421–30.
41. Bilgin B, Sendur MA, Akinci MB, et al. Targeting the PD-1 pathway: a new hope for gastrointestinal cancers. Curr Med Res Opin. 2017;33(4):749–59.
42. Wang J, Reiss KA, Khatri R, et al. Immune therapy in GI malignancies: a review. J Clin Oncol. 2015;33(16):1745–53.
43. Jacobs J, Smits E, Lardon F, et al. Immune checkpoint modulation in colorectal cancer: What's new and what to expect. J Immunol Res. 2015;2015:158038.
44. Reiss KA, Forde PM, Brahmer JR. Harnessing the power of the immune system via blockade of PD-1 and PD-L1: a promising new anticancer strategy. Immunotherapy. 2014;6(4):459–75.
45. Topalian SL, Hodi FS, Brahmer JR, et al. Safety, activity, and immune correlates of anti-PD-1 antibody in cancer. N Engl J Med. 2012;366(26):2443–54.
46. Robert C, Schachter J, Long GV, et al. Pembrolizumab versus Ipilimumab in Advanced Melanoma. N Engl J Med. 2015;372(26):2521–32.
47. Herbst RS, Baas P, Kim DW, et al. Pembrolizumab versus docetaxel for previously treated, PD-L1-positive, advanced non-small-cell lung cancer (KEYNOTE-010): a randomised controlled trial. Lancet. 2016;387(10027):1540–50.

48. Motzer RJ, Escudier B, McDermott DF, et al. Nivolumab versus Everolimus in Advanced Renal-Cell Carcinoma. N Engl J Med. 2015;373(19):1803–13.
49. Robert C, Long GV, Brady B, et al. Nivolumab in previously untreated melanoma without BRAF mutation. N Engl J Med. 2015;372(4):320–30.
50. Brahmer J, Reckamp KL, Baas P, et al. Nivolumab versus Docetaxel in Advanced Squamous-Cell Non-Small-Cell Lung Cancer. N Engl J Med. 2015;373(2):123–35.
51. Borghaei H, Paz-Ares L, Horn L, et al. Nivolumab versus Docetaxel in Advanced Nonsquamous Non-Small-Cell Lung Cancer. N Engl J Med. 2015;373(17):1627–39.
52. Inman BA, Sebo TJ, Frigola X, et al. PD-L1 (B7-H1) expression by urothelial carcinoma of the bladder and BCG-induced granulomata: associations with localized stage progression. Cancer. 2007;109(8):1499–505.
53. Lin Z, Xu Y, Zhang Y, et al. The prevalence and clinicopathological features of programmed death-ligand 1 (PD-L1) expression: a pooled analysis of literatures. Oncotarget. 2016;7(12):15033–46.
54. Herbst RS, Soria JC, Kowanetz M, et al. Predictive correlates of response to the anti-PD-L1 antibody MPDL3280A in cancer patients. Nature. 2014;515(7528):563–7.
55. Powles T, Eder JP, Fine GD, et al. MPDL3280A (anti-PD-L1) treatment leads to clinical activity in metastatic bladder cancer. Nature. 2014;515(7528):558–62.
56. Rosenberg JE, Hoffman-Censits J, Powles T, et al. Atezolizumab in patients with locally advanced and metastatic urothelial carcinoma who have progressed following treatment with platinum-based chemotherapy: a single-arm, multicentre, phase 2 trial. Lancet. 2016;387(10031):1909–20.
57. Balar AV, Galsky MD, Rosenberg JE, et al. Atezolizumab as first-line treatment in cisplatin-ineligible patients with locally advanced and metastatic urothelial carcinoma: a single-arm, multicentre, phase 2 trial. Lancet. 2017;389(10064):67–76.
58. Plimack ER, Bellmunt J, Gupta S, et al. Pembrolizumab (MK-3475) for advanced urothelial cancer: updated results and biomarker analysis from KEYNOTE-012. J Clin Oncol. 2015;33(suppl):abstr 4502.
59. Sharma P, Callahan MK, Bono P, et al. Nivolumab monotherapy in recurrent metastatic urothelial carcinoma (CheckMate 032): a multicentre, open-label, two-stage, multi-arm, phase 1/2 trial. Lancet Oncol. 2016;17(11):1590–8.

Radiotherapy in the Management of Testicular Cancers

7

Berna Akkus Yildirim and Cem Onal

Abstract

Testicular cancers are the most common solid malignancies affecting males between the ages of 15 and 35 years, although it accounts for only about 1% of all cancers in men. Approximately 95% of testicular tumors are germ cell tumors (GCT). At diagnosis, 1–2% of cases are bilateral and 80% of patients are diagnosed at stage I. The risk factors for testicular cancers are family history, cryptorchidism, altered hormonal environment, low fertility, abnormal sperm analysis, and immunosuppression. For treatment purposes, two broad categories are recognized: pure seminoma (no non-seminomatous elements present) and all others, which together are termed non-seminomatous germ cell tumors (NSGCT). Seminoma is highly sensitive to chemotherapy and radiotherapy (RT). The prognosis of patients is generally good; cure is an expected outcome in the majority of cases, even with metastatic disease.

7.1 Clinical Presentation

The clinical presentation is mostly a unilateral testicular mass lump or painless swelling detected incidentally. Testicular pain is seen in approximately 10% of cases at presentation. Since most of the patients are diagnosed at early stages, symptoms related to metastatic disease are observed very rarely. Additionally, gynecomastia is a rare presentation for embryonal carcinoma.

B.A. Yildirim, M.D. (✉) • C. Onal, M.D.
Department of Radiation Oncology, Adana Dr Turgut Noyan Research and Treatment Center, Başkent University, Adana, Turkey
e-mail: bernaakkus@yahoo.com

G. Ozyigit, U. Selek (eds.), *Principles and Practice of Urooncology*,
DOI 10.1007/978-3-319-56114-1_7

7.2 Diagnostic Work-Up

Although pure seminomas do not have any specific serum tumor markers, certain cases can produce a small amount of β-hCG (beta-human chorionic gonadotropin) [7]. The β-hCG-secreting seminoma is a rare form of pure seminoma with an incidence of about 10–20% [8]. Although an increase in serum β-hCG primarily reflects higher tumor burden, it does not reflect the metastatic potential [9]. β-hCG and alpha fetoprotein (α-FP), one or both, can be elevated in 80–85% of patients with disseminated NSGCT. Placental alkaline phosphatase (PALP) is another marker that may be elevated in 50% of patients with seminoma at presentation. The sensitivity and specificity of PALP were 50 and 90%, respectively. Therefore, it has a very limited capacity for initial evaluation and follow-up of patients. The half-lives of β-hCG, α-FP, and PALP were 18–24 h, 5 days, and 24 h, respectively.

7.3 Lymphatic Drainage

A well knowledge of the pathways of lymphatic nodal spread is essential for the radiation oncologist in the planning of the radiation treatment of the retroperitoneal region. Approximately 4 to 8 lymphatic collecting trucks drain from the hilum of the testes and accompanying the spermatic cord up to the internal ring. These lymphatic trucks continue cephalad with vessels to drain into retroperitoneal lymph nodes between T11 and L4; mostly concentrated at the level of L1 to L3. The first echelon of lymph nodes draining the right testis is located in the inter-aortocaval region, followed by the precaval and pre-aortic nodes [7]. For left-sided tumors, the first nodal stations include the para-aortic lymph nodes, around the left renal hilus and to the inter-aortocaval nodes. Clinically, contralateral spread is common with right-sided tumors but is rarely seen with left-sided tumors and is usually associated with bulky disease [10].

7.4 Treatment for Seminoma

High inguinal orchiectomy that allows accurate staging and histological diagnosis of the tumor while ensuring the best local control is the standard initial treatment for suspected testicular carcinoma [11]. Organ-sparing orchiectomy is an alternative option for patients with bilateral testicular tumors, lesions in a solitary testis, or metachronous contralateral tumors. This approach allows endocrinological, fertility, and psychological advantages for the patient, especially in younger patient population [2]. The German Testicular Cancer Intergroup have reported prospective data on partial orchiectomy for 73 patients with a solitary testis or bilateral testicular tumors with organ-confined disease with no infiltration of the rete testis, tumor of <2 cm in diameter, a negative surgical margins [2]. After a median follow-up of 91 months, 98.6% of patients had no evidence of disease, and only one patient died of systemic tumor progression.

7.4.1 Stage I Seminoma

Clinical stage I seminoma patients have a substantial risk of locoregional lymph node micrometastases with a 20% risk of disease progression if no adjuvant therapy is administered after radical orchiectomy. A primary tumor size of 4 cm or more and invasion of the rete testis have been identified as independent prognostic factors for relapse [12–14]. Stage I pure seminoma has an excellent prognosis, with almost 100% optimal cure rates that can be achieved with one of three treatment options [12, 15]:

- Active surveillance with treatment only in the case of relapse
- Adjuvant RT
- Adjuvant single-agent carboplatin

Taking into consideration of concerns about long-term complications of RT and chemotherapy, as well as the patient's ability to comply with intensive surveillance, decisions regarding the management of stage I seminoma in any individual are thus complex (Fig. 7.1).

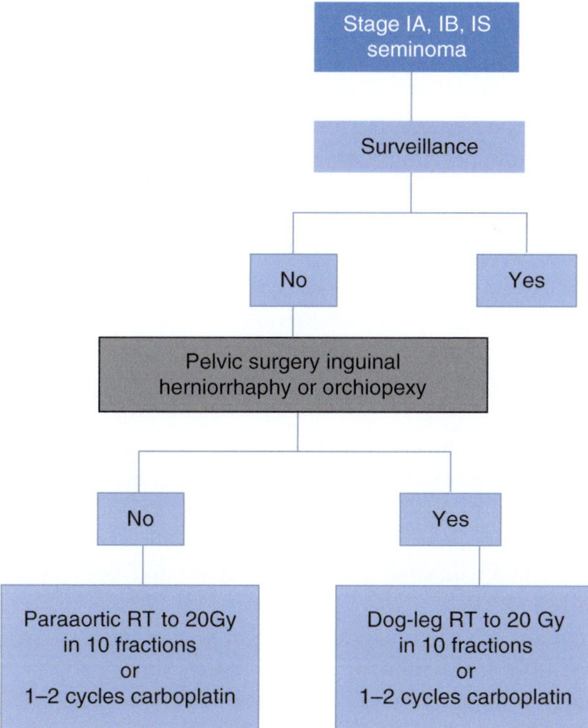

Fig. 7.1 Testicular seminoma treatment decision flow chart for clinical stage IA, IB, or IS disease

7.4.1.1 Active Surveillance

In current practice, together with the presence of highly effective RT and chemotherapy for salvage after relapse, post-orchiectomy surveillance is an alternative treatment approach [3, 16]. Surveillance policies offer the opportunity to detect relapsing patients early while avoiding the morbidities. Although no prospective studies compare surveillance alone versus adjuvant RT or chemotherapy, several large prospective nonrandomized studies of surveillance have been conducted over the past 15 years [12, 16–20]. Reports have demonstrated the feasibility of surveillance protocols, particularly when associated with effective salvage regimens. However, there are some practical difficulties in follow-up because of the lack of sensitivity of specific serum markers and accurate diagnostic tools [17–19]. Consensus guidelines and large groups accept surveillance as an option, which can be offered to stage I seminoma patients following orchiectomy [12, 21].

In British Columbia and Canada study, a total of 649 patients with clinical stage I (545 patients), stage II (87 patients), and stage III (17 patients) were analyzed [22]. For CSI, there was a progressive and marked decrease in the utilization of prophylactic radiation (RT) and increased use of active surveillance, from 10% in 1992 to 33% in 2002. A recent paper which analyzes retrospectively a total of 649 patients reports the evolution of treatment with an increased use of active surveillance for stage I disease (545 patients) without deaths related to seminoma [16].

According to numerous prospective nonrandomized studies, demonstrated relapse rate of stage I seminoma is 15–20% at 5 years, and usually of the relapses are first detected in infradiaphragmatic lymph nodes, and most patients are asymptomatic at the time of detection. Some studies suggested that tumor size (>4 cm) and rete testis invasion are predictive factors for relapse, but others demonstrated that these factors were not predictors of relapse. Retrospective studies on surveillance strategy analyze a total of 2483 patients with clinical stage I patients, 1139 CSI non-seminoma and 1344 CSI seminoma managed with active surveillance, and the majority treated between 1998 and 2010 [21, 22]. The cumulative relapse rate of 13% (173/1344) occurs during median 14 months (range 2–84) of follow-up.

The predominant site of relapse is in the para-aortic lymph nodes in the DATECA (Danish Testicular Carcinoma Study Group) and in the Princess Margaret Hospital retrospective studies; 41 of 49 relapses (82%) and 54 of 67 relapses (89%) occurred in the para-aortic lymph nodes, respectively, while other sites of relapse included the pelvic lymph nodes (approximately 3% overall) and, very rarely, the inguinal nodes and the lungs [18, 19].

Another advantage of active surveillance is the avoidance of secondary malignancy developed after irradiation of normal tissues during RT or chemotherapy, especially in men with early-stage seminoma who are expected to survive for decades following treatment [23–26]. Recently, Travis et al. [23] analyzed 40,576 1-year survivors of testicular cancer, with 2285 s solid cancers reported. The authors reported statistically significantly increased risks of solid cancers among patients treated with RT alone (RR = 2.0), chemotherapy alone (RR = 1.8), and both (RR = 2.9). For patients diagnosed with seminomas or non-seminomatous tumors at age 35 years, cumulative risks of solid cancer 40 years were 36 and 31%, respectively, compared with 23% for the general population. Data on the association of infradiaphragmatic RT with subsequent cardiovascular disease are conflicting [26–29].

Besides these advantages, the main drawback of surveillance is the need for intensive follow-up and repeated imaging for at least 5–10 years after radical orchiectomy. The main disadvantage of active surveillance is the absence of consensus regarding the optimum follow-up for these patients [13], which may potentially cause excessive imaging tests, radiation exposure during imaging, anxiety related to the risk of recurrence, and especially patient incompliance for follow-up [30, 31].

7.4.1.2 Radiation Therapy

Primary therapy for testicular seminoma involves radical inguinal orchiectomy. Seminoma cells are extremely radiosensitive, and RT has been widely used for more than 60 years and has an excellent long-term track record. This modality is still accepted as a standard management in pure seminomas [32]. For men with stage I disease that is confined to the testicle, approximately 80–85% require no further treatment [33]. Adjuvant RT improves the 5-year relapse-free survival rate up to 96% [33]. Within this long period, some changes are seen in RT techniques, irradiated fields, and RT doses.

Historically, RT was delivered using two parallel opposed anterior and posterior (AP-PA) fields that were defined with the help of bony landmarks. However, with this technique, high rates of geographic misses were reported [34, 35]. In order to diminish the marginal misses, CT-based RT planning is recommended [3]. There is a close spatial and developmental relationship between vasculature and lymphatics. So, blood vessels have been suggested as a landmark for the creation of a nodal clinical target volume (CTV) during RT planning [36, 37].

Patients with no history of pelvic or scrotal surgery before inguinal orchiectomy have traditionally been treated with opposed AP-PA fields from the top of the T11 vertebral body to the bottom of the L5 vertebral body [38] (Fig. 7.2). Para-aortic nodal irradiation alone is not sufficient in patients with a history of pelvic or scrotal surgery, since the primary lymphatic drainage has been altered and may no longer be confined to the para-aortic region. In these cases, inclusion of ipsilateral iliac and inguinal nodes in classic dogleg AP-PA fields is indicated [39]. In AP-PA para-aortic fields, the lateral borders have been placed at the tips of the transverse processes. For right-sided tumors, the treatment comprises the paracaval, precaval, and

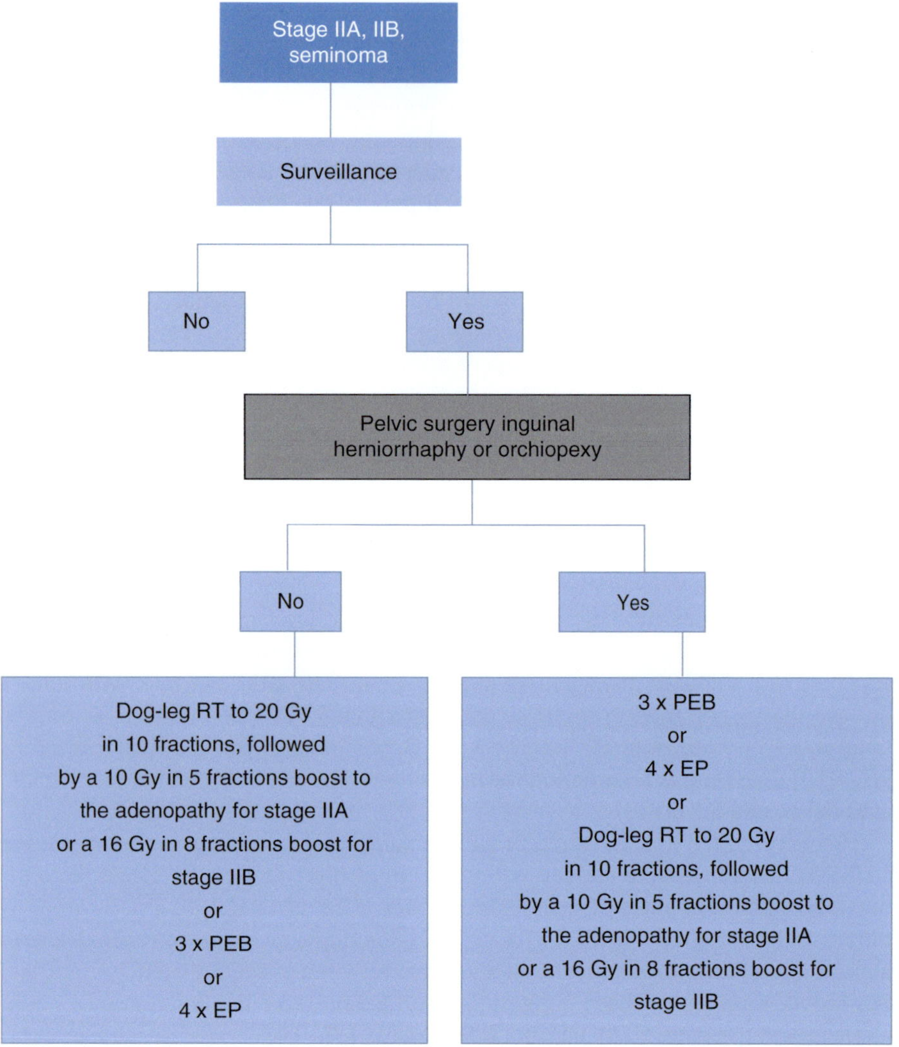

Fig. 7.2 (**a**) Anteroposterior, posteroanterior para-aortic radiotherapy field and dose distribution in (**b**) sagittal and (**c**) coronal computed tomography images

inter-aortocaval nodes. For left-sided seminomas, left renal hilus in AP-PA fields is additionally included. The inguinal orchiectomy scar and ipsilateral scrotal contents are not treated unless scrotal violation has occurred during surgery. Nodal mapping studies suggest that inclusion of left renal hilar nodes in a nodal CTV may be optional in a patient with a relatively lateral left kidney [39, 40].

Historically, the RT fields encompassed the para-aortic, ipsilateral external iliac lymph nodes and the orchiectomy scar with a total dose of 30 Gy delivered in 15 fractions. This technique was known as the “dogleg field or hockey stick field”

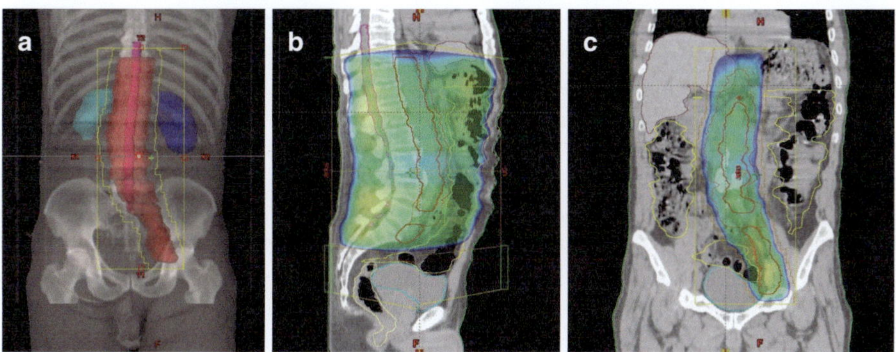

Fig. 7.3 (**a**) Anteroposterior, posteroanterior "dogleg" radiotherapy field and dose distribution in (**b**) sagittal and (**c**) coronal computed tomography images

(Fig. 7.3). The fields spread generally up to the superior aspect of T10 or T11 down to the inguinal ligament extending below the ischial tuberosities. This was the standard method until the beginning of the 1980s. Since the 1990s, following the low pelvic relapse rates reported in stage I tumors and increased gastrointestinal toxicities and secondary malignancy risk in long-term survivors, the indication for pelvic irradiation was challenged [41–43]. With omission of pelvic nodal irradiation, the preservation remaining testicular function will be possible, and the secondary cancer rates will be potentially decreased [44]. In Medical Research Council study, 478 stage I seminoma patients were randomized to dogleg field or para-aortic irradiation with a total dose of 30 Gy delivered in 15 fractions [38]. The relapse rates were 3.4% in the dogleg field irradiation arm, and all recurrences were localized above the diaphragm versus 4% in the para-aortic irradiation with 1.6% in the pelvis. In this study, the omission of pelvic field RT leads to reduction in acute toxicity and more rapid recovery of sperm count. Moreover, the linear dose-response model predicts that the aforementioned field reduction decreases second cancer risk by 45% [44]. In a prospective study with 675 patients with stage I seminoma conducted by the "German Testicular Cancer Study Group" (GTCSG), 5-year disease-free survival rate was 95.8% with a median follow-up of 61 months [34]. The reported isolated pelvic relapse rate was only 0.6%, without any "in-field" relapse. Nausea and diarrhea grade 3 were observed in 4.0 and 1.0% of the patients. Given a pelvic recurrence rate of approximately 2%, it is considered reasonable not to treat pelvic lymphatics and to treat para-aortic nodes only.

In order to decrease the toxicities and secondary malignancy risk, the RT dose is also reduced. Generally, the recommended dose is between 25 and 30 Gy delivered in 15–20 fractions. Several attempts have been introduced for dose reduction. The MRC TE18, "European Organization for Research and Treatment of Cancer Trial" (EORTC) 30942, is the only randomized study that evaluates a dose escalation, comparing 20 versus 30 Gy with conventional fractionation in 625 patients [45]. With a median follow-up of 61 months, 10 and 11 relapses, respectively, have been reported in the 30 and 20 Gy groups (hazard ratio, 1.11; 90% CI, 0.54–2.28). The absolute difference in 2-year relapse rates is 0.7%. The 20 Gy arm showed a slightly lower acute toxicity rate (moderate asthenia 5 vs 20%, work incapacity 28 vs 46%). In single-center or multicenter studies with a sufficient number of patients, the relapse rates were below 5%, and the relapses within the RT field were rare [45, 46].

7.4.2 Stage IIA/B Seminoma

Stage II seminoma is usually managed with RT or platinum-based combination chemotherapy regimens following orchiectomy. Surveillance is not an appropriate option for patients with stage II seminoma, and therapeutic retroperitoneal lymph node dissection has been largely RT and/or chemotherapy [11]. However, no prospective randomized trial has been published to date for the treatment of stage II seminoma. The optimal treatment depends on the spread of lymph node invasion. After orchiectomy, the treatment of stages IIA and IIB seminomas with less than 2.5 cm nodal involvement (N2 < 2.5 cm) classically consists of RT (Fig. 7.4) [11, 12]. These patients generally respond well to curative RT with favorable clinical outcomes. The need of chemotherapy for these patients is still a matter of debate. Platinum-based chemotherapeutics (PEB, cisplatin, etoposide, bleomycin for three cycles, or PE, cisplatin, etoposide for four cycles, if there are arguments against bleomycin) were also used in some centers [27, 37]. Prognosis remains good both with reported 5-year survival rates about 95–100% [12, 47, 48].

Patients with more advanced disease with more than 2.5 cm nodes (IB stage with N2 between 2.5 and 5 or IIC stage) respond better to combined chemotherapy, despite a greater risk of toxicity compared to RT [49]. In these patients and in patients refusing RT, three to four cycles of PEB or PE chemotherapy represent a valid option depending of the prognostic group [66]. Unlike stage I disease, a single-agent carboplatin chemotherapy is not proven to be efficient compared to combined cisplatin-based chemotherapy regimens. Therefore, CHT plays an important role in stages IIB and beyond.

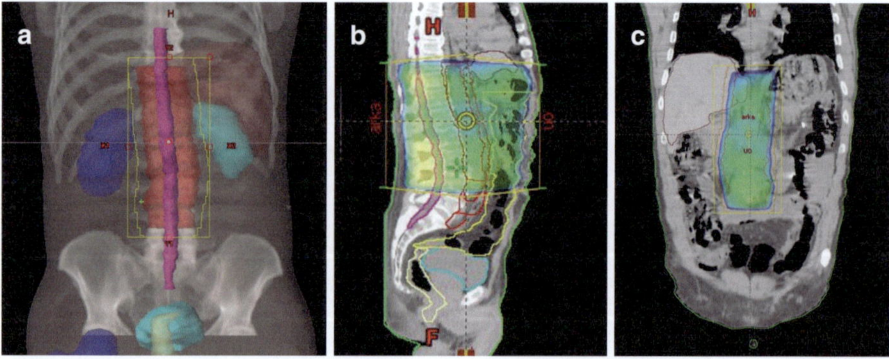

Fig. 7.4 Testicular seminoma treatment decision flow chart for clinical stage IIA and IIB disease

The standard radiation field includes para-aortic region and the ipsilateral iliac field; in stage IIB field, the lateral borders should include lymph nodes with a safety margin of 1.0–1.5 cm (Fig. 7.5). In initial phase, the RT doses were 20 Gy delivered in 10 fractions or 25.5 Gy delivered in 15 fractions [45]. The second phase (cone down) of treatment consists of daily 2 Gy fractions to a cumulative dose of 30 Gy for stage IIA and 36 Gy for selected patients with non-bulky stage IIB disease [47] (Fig. 7.6). In stage IIA and IIB seminoma, the RT dose is between 30 and 36 Gy, depending on the size of the positive nodes. The gross tumor volume (GTV) is defined on the planning CT scan. A first clinical target volume (CTV1) includes the GTV with a 0.5 cm margin, and a second (CTV2) includes the lymphatic risk areas (identical to CTV in stage I disease). The PTV should comprise both the CTV1 and CTV2 with a 0.5 cm margin. In patient with lymphadenopathy measuring more than 3 cm, the treatment of choice is chemotherapy, four cycles of etoposide and

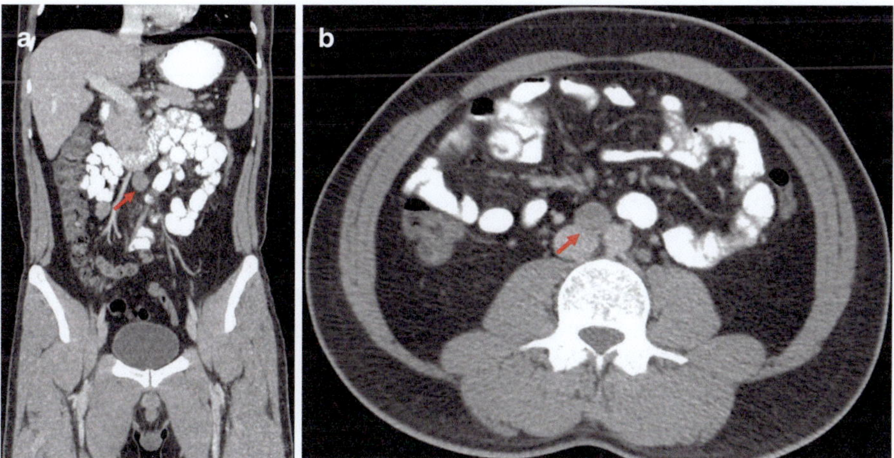

Fig. 7.5 (**a**) Coronal and (**b**) axial computed tomography images with a 2.3 cm lymphadenopathy at para-aortic area in a representative patient

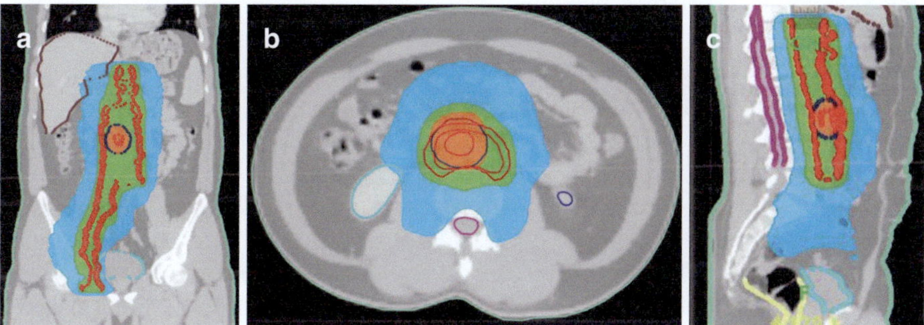

Fig. 7.6 Dose distribution of a representative patient with clinical stage IIB patients treated with tomotherapy with a 30 Gy total dose receiving para-aortic field and 36 Gy to lymphadenopathy

cisplatin (EP) or three cycles of bleomycin, etoposide, and cisplatin (PEB), rather than RT alone [41, 50, 51]. Also for patients with stage IIA disease with multiple lymphadenopathies, chemotherapy with four courses of EP or three courses of PEB is a treatment of choice.

7.4.3 Stage IIC and III Seminoma

All stage IIC and III seminomas are considered as good prognostic risk group except for patients with stage III disease with non-pulmonary visceral metastases, which is considered as intermediate risk. Chemotherapy with three cycles of PEB [52] or four cycles of EP [52, 53] has been the standard of treatment in good risk group patients. For patients with intermediate risk group, more intensive chemotherapy [four cycles of PEB or etoposide, cisplatin, ifosfamide (VIP) (in the case of contradictions to bleomycin)] is recommended.

7.5 Management of Relapse

Treatment of relapse depends on different parameters such as the nature of the initial treatment and the subsequent response, the localization, and the time since treatment. Most of the stage I seminoma patients who are under surveillance can be salvaged by RT or chemotherapy only, while surgery is not generally recommended. In case of relapse after RT, the recommended treatment scheme is a chemotherapy which is identical to that used in stage IIC and III. In selected cases, re-irradiation is also possible if the relapse is late and localized and represents a small volume, such as a solitary adenopathy. In relapse after chemotherapy, which occurs less than 3 months after one chemotherapy cycle, the disease is still considered to be sensitive to a platinum-based chemotherapy salvage treatment, and the chemosensitivity persists even after the second or third chemotherapy cycles. The most used first-line salvage protocols are the VIP (cisplatin, etoposide, ifosfamide), TIP (paclitaxel, ifosfamide, cisplatin), or VeIP (vinblastine, ifosfamide, cisplatin) schedules.

7.6 Follow-Up of After Treatment

After chemotherapy, the patients are generally evaluated with serum tumor markers and radiologic imaging (chest, abdomen, and pelvis). If marker level is normal and no residual mass or residual mass of ≤3 cm is observed, there is no need for further treatment. But, in case of residual tumor >3 cm and normal marker value, positron emission tomography (PET-CT) is recommended (Fig. 7.7). The PET-CT is usually performed at least 6 weeks after finishing chemotherapy. If technically dissected

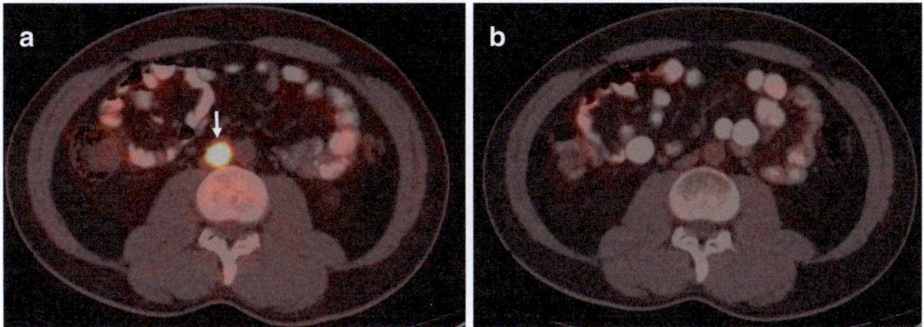

Fig. 7.7 (**a**) Positron emission tomography demonstrating lymph node metastasis (arrow) with maximum standardized value of 20.4. (**b**) Complete response demonstrated in positron emission tomography taken 3 months after completion of therapy

feasible, retroperitoneal lymph node dissection (RPLND) may be consider when a positive PET-CT [54, 55].

7.7 Non-seminoma

7.7.1 Stage I Non-seminoma

For initial evaluation, CT of the abdomen and pelvic is essential, because up to 30% of non-seminoma patients with clinical stage I disease have subclinical metastases. Adjuvant treatment options after inguinal orchiectomy include surveillance, chemotherapy, and RPLND.

7.7.1.1 Stage IA

Two adjuvant treatment options exist for patients with stage IA tumor after orchiectomy, surveillance and nerve-sparing RPLND. Although cure rates for each option is higher up to 95%, approximately 20–30% of patients experience relapse during surveillance. Approximately, 80% of these relapses occur in first year, 12% at second year, and 6% at third year and decrease to 1% thereafter [56–58]. Surveillance can be safely offered for patients with stage IA disease, as long as patients should agree to be compliant for follow-up [59, 60].

In case of no metastasis detected in lymph nodes after RPLND, no adjuvant treatment is required. However, if the dissected lymph nodes are metastatic, adjuvant chemotherapy may be required. While the patients with N1 disease are preferred for surveillance, the patient with N2 or N3 disease requires adjuvant chemotherapy regimens, either as EP or PEB. Two courses are recommended for patients with N1 or N2 disease. Chemotherapy with four courses of EP or three courses of PEB is recommended for patients with N3 disease [54, 61, 62].

7.7.1.2 Stage IB

Two adjuvant treatments such as nerve-sparing RPLND or chemotherapy options exist for patients with stage IB tumor after orchiectomy. In a randomized trial conducted by Albers et al. [63], one cycle of adjuvant BEP in patients with stage I non-seminoma paramount higher median 4.7 years recurrence-free survival compared to patients treated with RPLND only ($p = 0.01$). In other prospective nonrandomized trial, 5-year relapse rate was 3.2% for patient with lymphovascular invasion (LVI) who received one cycle of PEB and 1.6% for patients without LVI who allowed to choose between surveillance and one cycle of PEB [64]. After a median follow-up of 7.9 years, the relapse rate was 3.4% for those with LVI, and 1.3% for those without LVI. The authors suggested that one course of adjuvant PEB should be considered as a standard treatment in CS I non-seminoma with LVI. However, the role of primary diagnostic RPLND has lessened, because of higher rates of in-field recurrences and of complications [63].

7.7.1.3 Stage IS

Patient with stage IS disease display a persistent rise of tumor marker after orchiectomy, without no evidence of disease detected radiologically or clinically. According to NCCN guidelines, these patients may be treated with standard chemotherapy (either four course of EP or three course of PEB) or initial RPLND after orchiectomy.

7.7.2 Stage IIA/B

Treatment choice for patients with stage II non-seminoma is designed according to postsurgical tumor marker levels and radiological findings. Patient with normal post-orchiectomy tumor marker levels can be managed by primary RPLND or surveillance [65, 66]. If surveillance is preferred, first evaluation is performed after 6 weeks. A shrinking lesion is accepted as nonmalignant; on the contrary, a stable or growing lesion may address either teratoma or an undifferentiated malignant tumor. If the lesions grow with normal tumor markers (AFP, β-hCG), RPLND is required [65]. Patient with both enlarging lesion and elevated tumor marker indicates treatment with systemic chemotherapy [67, 68]. An alternative approach to RPLND in marker-negative patients with doubtful of a malign tumor is a CT-guided biopsy, if technically feasibly [52].

Adjuvant treatment options after inguinal orchiectomy include chemotherapy or RT encompassing para-aortic and ipsilateral iliac lymph nodes to a dose of 30 Gy delivered in 15 fractions for patients with stage IIA disease. The chemotherapy regimens include four courses of EP or three courses of PEB for patients with stage IIA. For patients with stage IIB disease with retroperitoneal lymph node metastases, two treatment options are available. First option is RPLN and adjuvant chemotherapy same as stage IIA disease. Second option is to treat with primary chemotherapy which includes four courses of EP or three courses of PEB, pursued by RPLND or surveillance. Moreover, RT with a dose of 36 Gy in selected non-bulky cases to include para-aortic and ipsilateral iliac lymph nodes may be used. Primary chemotherapy and primary RPLND have comparable treatment outcomes, but toxicity rates are different [69]. The relapse-free survival rate for either approach is close to 98% [65, 70, 71].

7.7.3 Advanced Metastatic (IIC–III) Non-seminoma

The management for patients with advanced metastatic non-seminoma is chemotherapy. Choice of chemotherapy regimen for these patients depends on the IGCCCG (International Germ Cell Consensus Classification) risk classification [72].

7.7.4 Late Relapse

Late relapse is defined as relapses observed >2 years after completion of primary treatment. The late relapse incidence is 3.2% of non-seminoma cases [73]. If technically feasible, all lesions in late relapsing non-seminoma cases should undergo surgical resection [52].

7.7.5 Brain Metastases

The prognosis of patients with brain metastases is poor [74]. If technically feasible, metastasectomy should be performed. For inoperable cases, RT and chemotherapy are accepted as treatment of choice [74–76].

7.7.6 Follow-Up of After Treatment

After chemotherapy, patients are evaluated with serum tumor markers and imaging investigation (chest, abdomen, and pelvis). PET-CT for residual disease has restrictive predictive value.

Conclusion

Two major categories are recognized, pure seminoma (no non-seminomatous elements present) and all others, which together are termed non-seminomatous germ cell tumors (NSGCT). Seminoma is highly sensitive to chemotherapy and radiotherapy. The prognosis of patients is generally good; cure is an expected outcome in the majority of cases, even with metastatic disease.

References

1. Siegel R, Ma J, Zou Z, Jemal A. Cancer statistics, 2014. CA Cancer J Clin. 2014;64(1):9–29. doi:10.3322/caac.21208.
2. Heidenreich A, Weissbach L, German Testicular Cancer I. Bilateral germ cell cancer of the testis: a report of 11 patients with a long-term follow-up. BJU Int. 2001;87(3):278–80.
3. Boujelbene N, Cosinschi A, Boujelbene N, Khanfir K, Bhagwati S, Herrmann E, et al. Pure seminoma: a review and update. Radiat Oncol. 2011;6:90. doi:10.1186/1748-717X-6-90.
4. Giannatempo P, Greco T, Mariani L, Nicolai N, Tana S, Fare E, et al. Radiotherapy or chemotherapy for clinical stage IIA and IIB seminoma: a systematic review and meta-analysis of patient outcomes. Ann Oncol. 2015;26(4):657–68. doi:10.1093/annonc/mdu447.
5. Pearce SM, Liauw SL, Eggener SE. Management of Low-Stage Testicular Seminoma. Urol Clin North Am. 2015;42(3):287–98. doi:10.1016/j.ucl.2015.04.003.
6. Mottet N, Culine S, Iborra F, Avances C, Bastide C, Lesourd A, et al. Testicular tumors. Prog Urol. 2007;17(6):1035–45.
7. Donohue JP, Zachary JM, Maynard BR. Distribution of nodal metastases in nonseminomatous testis cancer. J Urol. 1982;128(2):315–20.
8. Djeffal C, Demailly M, Tillou X, Saint F, Petit J. Place of serum HCG assay in the follow-up of non-HCG-secreting testicular seminomas. Prog Urol. 2008;18(10):654–6. doi:10.1016/j.purol.2008.04.024.
9. Hori K, Uematsu K, Yasoshima H, Yamada A, Sakurai K, Ohya M. Testicular seminoma with human chorionic gonadotropin production. Pathol Int. 1997;47(9):592–9.
10. Pizzocaro G, Nicolai N, Salvioni R. Evolution and controversies in the management of low-stage nonseminomatous germ-cell tumors of the testis. World J Urol. 1994;12(3):113–9.
11. Schmoll HJ, Jordan K, Huddart R, Pes MP, Horwich A, Fizazi K, et al. Testicular seminoma: ESMO Clinical Practice Guidelines for diagnosis, treatment and follow-up. Ann Oncol. 2010;21(Suppl 5):v140–6. doi:10.1093/annonc/mdq176.
12. Krege S, Beyer J, Souchon R, Albers P, Albrecht W, Algaba F, et al. European consensus conference on diagnosis and treatment of germ cell cancer: a report of the second meeting of the European Germ Cell Cancer Consensus group (EGCCCG): part I. Eur Urol. 2008;53(3):478–96. doi:10.1016/j.eururo.2007.12.024.
13. Warde P, Specht L, Horwich A, Oliver T, Panzarella T, Gospodarowicz M, et al. Prognostic factors for relapse in stage I seminoma managed by surveillance: a pooled analysis. J Clin Oncol. 2002;20(22):4448–52. doi:10.1200/JCO.2002.01.038.
14. Kamba T, Kamoto T, Okubo K, Teramukai S, Kakehi Y, Matsuda T, et al. Outcome of different post-orchiectomy management for stage I seminoma: Japanese multi-institutional study including 425 patients. Int J Urol. 2010;17(12):980–7. doi:10.1111/j.1442-2042.2010.02645.x.
15. Dieckmann KP, Bruggeboes B, Pichlmeier U, Kuster J, Mullerleile U, Bartels H. Adjuvant treatment of clinical stage I seminoma: is a single course of carboplatin sufficient? Urology. 2000;55(1):102–6.
16. Kollmannsberger C, Tyldesley S, Moore C, Chi KN, Murray N, Daneshmand S, et al. Evolution in management of testicular seminoma: population-based outcomes with selective utilization of active therapies. Ann Oncol. 2011;22(4):808–14. doi:10.1093/annonc/mdq466.
17. Warde P, Gospodarowicz MK, Panzarella T, Catton CN, Sturgeon JF, Moore M, et al. Stage I testicular seminoma: results of adjuvant irradiation and surveillance. J Clin Oncol. 1995;13(9):2255–62. doi:10.1200/jco.1995.13.9.2255.
18. Horwich A, Alsanjari N, A'Hern R, Nicholls J, Dearnaley DP, Fisher C. Surveillance following orchidectomy for stage I testicular seminoma. Br J Cancer. 1992;65(5):775–8.
19. von der Maase H, Specht L, Jacobsen GK, Jakobsen A, Madsen EL, Pedersen M, et al. Surveillance following orchidectomy for stage I seminoma of the testis. Eur J Cancer. 1993;29A(14):1931–4.
20. Ondrusova M, Ondrus D, Miskovska V, Kajo K, Szoldova K, Usakova V, et al. Management of clinical stage I testicular seminoma: active surveillance versus adjuvant chemotherapy. Int Urol Nephrol. 2015;47(7):1143–7. doi:10.1007/s11255-015-1002-4.

21. Cohn-Cedermark G, Stahl O, Tandstad T. Swenoteca. Surveillance vs. adjuvant therapy of clinical stage I testicular tumors – a review and the SWENOTECA experience. Andrology. 2015;3(1):102–10. doi:10.1111/andr.280.
22. Kollmannsberger C, Tandstad T, Bedard PL, Cohn-Cedermark G, Chung PW, Jewett MA, et al. Patterns of relapse in patients with clinical stage I testicular cancer managed with active surveillance. J Clin Oncol. 2015;33(1):51–7. doi:10.1200/JCO.2014.56.2116.
23. Travis LB, Fossa SD, Schonfeld SJ, McMaster ML, Lynch CF, Storm H, et al. Second cancers among 40,576 testicular cancer patients: focus on long-term survivors. J Natl Cancer Inst. 2005;97(18):1354–65. doi:10.1093/jnci/dji278.
24. Travis LB, Curtis RE, Storm H, Hall P, Holowaty E, Van Leeuwen FE, et al. Risk of second malignant neoplasms among long-term survivors of testicular cancer. J Natl Cancer Inst. 1997;89(19):1429–39.
25. Powles T, Robinson D, Shamash J, Moller H, Tranter N, Oliver T. The long-term risks of adjuvant carboplatin treatment for stage I seminoma of the testis. Ann Oncol. 2008;19(3):443–7. doi:10.1093/annonc/mdm540.
26. van den Belt-Dusebout AW, de Wit R, Gietema JA, Horenblas S, Louwman MW, Ribot JG, et al. Treatment-specific risks of second malignancies and cardiovascular disease in 5-year survivors of testicular cancer. J Clin Oncol. 2007;25(28):4370–8. doi:10.1200/JCO.2006.10.5296.
27. Huddart RA, Norman A, Shahidi M, Horwich A, Coward D, Nicholls J, et al. Cardiovascular disease as a long-term complication of treatment for testicular cancer. J Clin Oncol. 2003;21(8):1513–23. doi:10.1200/JCO.2003.04.173.
28. Haugnes HS, Aass N, Fossa SD, Dahl O, Klepp O, Wist EA, et al. Predicted cardiovascular mortality and reported cardiovascular morbidity in testicular cancer survivors. J Cancer Surviv. 2008;2(3):128–37. doi:10.1007/s11764-008-0054-1.
29. Haugnes HS, Wethal T, Aass N, Dahl O, Klepp O, Langberg CW, et al. Cardiovascular risk factors and morbidity in long-term survivors of testicular cancer: a 20-year follow-up study. J Clin Oncol. 2010;28(30):4649–57. doi:10.1200/JCO.2010.29.9362.
30. Buchholz TA, Walden TL, Prestidge BR. Cost-effectiveness of posttreatment surveillance after radiation therapy for early stage seminoma. Cancer. 1998;82(6):1126–33.
31. Clasen J, Schmidberger H, Souchon R, Weissbach L, Hartmann M, Hartmann JT, et al. What is the value of routine follow-up in stage I seminoma after paraaortic radiotherapy?: an analysis of the German Testicular Cancer Study Group (GTCSG) in 675 prospectively followed patients. Strahlenther Onkol. 2009;185(6):349–54. doi:10.1007/s00066-009-1958-z.
32. Krege S, Beyer J, Souchon R, Albers P, Albrecht W, Algaba F, et al. European consensus conference on diagnosis and treatment of germ cell cancer: a report of the second meeting of the European Germ Cell Cancer Consensus Group (EGCCCG): part II. Eur Urol. 2008;53(3):497–513. doi:10.1016/j.eururo.2007.12.025.
33. Mead GM, Fossa SD, Oliver RT, Joffe JK, Huddart RA, Roberts JT, et al. Randomized trials in 2466 patients with stage I seminoma: patterns of relapse and follow-up. J Natl Cancer Inst. 2011;103(3):241–9. doi:10.1093/jnci/djq525.
34. Classen J, Schmidberger H, Meisner C, Winkler C, Dunst J, Souchon R, et al. Para-aortic irradiation for stage I testicular seminoma: results of a prospective study in 675 patients. A trial of the German testicular cancer study group (GTCSG). Br J Cancer. 2004;90(12):2305–11. doi:10.1038/sj.bjc.6601867.
35. Martin JM, Joon DL, Ng N, Grace M, Gelderen DV, Lawlor M, et al. Towards individualised radiotherapy for Stage I seminoma. Radiother Oncol. 2005;76(3):251–6. doi:10.1016/j.radonc.2005.08.005.
36. Taylor A, Rockall AG, Reznek RH, Powell ME. Mapping pelvic lymph nodes: guidelines for delineation in intensity-modulated radiotherapy. Int J Radiat Oncol Biol Phys. 2005;63(5):1604–12. doi:10.1016/j.ijrobp.2005.05.062.
37. Shih HA, Harisinghani M, Zietman AL, Wolfgang JA, Saksena M, Weissleder R. Mapping of nodal disease in locally advanced prostate cancer: rethinking the clinical target volume for pelvic nodal irradiation based on vascular rather than bony anatomy. Int J Radiat Oncol Biol Phys. 2005;63(4):1262–9. doi:10.1016/j.ijrobp.2005.07.952.

38. Fossa SD, Horwich A, Russell JM, Roberts JT, Cullen MH, Hodson NJ, et al. Optimal planning target volume for stage I testicular seminoma: A Medical Research Council randomized trial. Medical Research Council Testicular Tumor Working Group. J Clin Oncol. 1999;17(4):1146. doi:10.1200/jco.1999.17.4.1146.
39. McMahon CJ, Rofsky NM, Pedrosa I. Lymphatic metastases from pelvic tumors: anatomic classification, characterization, and staging. Radiology. 2010;254(1):31–46. doi:10.1148/radiol.2541090361.
40. Dinniwell R, Chan P, Czarnota G, Haider MA, Jhaveri K, Jewett M, et al. Pelvic lymph node topography for radiotherapy treatment planning from ferumoxtran-10 contrast-enhanced magnetic resonance imaging. Int J Radiat Oncol Biol Phys. 2009;74(3):844–51. doi:10.1016/j.ijrobp.2008.09.026.
41. Detti B, Livi L, Scoccianti S, Gacci M, Lapini A, Cai T, et al. Management of Stage II testicular seminoma over a period of 40 years. Urol Oncol. 2009;27(5):534–8. doi:10.1016/j.urolonc.2008.07.034.
42. Hunter M, Peschel RE. Testicular seminoma. Results of the Yale University experience, 1964-1984. Cancer. 1989;64(8):1608–11.
43. Thomas GM. Is "optimal" radiation for stage I seminoma yet defined? J Clin Oncol. 1999;17(9):3004–5.
44. Zwahlen DR, Martin JM, Millar JL, Schneider U. Effect of radiotherapy volume and dose on secondary cancer risk in stage I testicular seminoma. Int J Radiat Oncol Biol Phys. 2008;70(3):853–8. doi:10.1016/j.ijrobp.2007.10.007.
45. Jones WG, Fossa SD, Mead GM, Roberts JT, Sokal M, Horwich A, et al. Randomized trial of 30 versus 20 Gy in the adjuvant treatment of stage I Testicular Seminoma: a report on Medical Research Council Trial TE18, European Organisation for the Research and Treatment of Cancer Trial 30942 (ISRCTN18525328). J Clin Oncol. 2005;23(6):1200–8. doi:10.1200/JCO.2005.08.003.
46. Coleman JM, Coleman RE, Turner AR, Radstone CR, Champion AE. The management and clinical course of testicular seminoma: 15 years' experience at a single institution. Clin Oncol (R Coll Radiol). 1998;10(4):237–41.
47. Classen J, Schmidberger H, Meisner C, Souchon R, Sautter-Bihl ML, Sauer R, et al. Radiotherapy for stages IIA/B testicular seminoma: final report of a prospective multicenter clinical trial. J Clin Oncol. 2003;21(6):1101–6. doi:10.1200/JCO.2003.06.065.
48. Patterson H, Norman AR, Mitra SS, Nicholls J, Fisher C, Dearnaley DP, et al. Combination carboplatin and radiotherapy in the management of stage II testicular seminoma: comparison with radiotherapy treatment alone. Radiother Oncol. 2001;59(1):5–11.
49. Arranz Arija JA, Garcia del Muro X, Guma J, Aparicio J, Salazar R, Saenz A, et al. E400P in advanced seminoma of good prognosis according to the international germ cell cancer collaborative group (IGCCCG) classification: the Spanish Germ Cell Cancer Group experience. Ann Oncol. 2001;12(4):487–91.
50. Domont J, Massard C, Patrikidou A, Bossi A, de Crevoisier R, Rose M, et al. A risk-adapted strategy of radiotherapy or cisplatin-based chemotherapy in stage II seminoma. Urol Oncol. 2013;31(5):697–705. doi:10.1016/j.urolonc.2011.04.004.
51. Garcia-del-Muro X, Maroto P, Guma J, Sastre J, Lopez Brea M, Arranz JA, et al. Chemotherapy as an alternative to radiotherapy in the treatment of stage IIA and IIB testicular seminoma: a Spanish Germ Cell Cancer Group Study. J Clin Oncol. 2008;26(33):5416–21. doi:10.1200/JCO.2007.15.9103.
52. Albers P, Albrecht W, Algaba F, Bokemeyer C, Cohn-Cedermark G, Fizazi K, et al. Guidelines on testicular cancer: 2015 update. Eur Urol. 2015;68(6):1054–68. doi:10.1016/j.eururo.2015.07.044.
53. van As NJ, Gilbert DC, Money-Kyrle J, Bloomfield D, Beesley S, Dearnaley DP, et al. Evidence-based pragmatic guidelines for the follow-up of testicular cancer: optimising the detection of relapse. Br J Cancer. 2008;98(12):1894–902. doi:10.1038/sj.bjc.6604280.
54. de Wit R, Collette L, Sylvester R, de Mulder PH, Sleijfer DT, ten Bokkel Huinink WW, et al. Serum alpha-fetoprotein surge after the initiation of chemotherapy for non-seminomatous testicular cancer has an adverse prognostic significance. Br J Cancer. 1998;78(10):1350–5.

55. Feldman DR, Motzer RJ, Bajorin DF. Is high-dose chemotherapy effective in patients with relapsed or refractory germ cell tumors? Nat Clin Pract Urol. 2008;5(2):78–9. doi:10.1038/ncpuro0999.
56. Daugaard G, Skoneczna I, Aass N, De Wit R, De Santis M, Dumez H, et al. A randomized phase III study comparing standard dose BEP with sequential high-dose cisplatin, etoposide, and ifosfamide (VIP) plus stem-cell support in males with poor-prognosis germ-cell cancer. An intergroup study of EORTC, GTCSG, and Grupo Germinal (EORTC 30974). Ann Oncol. 2011;22(5):1054–61. doi:10.1093/annonc/mdq575.
57. Oliver RT, Freedman LS, Parkinson MC, Peckham MJ. Medical options in the management of stages 1 and 2 (N0-N3, M0) testicular germ cell tumors. Urol Clin North Am. 1987;14(4):721–30.
58. Freedman LS, Parkinson MC, Jones WG, Oliver RT, Peckham MJ, Read G, et al. Histopathology in the prediction of relapse of patients with stage I testicular teratoma treated by orchidectomy alone. Lancet. 1987;2(8554):294–8.
59. Kollmannsberger C, Moore C, Chi KN, Murray N, Daneshmand S, Gleave M, et al. Non-risk-adapted surveillance for patients with stage I nonseminomatous testicular germ-cell tumors: diminishing treatment-related morbidity while maintaining efficacy. Ann Oncol. 2010;21(6):1296–301. doi:10.1093/annonc/mdp473.
60. Nichols CR, Roth B, Albers P, Einhorn LH, Foster R, Daneshmand S, et al. Active surveillance is the preferred approach to clinical stage I testicular cancer. J Clin Oncol. 2013;31(28):3490–3. doi:10.1200/JCO.2012.47.6010.
61. Schmoll HJ, Jordan K, Huddart R, Pes MP, Horwich A, Fizazi K, et al. Testicular non-seminoma: ESMO Clinical Practice Guidelines for diagnosis, treatment and follow-up. Ann Oncol. 2010;21(Suppl 5):v147–54. doi:10.1093/annonc/mdq177.
62. Sheinfeld J, Herr HW. Role of surgery in management of germ cell tumor. Semin Oncol. 1998;25(2):203–9.
63. Albers P, Siener R, Krege S, Schmelz HU, Dieckmann KP, Heidenreich A, et al. Randomized phase III trial comparing retroperitoneal lymph node dissection with one course of bleomycin and etoposide plus cisplatin chemotherapy in the adjuvant treatment of clinical stage I Nonseminomatous testicular germ cell tumors: AUO trial AH 01/94 by the German Testicular Cancer Study Group. J Clin Oncol. 2008;26(18):2966–72. doi:10.1200/JCO.2007.12.0899.
64. Tandstad T, Dahl O, Cohn-Cedermark G, Cavallin-Stahl E, Stierner U, Solberg A, et al. Risk-adapted treatment in clinical stage I nonseminomatous germ cell testicular cancer: the SWENOTECA management program. J Clin Oncol. 2009;27(13):2122–8. doi:10.1200/JCO.2008.18.8953.
65. Stephenson AJ, Bosl GJ, Motzer RJ, Bajorin DF, Stasi JP, Sheinfeld J. Nonrandomized comparison of primary chemotherapy and retroperitoneal lymph node dissection for clinical stage IIA and IIB nonseminomatous germ cell testicular cancer. J Clin Oncol. 2007;25(35):5597–602. doi:10.1200/JCO.2007.12.0808.
66. Frohlich MW, Small EJ. Stage II nonseminomatous testis cancer: the roles of primary and adjuvant chemotherapy. Urol Clin North Am. 1998;25(3):451–9.
67. Peckham MJ. Surveillance following orchiectomy for clinicaL stage I testicular germ-cell malignancy. Acta Urol Belg. 1985;53(2):283–98.
68. Horwich A, Norman A, Fisher C, Hendry WF, Nicholls J, Dearnaley DP. Primary chemotherapy for stage II nonseminomatous germ cell tumors of the testis. J Urol. 1994;151(1):72–7; discussion 7–8.
69. Chevreau C, Mazerolles C, Soulie M, Gaspard MH, Mourey L, Bujan L et al. Long-term efficacy of two cycles of BEP regimen in high-risk stage I nonseminomatous testicular germ cell tumors with embryonal carcinoma and/or vascular invasion. Eur Urol. 2004;46(2):209–14; discussion 14-–5. doi:10.1016/j.eururo.2004.03.022.
70. Davis BE, Herr HW, Fair WR, Bosl GJ. The management of patients with nonseminomatous germ cell tumors of the testis with serologic disease only after orchiectomy. J Urol. 1994;152(1):111–3; discussion 114.

71. Weissbach L, Bussar-Maatz R, Flechtner H, Pichlmeier U, Hartmann M, Keller L. RPLND or primary chemotherapy in clinical stage IIA/B nonseminomatous germ cell tumors? Results of a prospective multicenter trial including quality of life assessment. Eur Urol. 2000;37(5):582–94.
72. Mead GM, Stenning SP. The International Germ Cell Consensus Classification: a new prognostic factor-based staging classification for metastatic germ cell tumours. Clin Oncol (R Coll Radiol). 1997;9(4):207–9.
73. Oldenburg J, Alfsen GC, Waehre H, Fossa SD. Late recurrences of germ cell malignancies: a population-based experience over three decades. Br J Cancer. 2006;94(6):820–7. doi:10.1038/sj.bjc.6603014.
74. Motzer RJ, Bajorin DF, Bosl GJ. "Poor-risk" germ cell tumors: current progress and future directions. Semin Oncol. 1992;19(2):206–14.
75. Feldman DR, Sheinfeld J, Bajorin DF, Fischer P, Turkula S, Ishill N, et al. TI-CE high-dose chemotherapy for patients with previously treated germ cell tumors: results and prognostic factor analysis. J Clin Oncol. 2010;28(10):1706–13. doi:10.1200/JCO.2009.25.1561.
76. Baniel J, Roth BJ, Foster RS, Donohue JP. Cost and risk benefit in the management of clinical stage II nonseminomatous testicular tumors. Cancer. 1995;75(12):2897–903.

Systemic Therapies in the Management of Testicular Cancers

8

Mehmet Ali Nahit Şendur and Sercan Aksoy

Abstract

Testicular cancer has become one of the most curable of solid tumors due to the prominent treatment advances beginning in the last 2–3 decades; it only accounts 0.1% of cancer-related deaths. The availability of effective therapies and the development of risk prediction models have increased the cure rate for testicular germ cell tumors (GCT) to approximately 95%. Approximately 70–80% of patients with seminomas and 30–60% of patients with nonseminomatous GCTs (NSGCT) present with stage I disease, and about 80% of patients with stage I seminomas and 70% of NSGCTs are cured with radical orchiectomy alone. The aim of this chapter is to summarize systemic therapies for testicular cancer especially GCTs.

8.1 Introduction

Testicular cancer is the most common malignancy affecting men between ages 15 and 35. Although it accounts only 1% of all cancers in men, it accounts about 0.1% of cancer-related deaths. It is estimated that 8720 cases and 380 deaths occurred in the United States in 2016 [1]. Germ cell tumors (GCTs) account approximately 95% of testicular cancers. Sex cord-stromal tumors, gonadoblastomas, adnexal and paratesticular tumors, carcinoid tumors, lymphomas, and metastatic tumors comprise approximately the remaining 5% of testicular cancers [2].

M.A.N. Şendur, M.D. (✉)
Department of Medical Oncology, Ankara Atatürk Education and Research Hospital, Ankara Yıldırım Beyazıt University, Ankara, Turkey
e-mail: masendur@yahoo.com.tr

S. Aksoy, M.D.
Department of Medical Oncology, Hacettepe University Cancer Institute, Ankara, Turkey

G. Ozyigit, U. Selek (eds.), *Principles and Practice of Uroncology*,
DOI 10.1007/978-3-319-56114-1_8

Testicular cancer has become one of the most curable of solid tumors due to the prominent treatment advances beginning in last 2–3 decades; it only accounts 0.1% of cancer-related deaths [1]. Testicular germ cell tumors account most of the testicular cancers. Germ cell tumors consist of one predominant histologic pattern or mix of multiple histologic types. For treatment purposes, GCTs are divided into two categories: pure seminoma or nonseminoma. Nonseminomatous germ cell tumors (NSGCTs) consist of embryonal carcinoma, choriocarcinoma, yolk sac tumor (endodermal sinus tumor), teratoma, teratoma with malignant or somatic mutation, and mix germ cell tumors [3–5]. Nonseminoma tumors also include seminoma histology with elevated alpha fetoprotein (AFP) levels.

Most patients with testicular cancer usually present with painless testicular mass which is confirmed with scrotal ultrasonography. Preoperative and postoperative serum tumor markers such as beta subunit of human choriogonadotropin (β-HCG), AFP, and lactate dehydrogenase (LDH) levels should be measured. Treatment of the primary tumor is radical inguinal orchiectomy with removal of the testis, and ligation of the spermatic cord at the level of the internal ring is performed. After diagnosis, the extent of disease should be evaluated by chest x-ray, computed tomography of the abdomen and pelvis, and tumor markers. To determine the presence of lung, brain, and bone metastases, further radiologic evaluation should be performed if suspicious symptoms are present.

After histopathological evaluation of orchiectomy, clinical TNM (tumor-node-metastases) staging and risk evaluation should be done according to the International Germ Cell Cancer Consensus Group (IGCCCG) classification with post-orchiectomy tumor marker levels (Table 8.1). According to the this classification, prognostic factor-based staging system was developed, and easily applicable, clinically based,

Table 8.1 IGICC risk classification

Risk status	Seminoma	Nonseminoma
Good risk	Any primary site No non-pulmonary visceral metastases Normal AFP, any hCG, any LDH	Testis/retroperitoneal primary No non-pulmonary visceral metastases Good markers AFP < 1000 ng/mL hCG < 5000 iu/l LDH < 1.5 × ULN
Intermediate risk	Any primary site Non-pulmonary visceral metastases Normal AFP, any hCG, any LDH	Testis/retroperitoneal primary No non-pulmonary visceral metastases Intermediate markers AFP 1000–10,000 ng/mL hCG 5000–50,000 iu/I LDH 1.5×–10× ULN
Poor risk	No patients classified as poor prognosis	Mediastinal primary or non-pulmonary visceral metastases or poor markers AFP > 10,000 ng/mL or hCG > 50,000 iu/l or LDH > 10× ULN

ULN upper limit normal, *AFP* alpha fetoprotein, *hCG* human choriogonadotropin, *LDH* lactate dehydrogenase

prognostic classification for GCTs has been agreed to good, intermediate, and poor prognostic groups [6].

The aim of this chapter is to summarize systemic therapies for testicular cancer especially GCTs.

8.2 Management of Stage I Tumors

Most patients with stage I testicular tumors are cured with radical orchiectomy. Approximately 70–80% of patients with seminomas and 30–60% of patients with NSGCTs present with stage I disease, and about 80% of patients with stage I seminomas and 70% of NSGCTs are cured with radical orchiectomy alone [3, 7, 8].

In one retrospective study including data from 2483 clinical stage I GCTs managed with active surveillance, relapse was reported in 19% of NSGCTs and in 13% of seminoma patients [9]. Median time to relapse was 6 and 14 months in NSGCTs and seminomas, respectively. Ninety percent of relapses occurred within 2 years in NSGCT group; 92% of relapses occurred within 3 years in seminoma group. In one study involving 1954 patients with stage I seminoma who were followed by active surveillance for a median of 15.1 years, the incidence of relapse was 18.9% at a median of 13.7 months. The 15-year disease-specific survival rate was 99.3% [10]. In a long-term population-based cohort, the relapse rate after orchiectomy alone was 30.6% at 5 years in 1226 NSGCT patients managed with active surveillance [11]. The relapse risk was 50% in the presence of vascular invasion, embryonal carcinoma, and rete testis invasion, 12% without these three risk factors. Eighty percent of relapses were diagnosed within the first year after orchiectomy. The median time to relapse was 5 months, and the disease-specific survival at 15 years was 99.1%.

After diagnosing stage I seminoma, active surveillance or adjuvant radiotherapy or adjuvant chemotherapy can be offered. Cisplatin-based combination chemotherapy is the standard treatment for advanced testicular germ cell tumors for seminomas and NSGCTs. Single-agent carboplatin, rather than a cisplatin-based combination, has been used for stage I seminoma because it is associated with less toxicity than cisplatin-based regimens. According to the active surveillance data, risk of relapse was between 13% and 19% in stage I seminomas [9, 10]. In a phase III trial conducted by the European Organization for Research and Treatment of Cancer (EORTC), 1477 men with stage I seminoma were randomly assigned to adjuvant RT or a single course of carboplatin (AUC 7) [12]. The primary outcome relapse-free rates at 5 years were 94.7% and 96% for carboplatin and RT arms, respectively [13]. In addition to noninferiority of single agent of carboplatin to radiotherapy, reduction in the rate of contralateral GCTs was significantly reduced (carboplatin, $n = 2$; RT, $n = 15$; $P = 0.03$).

After diagnosing stage I NSGCT, active surveillance or retroperitoneal lymph node dissection (RPLND) or adjuvant chemotherapy can be offered. The risk of relapse was between 19% and 50% in stage I NSGCTs whether risk factors are present or not [9, 11]. In the longest-term population-based cohort, the risk of relapse was significantly associated with the presence of vascular invasion, the presence of embryonal carcinoma, and the presence of rete testes invasion [11]. In this cohort, 5-year relapse rate was 50% if all risk factors were present and only 12%, if none of the risk factors were present. In randomized phase III trial comparing RPLND with one course of bleomycin and etoposide plus cisplatin (BEP) chemotherapy in the adjuvant treatment of clinical stage I NSGCTs, 382 patients were randomly assigned to receive either RPLND (n = 191) or one course of BEP (n = 191) after orchidectomy [14]. The primary end point of the study was the rate of recurrence. Only two recurrences were observed in one course of BEP group, whereas 15 recurrences were observed in RPLND group with a median follow-up of 4.7 years ($P = 0.001$). Two-year recurrence-free survival rate were 99.46% and 91.87% in one course of BEP arms and RPLND arms, respectively. This study showed the superiority of one course of BEP over RPLND in the adjuvant treatment of clinical stage I NSGCT to prevent recurrence.

In the Swedish and Norwegian Testicular Cancer Group (SWENOTECA) trial which involved 745 patients with clinical stage I NSGCT, adjuvant BEP was recommended for patients according to the present high-risk disease or not [15]. During active surveillance, disease relapse was observed in 41% and 13.2% in patients with present lymphovascular invasion (LVI) and in patients who did not have LVI, respectively. In patients who received one cycle of BEP, disease relapse was observed only in 3.2% of patients who had LVI and 1.3% of the patients who did not have LVI. In the updated results of SWENOTECA with a median of 7.9-year follow-up, 5-year relapse rate in one course of BEP group was 3.2% and 1.6% for patients with LVI and without LVI [16].

Another option for stage I NSGCT is RPLND. The use of primary RPLND for clinical stage I NSGCT is both diagnostic and therapeutic. The main advantages of RPLND for patients with clinical stage I NSGST are the reduction for subsequent chemotherapy and the accurate staging. The relapse rate with RPLND is between 20% and 30% [14]. In clinical studies, pathological stage II disease is found in about 15–35% of patients as a result of RPLND [17, 18].

In summary, all treatment approaches have 99% of cancer-specific survival with different relapse rates in both stage I seminoma and NSGCT. Thus, active surveillance is a commonly recommended strategy for stage I seminoma. Surveillance is also recommended for stage IA (pT1 tumors; no vascular/lymphatic invasion and no invasion into the tunica vaginalis, spermatic cord, or scrotum) NSGCT patients who have a low risk for recurrence, whereas RPLND or 1–2 courses of BEP can be recommended to stage IB (pT2-4; vascular/lymphatic invasion or invasion into the tunica vaginalis, spermatic cord, or scrotum) [19–21].

8.3 Management of Stage II Tumors

Following orchiectomy, the optimal treatment for stage II disease depends upon the extent of lymph node involvement; stage IIA is defined as metastatic disease to lymph nodes, with a lymph node mass measuring less than 2 cm in diameter in greatest dimension on CT scan, whereas stage IIB is a disease measuring 2 to 5 cm in maximum diameter and stage IIC is a disease measuring more than 5 cm in maximum diameter [20].

Radiotherapy has been the mainstay of treatment in patients with low-volume stage IIA and IIB seminomas. In the final report of a prospective trial of RT (to para-aortic and high ipsilateral iliac lymph nodes; 30 Gy for stage IIA and 36 Gy for stage IIB disease) for stages IIA/B testicular seminoma, excellent tumor control was achieved; relapse-free survival rates at 6 years were 95.3% and 88.9% for stage IIA and IIB groups, respectively [22]. For selected patients with stage IIB seminoma, such as those with adenopathy measuring more than 3 cm, chemotherapy with four courses of etoposide and cisplatin (EP) or three cycles of BEP is an alternative to radiotherapy. In a risk-adapted strategy in patients with stage II seminoma, radiotherapy and cisplatin-based chemotherapy can be used. In a single-center study from Gustave Roussy, 3 cm was accepted as tumor size threshold above which individual patients were considered for chemotherapy in patients with stage II seminoma and relapses occurred in 30% and 27% of patients treated with radiotherapy and chemotherapy, respectively, with a median 9.4-year follow-up [23]. Five-year relapse-free survival rate was 71%, and 5-year overall survival (OS) rate was 97%. In a Spanish Germ Cell Cancer Group Study, 72 patients who had stage IIA ($n = 18$) or IIB ($n = 54$) disease were treated with four cycles of EP or three cycles of BEP [24]. Five-year PFS rates for patients with stage IIA or IIB disease were 100% and 87% with a median 71.5-month follow-up. For stage IIA and IIB seminoma patients, chemotherapy is a highly effective and a good alternative to RT. Patients with stage IIC seminoma are considered as good risk according to the IGCCCG and treated as good-risk stage III disease.

Residual masses can be detected on radiographic evaluation after chemotherapy. Residual masses smaller than 3 cm in diameter are usually not resected and are followed by observation. Masses larger than 3 cm carry a higher risk of containing seminoma, and 2–18 fluoro-deoxy-D-glucose positron emission tomography which is performed 6 weeks after completion of therapy is the best predictor of viable residual tumor in postchemotherapy seminoma residuals with higher specificity and sensitivity, positive predictive value, and negative predictive value compared to computed tomography evaluation [25].

Patients with a low-volume stage II NSGCTs (retroperitoneal lymph nodes <3 cm in diameter) and normal tumor marker levels after orchiectomy are generally treated with RPLND. Patients with higher-volume stage II disease or increasing levels of markers should receive chemotherapy (BEP for three cycles or EP for four cycles) if patients are in good-risk IGCCCG classification [26]. Cures are achieved in 95 to 99% of patients. Approximately 25% of patients with NSGCT have a residual mass, mostly in the retroperitoneum, after chemotherapy. Retroperitoneal lymph node dissection is the standard treatment after chemotherapy in patients with stage II or III disease who have had a serologic complete response but have persistently enlarged retroperitoneal lymph nodes ≥1 cm [27]. However, the management of small residual masses (≤1 cm) is controversial, with good outcomes reported with either RPLND or surveillance. A meta-analysis of RPLND after chemotherapy showed necrosis in 71% of patients, teratoma in 24%, and active cancer in 4% [28]. In these meta-analyses, the relapse rate was only 5% among patients who underwent surveillance and 3% among patients with RPLND only. The risk of relapse is approximately about 50% in patients with pathological N2 and N3 disease; thus, two cycles of EP can be recommended to patients with pathological N2 or N3. A treatment program of 50 patients that consists of two cycles of EP is effective in preventing relapses in patients with completely resected pathological stage N2 and N3 NSGCT [29].

8.4 Management of Stage III Tumors

For patients with advanced disease, the prognostic model that was developed by IGCCCG is very important to decide the treatment approach for both advanced seminoma and NSGCTs [6].

8.4.1 Seminoma

Patients with stage IIC seminomas are considered as good risk, and patients in stage III seminomas are considered as either good or intermediate risk. Patients with advanced seminomas are classified as having good risk if metastases are limited to the lungs and/or lymph nodes, regardless of the primary site, whereas patients with metastases at sites other than the lungs or lymph nodes are classified as having intermediate-risk disease. In a randomized 2 × 2 factorial design study of the European Organization for Research and Treatment of Cancer (EORTC) Genitourinary Tract Cancer Cooperative Group, the primary outcome 2-year PFS rates were 90.4% and 89.4% in three cycles and four cycles of BEP arms, respectively; thus, in conclusion, three cycles of BEP was equal to four cycles of BEP in good-prognosis germ cell cancer, and also the administration of the chemotherapy in 3 days or 5 days has similar effect on the effectiveness in the BEP regimen [30]. Thus, for patients with good risk, three cycles of BEP or four cycles of EP are recommended. In contrast, more intensive (four cycles of BEP) chemotherapy is recommended for those with intermediate-risk seminoma [20]. Pure seminomas are never classified as poor risk.

8.4.2 NSGCTs

The treatment approach for patients with advanced disease depends on the IGCCCG risk classification [6]. Patients with advanced NSGCTs are divided into good-, intermediate-, and poor-risk categories. In addition to stage IS disease, persistently elevated post-orchiectomy serum tumor markers with normal imaging studies indicate the presence of occult metastatic disease; therefore, these patients should be treated similarly with advanced (stage III) NSGCTs [31].

Approximately 60% of patients with NSGCTs present with good-risk disease. For patients with good-risk advanced GCTs, cisplatin-based combination therapy is recommended. In a randomized trial of BEP versus carboplatin, etoposide, and bleomycin (CEB) for patients with good-risk metastatic NSGCTs, relapse rate was 32% in carboplatin arm and 13% in cisplatin arm; thus, carboplatin should not replace cisplatin in patients with testicular cancer [32]. In a randomized study, for good-risk metastatic NSGCT, patients were randomly assigned to three cycles of BEP or four cycles of EP, and 4-year event-free survival rates were 91% and 86% in BEP and EP arms, respectively ($P = 0.13$); thus, both regimens are favorable and can be used for patients with metastatic good-risk NSGCTs [26].

Patients with intermediate-risk group include patients with nonseminomatous tumors with intermediate risk; poor-risk disease includes nonseminomatous germ cell tumors with non-pulmonary visceral metastases, poor-risk tumor markers, or primary mediastinal site [6]. For patients with intermediate- or poor-risk disease, four cycles of BEP was recommended rather than other platinum-based regimens [20]. There are no data to support the use of three rather than four cycles of BEP in this population. In addition, there are no data supporting the use of more than four cycles.

In a randomized clinical trial, 261 patients with disseminated GCTs were randomly assigned to four cycles of BEP or vinblastine, etoposide, and cisplatin (PVB) regimen [33]. Although similar OS was reported in two treatment arms, significantly higher complete response rate was reported in patients treated with BEP arm (77% vs 66%). Four cycles of BEP is the standard for patients with intermediate- and poor-risk NSGCTs, but to prevent lung toxicity of bleomycin in patients with lung metastases or underlying lung disease, the combination of ifosfamide, etoposide, and cisplatin (VIP) can be an alternative to BEP regimen [34–36].

In a randomized phase III trial of 219 patients with intermediate- or poor-risk GCTs randomly assigned to four cycles of BEP or two cycles of BEP followed by two cycles of high-dose chemotherapy (cyclophosphamide/etoposide/carboplatin) plus stem cell rescue [37]. The 1-year durable complete response rate was 52% after BEP plus stem cell rescue and 48% after BEP arm alone in patients with poor-prognosis GCTs ($P = 0.53$). In another randomized phase III EORTC 30974 trial comparing standard BEP with sequential high-dose VIP plus stem cell support in patients with poor-prognosis germ cell cancer, no failure-free survival and OS difference were reported [38]. Due to no additional benefit was observed with adding high-dose chemotherapy as part of first-line therapy, it is not recommended as first-line treatment for poor-risk NSGCTs.

In randomized phase III GETUG-13 (Groupe d'Etudes des Tumeurs Uro-Génitales) trial, the 203 men who had unfavorable decline in tumor markers (80%) after one cycle of standard BEP regimen were randomly assigned to treatment with three additional cycles of BEP or a dose-dense regimen that included paclitaxel, cisplatin, etoposide, oxaliplatin, and ifosfamide with continuous infusion bleomycin [39]. Three-year PFS rates were 59% in dose-dense regimen and 48% in standard BEP regimen ($P = 0.05$). Personalized treatment with dose-dense regimen intensification significantly reduced the risk of progression with no OS benefit.

Table 8.2 Summary of recommendations and outcomes for seminomas and NSGCTs

	Recommendation	Relapse risk
Seminoma		
Stage IA-IB	Active surveillance	13–19%
	One-cycle carboplatin (AUC 7)	5.3%
	RT (20 Gy)	4%
Stage IIA	RT (30–36 Gy)	5–30%
	Three-cycle BEP or four-cycle EP	
Stage IIB	RT 36 Gy (nodes <3 cm)	11–30%
	Three-cycle BEP or four-cycle EP	5–15%
Stage IIC	Three-cycle BEP or four-cycle EP	9–15%
Stage III good risk	Three-cycle BEP or four-cycle EP	9–15%
Stage III intermediate risk	Four-cycle BEP	25–35%
Nonseminoma		
Stage IA-IB	Active surveillance	19–50%
	RPLND	15–30%
	One-cycle BEP	1–5%
Stage IIA	RPLND	15–30%
	Three-cycle BEP or four-cycle EP	1–5%
Stage IIB	Three-cycle BEP or four-cycle EP	1–5%
	RPLND for selected cases	15–50%
Stage IIC	Three-cycle BEP or four-cycle EP	10–15%
Stage III good risk	Three-cycle BEP or four-cycle EP	10–15%
Stage III intermediate risk	Four-cycle BEP or four-cycle VİP	25–50%
Stage III poor risk	Four-cycle BEP or four-cycle VİP	40–60%

BEP bleomycin-etoposide-cisplatin, *EP* etoposide-cisplatin, *RPLND* retroperitoneal lymph node dissection, *RT* radiotherapy, *VİP* ifosfamide-etoposide-cisplatin

Treatment options and relapse risk are summarized in Table 8.2 according to the results of randomized trials and population-based cohorts.

8.5 Salvage Therapy for Relapsed and Refractory Germ Cell Tumors

According to the IGCCCG risk classification, the risk of relapse significantly increases with intermediate or poor risk [6]. Five-year PFS rates were 82% and 67% for good- and intermediate-risk seminomas, respectively, and 5-year PFS rates were 89%, 75%, and 41% for good-, intermediate-, and poor-risk NSGCTs, respectively [6]. Approximately 20% of patients with metastatic testicular GCTs will relapse after first-line chemotherapy [3].

The response to initial therapy (complete versus partial versus no response) and the duration of remission are important prognostic indicators. Progression of disease either during or within four weeks after completion of cisplatin-based chemotherapy is considered cisplatin-refractory disease. These patients have a very poor prognosis. A study from the International Prognostic Factors Study Group including 1984 patients with GCTs who progressed after at least three cycles of cisplatin-based chemotherapy and were treated with cisplatin-based conventional-dose or carboplatin-based high-dose salvage chemotherapy was retrospectively collected from 38 centers [40]. In this study, five prognostic subgroups of relapsed patients were identified on the basis of histology, primary tumor location, response to first-line therapy, tumor marker concentrations, and location of metastases (liver, brain, and bone). Patients with gonadal primary tumors and low concentrations of serum markers, previous complete remission, or partial remission with marker normalization had the best outcomes; 2-year PFS rates were 75% in very low-risk, 51% in low-risk, 40% in intermediate-risk, 26% in high-risk, and only 6% in very high-risk patients [40].

The optimal treatment of relapsed GCTs depends upon the response to prior therapy, the location and timing of the relapse, and tumor histology. Second-line therapy includes standard conventional chemotherapy or high-dose chemotherapy. Patients who are not previously treated with chemotherapy at the time of recurrence should be treated with a cisplatin-based combination regimen such as BEP or EP regimens. If patients were treated previously, the conventional-dose regimens are cisplatin and ifosfamide combined with either vinblastine or paclitaxel [35, 41, 42].

Conventional-dose chemotherapy and high-dose chemotherapy can be used successfully as salvage treatment for patients with metastatic GCTs after progression with first-line treatment. In a randomized phase III trial, 280 patients failing first-line platinum chemotherapy for advanced GCTs were randomly assigned to receive either four cycles of VİP or three such cycles followed by high-dose carboplatin, etoposide, and cyclophosphamide with hematopoietic stem cell support [43]. Similar response rates were observed in both treatment arms and high-dose salvage chemotherapy after three cycles of standard-dose chemotherapy had no effect on treatment outcomes. But complete responders with high-dose chemotherapy had significantly higher disease-free survival at 3 years (75 vs 55%, $P < 0.04$). In the retrospective comparison of conventional-dose chemotherapy and high-dose chemotherapy in which high-dose and standard-dose chemotherapy were compared, high-dose chemotherapy was associated with 10–40% higher 2-year PFS rates and 10–25% higher 5-year OS rates in almost all prognostic subgroups [44]. High-dose chemotherapy can be used as second-salvage treatment. The response rate was 55% with high-dose chemotherapy as second-salvage treatment in patients with multiple relapsed or refractory GCTs and remissions with a long-term survival rate was approximately 17% [45].

In patients who are resistant or refractory to cisplatin-based or high-dose salvage chemotherapy, several drugs such as gemcitabine, oxaliplatin, paclitaxel, and oral low-dose etoposide as single agent or combination were associated with response rates of up to 20–50% mostly based on data from phase II trials [3]. Gemcitabine plus paclitaxel and gemcitabine plus oxaliplatin are the most common preferred combinations for palliative treatment of metastatic refractory GCTs [46–48].

Conclusion

Single-agent carboplatin, rather than a cisplatin-based combination, has been used for stage I seminoma because it is associated with less toxicity than cisplatin-based regimens. The treatment approach for patients with advanced disease depends on the IGCCCG risk classification. Conventional-dose chemotherapy and high-dose chemotherapy can be used successfully as salvage treatment for patients with metastatic GCTs after progression with first-line treatment.

References

1. Siegel RL, Miller KD, Jemal A. Cancer statistics, 2016. CA Cancer J Clin. 2016;66(1):7–30.
2. Conkey DS, Howard GC, Grigor KM, et al. Testicular sex cord-stromal tumours: the Edinburgh experience 1988–2002, and a review of the literature. Clin Oncol (R Coll Radiol). 2005;17(5):322–7.
3. Rajpert-De Meyts E, McGlynn KA, Okamoto K, et al. Testicular germ cell tumours. Lancet. 2016;387(10029):1762–74.
4. Hanna NH, Einhorn LH. Testicular cancer–discoveries and updates. N Engl J Med. 2014;371(21):2005–16.
5. Hanna N, Einhorn LH. Testicular cancer: a reflection on 50 years of discovery. J Clin Oncol. 2014;32(28):3085–92.
6. International Germ Cell Consensus Classification: a prognostic factor-based staging system for metastatic germ cell cancers. International germ cell cancer collaborative group. J Clin Oncol. 1997;15(2):594–603.
7. Jones G, Arthurs B, Kaya H, et al. Overall survival analysis of adjuvant radiation versus observation in stage I testicular seminoma: a surveillance, epidemiology, and end results (SEER) analysis. Am J Clin Oncol. 2013;36(5):500–4.
8. Warde P, Specht L, Horwich A, et al. Prognostic factors for relapse in stage I seminoma managed by surveillance: a pooled analysis. J Clin Oncol. 2002;20(22):4448–52.
9. Kollmannsberger C, Tandstad T, Bedard PL, et al. Patterns of relapse in patients with clinical stage I testicular cancer managed with active surveillance. J Clin Oncol. 2015;33(1):51–7.
10. Mortensen MS, Lauritsen J, Gundgaard MG, et al. A nationwide cohort study of stage I seminoma patients followed on a surveillance program. Eur Urol. 2014;66(6):1172–8.
11. Daugaard G, Gundgaard MG, Mortensen MS, et al. Surveillance for stage I nonseminoma testicular cancer: outcomes and long-term follow-up in a population-based cohort. J Clin Oncol. 2014;32(34):3817–23.
12. Oliver RT, Mason MD, Mead GM, et al. Radiotherapy versus single-dose carboplatin in adjuvant treatment of stage I seminoma: a randomised trial. Lancet. 2005;366(9482):293–300.
13. Oliver RT, Mead GM, Rustin GJ, et al. Randomized trial of carboplatin versus radiotherapy for stage I seminoma: mature results on relapse and contralateral testis cancer rates in MRC TE19/EORTC 30982 study (ISRCTN27163214). J Clin Oncol. 2011;29(8):957–62.
14. Albers P, Siener R, Krege S, et al. Randomized phase III trial comparing retroperitoneal lymph node dissection with one course of bleomycin and etoposide plus cisplatin chemotherapy in the adjuvant treatment of clinical stage I Nonseminomatous testicular germ cell tumors: AUO trial AH 01/94 by the German Testicular Cancer Study Group. J Clin Oncol. 2008;26(18):2966–72.
15. Tandstad T, Dahl O, Cohn-Cedermark G, et al. Risk-adapted treatment in clinical stage I nonseminomatous germ cell testicular cancer: the SWENOTECA management program. J Clin Oncol. 2009;27(13):2122–8.
16. Tandstad T, Stahl O, Hakansson U, et al. One course of adjuvant BEP in clinical stage I nonseminoma mature and expanded results from the SWENOTECA group. Ann Oncol. 2014;25(11):2167–72.

17. Heidenreich A, Pfister D. Retroperitoneal lymphadenectomy and resection for testicular cancer: an update on best practice. Ther Adv Urol. 2012;4(4):187–205.
18. Chovanec M, Hanna N, Cary KC, et al. Management of stage I testicular germ cell tumours. Nat Rev Urol. 2016;13(11):663–73.
19. Oldenburg J, Fossa SD, Nuver J, et al. Testicular seminoma and non-seminoma: ESMO Clinical Practice Guidelines for diagnosis, treatment and follow-up. Ann Oncol. 2013;24(Suppl 6):vi125–32.
20. Motzer RJ, Jonasch E, Agarwal N, et al. Testicular cancer, version 2.2015. J Natl Compr Canc Netw. 2015;13(6):772–99.
21. Beard CJ, Gupta S, Motzer RJ, et al. Follow-up management of patients with testicular cancer: a multidisciplinary consensus-based approach. J Natl Compr Canc Netw. 2015;13(6):811–22.
22. Classen J, Schmidberger H, Meisner C, et al. Radiotherapy for stages IIA/B testicular seminoma: final report of a prospective multicenter clinical trial. J Clin Oncol. 2003;21(6):1101–6.
23. Domont J, Massard C, Patrikidou A, et al. A risk-adapted strategy of radiotherapy or cisplatin-based chemotherapy in stage II seminoma. Urol Oncol. 2013;31(5):697–705.
24. Garcia-del-Muro X, Maroto P, Guma J, et al. Chemotherapy as an alternative to radiotherapy in the treatment of stage IIA and IIB testicular seminoma: a Spanish germ cell cancer group study. J Clin Oncol. 2008;26(33):5416–21.
25. De Santis M, Becherer A, Bokemeyer C, et al. 2-18fluoro-deoxy-D-glucose positron emission tomography is a reliable predictor for viable tumor in postchemotherapy seminoma: an update of the prospective multicentric SEMPET trial. J Clin Oncol. 2004;22(6):1034–9.
26. Culine S, Kerbrat P, Kramar A, et al. Refining the optimal chemotherapy regimen for good-risk metastatic nonseminomatous germ-cell tumors: a randomized trial of the Genito-Urinary Group of the French Federation of Cancer Centers (GETUG T93BP). Ann Oncol. 2007;18(5):917–24.
27. Ehrlich Y, Brames MJ, Beck SD, et al. Long-term follow-up of Cisplatin combination chemotherapy in patients with disseminated nonseminomatous germ cell tumors: is a postchemotherapy retroperitoneal lymph node dissection needed after complete remission? J Clin Oncol. 2010;28(4):531–6.
28. Ravi P, Gray KP, O'Donnell EK, et al. A meta-analysis of patient outcomes with subcentimeter disease after chemotherapy for metastatic non-seminomatous germ cell tumor. Ann Oncol. 2014;25(2):331–8.
29. Motzer RJ, Sheinfeld J, Mazumdar M, et al. Etoposide and cisplatin adjuvant therapy for patients with pathologic stage II germ cell tumors. J Clin Oncol. 1995;13(11):2700–4.
30. de Wit R, Roberts JT, Wilkinson PM, et al. Equivalence of three or four cycles of bleomycin, etoposide, and cisplatin chemotherapy and of a 3- or 5-day schedule in good-prognosis germ cell cancer: a randomized study of the European Organization for Research and Treatment of Cancer Genitourinary Tract Cancer Cooperative Group and the Medical Research Council. J Clin Oncol. 2001;19(6):1629–40.
31. Klepp O, Flodgren P, Maartman-Moe H, et al. Early clinical stages (CS1, CS1Mk+ and CS2A) of non-seminomatous testis cancer. Value of pre- and post-orchiectomy serum tumor marker information in prediction of retroperitoneal lymph node metastases. Swedish-Norwegian Testicular Cancer Project (SWENOTECA). Ann Oncol. 1990;1(4):281–8.
32. Bokemeyer C, Kohrmann O, Tischler J, et al. A randomized trial of cisplatin, etoposide and bleomycin (PEB) versus carboplatin, etoposide and bleomycin (CEB) for patients with 'good-risk' metastatic non-seminomatous germ cell tumors. Ann Oncol. 1996;7(10):1015–21.
33. Williams SD, Birch R, Einhorn LH, et al. Treatment of disseminated germ-cell tumors with cisplatin, bleomycin, and either vinblastine or etoposide. N Engl J Med. 1987;316(23):1435–40.
34. Massard C, Plantade A, Gross-Goupil M, et al. Poor prognosis nonseminomatous germ-cell tumours (NSGCTs): should chemotherapy doses be reduced at first cycle to prevent acute respiratory distress syndrome in patients with multiple lung metastases? Ann Oncol. 2010;21(8):1585–8.
35. Nichols CR, Catalano PJ, Crawford ED, et al. Randomized comparison of cisplatin and etoposide and either bleomycin or ifosfamide in treatment of advanced disseminated germ cell

tumors: an Eastern Cooperative Oncology Group, Southwest Oncology Group, and Cancer and Leukemia Group B Study. J Clin Oncol. 1998;16(4):1287–93.
36. Hinton S, Catalano PJ, Einhorn LH, et al. Cisplatin, etoposide and either bleomycin or ifosfamide in the treatment of disseminated germ cell tumors: final analysis of an intergroup trial. Cancer. 2003;97(8):1869–75.
37. Motzer RJ, Nichols CJ, Margolin KA, et al. Phase III randomized trial of conventional-dose chemotherapy with or without high-dose chemotherapy and autologous hematopoietic stem-cell rescue as first-line treatment for patients with poor-prognosis metastatic germ cell tumors. J Clin Oncol. 2007;25(3):247–56.
38. Daugaard G, Skoneczna I, Aass N, et al. A randomized phase III study comparing standard dose BEP with sequential high-dose cisplatin, etoposide, and ifosfamide (VIP) plus stem-cell support in males with poor-prognosis germ-cell cancer. An intergroup study of EORTC, GTCSG, and Grupo Germinal (EORTC 30974). Ann Oncol. 2011;22(5):1054–61.
39. Fizazi K, Pagliaro L, Laplanche A, et al. Personalised chemotherapy based on tumour marker decline in poor prognosis germ-cell tumours (GETUG 13): a phase 3, multicentre, randomised trial. Lancet Oncol. 2014;15(13):1442–50.
40. International Prognostic Factors Study Group, Lorch A, Beyer J, et al. Prognostic factors in patients with metastatic germ cell tumors who experienced treatment failure with cisplatin-based first-line chemotherapy. J Clin Oncol. 2010;28(33):4906–11.
41. Loehrer PJ Sr, Lauer R, Roth BJ, et al. Salvage therapy in recurrent germ cell cancer: ifosfamide and cisplatin plus either vinblastine or etoposide. Ann Intern Med. 1988;109(7):540–6.
42. Kondagunta GV, Bacik J, Donadio A, et al. Combination of paclitaxel, ifosfamide, and cisplatin is an effective second-line therapy for patients with relapsed testicular germ cell tumors. J Clin Oncol. 2005;23(27):6549–55.
43. Pico JL, Rosti G, Kramar A, et al. A randomised trial of high-dose chemotherapy in the salvage treatment of patients failing first-line platinum chemotherapy for advanced germ cell tumours. Ann Oncol. 2005;16(7):1152–9.
44. Lorch A, Bascoul-Mollevi C, Kramar A, et al. Conventional-dose versus high-dose chemotherapy as first salvage treatment in male patients with metastatic germ cell tumors: evidence from a large international database. J Clin Oncol. 2011;29(16):2178–84.
45. Lorch A, Neubauer A, Hackenthal M, et al. High-dose chemotherapy (HDCT) as second-salvage treatment in patients with multiple relapsed or refractory germ-cell tumors. Ann Oncol. 2010;21(4):820–5.
46. De Giorgi U, G. Rosti, M. Aieta, et al. Phase II study of oxaliplatin and gemcitabine salvage chemotherapy in patients with cisplatin-refractory nonseminomatous germ cell tumor. Eur Urol. 2006;50(5):1032–8; discussion 1038–9.
47. Pectasides D, Pectasides M, Farmakis D, et al. Gemcitabine and oxaliplatin (GEMOX) in patients with cisplatin-refractory germ cell tumors: a phase II study. Ann Oncol. 2004;15(3):493–7.
48. Einhorn LH, Brames MJ, Juliar B, et al. Phase II study of paclitaxel plus gemcitabine salvage chemotherapy for germ cell tumors after progression following high-dose chemotherapy with tandem transplant. J Clin Oncol. 2007;25(5):513–6.

9 Post-chemotherapy Retroperitoneal Lymph Node Dissection in Advanced Germ Cell Tumors

Bülent Akdoğan and Mesut Altan

Abstract

Post-chemotherapy retroperitoneal lymph node dissection (PC-RPLND) is considered an important therapeutic and staging modality in advanced germ cell tumors (GCTs). An important step to better define the boundaries of PC-RPLND is to define the site of extra-template disease. Modified template RPLND causes less complications and better quality of life parameters; however, bilateral full template surgery accomplishes improved staging and better oncological outcomes. Recent data shows that minimally invasive PC-RPLND has several limitations, so it is not proven oncologically yet. It's one of the most challenging surgeries in urology practice. PC-RPLND should be performed only in experienced centers since it's not only a difficult surgery associated with major complications but also it often requires implementation of additional major procedures for complete removal of residual masses. PC-RPLND is an integral part of the multidisciplinary management. Residual tumor surgery for advanced stage testicular tumors ends up with viable tumors in about 50% of cases.

9.1 Introduction

Although rare, the incidence of testis tumor shows significant differences between geographical areas. Between 1970 and 2004, the worldwide incidence raised from 2.1 to 5.1 per 100,000 [1]. This rise was much more evident in seminoma and localized disease [2, 3]. Of all, 95% of testis tumors are germ cell tumors (GCT) and are basically classified as seminoma and non-seminoma. At presentation, stage III

B. Akdoğan, M.D. (✉) • M. Altan, M.D.
Department of Urology, Faculty of Medicine, Hacettepe University, Ankara, Turkey
e-mail: blntakdogan@yahoo.com

G. Ozyigit, U. Selek (eds.), *Principles and Practice of Urooncology*,
DOI 10.1007/978-3-319-56114-1_9

disease was detected in 33% of non-seminomas and 5% of seminomas [2]. One of the cornerstones in treatment of testis tumor is the discovery of cisplatin-based chemotherapy; survival rate has reached 70% even for poor prognostic patients [4, 5]. Besides effective chemotherapy, radiotherapy, successful risk stratification of patients according to the *International Germ Cell Cancer Collaborative Group* (IGCCCG), and post-chemo surgery, all have made a major impact on survival as a multidisciplinary team approach.

Improvement in PC-RPLND surgical technique, better understanding of retroperitoneal lymphatic drainage, enhanced comprehension of metastatic mechanisms, and clarification of indications, all those experiences caused reduced complications and improve oncological outcomes. For advanced GCTs, PC-RPLND maintains its worth and importance.

9.2 PC-RPLND for Advanced NSGCTs

Indications for PC-RPLND in NSGCTs are well defined and have significant advantages. One of the most important PC-RPLND arguments is the presence of about 15% live tumor after primary chemotherapy [6, 7] (Fig. 9.1). Live tumor in residual mass is an independent poor prognostic factor for recurrence-free survival [8]. In a study by Fizazi et al., better survival was associated with the presence of <10% live tumor, complete tumor resection, and IGCCCG low-risk group for patients with viable tumor after PC-RPLND [9]. Another study showed 5-year progression-free survival (PFS) rate for PC-RPLND patients was 65% [10]. Both studies emphasized that complete resection of residual masses was considered as significant prognostic parameter.

Post-chemo residual masses are teratomas in 40% of NSGCT cases [11]. In a study including 210 teratomas after PC-RPLND, the rate of mature teratomas, immature teratomas, and malignant transformation was 85, 7, and 8%, respectively [12]. Besides its chemo-resistant nature, teratomas are associated with debilitating

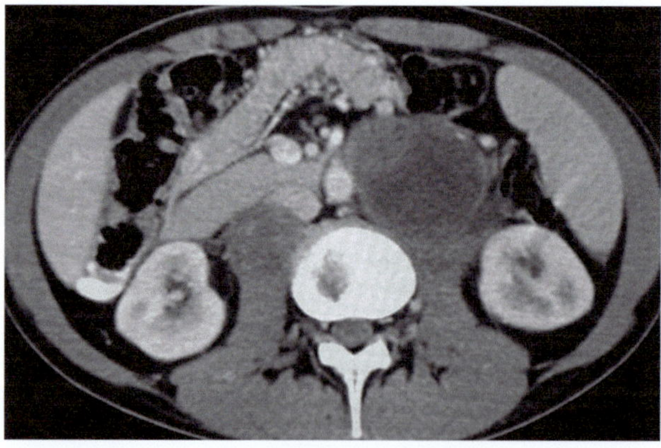

Fig. 9.1 Bilateral retroperitoneal metastasis of left testicular tumor, medializing aorta and vena cava

complications such as "growing teratoma syndrome" and malignant transformation. These findings and associated risks enlighten the importance of surgery [13–15].

Should we do PC-RPLND for all the patients? Computed tomography (CT) or magnetic resonance imaging (MRI) findings are inadequate to determine the presence of a viable tumor or teratoma [16, 17]. Kollmannsberger et al. evaluated residual mass viability in 85 masses in 45 patients and reported that FDG-PET scans had 59% sensitivity and 92% specificity [18]. A prospective study evaluated 60 residual tumors in 28 GCT patients after high-dose chemotherapy and concluded that PET seems useful in patients with stable disease or partial remission in CT/MRI and normal or marker-negative disease [19]. In another multicenter prospective study of 121 patients with stage IIC or III NSGCT, it was reported that sensitivity and specificity of FDG-PET were 70 and 48, respectively [20]. Prediction of tumor viability with FDG-PET was correct in 56% and was not better than the accuracy of CT (55%) or markers.

Various models were constructed to better decide usefulness of either immediate resection of a residual mass or follow-up. Steyerberg et al. developed a statistical model predicting the histology necrosis, mature teratoma, or cancer after chemotherapy. Predictors of necrosis were defined as the absence of teratoma elements in the primary tumor, pre-chemo normal alpha-fetoprotein (AFP), normal human chorionic gonadotropin (HCG) and elevated lactate dehydrogenase (LDH) levels, small pre- or post-chemotherapy mass, and large shrinkage of the mass during chemotherapy [21]. This model was updated in 2007 to select patients for surgery, particularly for patients with small residual masses and low predicted probabilities of benign tissue [22].

In NSGCTs, PET scan has no superiority over CT or tumor markers. Besides, the designed models are inadequate to predict histology. Of 276 post-chemo NSGCT patients, Kollmannsberger et al. reported that 161 achieved radiographic complete remission (CR) defined as minimal residual tissue ≤1 cm [23]. Eight of the ten relapses in the CR group were treated surgically for teratoma alone, whereas two required salvage chemotherapy. Disease-specific survival for the CR group was 100% after a median follow-up of 52 months. In another retrospective study, 141 NSGCT patients who achieved a CR to first-line chemotherapy were observed without further therapy [24]. Relapse was detected in 12 patients (9%) after a median 15.5-year follow-up. Six relapses were in the retroperitoneum. Of these 12 patients, only four died of the disease. The estimated 15-year recurrence-free survival (RFS) and cancer-specific survival rates were 90 and 97%, respectively. Toner et al. reported results of ≤1.5 cm residual retroperitoneal masses in 39 patients. They had only three residual viable tumors and five teratomas resected [16]. They've recommended RPLND for all patients with initial bulky retroperitoneal metastases (≥3 cm in diameter) irrespective of post-chemotherapy CT findings. On the contrary, Carver et al. analyzed the results of 532 post-chemo RPLND cases and reported 40% teratoma rate and 11% of them had post-chemo residual mass smaller than 1 cm [11].

For PC-RPLND, marker normalization is required first. The marker that is elevated after chemotherapy is directly related to the presence of viable tumor. However, the expected time for marker normalization may prolong in patients with very high HCG levels before chemotherapy. Marker decrease is expected in the presence of plateau marker after post-chemotherapy. Cystic teratoma may also cause elevated but stable marker level. In the presence of plateau but not rising marker levels after chemotherapy, RPLND is a treatment option [25].

Post-chemo residual tumor resection is performed for viable tumor or teratoma histologies in NSGCT. Those are detected in about 50% of stage IIC and higher stages. Today, there is no imaging or laboratory method predicting final pathology with a high accuracy. As a conclusion, post-chemo surgery is recommended to all residual masses larger than 1 cm [20, 26–28]. Another important data shows us that there is 6–9% relapse rate in masses smaller than 1 cm when observed [23, 24].

9.3 PC-RPLND for Advanced Seminoma

Although the risk of teratoma and malign transformation in seminomas is less worrying and in case of viable tumor the surgery is less effective on outcomes, PC-RPLND is still an important treatment option in seminoma treatment [29]. Similarly, post-chemo RT has no place in seminoma.

The tumor size in post-chemo seminoma has prognostic importance. Flechon et al. reported 13% of 79 patients had viable tumor on final pathology and all had residual masses larger than 3 cm in preoperative imaging [30]. Similarly Hofmockel et al. found one viable seminoma case in ten PC-RPLND patients whose residual mass was 5 cm in preoperative imaging [31]. Herr et al. studied 55 seminoma patients and noticed that only 30% (8/27) of patients with 3 cm or larger residual mass on CT had viable tumor (six seminomas and two teratomas) [32]. No viable tumor was detected in masses smaller than 3 cm. Although PC-RPLND lowers recurrence in cases with viable tumor, there is similar recurrence rate between both viable tumor and necrosis pathology. Puc et al. assessed 104 advanced seminoma patients who had achieved a complete response or partial response to induction cisplatin-based chemotherapy [33]. Their results on RPLND were assessed and correlated with pre-chemotherapy and post-chemotherapy characteristics. They found that two of 74 patients (3%) with residual masses less than 3 cm were considered site failures (had viable tumor on RPLND), compared with eight of 30 (27%) with residual masses > or = 3 cm.

Ganjoo et al. studied 29 advanced seminoma patients with post-chemotherapy residual masses and concluded that PET scans have no apparent benefit in PC evaluation of residual masses in bulky seminoma [34]. Another study analyzed the results of 37 seminoma patients and reported the cutoff point for PET scan to be 3 cm [35]. De Santis et al. analyzed the results of 56 patients with pure seminoma with post-chemo residual masses [36]. Only two patients with residual mass less than 3 cm had false-negative results. Positive predictive value was 100%. PET scans should be scheduled 6–8 weeks after chemotherapy. Three cm is the accepted cutoff size for PET scan. 2-18fluoro-deoxy-D-glucose FDG PET is the best predictor of viable residual tumor in post-chemotherapy seminoma residuals.

9.4 RPLND Borders

In the middle of the twentieth century, RPLND started having superiority over orchiectomy and RT [37]. In the 1960s, with the use of lymphangiography, it was shown that testis lymphatics drain to suprahilar LNs, and right testis lymphatics may drain to the left and vice versa [38]. Initially, extended dissection bypassed suprahilar LNs and included paracaval, precaval, para-aortic, preaortic, interaorta-caval, and common iliac regions. Ray and Whitmore retrospectively analyzed the location of retroperitoneal lymph node metastasis of 283 patients who underwent RPLND [39]. They found that lymphatic metastasis was to the left side of para-aortic area in case of left-sided tumor and to variable locations in case of right-sided tumor. Donohue et al., in their study of 104 stage II patients, demonstrated that lymphatic metastasis from right-sided tumor was to interaortacaval nodes followed by precaval and preaortic nodes while in case of left-sided tumors was to para-aortic and preaortic areas followed by interaortacaval [40]. Weissbach and Boedefeld evaluated 214 consecutive patients with stage II disease (excluding bulky disease) with respect to localization relative to the side of the relative testis [41]. Solitary nodes of the right-sided and left-sided tumors were primarily located in the interaortacaval and para-aortic areas, respectively. Testicular Tumor Study Group suggests specific template RPLND which includes paracaval, precaval, interaortacaval, preaortic, and ipsilateral ileac dissection for right-sided testis tumors and preaortic and para-aortic LND for left-sided tumors. These modified templates catch 95% of metastatic LNs. As these studies lack long-term results, it's hard to determine the true localization and ratio of recurrence. Here in the figure, you can see para-aortic and left parailiac metastasis of right testicular tumor (Fig. 9.2).

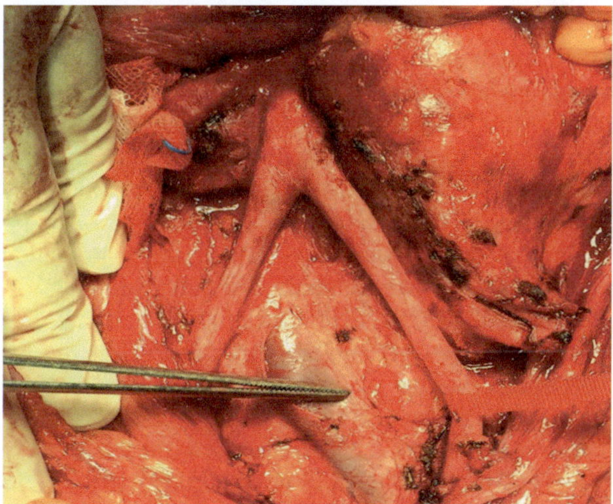

Fig. 9.2 Left parailiac and para-aortic metastasis of right testicular tumor

The sympathetic nerves originate from thoracic and upper lumbar areas synapse with paravertebral and hypogastric ganglions. Then, they spread to the pelvic organs along with the epigastric and presacral fibers. That's why ejaculation and fertility could be affected negatively by RPLND. In the early 1980s, Narayan et al. reported that 50% of patients had normal spontaneous ejaculation postoperatively [42]. This considered the start point for RPLND. In the same decade, Donohue et al. studied 75 patients, most of whom had stage I, and found that most of them had postoperative normal antegrade ejaculation [43]. Heidenreich et al. published the results of 152 PC-RPLND with median follow-up of 39 months [44]. Modified template RPLND was done to 98 patients with a mass less or equal to 5 cm in the primary landing zone. Radical template RPLND was done to the other 54 patients. Antegrade ejaculation was preserved in 85 and 25% of patients undergoing modified and bilateral PC-RPLND, respectively. Only one of the eight recurrences documented was in the modified group. Although short follow-up period and radical type being done to large masses limit these results, in well-defined masses, a modified template PC-RPLND does not interfere with oncologic outcome but decreases treatment-associated morbidity [45]. The main mechanism by which modified template RPLND prevents nerve injury is the limited dissection on the other side. The surgeon's effort to identify, dissect, and preserve sympathetic nerves is also essential. By this way, nerve-sparing intervention is a choice even for patients who undergo full template RPLND. Researchers suggested electrostimulation for intraoperative sympathetic nerve identification [46]. One should never forget about oncological principles while preserving nerves in testis cancer surgery.

9.5 Limitations of Modified Template RPLND

The most important argument for the use of modified templates is "the lower risk of other side lymphatic metastases, easier surgery when limited dissection, and lower complication rates." Most of these techniques were initially defined for stage I disease. Later, especially with the advance in effective chemotherapy, they've preferred for advanced stages too. The absence of long-term follow-up periods in mapping studies considered a major limitation for these techniques [39, 40]. If resected specimens are sent to pathology laboratories in different bags, it would be helpful for pathologists to correctly stage extra-template disease (Fig. 9.3).

Carver et al. studied 532 PC-RPLND cases [47]. Of all, 269 had either viable tumor or teratoma and 7–32% had extra-template disease. The most common extra-template area was interaortacaval and paracaval location for left-sided tumors and preaortic and para-aortic region for right-sided tumors. Residual mass size was reported to be the most significant indicator for extra-template disease. For residual masses larger than 5 cm, the incidence was as high as 25%. Another study including 500 cases has shown 1–11% and 5–33% risk of extra-template disease for pN1 and pN2/3 stages, respectively [48]. Extra-template disease risk for 191 pathological

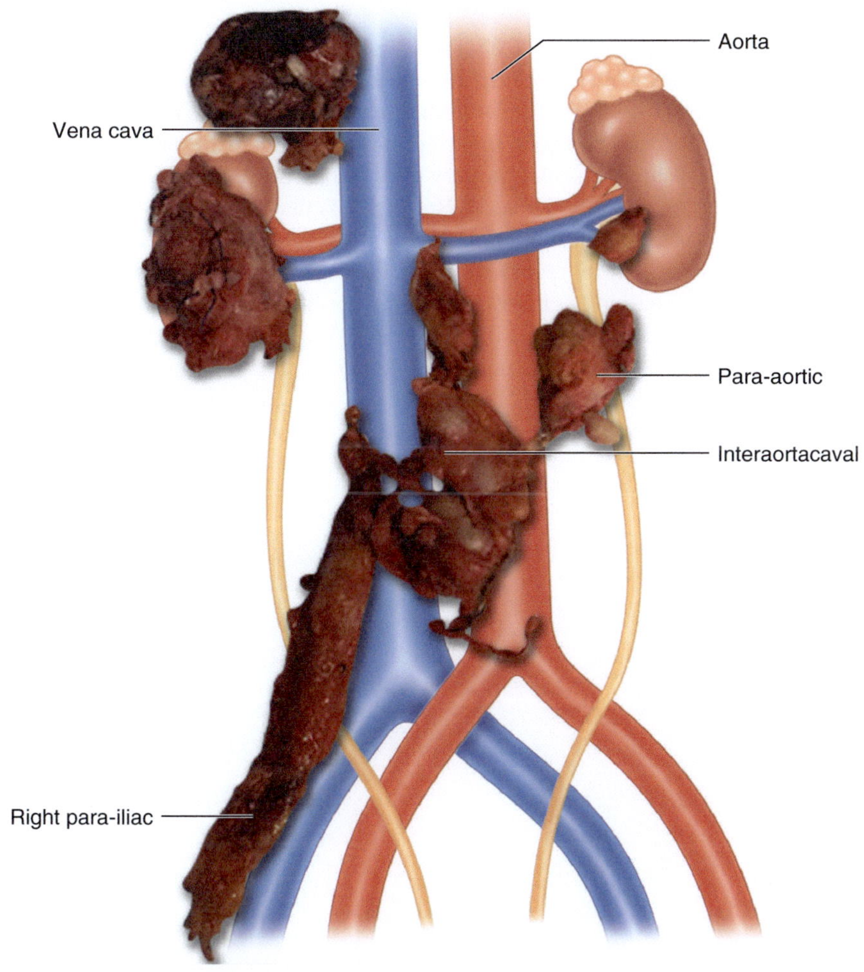

Fig. 9.3 Resected specimens sent to the pathology in different bags

stage II patients was reported to be 3–23%. The incidence was decreased to 2–3% by inclusion of para-aortic, preaortic, and right common iliac regions to right-side templates and by inclusion of interaortacaval, precaval, paracaval, and left common iliac regions to left-side templates.

Another important issue is the impact of size and number of excised lymph nodes on survival. Carver et al. found that increasing post-chemo nodal size and decreasing lymph node counts were significant predictors of recurrence in 628 PC-RPLND cases. The 2-year RFS rates for >10, >30, and >50 lymph nodes were 90, 95, and 97%, respectively [49].

9.6 Open PC-RPLND

Thoracoabdominal approach is a choice when easy access is required to reach suprahilar lymphatics. On the other hand, transabdominal approach is fast and relatively easy to do and offers good accessibility to both sides. In the last years, midline extraperitoneal approach has been reported in small number of patients. Donohue defined RPLND to be a vascular surgery [50]. After opening anterior abdominal wall and peritoneum, using a retractor (Bookwalter) may help getting a good look. After that, by opening the posterior peritoneum from inferior to IMA area, retroperitoneum anatomy will be revealed. Dissection in the defined borders is usually done by lymphatic ligation or clipping. For large residual masses or in case of surgical difficulties, IMA could be sacrificed in order to expose para-aortic and left renal hilus area. Here in the figure, the aorta and vena cava are demonstrated; the para-aortic lymph nodes are removed. Interaortocaval and paracaval lymph nodes are ready for excision (Fig. 9.4).

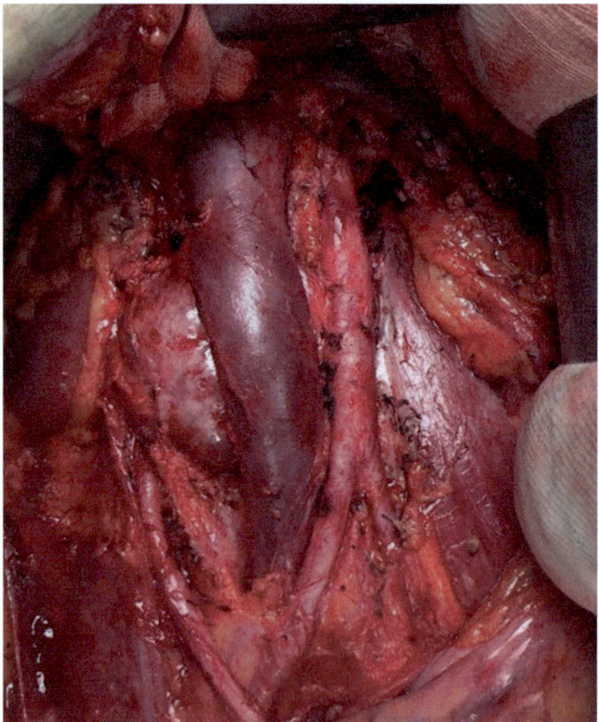

Fig. 9.4 Paracaval and interaortacaval lymph nodes ready for excision

9.7 Minimally Invasive PC-RPLND

Laparoscopic RPLND (L-RPLND) has been restricted since desmoplastic reaction caused by chemotherapy. Besides, instead of mass resection, bilateral templates are recommended techniques for RPLND that makes it much more complicated for laparoscopy. But it could be performed with acceptable results in low-stage tumors in experienced hands [51–53]. In a study including only seven patients, two cases were converted to open surgery, and three had major complications [54]. Rassweiler et al. reported seven conversions to open surgery in nine L-PC-RPLND cases [55]. As a result, L-PC-RPLND is not a self-proven technique and could only be done in large centers with experienced hands [56]. Robot-assisted primary RPLND is reported in limited number of cases [57].

9.8 Complications

Chemotherapy distorts the surgical plane between lymph nodes and surrounding tissues by causing desmoplastic reactions. In order to have a complete resection, there is 20–33% risk of additional procedure implementation that generally includes major vessel repair and nephrectomy [44, 58–61] (Fig. 9.5). Other additional surgeries are splenectomy, pancreatic resection, hepatic resection, and bowel resection with or without stoma. Nah et al. reported that of 848 PC-RPLND cases, 19% had en bloc nephrectomy, and of all 73% had prerenal structural

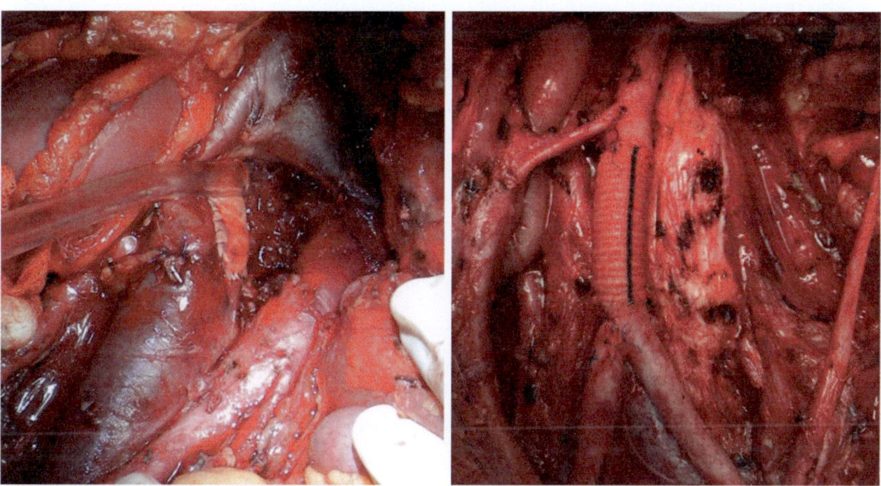

Fig. 9.5 Vena cava patch on left side and aortic graft distal to the inferior mesenteric artery on right side

involvement [61]. Nephrectomy risk is correlated with residual mass size and advanced stage disease.

Some studies reported that PC-RPLND compared with primary RPLND has longer surgical time, more bleeding, longer hospitalization time, and more additional procedure including nephrectomy, caval repair, bowel resection, and thrombectomy [62, 63]. These results are related mainly to the desmoplastic reaction; besides, primary RPLND is done in patients with lower stages.

Baniel et al. defined 144 complications established in 125 cases in their series of 603 PC-RPLND patients (20.7%). Of all, 93% had residual mass ≥ 5 cm, and overall mortality rate was 0.8% [64]. Pulmonary complications were most common because of bleomycin-related pulmonary toxicity and additional pulmonary procedures. Cary et al. reported 22.1% additional procedure and 3.7% complication rate [65]. Additional procedure rate was associated with mass size, high serum markers, and RPLND pathology.

Bleomycin toxicity-related ARDS is a mortal complication [66]. Another complication is chile ascites generally seen along with caval resection [67]. Meticulous clipping or ligation of lymphatic vessels is the most important approach to prevent this complication. Percutaneous drainage is required for symptomatic lymphoceles like compression-related hydronephrosis, bowel obstruction, pain, or infection.

In post-chemo seminomas incomplete resection rate is high due to the difficult dissection caused by the intense desmoplastic reaction [30, 68, 69]. In a study including 97 seminoma and 1269 NSGCT cases, additional procedure and complication rates were 38.1 and 24.7% in seminoma and 26.8 and 20.3% in NSGCTs [68].

The most important care to prevent complications is to perform surgery in experienced centers by expert hands. In a study of 993 patients who underwent PC-RPLND in different centers, those who were operated in higher volume centers had less complications, more transfusion rates, and higher cost [70]. These results may be attributed to the fact that more complex cases are seen in higher volume centers. Mosharafa et al. compared his PC-RPLND results in different time periods and reported that patients who underwent the procedure between 2000 and 2002 had fewer complications, fewer additional procedures, and shorter hospital stay than in the period between 1990 and 1992 [56].

9.9 PC-RPLND Pathology

PC-RPLND pathology has paramount importance for the prognosis and adjuvant treatment setting. The presence of viable tumor or teratoma in RPLND specimen is detected in about 50% of all cases. Carver et al. reported 49% fibrosis, 11% viable tumor (±teratoma), and 39% only teratoma in his 504 NSGCT cases [6]. Current literature reveals the rates of necrosis/fibrosis, viable malignancy (±teratoma), and only teratoma were identified in 25–52%, 9–31%, and 27–67%, respectively, in PC-RPLND pathology [26, 71–74]. Fizazi et al. studied prognostic factors in 238 viable tumor cases [9] and have shown that IGCCCG intermediate- or high-risk group, >10% viable tumor, and incomplete resection were independent poor prognostic factors. 5-year progression-free survival (PFS) rates for patients with no risk factors, with one risk factor, and with two or more risk factors were 100, 83, and 51%, respectively. Although the PFS was better in patients who received postoperative chemotherapy compared to the patients who had not, there was no significant difference in 5-year OS rates. These results were verified by a contemporary study published in 2008 [10]. With a median follow-up of 5.4 years, it was clear that postoperative chemotherapy patients did not have better OS compared to the patients under surveillance and treatment at relapse.

Fox et al. reported viable tumor was detected in 43 of 417 PC-RPLND cases [75]. Of 34 patients who had complete resection, 27 had adjuvant chemotherapy and 7 did not. The patients who had adjuvant chemo had 70% survival; however, all the patients who didn't have chemo recurred in a median 84-month follow-up.

After primary chemotherapy, 34 of 43 had complete resections, and 27 of the 34 received postoperative cisplatin-based chemotherapy. Nineteen of 27 (70%) were continuously disease-free. All seven who received no postoperative chemotherapy have relapsed.

There is no need for additional treatment in case of teratoma in PC-RPLND. But it usually recurs as mature/immature teratoma or sarcomatoid tumor, which usually has poor prognosis [71, 76]. Growing teratoma syndrome should be considered in case of negative tumor markers with enlarging residual mass during chemotherapy. Patients with incomplete resection in PC-RPLND have higher recurrence rates [77].

9.10 RPLND After Salvage Chemotherapy

Although the data about the role of RPLND in patients receiving salvage chemotherapy is conflicting, evidence suggests that complete resection would always cause finest staging and improved survival. Of all, 10% of advanced GCTs fail to respond primary chemotherapy [72, 74]. Viable tumor rates of patients who underwent RPLND after salvage chemotherapy were reported to be 50% [71, 75, 78]. Complete resection is possible in about 50–70% of cases, and 5-year survival rate is roughly 45–60% [28, 75, 79, 80].

Eggener et al. published the results of 71 patients who underwent RPLND after two or more chemotherapy regimens [80]. Viable tumor, teratoma, and fibrosis rates were 28, 21, and 51%, respectively. Patients who received taxane-containing salvage chemotherapy regimens had lower rates of viable tumor (14 vs. 42%; $p = 0.01$), higher rates of fibrosis (63 vs. 39%; $p = 0.04$), and similar rates of teratoma compared to regimens without taxane. It was found that second-line taxane-containing chemotherapy reduces viable tumor rates. The presence of large retroperitoneal mass (≥5 cm) and viable tumor were predictors of worse 10-year disease-specific survival (DSS) (70%). All these results support RPLND—with complete resection done as possible—in select patients after salvage chemotherapy.

9.11 Desperation Surgery

Desperation surgery is performed when tumor markers are rising in spite of chemotherapy. It's considered an important treatment choice especially in patients with retroperitoneal resectable disease without other visceral metastasis. Albers et al. reported overall persistent viable cancer, and teratomatous elements were identified in 64 and 11% of cases, respectively, in 30 patients [81]. Beck et al. performed desperation surgery in 114 patients with persistent serum tumor markers after second-line chemotherapy. Elevated markers, redo RPLND, and germ cell cancer in the resected specimen were identified as poor prognostic factors. 5-year overall survival was reported as 54% [82]. As a conclusion, surgery has critical importance especially in patients with solitary resectable tumors and rising markers despite salvage chemotherapy.

Conclusion

PC-RPLND is an essential treatment modality performed for all NSGCT and PET (+) seminoma residual masses with normal/plateau serum markers in multidisciplinary approach. Final pathology reveals viable tumor for NSGCT and seminoma in almost 15 and 10%, respectively. Desperation surgery for patients with rising serum markers despite multiple chemotherapy regimens promises reasonable survival rates. In case of teratoma, complete resection PC-RPLND is the curative treatment. Although modified templates cause less complications and less retrograde ejaculation, bilateral full templates promise better oncological outcomes. This challenging surgery necessitates implementation of additional procedures in one fifth of all procedures, so this should be done in only experienced centers. Although chemotherapy is the initial treatment modality for advanced stage testicular cancers, residual tumor surgery is the integral part and the last step in multimodal treatment.

References

1. Holmes L Jr, Escalante C, Garrison O, Foldi BX, Ogungbade GO, Essien EJ, et al. Testicular cancer incidence trends in the USA (1975–2004): plateau or shifting racial paradigm? Public Health. 2008;122(9):862–72.
2. Powles TB, Bhardwa J, Shamash J, Mandalia S, Oliver T. The changing presentation of germ cell tumours of the testis between 1983 and 2002. BJU Int. 2005;95(9):1197–200.
3. McGlynn KA, Devesa SS, Graubard BI, Castle PE. Increasing incidence of testicular germ cell tumors among black men in the United States. J Clin Oncol. 2005;23(24):5757–61.
4. Einhorn LH. Treatment of testicular cancer: a new and improved model. J Clin Oncol. 1990;8(11):1777–81.
5. van Dijk MR, Steyerberg EW, Habbema JD. Survival of non-seminomatous germ cell cancer patients according to the IGCC classification: an update based on meta-analysis. Eur J Cancer. 2006;42(7):820–6.
6. Carver BS, Serio AM, Bajorin D, Motzer RJ, Stasi J, Bosl GJ, et al. Improved clinical outcome in recent years for men with metastatic nonseminomatous germ cell tumors. J Clin Oncol. 2007;25(35):5603–8.

7. Spiess PE, Brown GA, Pisters LL, Liu P, Tu SM, Evans JG, et al. Viable malignant germ cell tumor in the postchemotherapy retroperitoneal lymph node dissection specimen: can it be predicted using clinical parameters? Cancer. 2006;107(7):1503–10.
8. Spiess PE, Brown GA, Liu P, Tannir NM, Tu SM, Evans JG, et al. Predictors of outcome in patients undergoing postchemotherapy retroperitoneal lymph node dissection for testicular cancer. Cancer. 2006;107(7):1483–90.
9. Fizazi K, Tjulandin S, Salvioni R, Germa-Lluch JR, Bouzy J, Ragan D, et al. Viable malignant cells after primary chemotherapy for disseminated nonseminomatous germ cell tumors: prognostic factors and role of postsurgery chemotherapy–results from an international study group. J Clin Oncol. 2001;19(10):2647–57.
10. Fizazi K, Oldenburg J, Dunant A, Chen I, Salvioni R, Hartmann JT, et al. Assessing prognosis and optimizing treatment in patients with postchemotherapy viable nonseminomatous germ-cell tumors (NSGCT): results of the sCR2 international study. Ann Oncol. 2008;19(2):259–64.
11. Carver BS, Bianco FJ Jr, Shayegan B, Vickers A, Motzer RJ, Bosl GJ, et al. Predicting teratoma in the retroperitoneum in men undergoing post-chemotherapy retroperitoneal lymph node dissection. J Urol. 2006;176(1):100–3; discussion 3–4.
12. Carver BS, Shayegan B, Serio A, Motzer RJ, Bosl GJ, Sheinfeld J. Long-term clinical outcome after postchemotherapy retroperitoneal lymph node dissection in men with residual teratoma. J Clin Oncol. 2007;25(9):1033–7.
13. Andre F, Fizazi K, Culine S, Droz J, Taupin P, Lhomme C, et al. The growing teratoma syndrome: results of therapy and long-term follow-up of 33 patients. Eur J Cancer. 2000;36(11): 1389–94.
14. El Mesbahi O, Terrier-Lacombe MJ, Rebischung C, Theodore C, Vanel D, Fizazi K. Chemotherapy in patients with teratoma with malignant transformation. Eur Urol. 2007;51(5):1306–11; discussion 11–2.
15. Donadio AC, Motzer RJ, Bajorin DF, Kantoff PW, Sheinfeld J, Houldsworth J, et al. Chemotherapy for teratoma with malignant transformation. J Clin Oncol. 2003;21(23):4285–91.
16. Toner GC, Panicek DM, Heelan RT, Geller NL, Lin SY, Bajorin D, et al. Adjunctive surgery after chemotherapy for nonseminomatous germ cell tumors: recommendations for patient selection. J Clin Oncol. 1990;8(10):1683–94.
17. Stomper PC, Kalish LA, Garnick MB, Richie JP, Kantoff PW. CT and pathologic predictive features of residual mass histologic findings after chemotherapy for nonseminomatous germ cell tumors: can residual malignancy or teratoma be excluded? Radiology. 1991;180(3): 711–4.
18. Kollmannsberger C, Oechsle K, Dohmen BM, Pfannenberg A, Bares R, Claussen CD, et al. Prospective comparison of [18F]fluorodeoxyglucose positron emission tomography with conventional assessment by computed tomography scans and serum tumor markers for the evaluation of residual masses in patients with nonseminomatous germ cell carcinoma. Cancer. 2002;94(9):2353–62.
19. Pfannenberg AC, Oechsle K, Bokemeyer C, Kollmannsberger C, Dohmen BM, Bares R, et al. The role of [(18)F] FDG-PET, CT/MRI and tumor marker kinetics in the evaluation of post chemotherapy residual masses in metastatic germ cell tumors--prospects for management. World J Urol. 2004;22(2):132–9.
20. Oechsle K, Hartmann M, Brenner W, Venz S, Weissbach L, Franzius C, et al. [18F] Fluorodeoxyglucose positron emission tomography in nonseminomatous germ cell tumors after chemotherapy: the German multicenter positron emission tomography study group. J Clin Oncol. 2008;26(36):5930–5.
21. Steyerberg EW, Keizer HJ, Fossa SD, Sleijfer DT, Toner GC, Schraffordt Koops H, et al. Prediction of residual retroperitoneal mass histology after chemotherapy for metastatic nonseminomatous germ cell tumor: multivariate analysis of individual patient data from six study groups. J Clin Oncol. 1995;13(5):1177–87.
22. Vergouwe Y, Steyerberg EW, Foster RS, Sleijfer DT, Fossa SD, Gerl A, et al. Predicting retroperitoneal histology in postchemotherapy testicular germ cell cancer: a model update and multicentre validation with more than 1000 patients. Eur Urol. 2007;51(2):424–32.

23. Kollmannsberger C, Daneshmand S, So A, Chi KN, Murray N, Moore C, et al. Management of disseminated nonseminomatous germ cell tumors with risk-based chemotherapy followed by response-guided postchemotherapy surgery. J Clin Oncol. 2010;28(4):537–42.
24. Ehrlich Y, Brames MJ, Beck SD, Foster RS, Einhorn LH. Long-term follow-up of Cisplatin combination chemotherapy in patients with disseminated nonseminomatous germ cell tumors: is a postchemotherapy retroperitoneal lymph node dissection needed after complete remission? J Clin Oncol. 2010;28(4):531–6.
25. Daneshmand S, Albers P, Fossa SD, Heidenreich A, Kollmannsberger C, Krege S, et al. Contemporary management of postchemotherapy testis cancer. Eur Urol. 2012;62(5):867–76.
26. Hartmann JT, Candelaria M, Kuczyk MA, Schmoll HJ, Bokemeyer C. Comparison of histological results from the resection of residual masses at different sites after chemotherapy for metastatic non-seminomatous germ cell tumours. Eur J Cancer. 1997;33(6):843–7.
27. Sheinfeld J. The role of adjunctive postchemotherapy surgery for nonseminomatous germ-cell tumors: current concepts and controversies. Semin Urol Oncol. 2002;20(4):262–71.
28. Hartmann JT, Schmoll HJ, Kuczyk MA, Candelaria M, Bokemeyer C. Postchemotherapy resections of residual masses from metastatic non-seminomatous testicular germ cell tumors. Ann Oncol. 1997;8(6):531–8.
29. Duchesne GM, Stenning SP, Aass N, Mead GM, Fossa SD, Oliver RT, et al. Radiotherapy after chemotherapy for metastatic seminoma–a diminishing role. MRC Testicular Tumour Working Party. Eur J Cancer. 1997;33(6):829–35.
30. Flechon A, Bompas E, Biron P, Droz JP. Management of post-chemotherapy residual masses in advanced seminoma. J Urol. 2002;168(5):1975–9.
31. Hofmockel G, Gruss A, Theiss M. Chemotherapy in advanced seminoma and the role of postcytostatic retroperitoneal lymph node dissection. Urol Int. 1996;57(1):38–42.
32. Herr HW, Sheinfeld J, Puc HS, Heelan R, Bajorin DF, Mencel P, et al. Surgery for a postchemotherapy residual mass in seminoma. J Urol. 1997;157(3):860–2.
33. Puc HS, Heelan R, Mazumdar M, Herr H, Scheinfeld J, Vlamis V, et al. Management of residual mass in advanced seminoma: results and recommendations from the Memorial Sloan-Kettering Cancer Center. J Clin Oncol. 1996;14(2):454–60.
34. Ganjoo KN, Chan RJ, Sharma M, Einhorn LH. Positron emission tomography scans in the evaluation of postchemotherapy residual masses in patients with seminoma. J Clin Oncol. 1999;17(11):3457–60.
35. De Santis M, Bokemeyer C, Becherer A, Stoiber F, Oechsle K, Kletter K, et al. Predictive impact of 2-18fluoro-2-deoxy-D-glucose positron emission tomography for residual postchemotherapy masses in patients with bulky seminoma. J Clin Oncol. 2001;19(17):3740–4.
36. De Santis M, Becherer A, Bokemeyer C, Stoiber F, Oechsle K, Sellner F, et al. 2-18fluoro-deoxy-D-glucose positron emission tomography is a reliable predictor for viable tumor in postchemotherapy seminoma: an update of the prospective multicentric SEMPET trial. J Clin Oncol. 2004;22(6):1034–9.
37. Patton JF, Hewitt CB, Mallis N. Diagnosis and treatment of tumors of the testis. JAMA. 1959;171:2194–8.
38. Busch FM, Sayegh ES. Roentgenographic visualization of human testicular lymphatics: a preliminary report. J Urol. 1963;89:106–10.
39. Ray B, Hajdu SI, Whitmore WF Jr. Proceedings: distribution of retroperitoneal lymph node metastases in testicular germinal tumors. Cancer. 1974;33(2):340–8.
40. Donohue JP, Zachary JM, Maynard BR. Distribution of nodal metastases in nonseminomatous testis cancer. J Urol. 1982;128(2):315–20.
41. Weissbach L, Boedefeld EA. Localization of solitary and multiple metastases in stage II nonseminomatous testis tumor as basis for a modified staging lymph node dissection in stage I. J Urol. 1987;138(1):77–82.
42. Narayan P, Lange PH, Fraley EE. Ejaculation and fertility after extended retroperitoneal lymph node dissection for testicular cancer. J Urol. 1982;127(4):685–8.
43. Donohue JP, Foster RS, Rowland RG, Bihrle R, Jones J, Geier G. Nerve-sparing retroperitoneal lymphadenectomy with preservation of ejaculation. J Urol. 1990;144(2 Pt 1):287–91; discussion 91–2.

44. Heidenreich A, Pfister D, Witthuhn R, Thuer D, Albers P. Postchemotherapy retroperitoneal lymph node dissection in advanced testicular cancer: radical or modified template resection. Eur Urol. 2009;55(1):217–24.
45. Beck SD, Foster RS, Bihrle R, Donohue JP, Einhorn LH. Is full bilateral retroperitoneal lymph node dissection always necessary for postchemotherapy residual tumor? Cancer. 2007;110(6):1235–40.
46. Recker F, Tscholl R. Monitoring of emission as direct intraoperative control for nerve sparing retroperitoneal lymphadenectomy. J Urol. 1993;150(5 Pt 1):1360–4.
47. Carver BS, Shayegan B, Eggener S, Stasi J, Motzer RJ, Bosl GJ, et al. Incidence of metastatic nonseminomatous germ cell tumor outside the boundaries of a modified postchemotherapy retroperitoneal lymph node dissection. J Clin Oncol. 2007;25(28):4365–9.
48. Eggener SE, Carver BS, Sharp DS, Motzer RJ, Bosl GJ, Sheinfeld J. Incidence of disease outside modified retroperitoneal lymph node dissection templates in clinical stage I or IIA nonseminomatous germ cell testicular cancer. J Urol. 2007;177(3):937–42; discussion 42–3.
49. Carver BS, Cronin AM, Eggener S, Savage CJ, Motzer RJ, Bajorin D, et al. The total number of retroperitoneal lymph nodes resected impacts clinical outcome after chemotherapy for metastatic testicular cancer. Urology. 2010;75(6):1431–5.
50. Donohue JP. Retroperitoneal lymphadenectomy: the anterior approach including bilateral suprarenal-hilar dissection. Urol Clin North Am. 1977;4(3):509–21.
51. Rassweiler JJ, Frede T, Lenz E, Seemann O, Alken P. Long-term experience with laparoscopic retroperitoneal lymph node dissection in the management of low-stage testis cancer. Eur Urol. 2000;37(3):251–60.
52. Bhayani SB, Allaf ME, Kavoussi LR. Laparoscopic RPLND for clinical stage I nonseminomatous germ cell testicular cancer: current status. Urol Oncol. 2004;22(2):145–8.
53. Hyams ES, Pierorazio P, Proteek O, Sroka M, Kavoussi LR, Allaf ME. Laparoscopic retroperitoneal lymph node dissection for clinical stage I nonseminomatous germ cell tumor: a large single institution experience. J Urol. 2012;187(2):487–92.
54. Palese MA, LM S, Kavoussi LR. Laparoscopic retroperitoneal lymph node dissection after chemotherapy. Urology. 2002;60(1):130–4.
55. Rassweiler JJ, Seemann O, Henkel TO, Stock C, Frede T, Alken P. Laparoscopic retroperitoneal lymph node dissection for nonseminomatous germ cell tumors: indications and limitations. J Urol. 1996;156(3):1108–13.
56. Mosharafa AA, Foster RS, Koch MO, Bihrle R, Donohue JP. Complications of post-chemotherapy retroperitoneal lymph node dissection for testis cancer. J Urol. 2004;171(5):1839–41.
57. Dogra PN, Singh P, Saini AK, Regmi KS, Singh BG, Nayak B. Robot assisted laparoscopic retroperitoneal lymph node dissection in testicular tumor. Urol Ann. 2013;5(4):223–6.
58. Djaladat H, Nichols C, Daneshmand S. Adjuvant surgery in testicular cancer patients undergoing postchemotherapy retroperitoneal lymph node dissection. Ann Surg Oncol. 2012;19(7):2388–93.
59. Winter C, Pfister D, Busch J, Bingol C, Ranft U, Schrader M, et al. Residual tumor size and IGCCCG risk classification predict additional vascular procedures in patients with germ cell tumors and residual tumor resection: a multicenter analysis of the German Testicular Cancer Study Group. Eur Urol. 2012;61(2):403–9.
60. Beck SD, Foster RS, Bihrle R, Koch MO, Wahle GR, Donohue JP. Aortic replacement during post-chemotherapy retroperitoneal lymph node dissection. J Urol. 2001;165(5):1517–20.
61. Nash PA, Leibovitch I, Foster RS, Bihrle R, Rowland RG, Donohue JP. En bloc nephrectomy in patients undergoing post-chemotherapy retroperitoneal lymph node dissection for nonseminomatous testis cancer: indications, implications and outcomes. J Urol. 1998;159(3): 707–10.
62. Macleod LC, Rajanahally S, Nayak JG, Parent BA, Ramos JD, Schade GR, et al. Characterizing the morbidity of postchemotherapy retroperitoneal lymph node dissection for testis cancer in a national cohort of privately insured patients. Urology. 2016;91:70–6.
63. Williams SB, McDermott DW, Dock W, Bahnson E, Berry AM, Steele GS, et al. Retroperitoneal lymph node dissection in patients with high risk testicular cancer. J Urol. 2009;181(5):2097–101; discussion 101–2.

64. Baniel J, Foster RS, Rowland RG, Bihrle R, Donohue JP. Complications of post-chemotherapy retroperitoneal lymph node dissection. J Urol. 1995;153(3 Pt 2):976–80.
65. Cary C, Masterson TA, Bihrle R, Foster RS. Contemporary trends in postchemotherapy retroperitoneal lymph node dissection: additional procedures and perioperative complications. Urol Oncol. 2015;33(9):389.e15–21.
66. Baniel J, Sella A. Complications of retroperitoneal lymph node dissection in testicular cancer: primary and post-chemotherapy. Semin Surg Oncol. 1999;17(4):263–7.
67. Baniel J, Foster RS, Rowland RG, Bihrle R, Donohue JP. Management of chylous ascites after retroperitoneal lymph node dissection for testicular cancer. J Urol. 1993;150(5 Pt 1):1422–4.
68. Mosharafa AA, Foster RS, Leibovich BC, Bihrle R, Johnson C, Donohue JP. Is post-chemotherapy resection of seminomatous elements associated with higher acute morbidity? J Urol. 2003;169(6):2126–8.
69. Ravi R, Ong J, Oliver RT, Badenoch DF, Fowler CG, Hendry WF. The management of residual masses after chemotherapy in metastatic seminoma. BJU Int. 1999;83(6):649–53.
70. Yu HY, Hevelone ND, Patel S, Lipsitz SR, Hu JC. Hospital surgical volume, utilization, costs and outcomes of retroperitoneal lymph node dissection for testis cancer. Adv Urol. 2012;2012:189823.
71. Hendry WF, Norman AR, Dearnaley DP, Fisher C, Nicholls J, Huddart RA, et al. Metastatic nonseminomatous germ cell tumors of the testis: results of elective and salvage surgery for patients with residual retroperitoneal masses. Cancer. 2002;94(6):1668–76.
72. de Wit R, Stoter G, Kaye SB, Sleijfer DT, Jones WG, ten Bokkel Huinink WW, et al. Importance of bleomycin in combination chemotherapy for good-prognosis testicular non-seminoma: a randomized study of the European Organization for Research and Treatment of Cancer Genitourinary Tract Cancer Cooperative Group. J Clin Oncol. 1997;15(5):1837–43.
73. Albers P, Weissbach L, Krege S, Kliesch S, Hartmann M, Heidenreich A, et al. Prediction of necrosis after chemotherapy of advanced germ cell tumors: results of a prospective multicenter trial of the German Testicular Cancer Study Group. J Urol. 2004;171(5):1835–8.
74. Debono DJ, Heilman DK, Einhorn LH, Donohue JP. Decision analysis for avoiding post-chemotherapy surgery in patients with disseminated nonseminomatous germ cell tumors. J Clin Oncol. 1997;15(4):1455–64.
75. Fox EP, Weathers TD, Williams SD, Loehrer PJ, Ulbright TM, Donohue JP, et al. Outcome analysis for patients with persistent nonteratomatous germ cell tumor in postchemotherapy retroperitoneal lymph node dissections. J Clin Oncol. 1993;11(7):1294–9.
76. Gelderman WA, Scraffordt Koops H, Sleijfer DT, Oosterhuis JW, Oldhoff J. Late recurrence of mature teratoma in nonseminomatous testicular tumors after PVB chemotherapy and surgery. Urology. 1989;33(1):10–4.
77. Carver BS, Sheinfeld J. Management of post-chemotherapy extra-retroperitoneal residual masses. World J Urol. 2009;27(4):489–92.
78. Rick O, Bokemeyer C, Weinknecht S, Schirren J, Pottek T, Hartmann JT, et al. Residual tumor resection after high-dose chemotherapy in patients with relapsed or refractory germ cell cancer. J Clin Oncol. 2004;22(18):3713–9.
79. Stenning SP, Parkinson MC, Fisher C, Mead GM, Cook PA, Fossa SD, et al. Postchemotherapy residual masses in germ cell tumor patients: content, clinical features, and prognosis. Medical Research Council Testicular Tumour Working Party. Cancer. 1998;83(7):1409–19.
80. Eggener SE, Carver BS, Loeb S, Kondagunta GV, Bosl GJ, Sheinfeld J. Pathologic findings and clinical outcome of patients undergoing retroperitoneal lymph node dissection after multiple chemotherapy regimens for metastatic testicular germ cell tumors. Cancer. 2007;109(3):528–35.
81. Albers P, Ganz A, Hannig E, Miersch WD, Muller SC. Salvage surgery of chemorefractory germ cell tumors with elevated tumor markers. J Urol. 2000;164(2):381–4.
82. Beck SD, Foster RS, Bihrle R, Einhorn LH, Donohue JP. Outcome analysis for patients with elevated serum tumor markers at postchemotherapy retroperitoneal lymph node dissection. J Clin Oncol. 2005;23(25):6149–56.

Histopathological Evaluation in Prostate Cancer

10

Funda Vakar-Lopez

Abstract

Prostate cancer (Pca) is one of the most common cancers diagnosed in men. Despite its prevalence, healthcare providers dealing with the disease still face challenges ranging from screening, diagnosis, to selection of patients for treatment and development of resistance to therapy. Over the years, with wide acceptance of screening practices, specifically with the use of serum PSA assays, the composition of the cohort of men who are newly diagnosed with prostate cancer (Pca) shifted from symptomatic men with clinically advanced disease to men where the diagnosis is based on a few neoplastic glands on a needle core biopsy. While histopathologic features of Pca have been well established, diagnosis of cancer on a limited number of neoplastic glands has presented new challenges. In this chapter we will review some of the diagnostic challenges as well as recent updates in grading and other pathologic parameters that aid management decisions.

10.1 Diagnosis of Prostate Cancer

One of the most powerful tools pathologists have when evaluating the biopsies for carcinoma is the immunohistochemical application of the antibodies against the basal cell layer, which is lost in carcinoma. These include antibodies against high molecular weight cytokeratins (clone 34BE12), p63, and cytokeratin 5/6. Addition of alpha methylacyl coA racemase (AMCR/P504S), most commonly in a cocktail

F. Vakar-Lopez, M.D.
Department of Pathology, University of Washington,
Box 359791, 325 Ninth Avenue, Seattle, WA 98104, USA
e-mail: fvakar@uw.edu

G. Ozyigit, U. Selek (eds.), *Principles and Practice of Uroncology*,
DOI 10.1007/978-3-319-56114-1_10

with basal cell markers, aids highlighting the carcinoma cells with increased cytoplasmic expression relative to nonneoplastic glands.

In the current urologic practice, nearly all Pca diagnosis is established in needle biopsies of prostate, in contrast to transurethral resections, which have been the main tissue source in the 1960s.

The needle biopsies obtained under ultrasound guidance mainly target the peripheral zone and only occasionally sample the transition zone; however, the resolution of the ultrasound is not sensitive or specific enough for only targeting the foci that would be suspicious for carcinoma. Starting in the 1980s more extensive sampling of the prostate with multiple needle cores became widely used [1]. Recently, the use of multiparametric magnetic resonance imaging (mpMRI) in conjunction with the ultrasound imaging (MRI/US fusion) to guide the prostate needle biopsies has increased the rate of detection rate of clinically significant cancer with fewer biopsy cores according to several studies [2]. The advantages of MRI-targeted biopsies include better representation of the tumor characteristics (i.e., tumor volume and Gleason grade), thus improving biopsy and radical prostatectomy (RP) Gleason score concordance enhancing the prognostic significance of findings of the biopsy.

The influence of specimen type on the diagnosis and grading of Pca may be minor but not trivial. The main difference between the needle core biopsies and transurethral resections of prostate (TURP) is the zone that they sample, peripheral zone for needle cores, and transition zone for TURPs. While most of the prostate cancers arise from the peripheral zone, the carcinomas arising from the transition zone have some distinct histologic features (see below) and tend to be of lower Gleason grade.

Regardless of how it is detected and diagnosed, most Pca is acinar carcinoma. But a number of histologic variants, some clinically relevant, have been described. These variants include foamy gland, mucinous (colloid), transition zone-like, ductal (previously known as endometrioid), atrophic, neuroendocrine (small cell), sarcomatoid, and adenosquamous carcinoma. Another example of clinically relevant histologic variants is transition zone-like carcinomas, which include mostly medium-sized glands of tall columnar cells with clear abundant cytoplasm and small, basally oriented nuclei. These tumors tend to involve the transition zone of the prostate thus mostly diagnosed in TURP specimens, appear to have lower frequency of TMPRSS2-erg fusion, and have a somewhat better outcome [3, 4]. At the other end of the spectrum are ductal, neuroendocrine, and sarcomatoid prostate carcinomas that have worse outcome than the typical acinar Pca. The ductal carcinomas comprise approximately 3% of all prostate cancers, and most of them occur as a component of typical acinar carcinomas. While large glands lined by tall, pseudostratified columnar neoplastic cells are the hallmark of ductal histology, variations in morphology including presence of large complex cribriform structures with slit-like spaces and papillary architecture create difficulties in clearly defining the unique features and thus diagnosis and recognition of ductal carcinoma variant. Clinical characteristics attributed to ductal carcinoma include low PSA levels relative to the tumor burden and visceral metastasis in addition to bone; however, like morphologic features, they are not uniform in all cases. At least partly due to lack of a unifying concept, little is known about the underlying molecular features of this histologic variant. In a recent study by Schweizer et al., in a cohort of ten cases of ductal carcinoma, 40% of cases had a mismatch repair gene alteration, and 75% of these cases had evidence of hypermutation [5]. Validation of these findings may provide a more clear definition of this subtype while presenting specific molecular targets for customized treatment options.

Similarly neuroendocrine (small cell) carcinomas may occur concomitantly with acinar carcinomas, either de novo or following systemic therapy. Histological diagnosis of this variant is mostly straightforward with the aid of immunohistochemical studies using antibodies against synaptophysin and chromogranin. The clinical significance of this subtype is reflected in selection of chemotherapeutic agents. Like its counterparts in other organ systems, neuroendocrine/small cell carcinomas respond better to cisplatin and etoposide combination therapy. In relatively rare cases where the morphology of prostate cancer is of a typical acinar carcinoma, expression of neuroendocrine markers can be demonstrated immunohistochemically. Whether these cases could be classified as neuroendocrine carcinomas or whether they would respond to the same therapeutic agents is not clear.

The most important aspect of these variant morphologies is the need for both the practicing pathologist and the treating physician to be aware of their presence and their correlation with specific clinical behaviors.

10.2 Grading Prostate Carcinoma

Gleason grading system, initially created in 1966 and expanded and updated with prognostic data in 1967 by Donald F. Gleason [6, 7], is one of the most enduring phenomena in medicine in that it is still the widely accepted grading system for prostate cancer throughout the world. However, many changes in the practice of urology, advances in and better understanding of the pathology, led to several modifications throughout the years, namely, in 1974 and 1977, in 2005, and most recently in 2014 (Figs. 10.1 and 10.2) [8–11].

Gleason grading system is based on the architectural patterns of the tumor, and taking in consideration of heterogeneity of prostate cancer, it includes the sum of the most common and the second most common patterns. The grading system encompasses grades from 1 to 5, from well circumscribed uniform glands (grade 1) to the poorly differentiated tumor composed of solid sheets and/or single cells or areas of central (comedo) necrosis (Fig. 10.1). Initial description of the system was based on a study of 270 patients from the Minneapolis Veterans Administration Hospital, and the study was expanded to 463 men in 1967 and 1032 men in 1974 [6–8]. These initial studies included men mostly with advanced disease with either extraprostatic extension or metastatic disease at the time of diagnosis. The strength of this grading system is that it is relatively simple and fairly easily applied with reasonable concordance (reproducibility). In addition, it is one of the most powerful prognostic predictors in Pca, predicting pathological findings in RP, biochemical

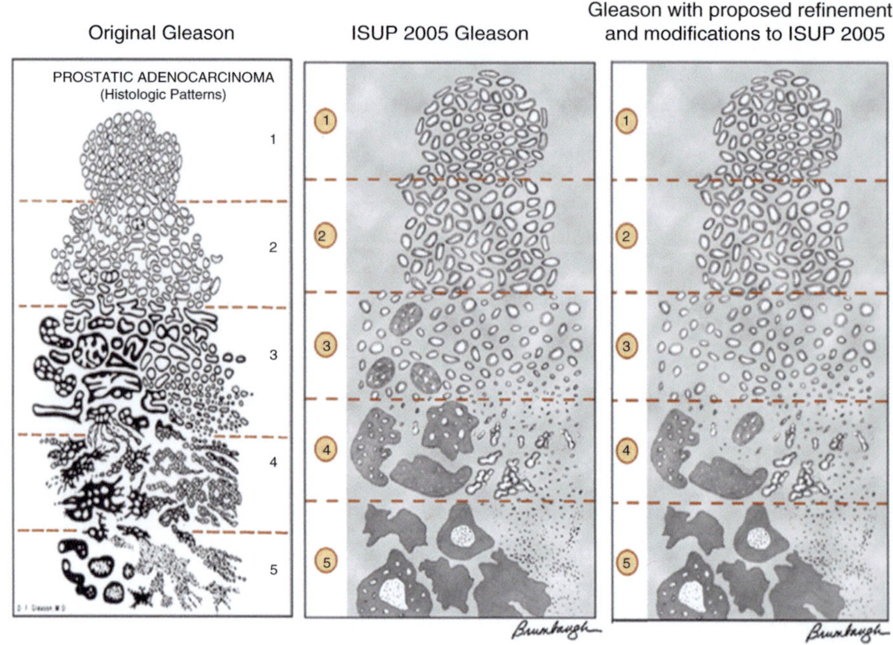

Fig. 10.1 Evolution of Gleason grading system

failure, local and distant metastasis after therapy, and Pca-specific mortality, and is one of the key parameters used in therapy planning, especially for decisions regarding active surveillance versus definitive therapy.

The current guidelines of the Gleason grading system, including the most recent updates which were introduced in 2014 at a meeting attended by pathologists with expertise in prostate pathology and groups of oncologists and urologists, include elimination of GS 2 (1 + 1) regardless of the specimen type and limiting GS 2–4 diagnosis to rare cases in which the cancer is diagnosed in transurethral resection (TURP) specimens where the circumscription of the tumor nodules can be observed [6] (Fig. 10.2).

It also includes expansion and better definition of Gleason grade 4 category. In Gleason's original descriptions, grade 4 group included only "large clear cells growing in a diffuse pattern resembling hypernephroma; may show gland formation" (Fig. 10.1). Later modifications included raggedly infiltrating fused glands and glands that are not single and separate but coalesce and branch. The 2005 consensus further expanded the category to include most cribriform glands (except "small cribriform glands with regular contour and round evenly distributed lumina" still regarded as Gleason grade 3) and ill-defined glands with poorly formed glandular lumens or "poorly formed" glands.

In 2014, all cribriform glands regardless of the shape and size and glands with glomeruloid architecture, considered a variant of cribriform architecture, were

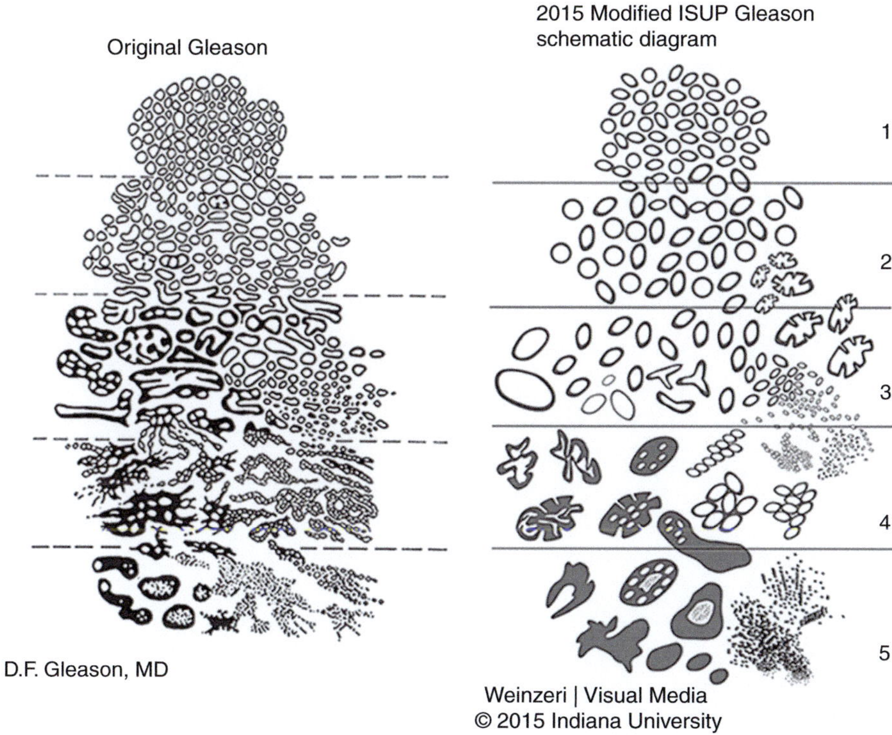

Fig. 10.2 Comparison of the original Gleason grading and the latest modifications (With permission, J Epstein et al. *Am J Surg Pathol* Volume 40, Number 2, February 2016)

added to the Gleason grade 4 category (Figs. 10.2 and 10.4). When compared with all the different patterns that make up Gleason grade 4 group, cribriform growth pattern has been shown to predict adverse clinical outcome parameters such as post-operative metastasis and disease-specific death [12, 13].

Distinguishing tangentially sectioned Gleason grade 3 glands that appear poorly formed from the truly poorly formed glands has been a great challenge for pathologists (Figs. 10.3 and 10.4). Although it was noted that "more than occasional poorly formed glands" must be seen for a tumor to be classified as Gleason grade 4 in the latest consensus meeting to avoid overcalling of tangentially cut glands, attempts have been made to determine the morphologic and quantitative criteria to overcome the ambiguity of "poorly formed" definition. Zhou et al. [14] studied interobserver reproducibility of diagnosing "poorly formed glands" on core needle biopsies among urologic pathologists and came up with recommendations to consider only cancer glands with no or rare luminal formation as "poorly formed" and to have at least ten "poorly formed glands" that are not immediately adjacent to well-formed glands to be considered Gleason pattern 4. This issue is of utmost important since presence of Gleason grade 4 pattern is among the criteria used to make decisions, namely, if a patient is going to be included in active surveillance programs or offered a definitive therapy,

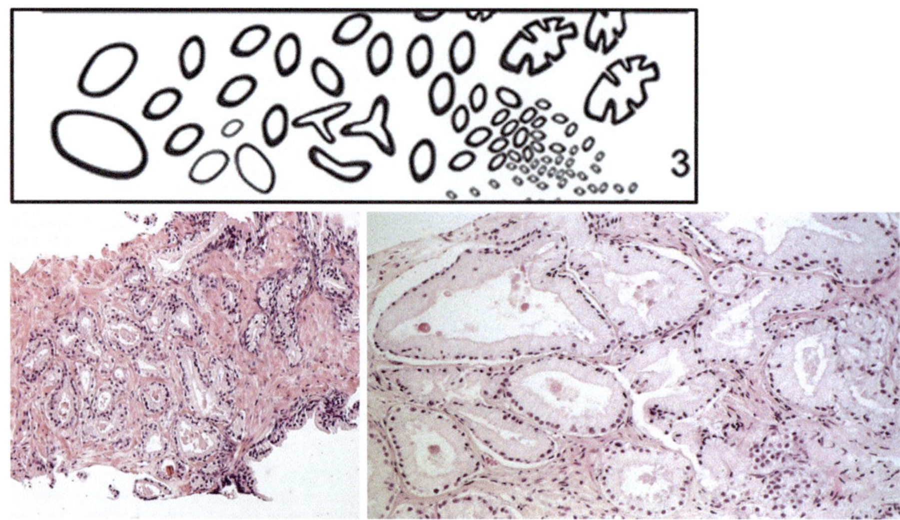

Fig. 10.3 Gleason grade 3 patterns

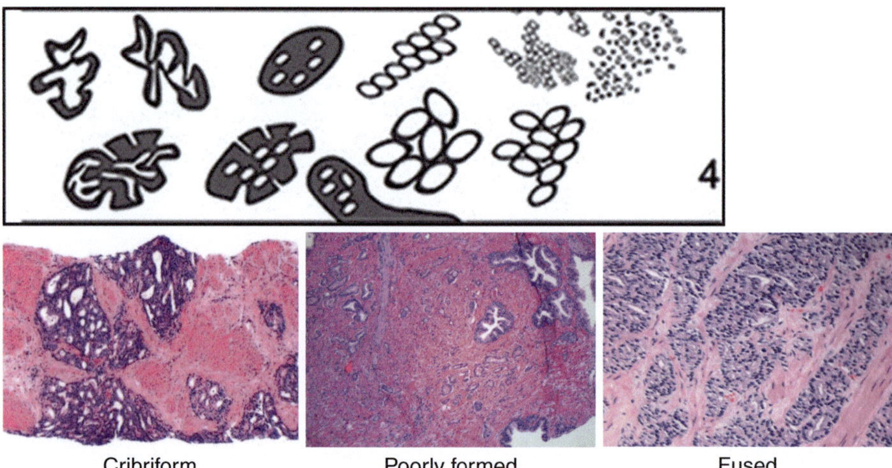

Fig. 10.4 Gleason grade 4 patterns

such as prostatectomy or radiation therapy. In a recent multi-institutional study involving an active surveillance cohort [15], the reproducibility of assigning a Gleason pattern 3 vs 4 or higher was worst for small foci with glands where the interpretation varied between tangentially sectioned Gleason pattern 3 vs poorly formed glands of Gleason pattern 4. The best interobserver agreement was in cribriform and glomeruloid Gleason 4 patterns [16] in a recent study among genitourinary pathologists. In line with the previous study by McKenney, hardly any consensus was reached on ill-formed and fused glands. More recent attempts to further optimize histologic grading

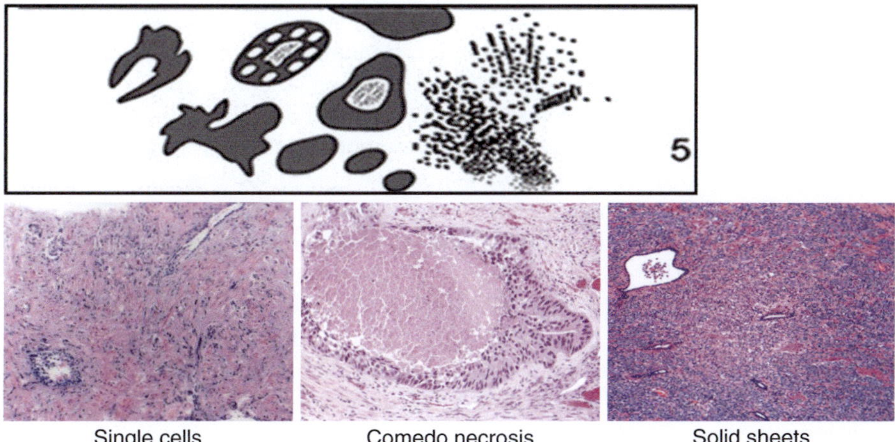

Fig. 10.5 Gleason grade 5 patterns

of prostatic adenocarcinoma to decrease interobserver variance and provide consistent and more accurate prognostic stratification for the individual patient include attempts of incorporating individual architectural patterns into the grading scheme and assessing their relative contribution to the prognostic strength [17].

Gleason grade 5 patterns include single cells, solid tumor sheets, and cords of cells without any glandular differentiation as well as central (comedo) necrosis (Fig. 10.5). They generally do not present diagnostic challenges, unless the amount of single cells/cords of cells is limited.

The most common practice is to give a Gleason score to each specimen of biopsy core(s) that is submitted in separate containers. For treatment algorithms, typically the highest Gleason score is used regardless of the volume of cancer in the particular core(s). In heterogeneous and multifocal tumors, this has the potential to overrepresent the high-grade component in the entire gland and place the patient in a higher-risk category. In a study by Aries-Stella et al., when using the highest biopsy Gleason score, the authors found that 60% of such patients had a downgraded Gleason score at prostatectomy [18]. As a result they concluded that a composite needle biopsy Gleason score combining relative proportions of each Gleason grade pattern in multiple contiguous positive biopsies correlated better with prostatectomy Gleason score in patients with heterogeneous needle biopsy Gleason scores (>2 different GSs or a two-step difference in GS between separate biopsies).

10.3 Grading Unusual Morphologies Variants of Pca

Overall the grading of histologic variants of Pca follows the conventional grading scheme, and except for the ductal carcinoma, most of these variants are assigned a Gleason score similar to the acinar carcinomas. Somewhat challenging patterns in this category include foamy gland and mucinous carcinomas and carcinomas with collagenous nodules and mucin extravasation. Previously, any carcinoma with extravasated mucin and mucinous (colloid) carcinomas (mucin extravasation occupying >25% of the tumor) were considered as Gleason grade 4. Recent studies have shown that mucinous carcinomas treated with RP are not aggressive and may even have better prognosis than the usual acinar carcinomas [19]. For these reasons, the latest consensus is that these carcinomas should be graded based on the pattern present after subtracting the mucinous component.

In contrast, all ductal carcinomas are graded as pattern 4 and pattern 5 if there is comedo necrosis. The ductal carcinoma component, even though it is mostly admixed with typical acinar carcinoma, is given a Gleason score of at least 8 (4 + 4) in keeping with the overall prognosis similar to other Gleason score 8 carcinomas.

Neither sarcomatoid nor small cell carcinomas should be graded due to their unique tumor biology and therapeutic implications, regardless of the amount of such components.

Intraductal carcinoma of the prostate (IDC-P), initially described by Kovi et al. in 1985 and McNeal in 1996, is described as dense cribriform glands with highly atypical epithelial cells that retain at least focally basal cells [20, 21]. Further studies, including by Guo and Epstein and Kimura et al., supported the adverse prognosis of IDC-P on biopsy and prostatectomy specimens and its association with high-grade invasive Pca [22–24]. Because of all the associations, some pathologists advocated grading of IDC-P; however, at the 2014 meeting it was the consensus not to grade it but to add a comment as to its invariable association with aggressive prostate cancer.

10.4 Tertiary Gleason Grade Pattern

The Gleason grading system is built on reporting the two most prevalent histological patterns as a sum score. More often than not, a tertiary or third most common pattern is encountered either in biopsies or prostatectomy specimens. Reporting this component especially if it is a higher-grade pattern may have different implications and purposes in needle biopsies and prostatectomies.

The current recommendation of including the higher tertiary grade component in the biopsies as the secondary grade is based on the assumption that the tumor has the biology of a higher-grade tumor, even though the amount of the higher-grade component is small in the biopsy, which may be due to a sampling error. The typical scenario of such a case is when the biopsy includes a tumor with a Gleason score 7, either 3 + 4 or 4 + 3 with a minor component of Gleason grade pattern 5. The final score in this case would end up being 8 (3 + 5) or 9 (4 + 5), respectively. This allows incorporation of the tertiary component in the risk stratification tools such as Partin tables and Kattan nomogram, which only allow primary and secondary patterns.

The presence of focal (less than 5% of the tumor volume) Gleason grade 5 has different implications in a prostatectomy since all tumor foci are available for review. It has been shown by Magi-Galuzzi et al. that in comparison the Gleason 7 (3 + 4) or 7 (4 + 3) with a tertiary pattern 5 was less likely to be organ confined and presented at a higher stage than the tumors with the same Gleason score but without the tertiary pattern 5 [25]. In these scenarios the Gleason score for the prostatectomy would be reported as 7 (4 + 3) with a tertiary 5, since the overall behavior of the tumor falls between Gleason 9 and 7.

10.5 Grade Groupings

With the modifications to the Gleason grading system, in recent years reporting of Gleason scores 2–5 has virtually vanished from general practice. This led to a shift in the grading system where originally the scores ranged from 2 to 10. Now the lowest score being 6 out of 10, giving the impression of the tumor to have intermediate prognosis, potentially causes patients unnecessary anxiety and overtreatment. There have been attempts to interpret the Gleason scores in groups of similar prognostic characteristics in the past; however, some of these groupings combined scores with wide variations in outcomes. For example, Gleason score 7 is considered as a homogenous group in many of these groupings, despite many studies showing a significantly worse prognosis for 4 + 3 than 3 + 4 [26–28]. In addition, combining scores 6 and 7, as some studies do, place tumors with almost uniformly excellent prognosis (3 + 3) and with a high likelihood of disease recurrence and progression (4 + 3) in the same prognostic category.

The newly accepted grade groupings that are included in the latest WHO 2016 edition of *Pathology and Genetics: Tumours of the Urinary System and Male Genital Organs* are proposed by Epstein based on data from Johns Hopkins Hospital [29]. It consists of five prognostically distinct grade groups, validated to accurately reflect prostate cancer biology. Grade group 1 in this new system includes cancers with Gleason score <6, with excellent prognosis, and now the grade designation of the tumor is better aligned with the lowest possible grade. Per consensus of the 2014 meeting, the new grades would, for the foreseeable future, be used in conjunction with the Gleason system [i.e., Gleason score 6 (3 + 3) (grade group 1)]. In a subsequent study of about 20,000 men from 5 different institutions who were treated by RP, grade groups strongly correlated with the risk of biological recurrence after surgery. In this study, large differences in recurrence rates between both Gleason 3 + 4 versus 4 + 3 and Gleason 8 versus 9 were found [30]. The proposed five-grade group system had the highest prognostic discrimination on both univariate and multivariate analysis. The major limitation was the use of PSA biochemical recurrence BCR as an end point as opposed to cancer-related death.

10.6 Prognostic Indicators

10.6.1 Volume

Prostate cancer is a heterogeneous disease with variable outcomes. One of the parameters suggested to be an important clinical predictor is the tumor volume. The assessment of tumor volume carries radically different implications in radical prostatectomy and needle biopsy. Whether tumor volume assessment in pathologically organ-confined (pT2) prostate cancer provides independent prognostic information beyond grade and stage is controversial. In early studies by Stamey and Humphrey, tumor volume correlated with metastasis, seminal vesicle invasion, extraprostatic extension (EPE), and grade [31, 32]. The latter study also showed that % of specimen involved by tumor independently predicted clinical recurrence. Since these studies have come out before PSA screening era, the mean tumor volume was fairly large 4.66 cc, and the mean Gleason score was 7.03 [31]. Nevertheless, in all the studies none of the tumor with volumes less than 0.5 cc progressed.

In the more contemporary studies, data on whether the tumor volume has independent prognostic significance in prostatectomy specimens are conflicting. One of the main reasons for this uncertainty is that there is not one agreed-upon method to estimate tumor volume. Among the presumably most precise methods used is the one that involves circling the tumor on glass slides and using computer-assisted planimetry or grid morphometric analysis to determine tumor volume. These methods are quite time consuming. Simpler methods such as visual estimation of tumor percentage and maximum tumor dimension (MTD) have the potential of wider use but due to their subjectivity and poor reproducibility fall short of providing uniform results. Other less frequently used methods include multiplying the largest tumor dimensions on the sections by the thickness of the tumor, using a grid to calculate tumor percentage, using number of blocks involved by tumor, calculating maximal area of the tumor, and determining the ratio of involved-to-uninvolved blocks. Another point of debate is whether to record the dominant tumor nodule(s) or total tumor volume. This point becomes more important in the tumors that would be in the clinically insignificant cancer category (less than 0.5 cc, no Gleason pattern 4, and organ confined) if only the largest of multiple small-volume tumors is reported as would be seen in a case with three separate tumor nodules (0.3, 0.2, and 0.1 cc) [33]. This variance in reporting total tumor volume may explain the variation in incidence of potentially insignificant cancers (ranging from 0.4–0.6% to 26–33%) in different institutions.

As a result of a consensus conference of the International Society of Urological Pathology, "some quantitative estimate of cancer volume should be undertaken" is recommended but "the nature of which being dependent on routine practice of with the pathology laboratory" [34].

Quantifying the amount of tumor in needle biopsies, on the other hand, provides one of the key data points used to make decisions on management options which increasingly in recent years includes active surveillance protocols. Given the importance of this parameter in management decisions, we should review the challenges associated with it. There are several ways to quantify cancer on biopsy. The simplest method is to estimate the percentage of the core(s) involved by carcinoma. While this assessment is easy, it is subjective and may be a cause for interobserver variability. Measuring cancer foci and total length of the biopsy cores may be more reproducible but also brings out other challenges such as how to measure two separate foci of carcinoma involving the same core but are separated by some amount of stroma. Among pathologists, there is no true consensus and there is variation in practice.

Some pathologists measure each focus separately without including the intervening stroma, while others measure from one end to the other including the stroma. Multiple studies suggest that inclusion of the benign prostatic tissue in between the foci correlates more closely with the amount of tumor in the prostatectomy [35, 36].

There is limited number of studies comparing different quantitative methods in predicting pathologic stage or outcome. In one of the later studies, percentage of carcinoma in all cores was significantly and consistently stronger than other measures in all comparisons. When combined with preoperative PSA and Gleason grade on multivariate analysis, this measure improved prediction of pT3 and was independent of preoperative PSA and Gleason grade for risk of biochemical recurrence [37].

It is recommended that at a minimum the number of positive cores along with at least one other more detailed measurement such as the % of core involvement or length of cancer should be included in a biopsy report.

10.6.2 Extraprostatic Extension

Even more informative than the total tumor volume in a prostatectomy specimen is the extent of tumor, i.e., if the tumor extends into extraprostatic tissue (extraprostatic extension) and/or into seminal vesicles. This information is reflected in the pathologic stage in the AJCC staging system as pT3a and pT3b, respectively. Extraprostatic extension is a well-established factor for adverse prognosis. However, definition and identification of extraprostatic extension can be challenging. Simply defined, extraprostatic extension is the tumor being present beyond the confines of the prostate gland [38]. This can be difficult to identify since the prostate gland lacks a discrete and microscopically well-defined prostate capsule. In addition, extraprostatic tissue present in different aspects of the prostate gland is different. For example, posterolateral soft tissue (superior neurovascular bundles), as the name implies, includes abundant adipose tissue (unless a nerve-sparing prostatectomy) with blood vessels and nerves, whereas anteriorly, especially in the apex, the prostatic parenchyma blends in with bundles of striated muscle and only occasionally may include some amount of adipose tissue. The determination of what constitutes "beyond the confines of prostate" can be difficult when carcinoma involves the muscle anteriorly and bulges into the adipose tissue or extends along with the fibrous fingerlike projections into the neurovascular bundle. While finding cancer glands among striated muscle bundles anteriorly does not constitute extraprostatic extension, the latter is considered to be diagnostic of extraprostatic extension by many pathologists.

10.6.3 Seminal Vesicle Invasion

Seminal vesicle invasion is defined as involvement of the wall of seminal vesicles by carcinoma and in most instances is straightforward diagnosis. There are three ways of seminal vesicle invasion: 1, spreading along the ejaculatory ducts; 2, direct extension at the base or extraprostatic extension into the superior neurovascular bundle and then invasion into seminal vesicle wall; and 3, discontinuous involvement, which is quite rare.

A point of debate especially before the ISUP consensus publications was if the involvement of the intraprostatic portion of seminal vesicles also qualified as a pT3b disease [39]. In one of the few available studies on this subject, invasion of only the intraprostatic portion of the seminal vesicle or ejaculatory ducts was correlated with better survival rate than for those with extraprostatic seminal vesicle invasion [40]. Currently, only invasion of the extraprostatic portion of seminal vesicle is considered for staging.

10.6.4 Margins

Involvement of margins of resection of prostatectomy specimens is among the most common reasons for biochemical recurrence and is a significant predictor of BCR-free survival (93.8% in margin negative versus 79.9% in margin positive cases) and prostate cancer-specific mortality (PCSM) in a univariate analysis [41, 42]. After adjusting other clinicopathological variables in a multivariate analysis, it remained moderately associated with PCSM, while RP Gleason score and pathologic stage were strong predictors [43, 44]. The most common site of margin positivity is the apex where there is not much extraprostatic tissue and surgically removable tissue is limited due to the anatomical restrictions [45]. In the posterolateral aspect of the prostate, the amount of extraprostatic tissue in a prostatectomy depends on the type of surgical procedure: nerve spearing versus non-nerve spearing; thus, a positive margin can be either in the setting of extraprostatic extension or incomplete removal of the entire prostatic tissue. As may be expected, efforts to preserve the neurovascular bundles increase the probability of incomplete excision of the prostate resulting in more frequent positive margins. Positive margins at bladder neck, which is relatively uncommon, and anterior are also correlated with BCR, but several studies with opposite conclusions are have also been published [46, 47]. The type of surgical intervention, i.e., open radical prostatectomy (ORP) versus laparoscopic radical prostatectomy (LARP), may influence the incidence and location of positive margins: lower incidence in LARP and apical region in both LARP and ORP [48].

For pathologists a positive margin is defined as having carcinoma cells at the margins where the surgeon has cut across the tissue planes, which are marked with a special ink during gross examination. Since carcinoma cells being at the inked surface are the diagnostic hallmark, care needs to be given by the pathologist to recognize surface irregularities and disruptions that may not reflect true resection margins. Good communication with the surgeon may clarify many of these irregularities. In cases where carcinoma cells are not actually touching the ink but are only a few cells away may be classified as "carcinoma abutting" the margin. In a study by True et al., these cases behaved as positive margins; however, in other studies, close distance to the margins did not appear to correlate with disease recurrence or residual cancer [49–51].

On the other hand, the extent of tumor at the surgical margin has been shown to be correlated with disease recurrence in several studies [52, 53]. Determining and reporting the linear extent of positive margin in mm is the most common way pathologist reports the extent, while some may also classify the extent as "focal" versus "extensive."

10.7 Treatment Effects on Histology

Prostate cancer treatments whether it be hormonal ablation or radiation therapy cause unique histologic changes in the carcinoma as well as the background non-neoplastic glandular tissue. Hormonal ablation causes, as expected, diffuse atrophy in the nonneoplastic glands with prominence of the basal cell layer (Fig. 10.6). Carcinomatous glands also shrink in size with vacuolization/clearing of the cytoplasm and nuclear pyknosis. Radiation therapy causes nuclear atypia and pleomorphism in addition to the diffuse atrophy in the nonneoplastic glands (Figs. 10.7 and 10.8). Stroma shows hyalinization and hypocellularity. Cancer glands become even more inconspicuous and appear mostly as single cells with vacuolated cytoplasm and eccentric nuclei or even empty spaces without any detectible nuclei.

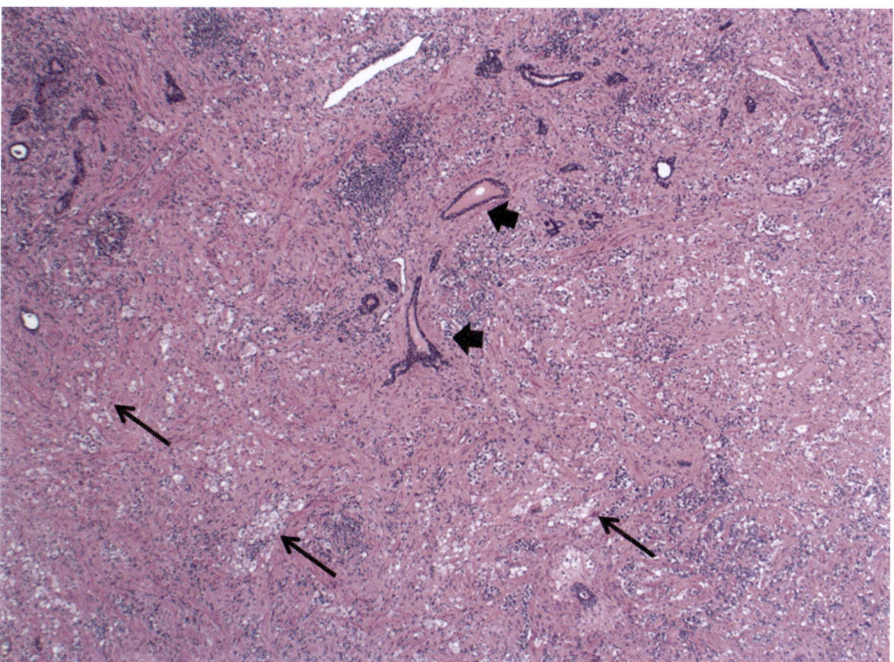

Fig. 10.6 Effects of hormonal ablation therapy on carcinoma and normal glands. Arrows = carcinoma glands; arrow heads = benign glands

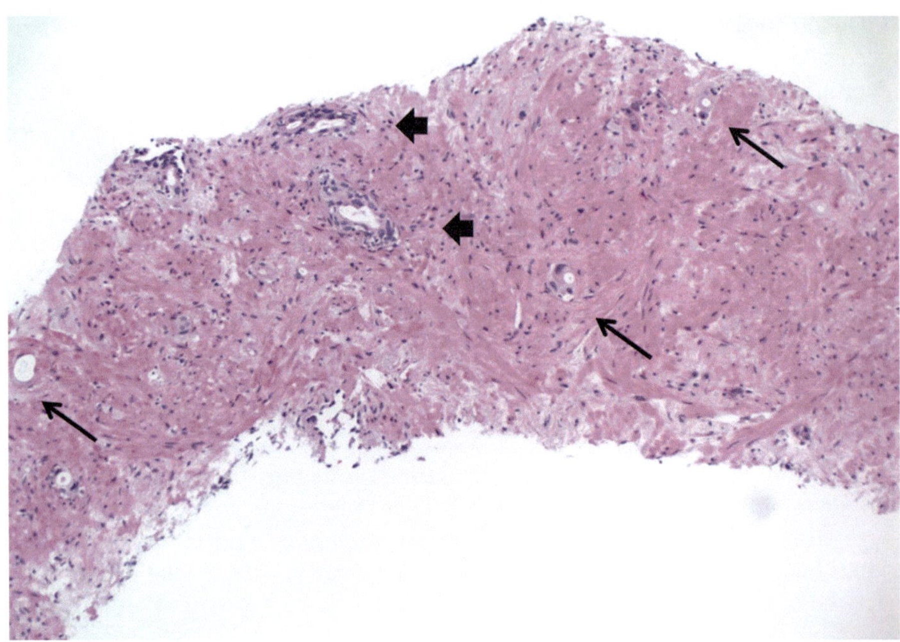

Fig. 10.7 Effects of radiation therapy on carcinoma and normal glands. Arrows = carcinoma glands; arrow heads = benign glands

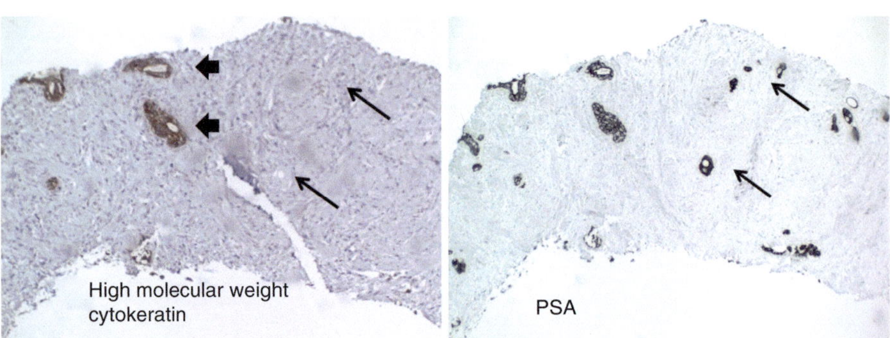

Fig. 10.8 Immunohistochemical profile of normal and carcinoma glands showing radiation therapy effect. Arrows = carcinoma glands; arrow heads = benign glands

Since all the described histologic changes in cancer are consistent with a high-grade morphology, Gleason grading no longer correlates with the disease severity and loses its prognostic prediction, and therefore by consensus no Gleason score is given to treated tumors. This creates a need for a new way of assessing the effect of therapy on the tumor and tumor burden, different than the volume estimation based on tumor area. One way is to assess the cellularity of the residual tumor. In a study by Murphy et al., the interobserver concordance was quite high for cellularity assessment in prostatectomies after treatment with abiraterone and enzalutamide, which may be a good candidate parameter to be measured if validation studies show that it correlates with the biology of the disease and the outcomes [54].

10.8 Biomarkers

Prostate cancer is a heterogeneous disease. Clinical presentation and behavior range from localized indolent to aggressive lethal disease. Currently the management is based on pathological (histologic grade, extent, etc.) and clinical parameters (PSA levels, clinical staging, etc.). For patients treated with surgery, pathological staging and surgical margin status are among the criteria used to stratify patients for further treatment and prognostic groups. None of these criteria adequately address the heterogeneity of the biologic behavior and response rates to available therapeutic regimens. Wider use of exome and whole genome sequencing identified genomic alterations that may both explain carcinogenesis and progression and potentially could be used as therapeutic targets [55, 56].

The most commonly encountered genomic alteration in prostate cancer are fusions of androgen-regulated gene promoters and E26 transformation-specific (ETS) family of oncogenes, which include ERG, ETV1, ETV4, and FLI1. Collectively these fusions occur in approximately 50% of prostate cancers; however, their clinical significance is still debated. While in some studies TMRSS2-ERG fusion is associated with worse outcome, the others failed to show any prognostic significance or reported a better outcome [57–60]. Other mutually exclusive mutations found in the TGCA cohort include mutations in SPOP, FOXA1, and IDH1 genes, yielding seven molecular subtypes. In the remaining 26% of tumors yet unknown, molecular alterations or epigenetic changes are presumed to occur. Of all the molecular changes, ETS fusions and SPOP mutations appear to be early events in the oncogenesis of Pca, while subclonal changes in CDKN1B, PTEN, and TP53 occur later and probably provide proliferative and survival advantage to cancer cells [61].

Despite emergence of newly identified molecular changes for potential therapy targets, androgen suppression is still the most commonly employed systemic therapy, taking advantage of prostate cancers' androgen dependence. Unfortunately, resistance to androgen blockade inevitably occurs resulting in a castration-resistant prostate cancer (CRPC). The mechanisms of resistance include a number of molecular changes including copy number alterations and mutations of AR or of its co-regulators and splice variants of AR and altered expression of AR pathway components that result in persistent AR-signaling. In case of splice variants, these truncated versions of AR permit constitutive activity of the receptor without presence of a cognate ligand. The most studied variant AR3 (also known as AR-V7) have been shown to be associated with resistance to abiraterone and enzalutamide both in Pca models and in patients [62–65]. Immunohistochemical detection of expression levels of ARV-7 in primary Pca and matched CRPC samples [66] demonstrated that levels are higher in advanced disease with the levels being the highest in tumors that have progressed on abiraterone and enzalutamide. Using the same antibody in an immunofluorescent assay, Scher et al. showed that ARV-7-positive CTCs have better overall survival with taxanes relative to AR-signaling inhibitors, highlighting the potential benefit of using splice variants as biomarkers that predict therapy response and assist physicians in individualizing treatment [67].

Another pathway with common genomic aberrations in up to 20–40% of Pcas is PI3K-AKT. Hyperactivity of PI3K-AKT pathway is frequently the result of PTEN inactivation, most commonly due to deletions but also through disruptive mutations and structural rearrangements. Immunohistochemical assay of PTEN expression has been recently validated by independent groups [68, 69]. In multiple studies, lack of PTEN expression is associated with poor prognosis [70] and poor overall survival and shorter time of response to abiraterone. In addition to predictive indicator of therapy response and prognosis, availability of compounds that are able to inhibit PI3K kinases made many clinical studies possible and promising. These studies include trials of mTOR inhibitors combined with androgen blockade and inhibitors of PI3K kinases and AKT in combination with AR-signaling inhibiting agents.

Most recently, some of the focus is shifted on the genetic mutations, both germline and somatic, of DNA repair genes found in approximately 12% of men who progress to advanced Pca and nearly 25% of CRPCs, respectively. Similar to breast carcinomas, men with germline mutations in genes involving homologous recombination (HR) like BRCA2 have been shown to be at greater risk of developing Pca [71, 72]. In this subset of patients with both germline and somatic aberrations in BRCA and other genes involved in HR DNA repair, a trial of olaparib, a poly-(adenosine diphosphate [ADP]-ribose) polymerase (PARP) inhibitor, showed antitumor activity which led to breakthrough designation of olaparib by the Food and Drug Administration (FDA) for accelerated approval for monotherapy in patients with BRCA1, BRCA2, or ATM-mutated metastatic CRPC. Other forms of DNA repair defects include mutations in mismatch (MM) repair genes that result in loss of MLH1, MLH2, PMS2, and MSH6 functions and are associated with microsatellite instability and high mutational load (hypermutated state) [73, 74]. Taking advantage of the correlation of high mutational load with increased numbers of tumor-specific neoantigens, novel immunotherapies activating cytotoxic T cell (CTL) are being tried [75].

10.9 Future Possibilities

10.9.1 The Third Dimension

The role of pathologists in diagnosing prostate cancer, providing useful information to predict its behavior and helping guide therapeutic management, is constantly evolving. One of the future directions of research involves alleviating limitations of light microscopy, which include the need for tissue fixation and limiting tissue analysis to two-dimensional images. By utilizing methods to clarify tissue (CLARITY) and specialized microscopy techniques such as light sheet fluorescence microscopy, structured illumination and confocal microscopy, and application of these methods to prostate tissue, it is possible to characterize the three-dimensional structure of prostate adenocarcinoma [76–78]. One immediate practical impact of these new tools will be on the Gleason grading system which is based on the structural arrangements of carcinoma glands on a two-dimensional plane. Using three-dimensional images may lead to reevaluation of the premises of grading prostate carcinoma, which are based on two-dimensionality.

10.9.2 Molecular Guides

Characterization of the molecular profiles of prostate cancer of different histologic types, grades, stages, and biologic states and of the genomes of both cancer-associated stroma and of the host has revealed potential new ways to manage and treat patients [55, 56]. For example, men with genomic microsatellite instability have a higher frequency of mutations in DNA repair genes. Phase I/II clinical trial data support the use of PARP inhibitors and DNA-damaging agents in this subgroup of patients, following success in using these drugs on other cancer types [79].

Some of the genes in CRPC differ from those in untreated primary prostate, i.e., monoamine oxidase A (MAOA) [56]. It has been shown that the expression of MAOA is induced by exposure to cytotoxic chemotherapy and, via increase in HIFα levels, contributes to docetaxel resistance. Since reversible competitive inhibitors with good selectivity for MAOA are approved for use as antidepressants, their potential use to enhance the effectiveness of already established therapies and to circumvent therapy resistance provides promising treatment options [80].

In addition, the stromal cells of primary prostate cancer secrete proteins, such as WNT16B, which increase chemoresistance and can potentially be targeted for augmenting the response to chemotherapeutic agents [81].

Conclusion

In this chapter we reviewed some of the challenges in prostate cancer diagnosis and prognostication from a pathologist's perspective. While there are many exciting and promising advancements in the field of prostate cancer research leading to new approaches to therapy such as "precision or personalized medicine" especially in academic and tertiary care centers, there is still room for improving the access of patients for these individualized therapies.

In an ideal scenario, the diagnosis of prostate cancer is enhanced through targeted sampling of the abnormal areas of the prostate gland detected by selective imaging. Pathologists, in addition to providing clinically significant information based on the morphology of the tumor, will report molecular features of the tumor which predict biologic behavior and guide the treatment choices with the goal of reducing suffering and mortality of men from prostate cancer.

References

1. Hodge KK, McNeal JE, Terris MK, et al. Random systematic versus directed ultrasound guided transrectal core biopsies of the prostate. J Urol. 1989;142:71–4.
2. Valerio M, Donaldson I, Emberton M, et al. Detection of clinically significant prostate cancer using magnetic resonance imaging-ultrasound fusion targeted biopsy: a systematic review. Eur Urol. 2015;68(1):8–19. doi:10.1016/j.eururo.2014.10.026.
3. Garcia JJ, Al-Ahmedie HA, Gopalan A, et al. Do prostatic transition zone tumors have a distinct morphology? Am J Surg Pathol. 2008;32:1709–14.
4. Al-Ahmedie HA, Tickoo SK, Olgac S, et al. Anterior predominant prostatic tumors: zone of origin and pathologic outcomes at radical prostatectomy. Am J Surg Pathol. 2008;32:229–35.
5. Schweizer MT, Cheng HH, Tretiakova MS, et al. Mismatch repair deficiency may be common in ductal adenocarcinoma of the prostate. Oncotarget. 2016;7(50):82504–10.
6. Gleason DF. Classification of prostatic carcinomas. Cancer Chemother Rep. 1966;50(3):125–8.
7. Mellinger GT, Gleason D, Bailar J III. The histology and prognosis of prostate cancer. J Urol. 1967;97:331–7.
8. Gleason DF, Mellinger GT. Prediction of prognosis for prostatic adenocarcinoma by combined histological grading and clinical staging. J Urol. 1974;11:58–64.
9. Mellinger GT. Prognosis of prostatic carcinoma. Recent Results Cancer Res. 1977;60:61–72.
10. Epstein JI, Allsbrook WC Jr, Amin MB, et al. ISUP grading committee. The 2005 international society of urological pathology (ISUP) consensus conference on Gleason grading of prostatic carcinoma. Am J Surg Pathol. 2005;29:1228–42.
11. Epstein JI, Egavad L, Amin MB, et al. The 2014 International Society of Urological Pathology (ISUP) consensus conference on Gleason grading of prostatic adenocarcinoma. Definition of grading patterns and proposal for a new grading system. Am J Surg Pathol. 2016;40(2):244–52.
12. Kweldam CF, Wildhagen MF, Steyerberg EW, et al. Cribriform growth is highly predictive for postoperative metastasis and disease-specific death in Gleason score 7 prostate cancer. Mod Pathol. 2015;28:457–64.
13. Dong F, Yang P, Wang C, et al. Architectural heterogeneity and cribriform pattern predict adverse clinical outcome for Gleason grade 4 prostatic adenocarcinoma. Am J Surg Pathol. 2013 Dec;37(12):1855–61.
14. Zhou M, Shah RB. Recent advances in prostate cancer pathology: Gleason grading and beyond. Pathol Int. 2016;66:260–72.
15. McKenney JK, Simko J, Bonham M, et al. The potential impact of reproducibility of Gleason grading in men with early stage prostate cancer managed by active surveillance: a multi-institutional study. J Urol. 2011 Aug;186(2):465–9.
16. Kweldam CF, Nieboer D, Algaba F, et al. Gleason grade 4 prostate adenocarcinoma patterns: an interobserver agreement study among genitourinary pathologists. Histopathology. 2016 Sep;69(3):441–9.
17. McKenney JK, Wei W, Hawley S, et al. Histologic grading of prostatic adenocarcinoma can be further optimized. Analysis of the relative prognostic strength of individual architectural patterns in 1275 patients from the Canary Retrospective Cohort. Am J Surg Pathol. 2016;40(11):1439–56.
18. Arias-Stella III, Shah AB, Montoya-Cerrillo D, et al. Prostate biopsy and radical prostatectomy Gleason score correlation in heterogeneous tumors. Proposal for a composite Gleason score. Am J Surg Pathol. 2015;39(9):1213–8.
19. Osunkaya AO, Nielsen ME, Epstein JI. Prognosis of mucinous adenocarcinoma of the prostate treated by radical prostatectomy: a study of 47 cases. Am J Surg Pathol. 2008;32(3):468–72.
20. Kovi J, Jackson MA, Heshmat MY. Ductal spread in prostatic carcinoma. Cancer. 1985;56(7):1566–73.
21. McNeal JE, Yemoto CE. Spread of adenocarcinoma within prostatic ducts and acini. Morphologic and clinical correlations. Am J Surg Pathol. 1996;20(7):802–14.

22. Guo CC, Epstein JI. Intraductal carcinoma of the prostate on needle biopsy: histologic features and clinical significance. Mod Pathol. 2006;19(12):1528–35.
23. Kimura K, Tsuzuki T, Kato M, et al. Prognostic value of intraductal carcinoma of the prostate in radical prostatectomy specimens. Prostate. 2014;74(6):680–7.
24. Kato M, Kimura K, Hirakawa A, et al. The presence of intraductal carcinoma of the prostate in needle biopsy is a significant prognostic factor for prostate cancer patients with distant metastasis at initial presentation. Mod Pathol. 2016;29(2):166–73.
25. Mosse CA, Magi-Galluzzi C, Tsuzuki T, et al. The prognostic significance of tertiary Gleason pattern 5 in radical prostatectomy specimens. Am J Surg Pathol. 2004;28(3):394–8.
26. Chan TY, Partin AW, Walsh PC, et al. Prognostic significance of Gleason score 3+4 versus Gleason score 4+3 tumor at radical prostatectomy. Urology. 2000;56:823–7.
27. Wright JL, Salinas CA, Lin DW, et al. Prostate cancer specific mortality and Gleason 7 disease differences in prostate cancer outcomes between cases with Gleason 4+3 and Gleason 3+4 tumors in a population based cohort. J Urol. 2009;182:2702–7.
28. Zumsteg ZS, Spratt DE, Pei I, et al. A new risk classification system for therapeutic decision making with intermediate-risk prostate cancer patients undergoing dose-escalated external-beam radiation therapy. Eur Urol. 2013;64(6):895–902. doi:10.1016/j.eururo.2013.03.033.
29. Moch H, Humphrey PA, Ulbright TM, Reuter V. WHO classification of tumours of the urinary system and male genital organs. Lyon, France: International Agency for Research on Cancer; 2016.
30. Ji E, Zelefsky MJ, Sjoberg D, et al. A contemporary prostate cancer grading system: a validated alternative to the Gleason score. Eur Urol. 2016;69(3):428–35.
31. Stamey TA, McNeal JE, Yemoto CM, et al. Biological determinants of cancer progression in men with prostate cancer. JAMA. 1999;281:1395–400.
32. Humphrey PA, Vollmer RT. Intraglandular tumor extent and prognosis in prostatic carcinoma: application of a grid method to prostatectomy specimens. Hum Pathol. 1990;21:799–804.
33. Epstein JI. Prognostic significance of tumor volume in radical prostatectomy and needle biopsy specimens. J Urol. 2011;186:790–7.
34. van der Kwast TH, Amin MB, Billis A, et al. International Society of Urologic Pathology (ISUP) Consensus Conference on Handling and Staging of Radical Prostatectomy Specimens. Working group 2: T2 substaging and prostate cancer volume. Mod Pathol. 2011;24:16–25.
35. Karram S, Trock BJ, Netto GJ, Epstein JI. Should intervening benign tissue be included in the measurement of discontinuous foci of cancer on prostate needle biopsy? Correlation with radical prostatectomy findings. Am J Surg Pathol. 2011;35:1351–5.
36. Epstein JI. Prognostic significance of tumor volume in radical prostatectomy and needle biopsy specimens. J Urol. 2011;186:790–7.
37. Quintal MM, Meirelles LR, Freitas LL, et al. Various morphometric measurements of cancer extent on needle prostate biopsies: which is predictive of pathologic stage and biochemical recurrence following radical prostatectomy? Int Urol Nephrol. 2011;43(3):697–705. doi:10.1007/s11255-011-9901-5.
38. Magi-Galuzzi C, et al. International Society of Urologic Pathology (ISUP) Consensus Conference on Handling and Staging of Radical Prostatectomy Specimens. Working group 3: extraprostatic extension, lymphovascular invasion and locally advanced disease. Mod Pathol. 2011;24:36–8.
39. Berney DM, et al. International Society of Urologic Pathology (ISUP) Consensus Conference on Handling and Staging of Radical Prostatectomy Specimens. Working group 4: seminal vesicles and lymph nodes. Mod Pathol. 2011;24:39–47.
40. Soh S, Arakawa A, Suyama K, et al. The prognosis of patients with seminal vesicle involvement depends upon the level of extraprostatic extension. J Urol. 1998;296A:159.
41. Tan PH, Cheng L, Srigley JR, et al. International Society of Urologic Pathology (ISUP) Consensus Conference on Handling and Staging of Radical Prostatectomy Specimens. Working group 5: surgical margins. Mod Pathol. 2011;24:48–57.

42. Alkhateeb S, Alibhai S, Fleshner N, et al. Impact of positive surgical margins after radical prostatectomy differs by disease risk group. J Urol. 2010;183:145–50.
43. Wright JL, Dalkin BL, True LD, et al. Positive surgical margins at radical prostatectomy predict prostate cancer specific mortality. J Urol. 2010;183:2213–8.
44. Chalfin HJ, et al. Impact of surgical margin status on prostate-cancer-specific mortality. BJU Int. 2012;110:1684–9.
45. Sooriakumaran P, Dev HS, Skarecky D, Ahlering T. The importance of surgical margins in prostate cancer. J Surg Oncol. 2016;113:310–5.
46. Aydin H, Tsuzuki T, Hernandez D, et al. Positive proximal (bladder neck) margin at radical prostatectomy confers greater risk of biochemical progression. Urology. 2004;64:551–5.
47. Pettus JA, Weight CJ, Thompson CJ, et al. Biochemical failure in men following radical retropubic prostatectomy: impact of surgical margin status and location. J Urol. 2004;172:129–32.
48. Smith JA Jr, Chan RC, Chang SS, et al. A comparison of the incidence and location of positive surgical margins in robotic assisted laparoscopic radical prostatectomy and open retropubic radical prostatectomy. J Urol. 2007;178:2385–9.
49. Izard JP, True LD, May P, et al. Prostate cancer that is within 0.1 mm of the surgical margin of a radical prostatectomy predicts greater likelihood of recurrence. Am J Surg Pathol. 2014;38(3):333–8.
50. Lu J, Wirth GJ, Wu S, et al. A close surgical margin after radical prostatectomy is an independent predictor of recurrence. J Urol. 2012;188(1):91–7.
51. Epstein JI, Sauvageot J. Do close but negative margins in radical prostatectomy specimens increase the risk of postoperative progression? J Urol. 1997;157:241–3.
52. Epstein JI, Partin AW, Sauvageot J, et al. Prediction of progression following radical prostatectomy. A multi-variate analysis of 721 men with long-term follow-up. Am J Surg Pathol. 1996;20:286–92.
53. Babaian RJ, Troncoso P, Bhadkamar VA, et al. Analysis of clinicopathologic factors predicting outcome after radical prostatectomy. Cancer. 2001;91:1414–22.
54. Murphy C, True L, Vakar-Lopez F, et al. A novel system for estimating residual disease and pathologic response to neoadjuvant treatment of prostate cancer. Prostate. 2016;76:1285–92.
55. The Cancer Genome Atlas Research Network. The molecular taxonomy of primary prostate cancer. Cell. 2015;163(4):1011–25.
56. Robinson D, Van Allen EM, Wu YM, et al. Integrative clinical genomics of advanced prostate cancer. Cell. 2015;161(5):1215–28.
57. Nam RK, Sugar L, Yang W, et al. Expression of the TMPRSS2:ERG fusion gene predicts cancer recurrence after surgery for localized prostate cancer. Br J Cancer. 2007;97:1690–5.
58. Demichelis F, Fall K, Perner S, et al. TMPRSS2:ERG gene fusion associated with lethal prostate cancer in a watchful waiting cohort. Oncogene. 2007;26:4596–9.
59. Pettersson A, Graff RE, Bauer SR, et al. The TMPRSS2:ERG rearrangement, ERG expression, and prostate cancer outcomes: a cohort study and meta-analysis. Cancer Epidemiol Biomark Prev. 2012;21:1497–509.
60. Gopalan A, Leversha MA, Satagopan JM, et al. TMPRSS2-ERG gene fusion is not associated with outcome in patients treated by prostatectomy. Cancer Res. 2009;69:1400–6.
61. Rodrigues DN, Boysen G, Sumanasuriya S, et al. The molecular underpinnings of prostate cancer: impacts of management and pathology practice. J Pathol. 2017;241(2):173–82.
62. Hu R, Lu C, Mostaghel EA, et al. Distinct transcriptional programs mediated by the ligand-dependent full-length androgen receptor and its splice variants in castration-resistant prostate cancer. Cancer Res. 2012;72:3457–62.
63. Mostaghel EA, Marck BT, Plymate SR, et al. Resistance to CYP17A1 inhibition with abiraterone in castration-resistant prostate cancer: induction of steroidogenesis and androgen receptor splice variants. Clin Cancer Res. 2011;17:5913–25.
64. Li Y, Chan SC, Brand LJ, et al. Androgen receptor splice variants mediate enzalutamide resistance in castration-resistant prostate cancer cell lines. Cancer Res. 2013;73:483–9.

65. Antonarakis ES, Lu C, Wang H, et al. AR-V7 and resistance to enzalutamide and abiraterone in prostate cancer. N Engl J Med. 2014;371:1028–38.
66. Welti J, Rodrigues DN, Sharp A, et al. Analytical validation and clinical qualification of a new immunohistochemical assay for androgen receptor splice variant-7 protein expression in metastatic castration-resistant prostate cancer. Eur Urol. 2016;70(4):599–608.
67. Scher HI, Lu D, Schreiber NA, Louw J, et al. Association of AR-V7 on circulating tumor cells as a treatment-specific biomarker with outcomes and survival in castration-resistant prostate cancer. JAMA Oncol. 2016 Nov 1;2(11):1441–9.
68. Lotan TL, Gurel B, Suttcliffe S, et al. PTEN protein loss by immunostaining: analytic validation and prognostic indicator for a high risk surgical cohort of prostate cancer patients. Clin Cancer Res. 2011;17:6563–73.
69. Ferraldeschi R, Nava Rodrigues D, Riisnaes R, et al. PTEN protein loss and clinical outcome from castration-resistant prostate cancer treated with abiraterone acetate. Eur Urol. 2015;67:795–802.
70. Ahearn TU, Pettersson A, Ebot EM, et al. A prospective investigation of PTEN loss and ERG expression in lethal prostate cancer. J Natl Cancer Inst. 2016;108:dvj346.
71. Struewing JP, Hartge P, Wacholder S, et al. The risk of cancer associated with specific mutations of BRCA1 and BRCA2 among Ashkenazi Jews. N Engl J Med. 1997;336:1401–8.
72. Gallagher DJ, Gaudet MM, Pal P, et al. Germline BRCA mutations denote clinicopathologic subset of prostate cancer. Clin Cancer Res. 2010;16:2115–21.
73. Mateo J, Carreira S, Sandhu S, et al. DNA-repair defects and olaparib in metastatic prostate cancer. N Engl J Med. 2015;373:1697–708.
74. Pritchard CC, Morrissey C, Kumar A, et al. Complex MSH2 and MSH6 mutations in hypermutated microsatellite unstable advanced prostate cancer. Nat Commun. 2014;5:4988.
75. Graff JN, Alumkal JJ, Drake CG, et al. Early evidence of anti-PD-1 activity in enzalutamide-resistant prostate cancer. Oncotarget. 2016; doi:10.18632/oncotarget.10547.
76. Chung K, Wallace J, Kim SY. Structural and molecular interrogation of intact biological systems. Nature. 2013;497(7449):332–7. doi:10.1038/nature12107.
77. Santi PA. Light sheet fluorescent microscopy: a review. J Histochem Cytochem. 2011;59(2):129–38. doi:10.1369/0022155410394857.
78. van Royen ME, Verhoef EI, Kweldam CF, et al. Three-dimensional microscopic analysis of clinical prostate specimens. Histopathology. 2016;69:985–92.
79. Mateo J, Boysen G, Barbieri CE, et al. DNA repair in prostate cancer: biology and clinical implications. Eur Urol. 2016; doi:10.1016/j.eururo.2016.08.037. pii:S0302-2838(16)30504-8
80. Gordon RR, Wu M, Huang C-Y, et al. Chemotherapy-induced monoamine oxidase expression in prostate carcinoma functions as a cytoprotective resistance enzyme and associates with clinical outcomes. PLoS. 2014;9(9):e104271.
81. Sun Y, Campisi J, Higano C, et al. Treatment-induced damage to the tumor microenvironment promotes prostate cancer therapy resistance through WNT16B. Nat Med. 2012;18(9):1359–68.

Prostate Cancer Risk Grouping and Selection Criteria Based on Radiation Oncology Perspective

11

Yasemin Bolukbasi, Duygu Sezen, and Ugur Selek

Abstract

Since many decades, TNM staging has been widely used for almost all the cancer-diagnosed cases, to ensure the common language among the literature and medicine, but specifically to prostate cancer, treatment decisions have been more driven by diagnostic findings such as pretreatment PSA, age, biopsy-based Gleason score, and treatment options as well as the TNM staging. The management of prostate cancer includes a variety of approaches starting from active surveillance for very early stage. Intermediate stages could be treated with either surgery, radiotherapy, or brachytherapy with definitive intent. More locally advanced stages need combination of hormonal treatment with radiotherapy and/or surgery. Following the several published surgical nomograms to differentiate the patients more suitable for surgery, various attempts to provide probability graphs, nomograms, lookup tables, and neural networks were published and also validated by various groups in order to clarify the heterogeneity among groups and to distinguish patient selections between surgery, external beam therapy, brachytherapy, and hormonal therapy. Among the published, more than 20 nomograms, NCCN, TNM, and D'Amico groupings are the well-known and

Y. Bolukbasi, M.D. (✉) • U. Selek, M.D.
Department of Radiation Oncology, Koc University, Istanbul, Turkey

Department of Radiation Oncology, The University of Texas MD Anderson Cancer Center, Houston, TX, USA
e-mail: yaseminb@amerikanhastanesi.org

D. Sezen, M.D.
Department of Radiation Oncology, Koc University, Istanbul, Turkey

G. Ozyigit, U. Selek (eds.), *Principles and Practice of Urooncology*,
DOI 10.1007/978-3-319-56114-1_11

mostly used evaluation systems. The traditional three-group and new five-group risk stratifications and the new prostate grade grouping 1–5 will be in use to predict the risk of PSA recurrence following surgery and radiotherapy. The aim of this chapter is to provide a scope on these nomograms and comparison to each other in clinical practice.

11.1 Introduction

Prostate cancer is the most common nonskin malignancy with low cancer-specific mortality rates [9]. The management of prostate cancer includes a variety of approaches in a great range starting from active surveillance for very early stage, continuing with surgery, radiotherapy, or brachytherapy for intermediate stages with definitive intent. More locally advanced stages need combination of hormonal treatment with radiotherapy and/or surgery. Chemotherapy is starting to get more roles in the treatment of locally advanced stage prostate cancer with lymph node-positive patients [9–12]. The most challenging step is to select the best treatment for the suitable patients because prostate cancer itself has heterogenic nature which is commonly seen in clinic. Since the last two decades, prostate-specific antigen (PSA) and Gleason score have been used for clinical decision guidance. Several other prognostic factors such as PSA velocity, tertiary Gleason score, and the presence of perineural invasion have been tried to use in patient stratification for the best treatment selection, but their roles have not been still clearly recognized [13–17]. More than 20 nomograms published, NCCN, TNM, and D'Amico groupings are the well-known and frequently used evaluation system for patient guidance [4, 9, 18, 19].

11.2 Staging

Worldwide-accepted TNM classification is used to stage prostate cancer along with almost all the cancer types [4]. This staging system structure uniforms the extent of the primary tumor (T stage), the spread to nearby lymph nodes (N stage), and the absence or presence of distant spread or metastasis (M stage). All information that has been obtained by laboratory results, radiological or nuclear imaging, and clinical examination before first definitive management may be used for clinical staging. Moreover, clinical stage provides information to distinguish the treatment options, such as watchful waiting, active surveillance, surgery, radiotherapy, chemotherapy, and/or palliative care. The pathological stage is grounded on the surgical removal and histological evaluation of the entire prostate gland, the seminal vesicles, and the surrounding structures and pelvic lymph nodes [4]. Regularly the American Joint Committee on Cancer (AJCC) and International Union Against Cancer (UICC) update the TNM classification system. The latest change was published in 2010; the previous 2003 prostate cancer staging principles were preserved except revising

Table 11.1 AJCC staging—prostate cancer

AJCC 7th Edition (2009) *Note*: new staging incorporates Gleason + PSA for risk group determination *Primary tumor*: T1—clinically inapparent tumor neither palpable nor visible by imaging T1a—incidental histologic finding in 5% or less of tissue resected T1b—incidental histologic finding in more than 5% of tissue resected T1c—identified by needle biopsy (e.g., because of elevated PSA) T2—confined within prostate T2a—involves one half of one lobe or less T2b—involves more than one half of one lobe but not both lobes T2c—involves both lobes T3—extends through the prostate capsule (note: invasion into the prostatic apex or into, but not beyond, the prostatic capsule is classified not as T3 but as T2) T3a—extracapsular extension (unilateral or bilateral) or microscopic invasion of bladder neck T3b—invades seminal vesicles T4—fixed or invades adjacent structures other than seminal vesicles: bladder, external sphincter, rectum, levator muscles, and/or pelvic wall (note: microscopic invasion of the bladder neck is pT3 and not pT4) Pathological staging: there is no pT1 classification *Regional lymph nodes:* N0—none N1—yes Regional lymph nodes: pelvic, hypogastric, obturator, iliac (internal, external), sacralDistant lymph nodes: aortic, common iliac, inguinal (deep), inguinal (superficial, femoral), supraclavicular, cervical, scalene, retroperitoneal *Distant metastases:* M0—none M1a—non-regional lymph nodes M1b—bone M1c—other sites
Changes from 6th Edition: New stage groupings incorporate Gleason + PSA Microscopic bladder neck invasion (previously T4) is now T3a

microscopic invasion of the bladder neck (previously T4) as T3a and including new anatomic stage/prognostic groups that incorporate both Gleason score and preoperative PSA. The 2010 AJCC/UICC staging system is summarized in Table 11.1, and the new anatomic stage/prognostic groups are outlined in Table 11.2 [4]. The grouping is warranted as prostate cancer management and depends on the prostate-specific marker biochemical information (e.g., prostate-specific antigen, PSA) and pathological information (e.g., Gleason score), where both provide proven prognostic information different from the other cancer types [2, 19, 20].

TNM staging stratification by itself presents a heterogeneous risk grouping several nomograms were statistically generated from outcome data on large groups of men with prostate cancer. They are used to describe to outcome of the disease using well-known diagnostic findings such as pretreatment PSA, age, Gleason score. Using various predictive factors such as T stage, Gleason score, PSA, and histology results, more accurate assessment of the risk of metastatic spread, lymph node

Table 11.2 NCCN 2010 stage grouping

NCCN stage grouping
Stage grouping: Note: the AJCC staging manual distinctly lists these as "groups" in contrast to other tumor sites where they are listed as "stage"
Group I
T1a–c N0 M0, PSA < 10, Gleason ≤ 6
T2a N0 M0, PSA < 10, Gleason ≤ 6
T1–2a N0 M0, PSA X, Gleason X
Group IIA
T1a–c N0 M0, PSA < 20, Gleason 7
T1a–c N0 M0, PSA ≥ 10 < 20, Gleason ≤ 6
T2a–b N0 M0, PSA < 20, Gleason 7 (corrected in erratum)
T2a N0 M0, PSA ≥ 10 < 20, Gleason ≤6 (added in erratum)
T2b N0 M0, PSA X, Gleason X
Group IIB
T2c N0 M0, any PSA, any Gleason
T1–2 N0 M0, PSA ≥ 20, any Gleason
T1–2 N0 M0, any PSA, Gleason ≥ 8
Group III
T3a–b N0 M0, any PSA, any Gleason
Group IV
T4 N0 M0, any PSA, any Gleason
N1, any PSA, any Gleason
M1, any PSA, any Gleason

Note: when either PSA or Gleason is not available, grouping should be determined by T stage and/or either PSA or Gleason as available

Correlation with risk groups for localized disease—I is "low risk" (PSA < 10, G ≤ 6), IIA is "intermediate risk" (roughly, PSA 10–20 or G7 and PSA < 20), and IIB is "high risk" (T2c or PSA ≥ 20 or G ≥ 8)

involvement, or recurrence following treatment has been achieved [19–21]. Especially, nomograms may be used by healthcare professionals in partnership with men with prostate cancer to aid decision-making, to help predict biopsy results, to help predict pathological stage, and to help predict risk of treatment failure [2].

To date, modern literature presented more than 20 pretreatment predictive models (probability graphs, nomograms, lookup tables, and neural networks), and mainly all were based on three classical prognostic factors (pretreatment PSA, biopsy-based Gleason score, T stage) [1, 22, 23].

11.3 PSA

PSA is a glycoprotein normally helping to dissolve semen and can be expressed in both benign and malign disorders where PSA leaks out to result an increased level in blood test. The potential benefits of PSA testing in clinic are detection of cancer before symptoms are occurring and/or spreading, diagnosis at early stage, and aid in prostate cancer treatment. The important disadvantage of using PSA as a surrogate marker is that elevated PSA levels may also found in benign prostate hyperplasia, prostatitis, ejaculation and increasing age besides adenocarcinoma [24].

PSA has been used as a useful marker for the diagnosis and follow-up of prostate cancer [24, 25]. The most significant tools for prostate cancer are PSA levels higher than 4 ng/mL and a suspicious digital rectal examination (DRE) even though PSA screening has a limitation of low specificity despite high sensitivity which could easily lead to false-positive diagnoses [25, 26]. The earliest described prognostic factor was pretreatment PSA level which notes that progressively worse biochemical and prostate cancer outcomes were increasing parallel to PSA level [19, 27]. RTOG studies demonstrated that a pretreatment PSA 20 ng/mL predicts a greater likelihood of distant failure [28]. A PSA of 20 ng/mL has been a biochemically alarming sign that was associated with a greater risk of prostate cancer death [18]. Early reports by Partin and colleagues and D'Amico and colleagues defined important PSA cut points of <10, 10.1–20, and >20 ng/mL that are still used to define prostate cancer risk stratification groups [2, 19].

11.4 Gleason Score

Gleason score was firstly described by a pathologist Donald Gleason in 1960 whom he categorized the intrinsic morphologic heterogeneity of prostate cancer into a histological grading system, and since then several studies have clearly established its prognostic value [29, 30]. It has been a standard in urological pathology and could be defined as the most important tool for oncological outcomes. A primary and a secondary pattern (the range of each is 1–5) of the glands defined by microscopy are defined and then summed to a total score. The newly diagnosed needle biopsy-detected prostate cancers are graded Gleason score 6 or above [30]. If a single pattern of disease is seen, it should be reported as both grades. In a radical prostatectomy, if a tertiary pattern is present, it is stated in comment section. Gleason score listing was given in Table 11.3. Recent studies have demonstrated that Gleason score was an extremely important prognostic factor for prostate cancer outcomes [31]. In an analysis of the Radiation Therapy Oncology Group (RTOG), consisting of more than 1500 men included on prospective randomized trials, Gleason score was found to be the only most important predictor of death from prostate cancer [28, 31]. At the diagnostic pathology, Gleason score has to be defined and taken into consideration for patient personalized treatment selection.

Table 11.3 Gleason scoring system

Score	Definition
Gleason X	Gleason score cannot be processed
Gleason 6	Well differentiated (slight anaplasia)
Gleason 7	Moderately differentiated (moderate anaplasia)
Gleason 8–10	Poorly differentiated/undifferentiated (marked anaplasia)

11.5 T Stage

The T stage involves the evaluation of the local extent of the primary tumor in the prostate and its association to adjacent structures. The digital rectal examination (DRE) is still accepted as the "gold standard" for staging which provides almost nonsensitive information for extracapsular extension and depends on the examiner's experience [32]. Imaging is usually warranted to distinguish between T2 and T3/T4 (spread outside the prostate) cancers where MRI is the commonly used imaging technique for T staging of prostate cancer [33, 34].

AJCC TNM staging system subdivides pT2 disease into three categories pT2a, pT2b, and pT2c as determined by involvement of one half of one side and more than one half of one side and involvement of both sides of the prostate gland. The importance of this subdividing is the representation of the volume of cancer. pT3 disease has been categorized by two sections depending on the presence of extracapsular invasion in any location and presence of seminal vesical invasion with or without extracapsular invasion. Four large retrospective analyses have addressed that microscopic involvement of the bladder neck tissue by prostate cancer does not predict a significantly worse prognosis than extracapsular extension which has been expressed in the new version of staging and revised as pT3a [4].

11.6 Surgical Nomograms

Partin's table was established as the first nomogram that helps to predict the risk of post-prostatectomy, seminal vesicle invasion, and lymph node positivity after radical prostatectomy as a function of initial PSA, Gleason score, and clinical T stage based on a cohort of 2953 patients [27]. The following important surgical analytical models were published by Kattan and Stephenson (Fig. 11.1 and Table 11.4) [21, 35]. Kattan nomogram relates the classical prognostic factors with biochemical recurrence outcome, whereas the lately stated Stephenson nomogram relates the three classical prognostic factors to 15-year cancer-specific mortality with validation of 82% accuracy in a cohort of 12,677 radical prostatectomy patients [21, 36]. All nomograms described above were surgical nomograms that were developed by urologists.

11.7 Treatment Decision-Derived Nomograms

In 1998, D'Amico and colleagues first suggested a three-group risk stratification system to predict posttreatment biochemical failure after radical prostatectomy or external beam radiotherapy [19]. This system separated nonmetastatic patients into low, intermediate, and high risk grounded on initial PSA, clinical T stage, and biopsy Gleason score. Categories were as follows: low-risk prostate cancer as having 1992 AJCC T1/T2a and PSA $\leq$ 10 ng/mL and Gleason score $\leq$ 6, intermediate-risk prostate cancer as having 1992 AJCC T2b and/or PSA 10–20 ng/mL and/or

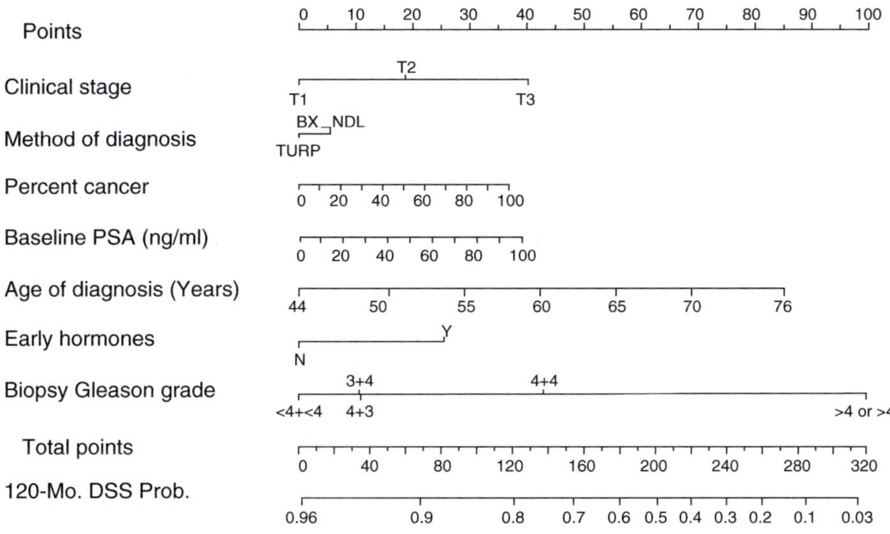

Fig. 11.1 Kattan nomogram. *Source*: M. Kattan et al., Cancer 112: 69–74, 2008

Table 11.4 Stephenson nomogram: pretreatment risk stratification for prostate cancer

Risk group	Clinical stage	Gleason score	Serum PSA
Standard risk groups			
Low risk	T1c–T2a	≤6	<10 ng/mL
Intermediate risk	T2b	7	10–20 ng/mL
High risk	T2c, T3	8–10	>20 ng/mL
Risk groupings used by Memorial Sloan Kettering and Seattle groups [1, 2]			
Low risk	≤T2a	≤6	<10 ng/mL
Intermediate risk	One elevated risk factor		
	One elevated risk factor: clinical stage ≥T2a disease, Gleason score ≥7, PSA ≥10 ng/mL		
High risk	Two elevated risk factors		

T1c tumor identified by needle biopsy (e.g., because of elevated PSA), *T2a* tumor which involves one half of one lobe or less, *T2b* tumor which involves more than one half of one lobe but not both lobes, *T2c* tumor involving both lobes

Gleason 7 disease, and high-risk disease as having any one of the following high-risk features—1922 AJCC ≥T2c, PSA >20 ng/mL, or Gleason 8–10 disease [19]. Although this system has been defined for patient selection for radiotherapy, it has been validated in surgical series [37].

In 2001, The Genito-Urinary Radiation Oncologists of Canada (GUROC) issued the consensus on the prostate cancer topics of risk evaluation, conformal radiotherapy, and brachytherapy and combined hormonal therapy [38]. A consensus of risk stratification for prostate cancer around three categories was defined: (1) low, 1997 AJCC T1–T2a, PSA ≤10 ng/mL, and Gleason ≤6; (2) intermediate, 1997 AJCC

T1–T2, PSA ≤20 ng/mL, and Gleason ≤7 not otherwise low risk; and (3) high risk, 1997 AJCC T3–T4 or PSA >20 ng/mL or Gleason 8–10 [38]. In 2013, Rodrigues et al. validated the published three-group risk stratification system in a database that consists of 7974 patients from four Canadian institutions. Additionally, to improve the selection capability, recursive partitioning analysis was developed to determine the sub-stratification of groups defined in 2001 which suggested six separate and statistical unique groups [39]. GUROC low-risk patients were classified as favorable low and low-risk groups based on PSA ≤ 6 and PSA > 6. Additionally GUROC intermediate-risk patients were subclassified into low-intermediate and high-intermediate groups which were intersected by PSA ≥ 10 and either T2b/T2c disease or T1–T2a disease with Gleason 7. An additional extreme-risk group (GUROC high-risk and positive cores ≥ 87.5% or PSA > 30) was added to the GUROC high-risk patient categorization [39]. The GUROC has published a project to revise appropriate definitions of low-intermediate, high-intermediate, and high-risk prostate cancer using a multi-institutional database to using new candidate factors as amount of high-grade cancer, Gleason pattern 3 + 4 versus 4 + 3, percentage of positive biopsy cores, and T stage (i.e., presence of T2b/T2c disease). Available Canadian databases considered for combined analysis will include the British Columbia Cancer Agency prostate cancer database, the National Cancer Institute of Canada PR5 intermediate-risk dose (and dose per fraction) fractionation study, as well as the Princess Margaret Hospital prostate cancer dose escalation and brachytherapy clinical databases [1]. In this project, up to six categories (very low risk, low risk, low-intermediate risk, high-intermediate risk, high risk, and extreme risk) will be defined and characterized in terms of ASTRO BFFS and overall survival. In addition, the ProCaRS database will be used to perform direct propensity score matched-pair analyses of various interventions (e.g., brachytherapy vs. external beam radiation therapy) [1]. Gabriele et al. has published a new classification with a combination of age, pretreatment PSA' clinical-radiological staging, Gleason score, and percentage of positive cores at biopsy. EUREKA-2 retrospective multicentric database has been used to create "Candiolo" risk classes which are the subgroups of all defined variables and compared to D'Amico staging for progression-free survival and prostate cancer-specific survival and revealed that this system stratifies patients better for these oncological outcomes. Five-year progression-free survival was 94% for very low-risk and 43% for very high-risk group (Fig. 11.2). The major difference from the D'Amico system was the cutoff level of pretreatment PSA level as in this new system defined as 7 ng/mL and 15 ng/mL. Also T2 staging was not divided into subgroups as T2a, T2b, or T2c [40]. External validation studies were warranted to be accepted as a clinical decision-making tool.

TNM staging stratification which has been the most commonly used disease stratification system provides a heterogeneous risk grouping in clinical daily routine for prostate cancer. After Roach et al. demonstrated that clinical outcome reflection of three classical prognostic factor systems versus one based on T stage classification alone was superior. The AJCC and UICC have implemented initial PSA level and Gleason score into the staging system [41]. This grouping was generally parallel to the D'Amico classification except previous editions of local advanced stages

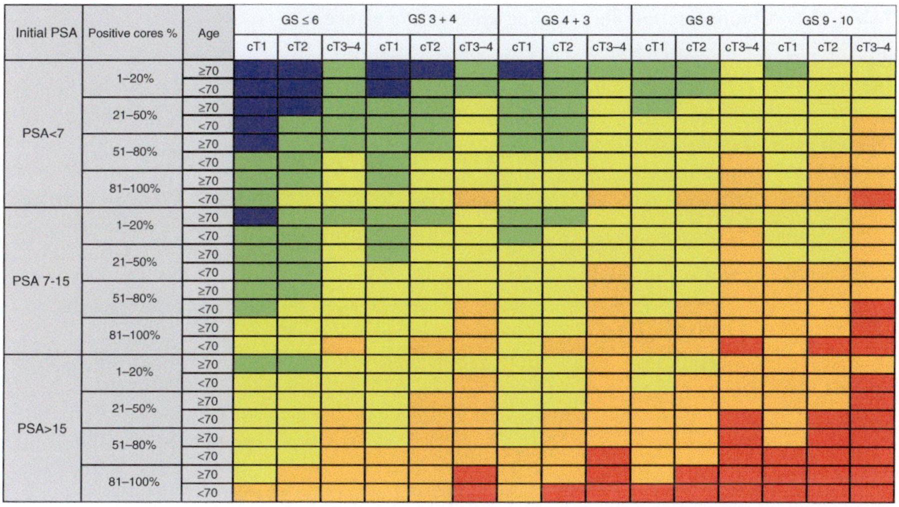

Initial PSA	Positive cores %	Age	GS ≤ 6			GS 3 + 4			GS 4 + 3			GS 8			GS 9 - 10		
			cT1	cT2	cT3–4	cT1	cT2	cT3–4	cT1	cT2	cT3–4	cT1	cT2	cT3–4	cT1	cT2	cT3–4
PSA<7	1–20%	≥70															
		<70															
	21–50%	≥70															
		<70															
	51–80%	≥70															
		<70															
	81–100%	≥70															
		<70															
PSA 7-15	1–20%	≥70															
		<70															
	21–50%	≥70															
		<70															
	51–80%	≥70															
		<70															
	81–100%	≥70															
		<70															
PSA>15	1–20%	≥70															
		<70															
	21–50%	≥70															
		<70															
	51–80%	≥70															
		<70															
	81–100%	≥70															
		<70															

Fig. 11.2 Candiolo classifier table. Very low risk, *blue*; low risk, *green*; intermediate risk, *yellow*; high risk, *orange*; and very high risk, *red*

3 and 4 which were used. In 2010, the NCCN guidelines currently include risk categories from very low-risk (T1c and Gleason score ≤ 6, PSA ≤10 ng/mL, <3 positive biopsy cores each ≤50% involved, and PSA density of <0.15 ng/mL/g) to very high-risk (T3b–T4) subdivision (Table 11.2) [4] which is clinically useful with distinct five subgroups.

The Radiation Therapy Oncology Group (RTOG) also proposed a validated four-group risk stratification system, as a low-risk cohort (T1–T2 and GS2–GS6 with no PSA cutoffs) followed with higher-risk cohorts (RTOG 2—T1T2GS7 or T3GS2–6; RTOG 3—T1–T2GS8–10 or T3GS7; and RTOG 4—T3GS8–10) [28]. This grouping has been validated in Japan study group database which consists of 15,259 patients [42]. Five-year overall survival in prognostic groups starting from group I to IV was as follows: 90, 88.3, 84.4, 80.6, and 57.1%, respectively. The concordance index of prognostic grouping has defined 0.670 and revealed that even hormonal therapy was prescribed, the stratification power has been validated.

A part from the previous grouping systems, Williams and Beasley have published validation analyses regarding a five-group risk stratification system including low (PSA <7.5, Gleason score ≤6), low-intermediate (PSA 7.5–15, Gleason score ≤ 6), high-intermediate (PSA 15–20, Gleason score ≤ 6 or PSA ≤10, Gleason score ≥ 7), high (PSA 20–30, Gleason score ≤ 6 or PSA 10–20, Gleason score ≥7), and extreme (PSA >20, Gleason score ≥7 or PSA >30, Gleason score ≤6) groups [21, 43, 44]. Using all GS 7–10 tumors as intermediate or high risk showed improved discrimination but still have a lesser significant projection in the intermediate-risk region.

In the light of several clinical nomograms, comparisons were performed (Table 11.5). Kattan et al. compared previous five-group recursive partitioning

Table 11.5 Comparisons of the grouping systems at a glance

Group name	Low risk	Intermediate risk	High risk
NCCN	PSA < 10, G ≤ 6	PSA 10–20 or G7 and PSA < 20	T2c or PSA ≥ 20 or G ≥ 8
D'Amico	1992 AJCC T1/T2a, and PSA ≤10 ng/mL, and Gleason score ≤6	1992 AJCC T2b and/or PSA 10–20 ng/mL and/or Gleason 7 disease	Any one of the following high-risk features: 1922 AJCC ≥T2c, PSA > 20 ng/mL, or Gleason 8–10 disease
GUROC	1997 AJCC T1–T2a, PSA ≤ 10 ng/mL and Gleason ≤ 6	1997 AJCC T1–T2, PSA ≤20 ng/mL and Gleason ≤7 not otherwise low risk	1997 AJCC T3–T4 or PSA >20 ng/mL or Gleason 8–10
Williams and Beasley	Low (PSA < 7.5, Gleason score ≤ 6)	Low-intermediate (PSA 7.5–15, Gleason score ≤6), high-intermediate (PSA 15–20, Gleason score ≤ 6 or PSA ≤ 10, Gleason score ≥ 7)	High (PSA 20–30, Gleason score ≤6 or PSA 10–20, Gleason score ≥ 7), extreme (PSA >20, Gleason score ≥ 7 or PSA > 30, Gleason score ≤ 6) groups
RTOG	T1–T2 and GS2–GS6 with no PSA cutoffs	RTOG 2–T1T2GS7 or T3GS2–6	RTOG 3–T1–T2GS8–10 or T3GS7 RTOG 4–T3GS8–10

analysis-based system to the contemporary NCCN three-group risk stratification system and the Kattan nomogram to evaluate and validate using Memorial Sloan Kettering Cancer Center prostate cancer data [21]. This comparison was aimed to predict biochemical failure defined as three consecutive rises of serum PSA. This five-group system was found to be superior when compared to the other systems; even, there was difficulty in the discrimination of the intermediate-risk groups [21]. The use of hormonal therapy has been more often prescribed for this subgroup of patients based on the result of several randomized trials which has not been usually accounted in the nomograms. Beasley et al. assessed the impact of hormonal therapy and the five-group model to determine if any subgroups would benefit from combined hormonal therapy with external beam radiotherapy [44]. A prospective nonrandomized data set of 1423 men treated at the British Columbia Cancer Agency was evaluated for the primary end point of biochemical control (bNED) with the RTOG-ASTRO "phoenix" definition (lowest PSA to date + 2 ng/mL), both with and without adjuvant ADT. Despite no bNED benefit for ADT in the low or low-intermediate groups where the Gleason score is 6 or less and PSA is 15 or less, a statistically significant bNED benefit in the high intermediate-, high-, and extreme-risk groups was demonstrated. These results have suggested that current risk stratification systems should be modified intermediate risk into two groups [44].

To differentiate the patient subgroups, five-section grouping systems seem to be more accurate. For example, the NCCN grouping has defined the inclusion of a very low-risk category to identify patients that may be entered into observation/surveillance protocols should be considered [4]. Because there are more unreliable results for intermediate risk as this group covers more a heterogeneous group of patients in terms of outcome and treatment management, a subdivision of the intermediate-risk group into a low-intermediate- and a high intermediate-risk group could be proper as given the reflection of hormonal therapy for the higher-risk group [44]. Yet, five-group stratification system did not compensate the amount of high-grade cancer, Gleason pattern 4 + 3 versus 3 + 4, and percentage positive biopsy cores nor tertiary pattern five.

11.8 Prostate Cancer Grading Grouping System

A new Gleason grading system in prostate cancer has been discussed since the International Society of Urological Pathology (ISUP) consensus meeting in 2014 gathered many prostate cancer pathology experts, as well as clinicians in urology, radiation, and medical oncology [5]. As the lowest current score is 6 in the Gleason grading system ranging from 2 to 10, this assigned score terrifies the patients being told, implying that a score 6 out of 10 carries an intermediate prognosis of an aggressive cancer. Besides, current incorrect groupings such as Gleason score 7 without any distinctive 3 + 4 versus 4 + 3 information might blur the outcome data. Therefore, a broad consensus was built to be adopted to simplify stratification as grade groups 1–5 (defined as Gleason grades ≤6, 3 + 4, 4 + 3, 8, and >8, respectively) which will be used in conjunction with Gleason score such as Gleason score 3 + 3 = 6 and grade group 1; and this terminology was accepted by the World Health Organization for the 2016 edition [5].

Rubin et al. sought genomic support in radical prostatectomy data of 426 clinically localized prostate cancer patients for new prostate grading group (PGG) system using whole-exome and whole-genome sequencing data [7]. They have pointed out a significant frequency increase with increasing PGG in genomic amplifications and deletions and in nonsynonymous point mutations entirely haploid in low-risk PGG1 but increasing polyploidy frequency in PGG2 to PGG5 and revealed distinct classes based on genomic profiles for PGG1, PGG2, and PGG3 and genomic similarity for PGG4 and PGG5. Rubin et al., with the largest to date prostate cancer genomic data set, demonstrated increasing genomic alterations with increasing PGG and molecular support for new five-tiered PGG system [7]. Epstein et al. tried to verify the accuracy of new grading group system in a multi-institutional and multimodal therapy data; [8] data from five academic institutions including 20,845 men treated by radical prostatectomy and from two academic institutions including 5501 men treated with radiotherapy was analyzed. The five-grade grouping system was demonstrated for all cohorts to have the highest prognostic discrimination on both uni- and multivariable analysis [8]. Loeb et al. evaluated the performance of PGG in National Prostate Cancer Register of Sweden with 5880 men (between 2005 and 2007: 4325, radical prostatectomy; 1555, radiation therapy) [6]. They have documented PGG as significant independent predictors of biochemical recurrence both after radical prostatectomy and radiation therapy based on adjustments for preoperative PSA, biopsy PGG, and clinical stage; biochemical recurrence-free survival rates for PGG 1–5, respectively, at 4 years by surgery were 89, 82, 74, 77, and 49% on biopsy and 92, 85, 73, 63, and 51% for prostatectomy and by radiation therapy were 95, 91, 85, 78, and 70% [6].

The new PGGs 1–5 sound to provide a plain user-friendly classification system to independently predict the risk of PSA recurrence following surgery and radiotherapy [5–8].

Conclusion

Multiple studies of prognostic factors have been accomplished to create currently applied prostate cancer risk stratification systems. The traditional three-group and new five-group risk stratifications in addition to the new pathology grade grouping 1–5 will be in play to predict the risk of PSA recurrence following surgery and radiotherapy. Eventually, in the era of individualization along with the multidisciplinary care and consensus, treatment approaches linked to current practice patterns are evolving, and we need to stratify our patients as accurate as possible between the risk groups to finalize their treatment recommendations.

References

1. Rodrigues G, Lukka H, Warde P, Brundage M, Souhami L, Crook J, Cury F, Catton C, Mok G, Martin AG, et al. The prostate cancer risk stratification project: database construction and risk stratification outcome analysis. J Natl Compr Cancer Netw. 2014;12(1):60–9.
2. Kattan MW, Eastham JA, Wheeler TM, Maru N, Scardino PT, Erbersdobler A, Graefen M, Huland H, Koh H, Shariat S, et al. Counseling men with prostate cancer: a nomogram for predicting the presence of small, moderately differentiated, confined tumors. J Urol. 2003;170(5):1792–7.
3. AJCC. Cancer staging handbook. 7th ed. Chicago, IL: American Joint Committee on Cancer; 2010.
4. Epstein JI, Egevad L, Amin MB, Delahunt B, Srigley JR, Humphrey PA. The 2014 International Society of Urological Pathology (ISUP) consensus conference on Gleason grading of prostatic carcinoma: definition of grading patterns and proposal for a new grading system. Am J Surg Pathol. 2016;40(2):244–52.
5. Loeb S, Folkvaljon Y, Robinson D, Lissbrant IF, Egevad L, Stattin P. Evaluation of the 2015 Gleason Grade Groups in a Nationwide Population-based Cohort. Eur Urol. 2016;69(6):1135–41.
6. Rubin MA, Girelli G, Demichelis F. Genomic correlates to the newly proposed grading prognostic groups for prostate cancer. Eur Urol. 2016;69(4):557–60.
7. Epstein JI, Zelefsky MJ, Sjoberg DD, Nelson JB, Egevad L, Magi-Galluzzi C, Vickers AJ, Parwani AV, Reuter VE, Fine SW, et al. A contemporary prostate cancer grading system: a validated alternative to the Gleason score. Eur Urol. 2016;69(3):428–35.
8. Aizer AA, Paly JJ, Efstathiou JA. Multidisciplinary care and management selection in prostate cancer. Semin Radiat Oncol. 2013;23(3):157–64.
9. Markowski MC, Carducci MA. Early use of chemotherapy in metastatic prostate cancer. Cancer Treat Rev. 2016. doi:10.1016/j.ctrv.2016.09.017.
10. Crook J, Ots AF. Prognostic factors for newly diagnosed prostate cancer and their role in treatment selection. Semin Radiat Oncol. 2013;23(3):165–72.
11. Carthon BC, Antonarakis ES. The STAMPEDE trial: paradigm-changing data through innovative trial design. Transl Cancer Res. 2016;5(3 Suppl):S485–90.
12. D'Amico AV, Renshaw AA, Sussman B, Chen MH. Pretreatment PSA velocity and risk of death from prostate cancer following external beam radiation therapy. JAMA. 2005;294(4):440–7.
13. Lotan Y, Shariat SF, Khoddami SM, Saboorian H, Koeneman KS, Cadeddu JA, Sagalowsky AI, McConnell JD, Roehrborn CG. The percent of biopsy cores positive for cancer is a

predictor of advanced pathological stage and poor clinical outcomes in patients treated with radical prostatectomy. J Urol. 2004;171(6 Pt 1):2209–14.
14. Freedland SJ, Aronson WJ, Terris MK, Kane CJ, Amling CL, Dorey F, Presti JC Jr. Percent of prostate needle biopsy cores with cancer is significant independent predictor of prostate specific antigen recurrence following radical prostatectomy: results from SEARCH database. J Urol. 2003;169(6):2136–41.
15. Lee JT, Lee S, Yun CJ, Jeon BJ, Kim JM, Ha HK, Lee W, Chung MK. Prediction of perineural invasion and its prognostic value in patients with prostate cancer. Korean J Urol. 2010;51(11):745–51.
16. Patel AA, Chen MH, Renshaw AA, D'Amico AV. PSA failure following definitive treatment of prostate cancer having biopsy Gleason score 7 with tertiary grade 5. JAMA. 2007;298(13):1533–8.
17. Aus G, Abbou CC, Bolla M, Heidenreich A, Schmid HP, van Poppel H, Wolff J, Zattoni F. EAU guidelines on prostate cancer. Eur Urol. 2005;48(4):546–51.
18. D'Amico AV, Whittington R, Malkowicz S, et al. BIochemical outcome after radical prostatectomy, external beam radiation therapy, or interstitial radiation therapy for clinically localized prostate cancer. JAMA. 1998;280(11):969–74.
19. Sebo TJ, Cheville JC, Riehle DL, Lohse CM, Pankratz VS, Myers RP, Blute ML, Zincke H. Predicting prostate carcinoma volume and stage at radical prostatectomy by assessing needle biopsy specimens for percent surface area and cores positive for carcinoma, perineural invasion, Gleason score, DNA ploidy and proliferation, and preoperative serum prostate specific antigen: a report of 454 cases. Cancer. 2001;91(11):2196–204.
20. Kattan MW, Zelefsky MJ, Kupelian PA, Scardino PT, Fuks Z, Leibel SA. Pretreatment nomogram for predicting the outcome of three-dimensional conformal radiotherapy in prostate cancer. J Clin Oncol. 2000;18(19):3352–9.
21. Eifler JB, Feng Z, Lin BM, Partin MT, Humphreys EB, Han M, Epstein JI, Walsh PC, Trock BJ, Partin AW. An updated prostate cancer staging nomogram (Partin tables) based on cases from 2006 to 2011. BJU Int. 2013;111(1):22–9.
22. Gnanapragasam VJ, Lophatananon A, Wright KA, Muir KR, Gavin A, Greenberg DC. Improving clinical risk stratification at diagnosis in primary prostate cancer: a prognostic modelling study. PLoS Med. 2016;13(8):e1002063.
23. Kirby R. The role of PSA in detection and management of prostate cancer. Practitioner. 2016;260(1792):17–21, 3.
24. Dinnes J, Hewison J, Altman DG, Deeks JJ. The basis for monitoring strategies in clinical guidelines: a case study of prostate-specific antigen for monitoring in prostate cancer. CMAJ. 2012;184(2):169–77.
25. Kim JS, Ryu J-G, Kim JW, Hwang EC, Jung SI, Kang TW, Kwon D, Park K. Prostate-specific antigen fluctuation: what does it mean in diagnosis of prostate cancer? Int Braz J Urol. 2015;41(2):258–64.
26. Partin AW, Kattan MW, Subong EN, Walsh PC, Wojno KJ, Oesterling JE, Scardino PT, Pearson JD. Combination of prostate-specific antigen, clinical stage, and Gleason score to predict pathological stage of localized prostate cancer. A multi-institutional update. JAMA. 1997;277(18):1445–51.
27. Roach M, Lu J, Pilepich MV, Asbell SO, Mohiuddin M, Terry R, Grignon D. Four prognostic groups predict long-term survival from prostate cancer following radiotherapy alone on Radiation Therapy Oncology Group clinical trials. Int J Radiat Oncol Biol Phys. 2000;47(3):609–15.
28. Pierorazio PM, Walsh PC, Partin AW, Epstein JI. Prognostic Gleason grade grouping: data based on the modified Gleason scoring system. BJU Int. 2013;111(5):753–60.
29. Gordetsky J, Epstein J. Grading of prostatic adenocarcinoma: current state and prognostic implications. Diagn Pathol. 2016;11:25.
30. Roach M 3rd, Lu J, Pilepich MV, Asbell SO, Mohiuddin M, Terry R, Grignon D. Long-term survival after radiotherapy alone: radiation therapy oncology group prostate cancer trials. J Urol. 1999;161(3):864–8.

31. Lee HW, Seo SI, Jeon SS, Lee HM, Choi HY. Can we predict real T3 stage prostate cancer in patients with clinical T3 (cT3) disease before radical prostatectomy? Yonsei Med J. 2010;51(5):700–7.
32. Bonekamp D, Jacobs MA, El-Khouli R, Stoianovici D, Macura KJ. Advancements in MR imaging of the prostate: from diagnosis to interventions. Radiographics. 2011;31(3):677–703.
33. Yoo S, Kim JK, Jeong IG. Multiparametric magnetic resonance imaging for prostate cancer: a review and update for urologists. Korean J Urol. 2015;56(7):487–97.
34. Stephenson AJ, Scardino PT, Eastham JA, Bianco FJ, Dotan ZA, Fearn PA, Kattan MW. Preoperative nomogram predicting the 10-year probability of prostate cancer recurrence after radical prostatectomy. J Natl Cancer Inst. 2006;98(10):715–7.
35. Brockman JA, Alanee S, Vickers AJ, Scardino PT, Wood DP, Kibel AS, Lin DW, Bianco FJ, Rabah DM, Klein EA, et al. Nomogram predicting prostate cancer–specific mortality for men with biochemical recurrence after radical prostatectomy. Eur Urol. 2015;67(6):1160–7.
36. Dorin RP, Daneshmand S, Lassoff MA, Cai J, Skinner DG, Lieskovsky G. Long-term outcomes of open radical retropubic prostatectomy for clinically localized prostate cancer in the prostate-specific antigen era. Urology. 2012;79(3):626–31.
37. Lukka H, Warde P, Pickles T, Morton G, Brundage M, Souhami L. Controversies in prostate cancer radiotherapy: consensus development. Can J Urol. 2001;8(4):1314–22.
38. Rodrigues G, Lukka H, Warde P, Brundage M, Souhami L, Crook J, Cury F, Catton C, Mok G, Martin AG, et al. The prostate cancer risk stratification (ProCaRS) project: recursive partitioning risk stratification analysis. Radiother Oncol. 2013;109(2):204–10.
39. Gabriele D, Jereczek-Fossa BA, Krengli M, Garibaldi E, Tessa M, Moro G, Girelli G, Gabriele P, EUREKA-2 Consortium. Beyond D'Amico risk classes for predicting recurrence after external beam radiotherapy for prostate cancer: the Candiolo classifier. Radiat Oncol. 2016;11:23.
40. Roach M 3rd, Weinberg V, Sandler H, Thompson I. Staging for prostate cancer: time to incorporate pretreatment prostate-specific antigen and Gleason score? Cancer. 2007;109(2):213–20.
41. Kimura T, Onozawa M, Miyazaki J, Kawai K, Nishiyama H, Hinotsu S, Akaza H. Validation of the prognostic grouping of the seventh edition of the tumor-nodes-metastasis classification using a large-scale prospective cohort study database of prostate cancer treated with primary androgen deprivation therapy. Int J Urol. 2013;20(9):880–8.
42. Williams SG, Duchesne GM, Gogna NK, Millar JL, Pickles T, Pratt GR, Turner S. An international multicenter study evaluating the impact of an alternative biochemical failure definition on the judgment of prostate cancer risk. Int J Radiat Oncol Biol Phys. 2006;65(2):351–7.
43. Beasley M, Williams SG, Pickles T. Expanded risk groups help determine which prostate radiotherapy sub-group may benefit from adjuvant androgen deprivation therapy. Radiat Oncol. 2008;3:8.

Robotic Surgery in Prostate Cancer

12

Ömer Acar and Tarık Esen

Abstract

Prostate cancer is the second most common malignancy in men (excluding skin cancer) behind lung cancer, with more than one million cases estimated to be diagnosed worldwide in 2016. Radical prostatectomy (RP) has been the most widely used approach for the treatment of organ-confined prostate cancer. However, the high incidence of perioperative morbidities and functional derangements related with open radical retropubic prostatectomy (RRP) has led to the search for less invasive treatments to improve oncological outcomes and quality of life issues. Binder and Kramer were the first to report the feasibility of robot-assisted laparoscopic radical prostatectomy in 2001, and the Vattikuti Urology Institute at Henry Ford Hospital in Detroit, Michigan, USA, pioneered the establishment of urologic robotic surgery programs worldwide. The application of robotic technology in surgical practice has developed tremendously over the past three decades. Urologists in particular have embraced surgical robots throughout their evolution, and robot-assisted urologic surgeries have matured into everyday clinical practice in many parts of the world. Herein, we will review the available literature data about robotic surgery in prostate cancer concentrating mainly on the evolution and adaptation of robot-assisted radical prostatectomy (RARP), its perioperative/functional/oncological outcomes, results of comparative studies with open/laparoscopic RP, and relevant future directions related with optimization of RARP outcomes.

Ö. Acar, M.D. (✉)
Department of Urology, School of Medicine, Koc University, Istanbul, Turkey
e-mail: oacar@kuh.ku.edu.tr

T. Esen, M.D.
Department of Urology, School of Medicine, Koc University, Istanbul, Turkey

Department of Urology, VKF American Hospital, Istanbul, Turkey

G. Ozyigit, U. Selek (eds.), *Principles and Practice of Urooncology*,
DOI 10.1007/978-3-319-56114-1_12

12.1 Robot-Assisted Radical Prostatectomy

Prostate cancer remains the second most commonly diagnosed cancer in men [1]. Radical prostatectomy, which represents the removal of prostate together with seminal vesicles, can be employed in the setting of organ confined disease. Selected patients with locally advanced and oligometastatic prostate cancer can also be managed via radical prostatectomy as the first step of a multimodal treatment approach. The first radical prostatectomy was performed by the perineal approach in 1903 by Young [4], followed by the description of the retropubic technique by Millin [5] in 1947. The current concept of retropubic radical and "nerve-sparing" prostatectomy was established by Patrick Walsh et al. in 1982 [6]. Laparoscopic surgeries were initiated in the 1990s, and the robotic approach in radical prostatectomy was introduced in 2001 [2], and at that time, only a few case reports or series were published, none of which being able to demonstrate any clinical benefit [7–9].

Surgical techniques requiring microsurgical precision and advanced reconstructive skills, as well as inaccessible operative fields, can be made amenable with robotic surgery. Advanced robotic surgical systems such as da Vinci are equipped with three-dimensional, high-definition visualization, improved dexterity, seven degrees of freedom, ergonomic position, elimination of tremors, and ability to scale motions and have effectively overcome several limitations of conventional laparoscopy. Hence, open surgeons had the option to adapt a minimally invasive approach with a relatively simpler and faster learning curve when compared with its "pure" laparoscopic counterpart [10].

Since its introduction to the urological armamentarium, robot-assisted radical prostatectomy (RARP) carried out using the da Vinci Surgical System TM (Intuitive Surgical, Sunnyvale, CA, USA) has been rapidly accepted as a safe and efficacious surgical treatment option for localized prostate cancer [11]. Radical prostatectomy (RP) represents the most widely performed surgical applications in the context of minimally invasive urooncological surgery [11]. Almost 80% of the RARPs performed in the USA are being carried out via the robotic approach [10]. Noteworthy, this trend has occurred despite the lack of high-quality evidence to support the superiority of RARP, which will be discussed further in detail in the following sections of this chapter.

Indications for RARP are the same as for RRP and laparoscopic radical prostatectomy (LRP), and any of these surgical approaches can be offered to a patient who is a candidate for radical prostatectomy. The European Association of Urology (EAU) advocates RP to be offered to patients with low- and intermediate-risk prostate cancer and a life expectancy exceeding 10 years. Additionally, those with high-risk localized or locally advanced (cT3a) disease together with a life expectancy of >10 years can also be candidates for RP as the initial step of a multimodal treatment approach. Lastly, highly selected cases with more locally advanced disease (cT3b-T4 N0 or any T N1) can also be considered for RP again in the context of a multidisciplinary team approach involving the participation of medical and radiation oncologists [12].

12.2 Overview of the Surgical Steps of RARP

We have been performing RARPs since May 2010 in our clinic. The same surgeon (T.E.), who has made a direct transition from open to robotic surgery, has carried out all of these operations. Herein, we will review our technique of RARP using the da Vinci(si) surgical system (Intuitive Surgical, Sunnyvale, CA, USA), highlighting some of the basic steps of the procedure.

We use a transperitoneal antegrade approach and place a total of six abdominal ports (four for the robotic arms and two for the bedside assistant) after creating pneumoperitoneum via the Hasson technique [13]. Bilateral extended pelvic lymph node dissection (ePLND), which includes the removal of obturator, external iliac, internal iliac, presacral, and common iliac LNs, is performed in intermediate- or high-risk patients and in those with ≥5% risk of pelvic lymph node involvement according to Partin tables [14] or Briganti nomogram [15].

Initially, the thin fascial layer over the seminal vesicles and vasa is opened (Fig. 12.1). Both vasa are then incised and their inferior portions are retracted to aid in dissection (Fig. 12.2). The vas is then followed posteriorly to expose the tips of the seminal vesicles. Seminal vesicles are dissected all the way to the base to allow for appropriate elevation of the prostate and identification of posterior

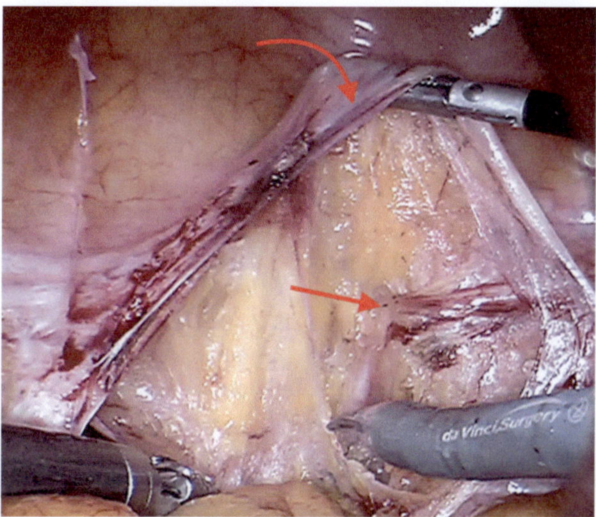

Fig. 12.1 Fascial coverings (*curved arrow*) over vasa deferentia (*straight arrow*) are released

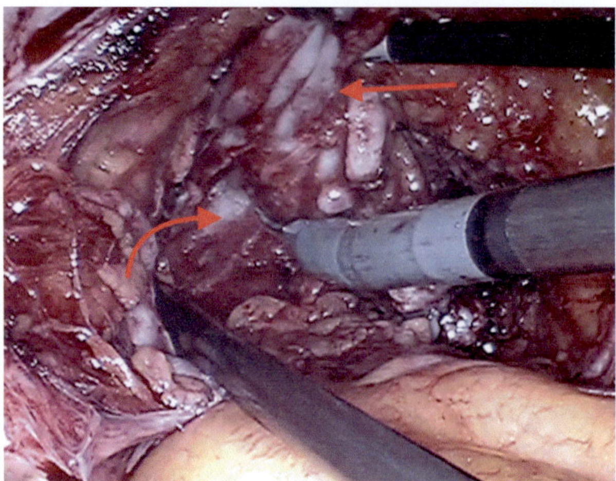

Fig. 12.2 Vas deferens and seminal vesicle being retracted (*straight arrow*) to develop the plane of dissection (*curved arrow*)

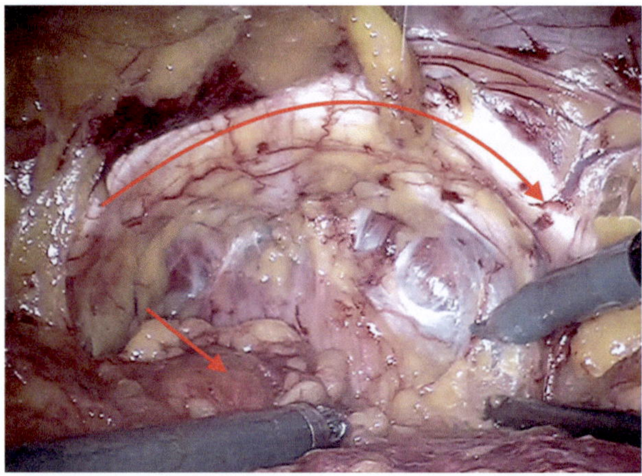

Fig. 12.3 Prevesical space (the space of Retzius or retropubic space), pubic arc (*curved arrow*), and bladder (*straight arrow*)

Denonvilliers' fascia. We avoid using electrocautery particularly at the tip of the seminal vesicles in order not to damage the neurovascular bundles and use nonabsorbable endoclips. For the posterior dissection, we try to stay on the plane between Denonvilliers' fascia and the prostatic capsule.

After completing the posterior dissection, the peritoneum is incised transversally through the medial umbilical ligament. The incision is extended on both sides in an inverted U fashion to develop the space of Retzius (Fig. 12.3). Then the endopelvic fascia is opened from the base of the prostate to the reflection of puboprostatic ligaments bilaterally using cold scissors (Fig. 12.4). After incising puboprostatic

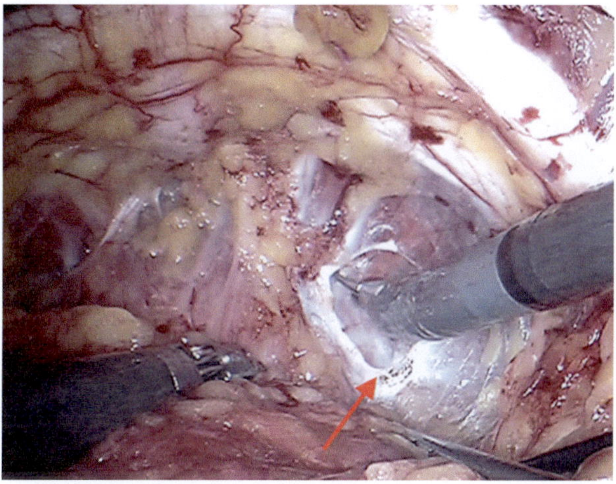

Fig. 12.4 Endopelvic fascia (*arrow*) incised with scissors

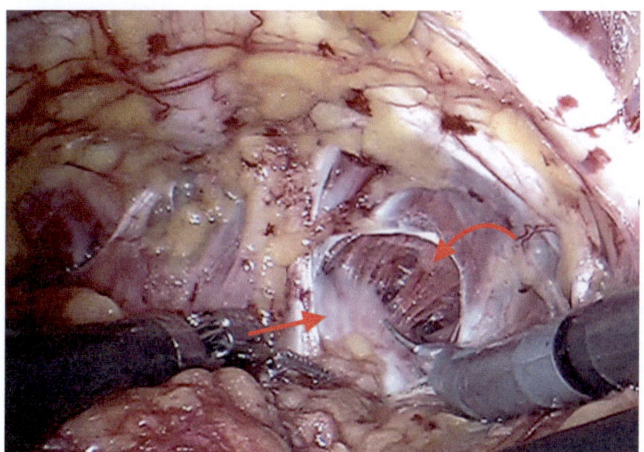

Fig. 12.5 Fibers of levator ani (*curved arrow*) are being pushed away from the prostatic surface (*straight arrow*)

ligaments (Fig. 12.5), the levator fibers are pushed away from the prostate (Fig. 12.6) until the dorsal venous complex (DVC) and urethra are visualized which is necessary to get in a good and reliable DVC stitch.

In order to ligate the DVC, robotic needle drivers are introduced, and the needle of an absorbable suture (zero polyglycolic acid) material is placed in the groove between the urethra and DVC (Fig. 12.7). The suture strength needs to be sufficient to allow the needle holders to pull up and perform a slip knot, which prevents the suture from loosening once it is tied (Fig. 12.8).

After identifying the bladder neck via pulling on the urethral catheter and visualizing the balloon, the bladder is dissected off the prostate in the midline using a

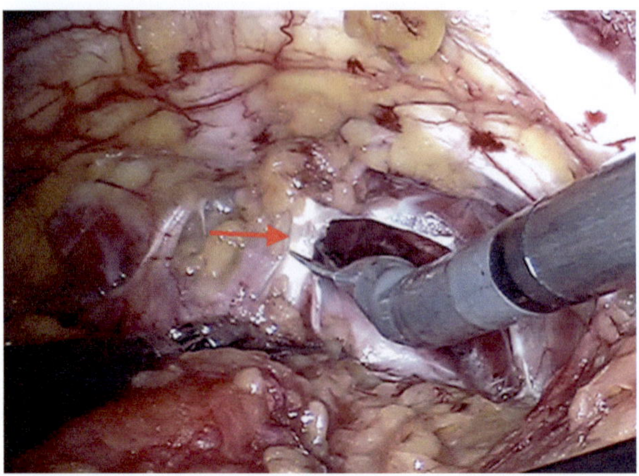

Fig. 12.6 Puboprostatic ligament (*arrow*) is being incised by scissors

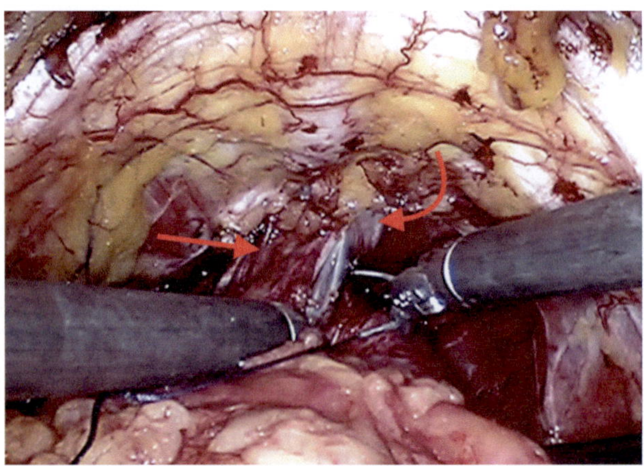

Fig. 12.7 Dorsal venous complex (DVC) stitch is being placed into the groove between the urethra (*curved arrow*) and DVC (*straight arrow*)

sweeping motion of the monopolar scissor. Once the anterior bladder neck is opened in the midline, bladder neck dissection begins on both sides. Afterward, the anterior urethra is divided, and the Foley catheter is retracted out of the bladder to apply upward traction (Fig. 12.9) which will be helpful while controlling the pedicle and exposing the posterior bladder neck.

Remaining peripheral bladder attachments are divided (Fig. 12.10) to flatten out the area of the posterior bladder neck, full thickness of which should be incised at the junction between the prostate and bladder. After grasping and applying traction to the lip of posterior bladder neck, the natural plane of dissection, which should be directed posteriorly and cranially, is appreciated more easily. This dissection should be carried out once the seminal vesicles are exposed.

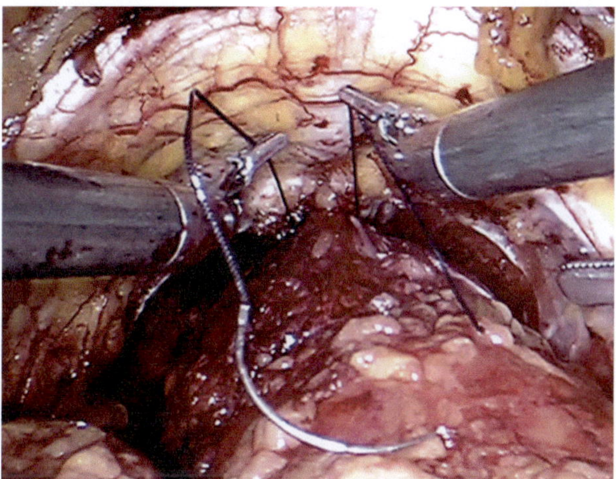

Fig. 12.8 Estimating the suture strength before applying the knot

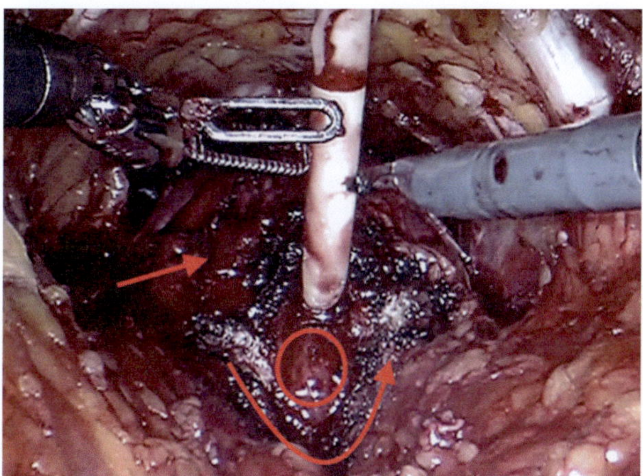

Fig. 12.9 The plane between the prostate (*straight arrow*) and anterior bladder neck (*curved arrow*) is developed, exposing the Foley catheter and the bladder mucosa (*oval area*)

We usually opt for an interfascial nerve-sparing pedicle dissection in an antegrade manner during RARP, if it is oncologically feasible to do so. For this purpose, the periprostatic fascia is incised, and then the tissue on the lateral aspect of the prostate is gently spread in order to identify prostatic capsule and the neurovascular bundle (NVB). No thermal energy is used during NVB dissection or ligation of the pedicle, and since the plane between the NVB sheath and the prostate capsule is relatively avascular, there should be minor bleeding once you are in the correct route. The NVB is then released in an antegrade fashion toward the apex (Fig. 12.11). The prostate pedicle can then be thinned out with sharp dissection, and this separation will allow safe placement of clip(s) on the pedicle away from the NVB.

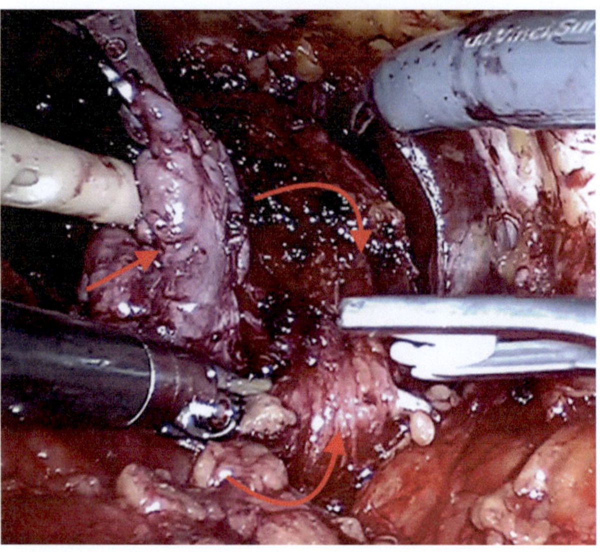

Fig. 12.10 Peripheral bladder attachments (*curved arrow facing up*) are being divided via clips. Note the dissection plane between the bulk of seminal vesicles (*straight arrow*) and prostate (*curved arrow facing down*) and bladder attachments

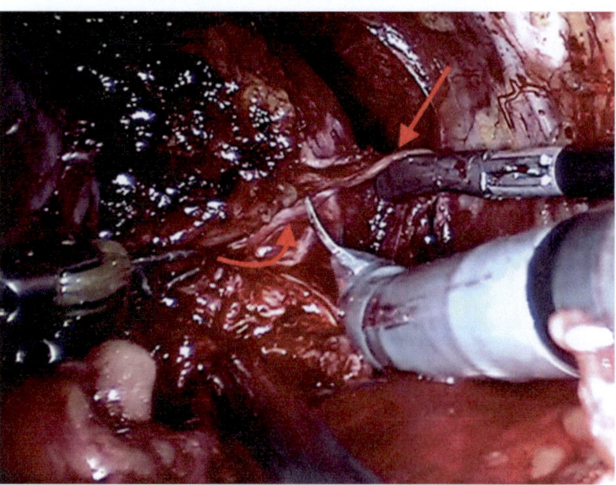

Fig. 12.11 Neurovascular bundle (NVB) (*straight arrow*) is released off the prostate capsule and prostatic fascia (*curved arrow*) via gentle sharp dissection

Cold scissors are used to divide the DVC and a long urethral stump is developed (Fig. 12.12). The urethra is then incised at the apex of the prostate to completely liberate the prostate (Fig. 12.13). In case of large prostate volume, large median lobe, or in patients with previous TURP, bladder neck reconstruction via application

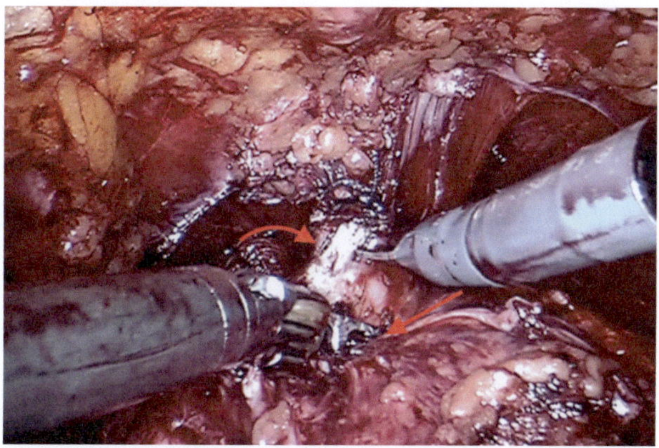

Fig. 12.12 Urethra (*curved arrow*) is being divided at the level of prostatic apex (*straight arrow*)

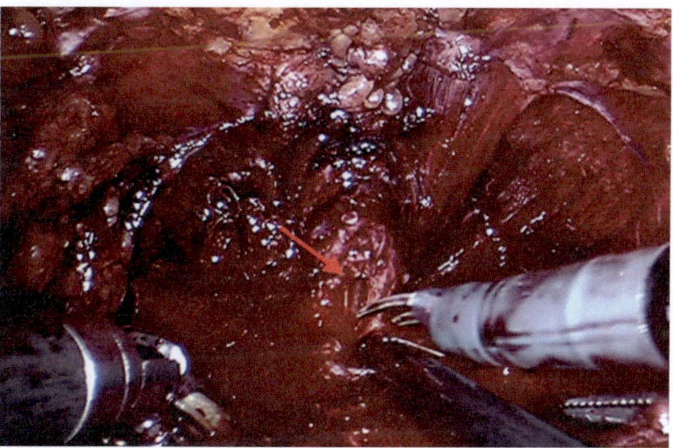

Fig. 12.13 Urethra is divided anteriorly; urethral lumen (*arrow*) becomes visible. Transection proceeds with the posterior aspect of the urethral circumference

of transverse plication sutures can be necessary. Otherwise we usually attempt to preserve the bladder neck.

After the specimen is extracted and the hemostatic measures are taken, the next step will be vesicourethral anastomosis. Before doing so, we usually apply the technique that has been proposed by Rocco et al. in 2006 [16], which includes restoration of the posterior aspect of the rhabdosphincter by reconstruction of the surrounding musculofascial plate in an attempt to fasten the recovery of continence post-RARP.

The urethra and bladder are reapproximated using running sutures as described by Van Velthoven [17]. Two 3/0 barbed sutures are used for this purpose, and first the posterior anastomosis is completed in a clockwise direction which is followed by the anterior anastomosis which is conducted in a counterclockwise fashion

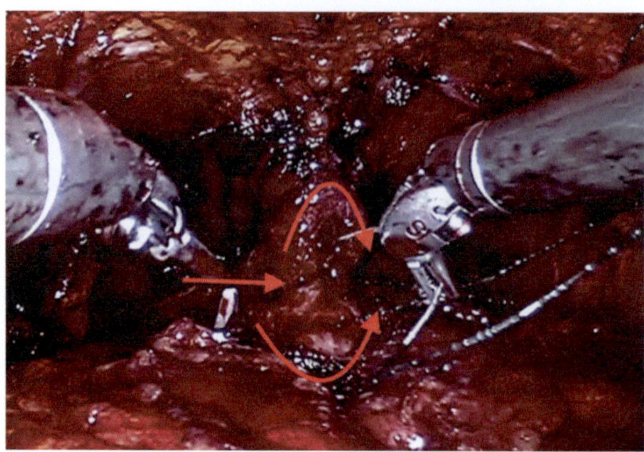

Fig. 12.14 Urethral stump (*curved arrow facing down*) is being anastomosed with the bladder neck (*curved arrow facing up*) via continuous sutures. Posterior lips of the two ends have been joined (*straight arrow*)

(Fig. 12.14). Then a Foley catheter (Chap. 22) is placed, and saline irrigation is done to confirm the watertightness of the anastomosis. Following this confirmation, a Jackson-Pratt drain is placed around the anastomosis, and all the trocars are removed under direct vision. Foley catheter is removed after 7 days without the routine need of a cystography.

A total of 121 patients have undergone RARP in our clinic between May 2010 and August 2016. Mean patient age and mean pre-biopsy serum PSA level were 60.2 years (range, 40–76) and 6.6 ng/mL (range, 1–40), respectively. Mean ASA (American Society of Anesthesiologists) score and mean BMI (body mass index) of the patients were 1.6 (range, 1–3) and 28.2 kg/m^2 (range, 22–37), respectively. Operations lasted 202.2 min (range, 115–440) on average, and mean estimated blood loss amount was 153.6 mL (range, 50–900). A total of four patients (3.3%) have received blood transfusions. Open conversion rate was 1.6% (*n*, 2). Sixteen complications that were of Clavien grade 2 and higher were recorded during the perioperative period of 11 patients. Distribution of the complications were as follows: grade 2 (*n*, 7 in seven patients), grade 3a (*n*, 2 in two patients), grade 3b (*n*, 6 in five patients), and grade 4 (*n*,1 in one patient). Mean duration of hospitalization was 4.5 days (range, 2–10). Overall positive surgical margin rate was 4.9% (*n*, 6). Distribution of the RP Gleason scores were as follows: 3 + 3 (3.9%), 3 + 4 (45.5%), 4 + 3 (11.8%), 4 + 4 (1.9%), 4 + 5 (3.9%), and 5 + 4 (2.9%). Mean tumor volume in the RP specimens was 2.89 cm^3 (range, 0.2–18.5). After a mean follow-up duration of 13.8 months, biochemical recurrence was detected in a total of 12 patients (9.9%).

12.3 Perioperative Outcomes

Novara et al. has reported the perioperative outcomes and complications after robot-assisted radical prostatectomy in their systematic review and meta-analysis of the literature focusing on 110 papers published between January 1, 2008 and August

2011 [18]. Overall, mean operative time, mean blood loss, and mean transfusion rate were 152 min (range, 90–291), 166 mL (range, 69–534), and 2% (range, 0.5–5%), respectively. Mean duration of catheterization was 6.3 days (range, 5–8.6), and patients were hospitalized for a mean period of 1.9 days (range, 1–6). They additionally evaluated the outcomes in "difficult-to-treat" patient subpopulations. Higher BMI, higher prostate volume, prior BPH surgery, and the presence of median lobe were found to be associated with longer operative times. Larger prostates also lead to higher amount of blood loss, longer catheterization time, and longer length of hospitalization [18]. In the same study, the mean complication rate was calculated as 9% with the majority being of low grade (grades 1–3 according to the Martin criteria [19]), and the most prevalent complications were lymphocele/lymphorrhea (3.1%), urine leak (1.8%), and reoperation (1.6%).

Cumulative analyses of the studies comparing open RP versus robotic RP yielded that rates for blood loss and transfusion were in favor of RARP. On the other hand, operative duration and overall complication rates were similar between the two approaches. Considering the comparison between laparoscopic RP and robotic RP, transfusion rate, which was significantly lower in RARP, was the only parameter that showed a statistically significant difference. The authors denoted the impossibility of meta-analyses in terms of catheterization time and length of hospital stay [18].

Another systematic review and meta-analysis of the perioperative outcomes have revealed significantly less complications following RARP as compared to RRP and LRP [20]. Perioperative results of some of the most contemporary RARP series with available data are summarized in Table 12.1.

12.4 Functional Outcomes

12.4.1 Erectile Function

Ficarra et al. have published a systematic review and meta-analysis of the studies that have reported outcomes related with erectile function in 2012 [28]. The 12- and 24- month potency rates ranged from 54 to 90% and 63 to 94%, respectively. In this paper, they have covered the RARP series that were published between 2008 and 2011 and included more than 100 patients. Age, baseline erectile function (International Index of Erectile Function (IIEF)-5 score), comorbidities (Charlson score), and extension of the nerve-sparing procedure represented the most important predictors of the risk of postoperative erectile dysfunction.

Furthermore, combination of these variables (age, IIEF score, and Charlson score) within the context of Briganti risk group stratification made it possible to provide a better overview to the patients about what to be expected after RARP in terms of erectile function recovery according to their individual risk category. Low-risk patients' (age ≤ 60 year, baseline IIEF-6 > 21, and Charlson score ≤ 1) potency rates were 81.9% at 12 months, while the same rate was calculated to be 28.6% among high-risk individuals (age > 70, baseline IIEF-6 score ≤ 10, and Charlson score ≤ 2) [29].

Table 12.1 Perioperative outcomes of selected RARP series

Study	N	Median/mean operative time, min	Median/mean blood loss, mL	Transfusion rate, %	Catheterization time, days	Length of hospitalization, days	Overall complication rate, %
Menon et al. [21]	30	288	329	7	11	1.5	6
Tewari et al. [22]	200	160	153	0	7	1.2	3
Ahlering et al. [23]	60	231	103	0	7	1	6.7
Rocco et al. [24]	120	215	200	NA	6	3	NA
Krambeck et al. [25]	286	236	NA	5.1	NA	NA	4.8
Rozet et al. [26]	133	166	609	3	9.2	5.4	19.4
Drouin et al. [27]	71	199	310	NA	8.1	4.4	8.4

NA not available

Among the clinical series that included only the bilateral nerve-sparing procedures, 3-, 6-, 12-, and 24-month potency rates were 56%, 69% (50–86%), 74% (62–90%), and 82% (69–94%), respectively [28]. (A)thermal dissection of the neurovascular bundles [30], cold dissection of the cavernous nerve [31], countertraction during the nerve-sparing dissection [32], and the boundaries of the nerve-sparing dissection (intrafascial, interfascial, and extrafascial) represent the most common technical modifications that have been tested in terms of their potential beneficial role regarding postoperative erectile function recovery. Mean potency rates at 3, 6, and 12 months were 44, 50, and 66% (62–75%), respectively, in the clinical series using cautery (monopolar or bipolar) dissection and 52%, 78% (70–86%), and 81% (62–90%), respectively, in the studies using the athermal dissection [28]. Available data seem to support the use of cautery-free dissection or the use of pinpointed low-energy cauterization.

Despite the absence of high-quality level of evidence within this context, cumulative analyses showed better 12-month potency rates after RARP in comparison with RRP (odds ratio [OR], 2.84; 95% confidence interval [CI], 1.46–5.43; $p = 0.002$). On the other hand, the difference between RARP and LRP remained statistically insignificant (OR, 1.89; $p = 0.21$) [28].

In the recently published prospective randomized study comparing the outcomes of open versus robotic RP, which represent the relevant paper with the highest level of evidence so far, sexual function scores (sexual domain of EPIC and IIEF) did not differ significantly between the RRP group and the RARP group at 6 weeks postsurgery (30.70 vs. 32.70; $p = 0.45$) or 12 weeks postsurgery (35.00 vs. 38.90; $p = 0.18$) [33].

12.4.2 Continence

In their systematic review, Ficarra et al. have analyzed 51 articles that reported on urinary continence rates after RARP [34]. If urinary continence was defined more strictly as using no pads at all, the 12-month urinary incontinence rates ranged from 4 to 31%, with a mean value of 16%. However, if the definition was extended to involve a safety pad, then the incidence ranged from 8 to 11%, with a mean value of 9%. Age, body mass index, comorbidity index, lower urinary tract symptoms, and prostate volume were the most important preoperative parameters that influenced the risk of urinary incontinence after RARP. When different surgical approaches were compared in terms of continence recovery, RARP outperformed open (OR, 1.53; $p = 0.03$) and laparoscopic RP (OR, 2.39; $p = 0.006$) with a significantly better 12-month continence rate [34]. Approaching extra- or transperitoneally [35], bladder neck preservation [36], hypothermic nerve-sparing dissection using cold irrigation [31], dividing dorsal venous complex via athermal techniques initially and then selectively suture ligating prior to anastomosis [36], barbed versus monofilament sutures for urethrovesical anastomosis [37], and posterior/anterior reconstructions [38] represent the most commonly utilized/tested technical modifications that were employed in an effort to optimize continence

Table 12.2 Continence outcomes of selected RARP series

Study	N	Assessment method	Criterion	6 months, %	12 months, %	24 months, %
Krambeck et al. [25]	286	NVQ	No leak	NA	91.8	NA
Di Pierro et al. [40]	75	NVQ	No leak	NA	89	NA
Geraerts et al. [41]	64	Physician reported	No leak	90.3	89.8	NA
Rocco et al. [24]	120	Interview	No pad/one safety pad	93	97	NA
Son et al. [42]	146	NVQ	No pad	87.5	94.5	95.2
Joseph et al. [43]	50	Physician reported	No pad	90	NA	NA

NA not available, *NVQ* nonvalidated questionnaire

Table 12.3 Potency outcomes of selected RARP series

Study	N	Assessment method	Criterion	3 months, %	12 months, %	24 months, %
Krambeck et al. [25]	286	NVQ	Intercourse	NA	70	NA
Di Pierro et al. [40]	75	NVQ	Presence of erection	26	55	NA
Joseph et al. [43]	50	IIEF	Erection sufficient for intercourse	46	NA	NA
Rocco et al. [24]	120	Interview	Intercourse	31	43	61

NA not available

recovery post-RARP. Available literature data seems in favor of total reconstruction with a significantly better continence outcome early postoperatively when compared with those who did not undergo such a reconstruction. However, it should be noted that beyond 6 months postoperatively continence rates of those who were reconstructed or not started to overlap.

A recent, prospective, controlled, nonrandomized, multi-institutional trial, comparing open and robotic approaches, showed that continence rates did not differ at 12 months postoperatively [39]. Yaxley et al. reported nonsignificant differences between the urinary function scores (urinary domain of EPIC) of open versus robotic RP at 6 (74.50 vs. 71.10; $p = 0.09$) and 12 weeks (83.80 vs. 82.50; $p = 0.48$) postoperatively in their randomized controlled phase 3 study [33]. Functional results of some of the most contemporary RARP series with available data are summarized in Tables 12.2 and 12.3.

12.5 Oncological Outcomes

Long-term data from RARP series has shown that the actuarial biochemical recurrence-free survival, metastasis-free survival, and cancer-specific survival rates at 10 years were 73.1, 97.5, and 98.8%, respectively. The overall incidence of

Table 12.4 Oncological outcomes of selected RARP series

Study	N	Overall PSM, %	pT2 PSM, %	pT3 PSM, %
Menon et al. [21]	30	26	NA	NA
Tewari et al. [22]	200	6	NA	NA
Krambeck et al. [25]	286	15.6	NA	NA
Di Pierro et al. [40]	75	16	8.3	42.8
Drouin et al. [27]	71	15.4	9.8	60
Harty et al. [47]	152	50	12	79
Rozet et al. [26]	133	19.5	20	NA

NA not available

biochemical recurrence and positive surgical margins (PSM) following RARP were 22.4 and 9–15%, respectively [18, 44]. These results are comparable to contemporary open RP cohorts.

In the systematic review conducted by Novara et al., the mean PSM rates after RARP in pT2, pT3, and pT4 disease were 9, 37, and 50%, respectively. Serum PSA level, pT stage, Gleason score, prostate volume, surgeon experience, type of nerve-sparing approach, and technique of DVC control were among the most important factors that predicted the likelihood of PSMs [18].

Despite considerable methodological flaws and uncertainties, a recent systematic review demonstrated that RARP was associated with lower perioperative morbidity and a reduced risk of positive surgical margins compared with its pure laparoscopic counterpart [45].

De Carlo et al. have compared retropubic, laparoscopic, and robotic radical prostatectomy in terms of their oncological outcomes in their recent systematic review covering 44 relevant articles published between 1999 and 2013 [46]. As a result, mean overall PSM rate of RARP was 21.14%, whereas LRP and RRP yielded PSM rates of 22.04 and 22.45%, respectively. When only the pT2 tumors were considered, PSM rates were calculated to be 10.53, 17.44, and 16.64%, respectively, for RARP, LRP, and RRP. Among pT3 cancers, PSM rates were 53.37, 49.61, and 46.75%, respectively. According to the results of cumulative analyses, PSM rates were similar for RRP versus LRP. However, statistical analyses of the comparative studies reporting data on RRP and LRP versus RARP margin status indicated a significant difference in favor of RARP [46]. Oncological results of some of the most contemporary RARP series with available data are summarized in Table 12.4.

12.6 RARP in High-Risk Prostate Cancer

There has been a recent trend toward performing RP in high-risk prostate cancer, and based on the current literature, RARP seems to have similar oncological outcomes including surgical margin positivity, biochemical recurrence and recurrence-free survival rates, additional treatment requirements, and lymph node (LN) yields with similar complication rates compared to open surgery in this particular patient group. Moreover, decreased blood loss, lower transfusion rates, and shorter length of hospitalization seem to be the advantages of robotic surgery in this context [48].

Tissue characteristics and intraoperative findings may make dissection more difficult and increase the likelihood of perioperative complication in high-risk patients: bulky and adherent disease, seminal vesicle and/or bladder neck involvement, extracapsular extension of the tumor especially in the apical region, loss of tissue planes between the prostate and rectum, etc. In order to perform RARP without compromising oncological efficiency in such high-risk and/or locally advanced cases, one should have gained sufficient expertise in low-risk cases.

Preoperative multiparametric MRI might be helpful for the surgeon and tailor the surgical management strategy by delineating the risk, extent, and location of extracapsular disease, presence/absence of seminal vesicle invasion, and extent of pelvic lymph node involvement.

12.7 RARP in the Salvage Setting

Salvage RP is a surgically challenging but effective secondary local treatment of prostate cancer that recurred after radiotherapy with curative intent. In salvage RP for radiorecurrent prostate cancer, tissue planes are often obscured, and there is adherence of adjacent structures such as the rectum, pubic bone, and bladder. Healing and recovery are also delayed following energy destruction of tissue.

Considering the robotic approach in salvage RP, pneumoperitoneum may contribute to reduced blood loss compared to open salvage RP with EBL and transfusion requirements that do not appear to exceed that of primary RARP. However, all of these advantages may be offset by the lack of tactile feedback, which is a major concern in this setting. Future improvements in haptic feedback technology are especially important in salvage surgeries where tissue planes are harder to discern.

Despite the fact that complications were not reported in a standardized categorical manner, the majority of them were of high importance as they required procedural intervention for bladder neck contracture, artificial urinary sphincter, or penile prosthesis.

Zargar et al. have recently conducted a systematic review and reported on ten case series including 197 men undergoing salvage RARP (sRARP) after varying modalities of radiotherapy. The majority of the patients (>2/3) were recurrence-free at the time of follow-up. However, continence and potency rates of 60 and 26%, respectively, deserved attention to the increased likelihood of functional deterioration after such salvage surgery attempts irrespective of the minimally invasive nature of the intervention [49].

One of the largest sRARP series has been published by Yuh et al. who have reported the outcome of 51 consecutive patients who underwent sRARP after previous failed local radiotherapy. Median operative time and estimated blood loss amount were 179 min and 175 mL, respectively. Positive surgical margin rate was 31%. After a median follow-up of 36 months, their estimated 3-year biochemical recurrence or progression-free survival was 57%. Noteworthy, they reported significant complication (47%) rates. Potency was maintained in 23% of preoperatively potent men, and spontaneous return of urinary continence was achieved in 23 patients (45%) with a median time to continence of 6 months [50]. Nevertheless, they emphasized the importance of proper patient counseling and selection before sRARP.

Available data about salvage RARP is consisting of small case series with limited follow-up. Larger series with a longer follow-up are necessary to make definitive conclusions about the oncological and functional outcomes.

12.8 The Concepts of "Trifecta" and "Pentafecta"

Salomon et al. were the first to report functional and oncological outcomes of their series consisting of open, laparoscopic, and perineal prostatectomy in 2003 [51]. Afterward, innumerous case series, comparative studies, and reviews concentrating on the outcome of RARP have been published. The term "trifecta," which includes the description of concomitant oncological, continence, and potency outcomes in a patient who has undergone RP, was introduced at the Challenges in Laparoscopy Conference in 2004 [52]. Trifecta simply denotes freedom from biochemical recurrence in a potent and continent patient s/p RP. However, the definitions of continence and potency within this context are not universally agreed upon, which definitely affects the success numbers that have been reported. Trifecta rates in preoperatively potent and continent men following RARP may show considerable variations throughout the literature, with as low as 37.3% or as high as 86% which were found to be fulfilling the criteria at 12 months in different series [53]. Age at surgery, initial PSA level, nerve-sparing status (uni- and bilateral or none), and preoperative functional assessment were found to be influencing the trifecta outcome [54].

In 2011, Patel et al. introduced the term "pentafecta" which includes the addition of the absence of postoperative complications and negative surgical margins to the established trifecta criteria. They have reported the pentafecta outcomes of 332 preoperatively potent men who underwent RARP with bilateral nerve sparing. At 3-, 6-, and 12-month follow-up, 51.8, 66.9, and 70.8% of this cohort, respectively, achieved pentafecta. The most common reasons for pentafecta failure were erectile dysfunction (35.0%) and positive surgical margins (31.9%). Age at surgery was the only parameter that showed a significant association with pentafecta on multivariable analyses [55].

12.9 Robot-Assisted Pelvic Lymph Node Dissection

The lymph nodes that drain the lymphatic outflow of the prostate are external iliac-obturator (38%), internal iliac (25%), common iliac (16%), para-aortic/para-caval (12%), presacral (8%), and inguinal (1%) [56]. Indications for pelvic lymph node dissection (PLND) do not differ between robotic, laparoscopic, and open RPs.

Therefore, if a PLND is indicated, then it should be done in the context of every RP, no matter what the surgical approach is. In other words, surgical approach preference should not preclude a PLND from being properly done in a patient who actually deserves it. EAU recommends an extended PLND in those intermediate-risk patients (cT2a, PSA 10–20 ng/mL, biopsy Gleason score 7) whose probability of lymph node involvement exceeds 5% on the Briganti nomogram and all high-risk patients (≥cT2b, PSA > 20 ng/mL, biopsy Gleason score ≥ 8) [12]. Extended PLND dissection field is bounded by the external iliac artery anteriorly, the pelvic side wall laterally, the bladder wall medially, the floor of the pelvis posteriorly, Cooper ligament distally, and the common iliac artery/ureter crossing proximally [57]. Several authors have reported the feasibility of an extended PLND during the course of RARP with a mean number of 12–19 lymph nodes being extracted and the positive node rates ranging from 11 to 24% [58, 59]. Transperitoneal and extraperitoneal RARP yielded similar results in terms of the lymph node yield. However, the risk of postoperative symptomatic lymphocele is higher with the extraperitoneal approach [35].

12.10 The Pasadena Consensus Panel

The Robotic Urology Section of the European Association of Urology organized a consensus conference in Pasadena, California, gathering the 17 world leaders in prostate cancer and radical prostatectomy. Aims were to review the available literature data on RARP, critically assess surgical techniques, and describe best practice recommendations [57]. According to the Pasadena Consensus Panel (PCP), indications of RARP should principally be the same as LRP or RRP. Additionally, it is the panel's advice that only the (very) experienced robotic surgeons should operate on special patient subgroups such as those with a body mass index > 30, prostate volume > 70 cm^3, history of prior TURP, presence of median lobe, high-risk features necessitating extended pelvic lymph node dissection, history of previous pelvic surgery, and recurrent disease after radiation therapy, cryotherapy, or HIFU requiring salvage RARP [57].

Considering relatively young sexually active men without significant comorbidities and low-risk disease, every effort should be made in order to maximally preserve cavernous nerves by following the plane between the prostate capsule and prostatic fascia (intrafascial). Those with intermediate- or high-risk localized disease, intact preoperative erectile function and absence of significant comorbidities should be candidate for a "partial" nerve-sparing approach which denotes the plane within the multilayer tissue of the prostatic fascia (interfascial). The preoperative erectile dysfunction, the lack of interest in sexual activity, and the presence of significant comorbidities were accepted as the indications for a "minimal" nerve-sparing strategy in which only the nervous structures that run at the posterolateral aspect of the prostate are spared while staying extrafascial [57].

The PCP confirmed that the well-established indications of pelvic lymph node dissection in prostate cancer can safely be applied in the robotic setting once the decision to proceed with radical surgery has been settled down. Considering high-risk cases, the PCP advocated the safe and effective utility of RARP along the later steps of the learning curve.

12.11 Technical Modifications and Novelties Related with RARP

The surgical technique of RARP has evolved over the last 15 years. Initial surgical technique imitated a laparoscopic approach, which started posteriorly to dissect the seminal vesicles and vasa deferentia, followed by mobilization of the bladder in order to approach the bladder neck. Patel et al. have proposed their "VIP" technique, whereby the prostate is approached anteriorly, starting with the bladder takedown, followed by the bladder neck, and then dissecting the seminal vesicles and vasa deferentia. This modification enabled the robotic approach to be applied on "difficult-to-treat" patient subpopulations, such as those with higher BMI [3]. Furthermore, anatomic studies revealed that the NVB spread over a wider surface of the prostatic fascia, not merely the posterolateral aspect [60, 61]. The preserved neural tissue of the anterolateral aspects of the periprostatic fascial layer (Veil of Aphrodite) could potentially allow for greater nerve preservation [62] and hence optimize functional outcomes. Preserving these "anterolateral" neural structures in addition to their posterolateral counterparts resulted in better recovery of postoperative erectile function and a higher percentage of erections firm enough for intercourse at 12 months postoperatively, compared to men undergoing a "conventional" bilateral nerve-sparing technique [63].

Ko et al. compared antegrade vs. retrograde nerve-sparing dissection during RARP in terms of their effect on functional recovery. They evaluated 501 potent men who underwent bilateral nerve-sparing RARP and had eligible follow-up data. Potency rates were significantly higher in the retrograde approach at all time points. On multivariate analyses, nerve-sparing approach was found to be an independent predictor for potency recovery, and the hazard ratio for the retrograde approach was higher than the antegrade technique [64].

Double-layered urethrovesical anastomosis (UVA), which implies the combination of posterior rhabdosphincteric reconstruction and anterolateral reconstruction, was expected to enhance continence recovery. However, neither early continence recovery nor long-term continence rates were significantly affected in a randomized controlled trial comparing double-layered vs. single-layered UVA [65, 66]. However, double-layered UVA did show a significant decrease in cystographic leaks compared to single-layered UVA [67].

Urinary diversion after UVA can alternatively be achieved with the aid of a suprapubic tube (SPT) instead of the conventional urethral Foley catheter [68]. The proposed benefits of the SPT are less catheter-related discomfort, decreased need for anticholinergic medications due to foreign body-induced uninhibited bladder contractions leading to distressing lower urinary tract symptoms, and reduced risk of strictures (urethral, meatal, and bladder neck) [69].

The Food and Drug Administration (FDA) approved the polyglyconate-barbed suture for soft tissue approximation in 2010 [70]. The barbed suture reduced the anastomotic time by 26% without compromising outcomes, compared with the conventional monofilament double-armed suturing technique.

GelPOINT (Applied Medical, Rancho Santa Margarita, CA, USA) has been applied for real-time bedside bimanual examination of the specimen and for regional hypothermia by introducing ice slush, the introcorporeal cooling and extraction (ICE) technique [71]. By applying the ICE technique with the use of the GelPOINT, and real-time bimanual examination, the absolute risk of PSM in pT3a disease was reduced by 26.6%. The impact of regional hypothermia by cooling the neurovascular bundle is currently under investigation.

In 2012, Schlomm et al. have described the efficacy and oncologic safety of neurovascular structure-adjacent frozen-section examination (NeuroSAFE) in their retrospective study including over 11.000 consecutive open and robotic RPs. NeuroSAFE, which included the whole laterorectal circumference of the prostate, enabled the secondary resection of the ipsilateral neurovascular tissue if margins were positive at the neurovascular tissue-corresponding prostatic surface. When NeuroSAFE RPs were compared with their matched non-NeuroSAFE counterparts, the frequency of nerve sparing was significantly higher, and PSM rates were significantly lower, irrespective of the pathological T stage. Furthermore, it was found to have no negative impact on biochemical recurrence rates [72].

Manny et al. reported on their experience about fluorescence-enhanced robotic radical prostatectomy (FERRP) using real-time lymphangiography and tissue marking with percutaneous injection of unconjugated indocyanine green in order to identify sentinel lymphatic drainage and optimize LND during RARP. Sentinel nodes were identified in 76% of patients after a mean time period of 30 minutes postinjection. FERRP had 100% sensitivity, 75.4% specificity, 14.6% positive predictive value, and 100% negative predictive value for the detection of nodal metastasis in this cohort of 50 patients [73].

Conclusions

What has been offered by the robot made adaptation of minimally invasive surgery in prostate cancer more feasible, such that proficient open surgeons were able to adapt robotic radical prostatectomy into their clinical practice without struggling in the steep learning curve of laparoscopic RP. Robotic surgery in prostate cancer consists mainly of radical prostatectomy +/− pelvic lymphadenectomy performed due to localized or locally advanced/high-risk localized primary disease. The indications of radical prostatectomy and pelvic lymph node dissection do not differ between surgical approach alternatives. Robotic radical prostatectomy has gained considerable popularity throughout the globe, and in certain countries it is “the” method of choice when there is an indication to proceed with radical surgery in a patient diagnosed with prostate cancer. The statements of the Pasadena Consensus Panel can be followed if RARP is going to be performed. RARP provides comparable early and midterm oncological and functional outcomes when compared with its open and laparoscopic counterparts. Less need for transfusion and shorter hospitalization are its proposed advantages in terms of the perioperative outcomes. There is limited and low-quality evidence in order to promote one surgical approach alternative to another based on the available literature data. Oncological priorities and individual tumor-related parameters, the need/request to preserve functional status, surgeon preference and experience, and technical availabilities are the main factors that lead the shared discussion with the patient upon deciding on how to do his radical prostatectomy. Technical modifications and novel adaptations of the robotic armamentarium may help to optimize functional and oncological outcomes.

References

1. Ferlay J, Soerjomataram I, Ervik M, et al. GLOBOCAN 2012 v1.0, Cancer incidence and mortality worldwide: IARC CancerBase No. 11. 2012. http://globocan.iarc.fr/Pages/fact_sheets_cancer.aspx. Accessed 22 July 2016.
2. Binder J, Kramer W. Robotically-assisted laparoscopic radical prostatectomy. BJU Int. 2001;87:408–10.
3. Jeong W, Kumar R, Menon M. Past, present and future of urological robotic surgery. Investig Clin Urol. 2016;57:75–83.
4. Young HH. VIII. Conservative perineal prostatectomy: the results of two years' experience and report of seventy-five cases. Ann Surg. 1905;41:549–57.
5. Millin T. Retropubic prostatectomy; a new extravesical technique; report of 20 cases. Lancet. 1945;2:693–6.
6. Walsh PC, Lepor H, Eggleston JC. Radical prostatectomy with preservation of sexual function: anatomical and pathological considerations. Prostate. 1983;4:473–85.
7. Abbou CC, Hoznek A, Salomon L, Lobontiu A, Saint F, Cicco A, et al. Remote laparoscopic radical prostatectomy carried out with a robot: report of a case. Prog Urol. 2000;10:520–3.
8. Abbou CC, Hoznek A, Salomon L, Olsson LE, Lobontiu A, Saint F, et al. Laparoscopic radical prostatectomy with a remote controlled robot. J Urol. 2001;165(6 Pt 1):1964–6.
9. Pasticier G, Rietbergen JB, Guillonneau B, Fromont G, Menon M, Vallancien G. Robotically assisted laparoscopic radical prostatectomy: feasibility study in men. Eur Urol. 2001;40:70–4.
10. Piechaud P. State of the art: urologic surgery. J Visc Surg. 2011;148(5 Suppl):e27–9. doi:10.1016/j.jviscsurg.2011.08.004. Review
11. Patel VR, Coelho RF, Chauhan S, Orvieto MA, Palmer KJ, Rocco B, Sivaraman A, Coughlin G. Continence, potency and oncological outcomes after robotic-assisted radical prostatectomy: early trifecta results of a high-volume surgeon. BJU Int. 2010 Sep;106(5):696–702. doi:10.1111/j.1464-410X.2010.09541.x.
12. Mottet N, Bellmunt J, Bolla M, Briers E, Cumberbatch MG, De Santis M, Fossati N, Gross T, Henry AM, Joniau S, Lam TB, Mason MD, Matveev VB, Moldovan PC, van den Bergh RC, Van den Broeck T, van der Poel HG, van der Kwast TH, Rouvière O, Schoots IG, Wiegel T, Cornford P. EAU-ESTRO-SIOG guidelines on prostate cancer. Part 1: screening, diagnosis, and local treatment with curative intent. Eur Urol. 2016; doi:10.1016/j.eururo.2016.08.003. pii:S0302–2838(16)30470–5. [Epub ahead of print] PubMed.
13. Hasson HM. A modified instrument and method for laparoscopy. Am J Obstet Gynecol. 1971;110(6):886–7.
14. Partin AW, Mangold LA, Lamm DM, Walsh PC, Epstein JI, Pearson JD. Contemporary update of prostate cancer staging nomograms (Partin Tables) for the new millennium. Urology. 2001;58(6):843–8.
15. Briganti A, Joniau S, Gontero P, et al. Identifying the best candidate for radical prostatectomy among patients with high-risk prostate cancer. Eur Urol. 2012;61:584–92.

16. Rocco F, Carmignani L, Acquati P, Gadda F, Dell'Orto P, Rocco B, Bozzini G, Gazzano G, Morabito A. Restoration of posterior aspect of rhabdosphincter shortens continence time after radical retropubic prostatectomy. J Urol. 2006;175(6):2201–6.
17. Van Velthoven RF, Ahlering TE, Peltier A, Skarecky DW, Clayman RV. Technique for laparoscopic running urethrovesical anastomosis:the single knot method. Urology. 2003;61(4):699–702.
18. Novara G, Ficarra V, Rosen RC, Artibani W, Costello A, Eastham JA, Graefen M, Guazzoni G, Shariat SF, Stolzenburg JU, Van Poppel H, Zattoni F, Montorsi F, Mottrie A, Wilson TG. Systematic review and meta-analysis of perioperative outcomes and complications after robot-assisted radical prostatectomy. Eur Urol. 2012;62(3):431–52.
19. Martin RC, Brennan MF, Jaques DP. Quality of complication reporting in the surgical literature. Ann Surg. 2002;235:803–13.
20. Tewari A, Sooriakumaran P, Bloch DA, et al. Positive surgical margin and perioperative complication rates of primary surgical treatments for prostate cancer: a systematic review and meta-analysis comparing retropubic, laparoscopic, and robotic prostatectomy. Eur Urol. 2012;62(1):1–15.
21. Menon M, Tewari A, Baize B, Guillonneau B, Vallancien G. Prospective comparison of radical retropubic prostatectomy and robot-assisted anatomic prostatectomy: the Vattikuti Urology Institute experience. Urology. 2002;60:864–8.
22. Tewari A, Srivasatava A, Menon M. A prospective comparison of radical retropubic and robot-assisted prostatectomy: experience in one institution. BJU Int. 2003;92:205–10.
23. Ahlering TE, Woo D, Eichel L, Lee DI, Edwards R, Skarecky DW. Robot-assisted versus open radical prostatectomy: a comparison of one surgeon's outcomes. Urology. 2004;63:819–22.
24. Rocco B, Matei DV, Melegari S, Ospina JC, Mazzoleni F, Errico G, Mastropasqua M, Santoro L, Detti S, De Cobelli O. Robotic vs. open prostatectomy in a laparoscopically naïve centre: a matched-pair analysis. BJU Int. 2009;104:991–5.
25. Krambeck AE, DiMarco DS, Rangel LJ, et al. Radical prostatectomy for prostatic adenocarcinoma: a matched comparison of open retropubic and robot-assisted techniques. BJU Int. 2009;103:448–53.
26. Rozet F, Jaffe J, Braud G, et al. A direct comparison of robotic assisted versus pure laparoscopic radical prostatectomy: a single institution experience. J Urol. 2007;178:478–82.
27. Drouin SJ, Vaessen C, Hupertan V, Comperat E, Misraï V, Haertig A, Bitker M-C, Chartier-Kastler E, Richard F, Rouprêt M. Comparison of mid-term carcinologic control obtained after open, laparoscopic, and robot-assisted radical prostatectomy for localized prostate cancer. World J Urol. 2009;27:599–605.
28. Ficarra V, Novara G, Ahlering TE, et al. Systematic review and meta- analysis of studies reporting potency rates after robot-assisted radical prostatectomy. Eur Urol. 2012;62(3):418–30.
29. Novara G, Ficarra V, D'Elia C, et al. Preoperative criteria to select patients for bilateral nerve-sparing robotic-assisted radical prostatectomy. J Sex Med. 2010;7:839–45.
30. Ahlering TE, Rodriguez E, Skarecky DW. Overcoming obstacles: nerve-sparing issues in radical prostatectomy. J Endourol. 2008;22:745–50.
31. Finley DS, Osann K, Chang A, Santos R, Skarecky D, Ahlering TE. Hypothermic robotic radical prostatectomy: impact on continence. J Endourol. 2009;23:1443–50.
32. Kowalczyk KJ, Huang AC, Hevelone ND, et al. Stepwise approach for nerve sparing without countertraction during robot-assisted radical prostatectomy: technique and outcomes. Eur Urol. 2011;60:536–47.
33. Yaxley JW, Coughlin GD, Chambers SK, Occhipinti S, Samaratunga H, Zajdlewicz L, Dunglison N, Carter R, Williams S, Payton DJ, Perry-Keene J, Lavin MF, Gardiner RA. Robot-assisted laparoscopic prostatectomy versus open radical retropubic prostatectomy: early outcomes from a randomised controlled phase 3 study. Lancet. 2016 Sep 10;388(10049):1057–66.
34. Ficarra V, Novara G, Rosen RC, et al. Systematic review and meta- analysis of studies reporting urinary continence recovery after robot- assisted radical prostatectomy. Eur Urol. 2012;62(3):405–17.

35. Chung JS, Kim WT, Ham WS, et al. Comparison of oncological results, functional outcomes, and complications for transperitoneal versus extraperitoneal robot-assisted radical prostatectomy: a single surgeon's experience. J Endourol. 2011;25:787–92.
36. Lei Y, Alemozaffar M, Williams SB, et al. Athermal division and selective suture ligation of the dorsal vein complex during robot- assisted laparoscopic radical prostatectomy: description of technique and outcomes. Eur Urol. 2011;59:235–43.
37. Sammon J, Kim TK, Trinh QD, et al. Anastomosis during robot-assisted radical prostatectomy: randomized controlled trial comparing barbed and standard monofilament suture. Urology. 2011;78:572–9.
38. Woo JR, Shikanov S, Zorn KC, Shalhav AL, Zagaja GP. Impact of posterior rhabdosphincter reconstruction during robot-assisted radical prostatectomy: retrospective analysis of time to continence. J Endourol. 2009;23:1995–9.
39. Haglind E, et al. Urinary incontinence and erectile dysfunction after robotic versus open radical prostatectomy: a prospective, controlled, nonrandomised trial. Eur Urol. 2015;68:216.
40. Di Pierro GB, Baumeister P, Stucki P, Beatrice J, Danuser H, Mattei A. A prospective trial comparing consecutive series of open retropubic and robot-assisted laparoscopic radical prostatectomy in a centre with a limited caseload. Eur Urol. 2011;59:1–6.
41. Geraerts I, Van Poppel H, Devoogdt N, Van Cleynenbreugel B, Joniau S, Van Kampen M. Prospective evaluation of urinary incontinence, voiding symptoms and quality of life after open and robot-assisted radical prostatectomy. BJU Int. 2013;112:936–43.
42. Son SJ, Lee SC, Jeong CW, Jeong SJ, Byun SS, Lee SE. Comparison of continence recovery between robot-assisted laparoscopic prostatectomy and open radical retropubic prostatectomy: a single surgeon experience. Korean J Urol. 2013;54:598–602.
43. Joseph JV, Vicente I, Madeb R, Erturk E, Patel HR. Robot-assisted versus pure laparoscopic radical prostatectomy: are there any differences? BJU Int. 2005;96:39–42.
44. Diaz M, Peabody JO, Kapoor V, et al. Oncologic outcomes at 10 years following robotic radical prostatectomy. Eur Urol. 2014; doi:10.1016/j.eururo.2014.06.025.
45. Ramsay C, et al. Systematic review and economic modelling of the relative clinical benefit and cost-effectiveness of laparoscopic surgery and robotic surgery for removal of the prostate in men with localised prostate cancer. Health Technol Assess. 2012;16:1.
46. De Carlo F, Celestino F, Verri C, Masedu F, Liberati E, Di Stasi SM. Retropubic, laparoscopic, and robot-assisted radical prostatectomy: surgical, oncological, and functional outcomes: a systematic review. Urol Int. 2014;93(4):373–83.
47. Harty NJ, Kozinn SI, Canes D, Sorcini A, Moinzadeh A. Comparison of positive surgical margin rates in high risk prostate cancer: open versus minimally invasive radical prostatectomy. Int Braz J Urol. 2013;39:639–46.
48. Canda AE, Balbay MD. Robotic radical prostatectomy in high-risk prostate cancer: current perspectives. Asian J Androl. 2015;17(6):908–15. doi:10.4103/1008-682X.153541. discussion 913.
49. Zargar H, Lamb AD, Rocco B, Porpiglia F, Liatsikos E, Davis J, Coelho RF, Pow-Sang JM, Patel VR, Murphy DG. Salvage robotic prostatectomy for radio recurrent prostate cancer: technical challenges and outcome analysis. Minerva Urol Nefrol. 2017;69(1):26–37.
50. Yuh B, Ruel N, Muldrewetal S. Complications and outcomes of robot-assisted salvage radical prostatectomy—a single institution experience. BJU Int. 2014;113(5):769–76.
51. Salomon L, Saint F, Anastasiadis AG, Sebe P, Chopin D, Abbou CC. Combined reporting of cancer control and functional results of radical prostatectomy. Eur Urol. 2003 Dec;44(6):656–60.
52. Pierorazio PM, Spencer BA, McCann TR, McKiernan JM, Benson MC. Preoperative risk stratification predicts likelihood of concurrent PSA-free survival, continence, and potency (the trifecta analysis) after radical retropubic prostatectomy. Urology. 2007 Oct;70(4):717–22.
53. Shikanov SA, Zorn KC, Zagaja GP, Shalhav AL. Trifecta outcomes after robotic-assisted laparoscopic prostatectomy. Urology. 2009 Sep;74(3):619–23.
54. Xylinas E, Durand X, Ploussard G, Campeggi A, Allory Y, Vordos D, Hoznek A, Abbou CC, de la Taille A, Salomon L. Evaluation of combined oncologic and functional outcomes after

robotic-assisted laparoscopic extraperitoneal radical prostatectomy: trifecta rate of achieving continence, potency and cancer control. Urol Oncol. 2013;31(1):99–103. doi:10.1016/j.urolonc.2010.10.012.
55. Patel VR, Sivaraman A, Coelho RF, Chauhan S, Palmer KJ, Orvieto MA, Camacho I, Coughlin G, Rocco B. Pentafecta: a new concept for reporting outcomes of robot-assisted laparoscopic radical prostatectomy. Eur Urol. 2011;59(5):702–7. doi:10.1016/j.eururo.2011.01.032.
56. Mattei A, Fuechsel FG, Bhatta Dhar N, Warncke SH, Thalmann GN, Krause T, Studer UE. The template of the primary lymphatic landing sites of the prostate should be revisited: results of a multimodality mapping study. Eur Urol. 2008;53(1):118–25.
57. Montorsi F, Wilson TG, Rosen RC, Ahlering TE, Artibani W, Carroll PR, Costello A, Eastham JA, Ficarra V, Guazzoni G, Menon M, Novara G, Patel VR, Stolzenburg JU, Van der Poel H, Van Poppel H, Mottrie A, Pasadena Consensus Panel. Best practices in robot-assisted radical prostatectomy: recommendations of the Pasadena consensus panel. Eur Urol. 2012;62(3):368–81.
58. Feicke A, Baumgartner M, Talimi S, Schmid DM, Seifert HH, Müntener M, Fatzer M, Sulser T, Strebel RT. Robotic-assisted laparoscopic extended pelvic lymph node dissection for prostate cancer: surgical technique and experience with the first 99 cases. Eur Urol. 2009;55(4):876–83.
59. Ham WS, Park SY, Rha KH, Kim WT, Choi YD. Robotic radical prostatectomy for patients with locally advanced prostate cancer is feasible: results of a single-institution study. J Laparoendosc Adv Surg Tech A. 2009 Jun;19(3):329–32.
60. Kiyoshima K, Yokomizo A, Yoshida T, Tomita K, Yonemasu H, Nakamura M, et al. Anatomical features of periprostatic tissue and its surroundings: a histological analysis of 79 radical retropubic prostatectomy specimens. Jpn J Clin Oncol. 2004;34(8):463.
61. Costello AJ, Brooks M, Cole OJ. Anatomical studies of the neurovascular bundle and cavernosal nerves. BJU Int. 2004;94:1071–6.
62. Kaul S, Bhandari A, Hemal A, Savera A, Shrivastava A, Menon M. Robotic radical prostatectomy with preservation of the prostatic fascia: a feasibility study. Urology. 2005;66:1261–5.
63. Menon M, Kaul S, Bhandari A, Shrivastava A, Tewari A, Hemal A. Potency following robotic radical prostatectomy: a questionnaire based analysis of outcomes after conventional nerve sparing and prostatic fascia sparing techniques. J Urol. 2005;174:2291–6.
64. Ko YH, Coelho RF, Sivaraman A, Schatloff O, Chauhan S, Abdul-Muhsin HM, Carrion RJ, Palmer KJ, Cheon J, Patel VR. Retrograde versus antegrade nerve sparing during robot-assisted radical prostatectomy: which is better for achieving early functional recovery? Eur Urol. 2013;63(1):169–77.
65. Tewari AK, Bigelow K, Rao S, Takenaka A, El-Tabi N, Te A, et al. Anatomic restoration technique of continence mechanism and preservation of puboprostatic collar: a novel modification to achieve early urinary continence in men undergoing robotic prostatectomy. Urology. 2007;69:726–31.
66. Menon M, Muhletaler F, Campos M, Peabody JO. Assessment of early continence after reconstruction of the periprostatic tissues in patients undergoing computer assisted (robotic) prostatectomy: results of a 2 group parallel randomized controlled trial. J Urol. 2008;180:1018–23.
67. Sammon JD, Muhletaler F, Peabody JO, Diaz-Insua M, Satya- naryana R, Menon M. Long-term functional urinary outcomes comparing single- vs double-layer urethrovesical anastomosis: two-year follow-up of a two-group parallel randomized con- trolled trial. Urology. 2010;76:1102–7.
68. Krane LS, Bhandari M, Peabody JO, Menon M. Impact of percutaneous suprapubic tube drainage on patient discomfort after radical prostatectomy. Eur Urol. 2009;56:325–30.
69. Sammon JD, Trinh QD, Sukumar S, Diaz M, Simone A, Kaul S, et al. Long-term follow-up of patients undergoing percutaneous suprapubic tube drainage after robot-assisted radical prostatectomy (RARP). BJU Int. 2012;110:580–5.
70. Kaul S, Sammon J, Bhandari A, Peabody J, Rogers CG, Menon M. A novel method of urethrovesical anastomosis during robot-assisted radical prostatectomy using a unidirectional barbed wound closure device: feasibility study and early out- comes in 51 patients. J Endourol. 2010;24:1789–93.

71. Jeong W, Sood A, Ghani KR, Pucheril D, Sammon JD, Gupta NS, et al. Bimanual examination of the retrieved specimen and regional hypothermia during robot-assisted radical prostatectomy: a novel technique for reducing positive surgical margin and achieving pelvic cooling. BJU Int. 2014;114:955–7.
72. Schlomm T, Tennstedt P, Huxhold C, Steuber T, Salomon G, Michl U, Heinzer H, Hansen J, Budäus L, Steurer S, Wittmer C, Minner S, Haese A, Sauter G, Graefen M, Huland H. Neurovascular structure-adjacent frozen-section examination (NeuroSAFE) increases nerve-sparing frequency and reduces positive surgical margins in open and robot-assisted laparoscopic radical prostatectomy: experience after 11,069 consecutive patients. Eur Urol. 2012;62(2):333–40.
73. Manny TB, Patel M, Hemal AK. Fluorescence-enhanced robotic radical prostatectomy using real-time lymphangiography and tissue marking with percutaneous injection of unconjugated indocyanine green: the initial clinical experience in 50 patients. Eur Urol. 2014 Jun;65(6):1162–8.

Retropubic Radical Prostatectomy 13

Bulent Akdogan, Mesut Altan, and Haluk Ozen

Abstract

The interest in performing radical prostatectomy (RP) for the treatment of localized prostate cancer started next to the widespread use of PSA and then grew with Walsh's technical definitions. Increasing experience on the technique and stage migration by the use of PSA triggered excellent oncological and functional outcomes. However, unlike other surgeries, RP may result in a very wide satisfaction spectrum since many factors such as patient comorbidities, tumor stage, and surgeon's experience may affect results. In this section, diagnosis, patient selection, RP technique, complications, and postoperative follow-up will be discussed briefly.

13.1 Introduction

Although radical prostatectomy (RP) was first performed in 1867, for long period, it was abandoned because of early and late complications. Besides excessive intraoperative bleeding rates, severe incontinence and erectile dysfunction rates were detected almost for every case. Nevertheless, on the definition of anatomical RP by Walsh in the 1970s, this surgery has become the gold standard treatment modality with acceptable oncological and improved functional outcomes [1–3]. One of the most important concerns to get better outcomes is surgeon volume. A very high number of patients are required for excellent results in the learning curve. Careful "extirpative" manipulations in bloody surgical area affect oncological outcomes. Likewise, meticulous "reconstructive" handling for bladder neck and urethra is required for good functional outcomes. All those vigilant steps are considered absolutely necessary for an efficacious surgery.

B. Akdogan, M.D. • M. Altan, M.D. • H. Ozen, M.D. (✉)
Department of Urology, Hacettepe University, Ankara, Turkey
e-mail: hozen@hacettepe.edu.tr

G. Ozyigit, U. Selek (eds.), *Principles and Practice of Urooncology*,
DOI 10.1007/978-3-319-56114-1_13

13.2 Patient Selection

Though prostate cancer is the most frequent cancer in men, it has a low disease-specific mortality since most patients die from other causes. In 2008 AAC reported 16.7% incidence and 2.57% mortality rate of prostate cancer. First, it's necessary to evaluate all factors about the patient, tumor, surgeon, and current available treatment alternatives at that particular hospital. Then discuss with the patient the best alternative strategy. In order to attain finest decision, besides patient age and comorbidities, tumor features, ability of the surgeon, and patient expectations carry paramount importance. To predict recurrence and progression after surgery, patients are stratified into prognostic risk groups based on preoperative clinical stage, Gleason score, and PSA level (Table 13.1). However every single patient has unique properties and should be evaluated at his own setting. Similarly every surgeon has different experiences and facilities in his hospital. So, treatment decision should vary in dissimilar conditions for each particular patient.

RP, compared to watchful waiting (WW), had better survival rates in prospective randomized Scandinavian Prostate Cancer Group Study [4]. The benefit of RP on disease-specific mortality and metastasis rates was persistent beyond 10 years [5]. Overdiagnosis has been a fulcrum for follow-up. Despite the reported 50% overdiagnosis rate, recent other studies estimated this rate to be 23–28% [6, 7]. On the other hand, clinicopathological studies interestingly reported an overdiagnosis rate of 7–20% and claimed that underdiagnosis occurs more frequently than overdiagnosis [8, 9]. These results showed that overdiagnosis rates are much less than what's believed. Currently there is no method to diagnose clinically insignificant prostate cancer, and in order to lower cancer-related deaths, it's essential to ignore the low overdiagnosis rates.

An ideal candidate for RP is the one with a life expectancy of at least 10–15 years and with less comorbidity. Complete surgical resection is a must for an effective surgery. A palpable nodule on examination, positive imaging findings, and high percentage of positive biopsy cores are significant risk factors for extracapsular extension (ECE) [10, 11]. RP offers excellent progression-free survival rates when the tumor is organ confined even for the patients with high Gleason scores [12]. Excellent continence and erectile function rates are feasible with adequate experience. Furthermore, RP improves lower urinary tract symptoms and quality of life (QoL) parameters [13].

Table 13.1 Risk classification in localized prostate cancer

Low risk	Intermediate risk	High risk
Clinical T1–T2a and Gleason <7 and PSA <10 ng/mL	Clinical T2b or Gleason 7 or PSA 10–20 ng/mL	Clinical T2c, T3a-b or Gleason 8–10 or PSA > 20 ng/mL
Localized		Locally advanced

13.3 Indications of Nerve-Sparing (NS) Approach

Preoperative erectile function is the most important denominator of postoperative erection. Meticulous bilateral nerve-sparing approach in a young patient would result in satisfactory erections postoperatively. Walsh et al. were the first to show the possibility of sparing neurovascular bundle (NVB) that contains the cavernous nerves. Recently, many authors reported their outcomes about this technique [14].

Although NS technique can safely be performed in localized disease, indications of nerve-sparing RP are still debatable [15]. Preserving cavernous nerves without jeopardizing oncological principles may only be possible with a sufficient learning curve. For the beginner surgeons at the onset of this curve, clinicopathological risk factors demonstrating ECE may guide them to better select candidates. Nowadays certain nomograms are widely used in order to predict ECE [16–19]. Similarly new-generation MRI technology may give an insight to predict ECE and locally advanced disease [20–22], although MRI is not sensitive enough to find all tumors with extra-prostatic growth or microscopic ECE [23, 24]. The use of MRI in low-risk patients has no benefits either [25, 26].

Undoubtedly the most critical decision to perform NS approach is made during the surgery. When the tumor extends beyond the capsule, it's possible to resect the prostate with negative surgical margin by interfascial dissection [27]. But NVB must be resected in case of invasion or suspicion of residual tumor inside it on palpation.

13.4 Steps in Retropubic Radical Prostatectomy

An 8–10 cm midline incision is made through subcutaneous tissues between the umbilicus and pubis symphysis. After dissecting the rectus muscles, the transverse fascia will sharply be opened at midline (Fig. 13.1). Blunt dissection starting laterally the peritoneum will be released cranially up to iliac vessels. The fat anterior and lateral to the prostate is teased away to expose the underlying anatomy. Endopelvic fascia is incised laterally between the prostate and the levator ani muscles (Fig. 13.2).

In most patients, an opening is found in the endopelvic fascia laterally of the puboprostatic ligaments. An incision is made from that opening throughout the lowest point of the fascia. The puboprostatic ligaments can then be sharply incised at their attachment to the pubic bone, with care taken to not damage the dorsal vein complex (DVC) (Fig. 13.3). A figure-of-eight suture is then placed approximately 1 cm cephalad to the anterior bladder neck, to ligate the superficial DVC. This suture helps identifying the proper location to divide the bladder neck later in the surgery and also to minimize backflow bleeding (Fig. 13.4). The deep DVC is ligated distally after the DVC is isolated from the urethra just beyond the apex of the

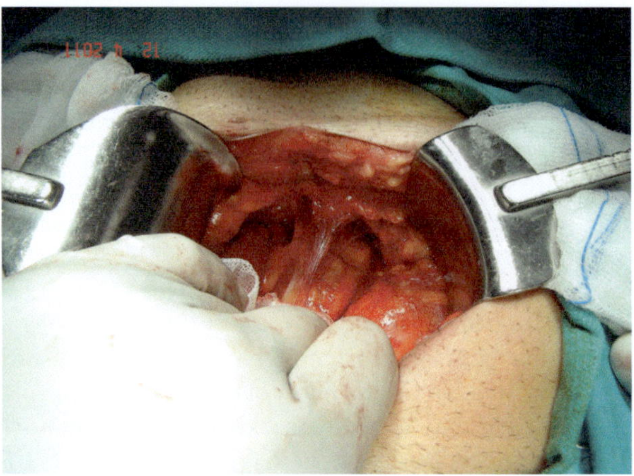

Fig. 13.1 Midline incision and exposure of retzius space

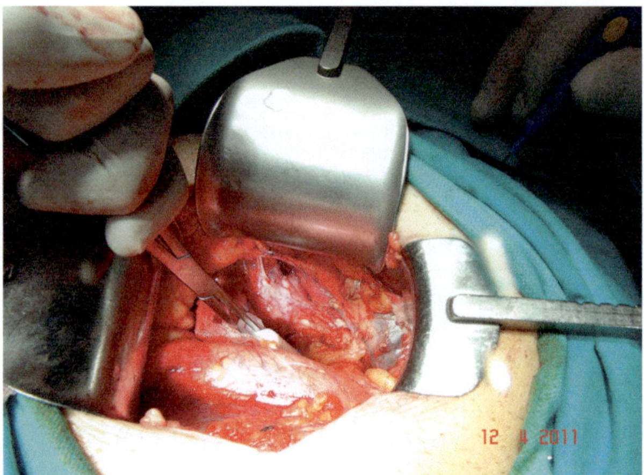

Fig. 13.2 Endopelvic fascia is incised

prostate (Fig. 13.5). The fascial layer surrounding the DVC and urethra is bluntly ruptured with the index finger, allowing the surgeon to appreciate a sulcus between the most distal part of urethra and the DVC. Gentle traction on the Foley catheter may help identify the urethra. A long, blunt-tipped right-angle clamp is passed between the DVC and the urethra and is used to grasp stainless steel wire. The wire loop will be used as a guide transecting the DVC, after the distal suture ligature is placed through the DVC, a few millimeters dorsal and caudal to the wire (Fig. 13.6). The suture is anchored through the posterior periosteum of the pubis and tied securely, controlling bleeding from the DVC when it is divided. After releasing the urethra from the fibrous fibers adjacent to the urogenital diaphragm posteriorly and

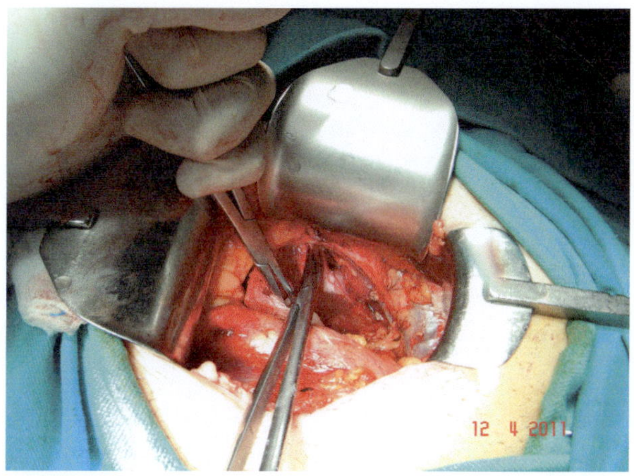

Fig. 13.3 Puboprostatic ligament is cut

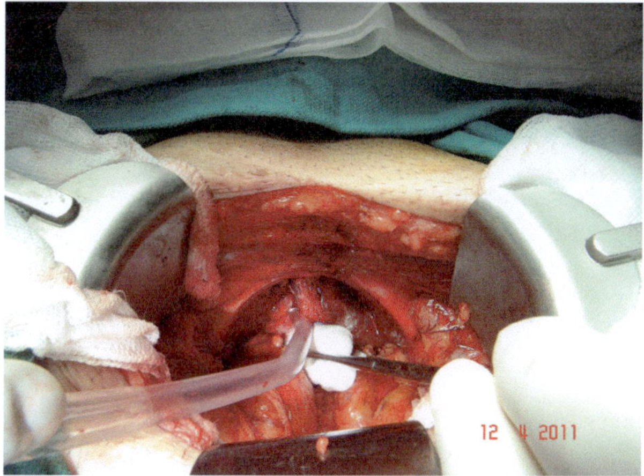

Fig. 13.4 Dorsal vein complex

lifting it with a right-angle clamp, the urethra is cut 270° (Fig. 13.7). Then, 3.0 Vicryl anastomotic stitches are placed at 1 and 11 o'clock positions. Then bilateral 3, 5, 7, and 9 o'clock sutures are placed (Fig. 13.8). After passing six stitches from the urethra, the catheter is held with a thick clamp and cut off, the distal part is removed from the urethra, and the proximal part is directed cranially without excessive traction. At this point, the posterior 90° part of the urethra is cut off, and the urethra is completely separated. Subsequently, rectourethral fascia (posterior striated sphincter) will be dissected. This stage is extremely important because finding the exact plane is essential both for the negative surgical margin and for preventing rectal injury.

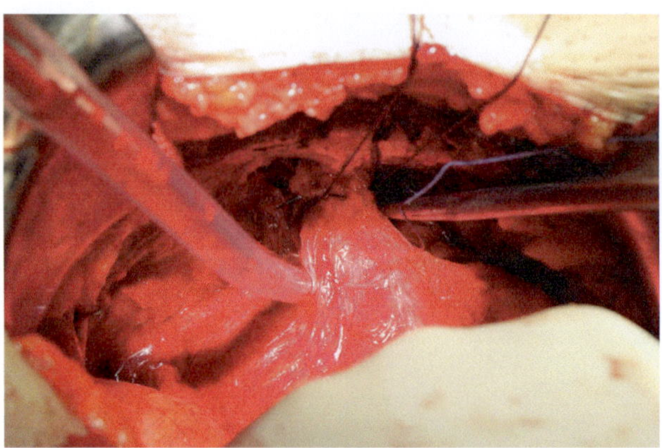

Fig. 13.5 Dorsal vein complex is ligated

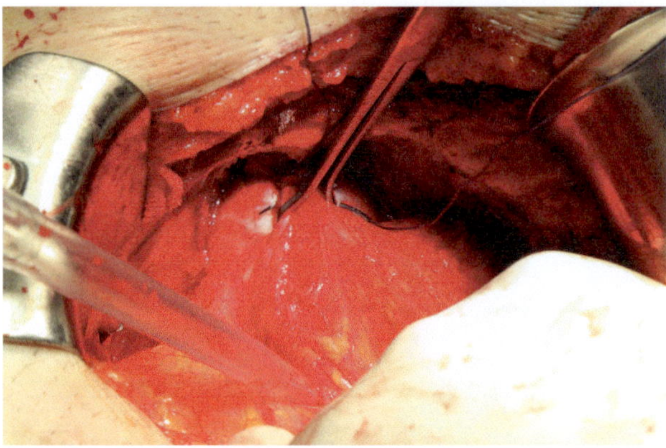

Fig. 13.6 Backflow suture

The cavernous nerve passes laterally to the rectourethral fascia. Without dissecting this tissue, which is relatively thin in some patients and scarred in others due to the possible desmoplastic reaction, the posterior part of the prostate will not be liberal. The correct depth for the dissection border can be defined as the appearance of pararectal fat tissue (Fig. 13.9). Seminal vesicles will appear when the lateral pedicle is fully ligated. A single clamp cannot control the lateral pedicle. The lateral pedicles are separated after multiple ligations of the vascular and fibrous ligaments with individual clips or via clamps. The lateral dissection is continued until the junction of the seminal vesicle with the prostate floor. Opening the bands between the rectum and the Denonvilliers' fascia covering the seminal vesicle continues the dissection. At this point, both the vas deferens and seminal

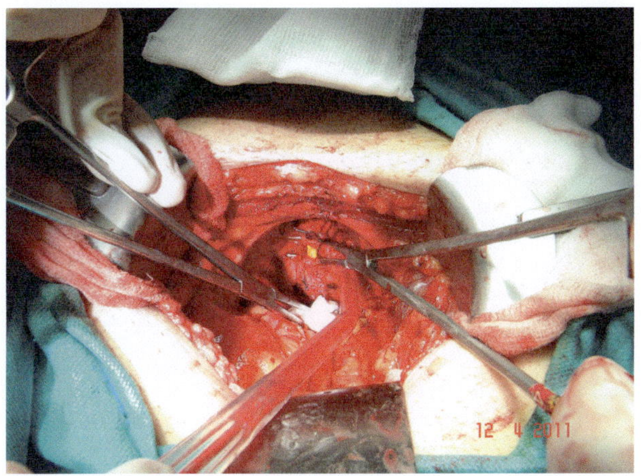

Fig. 13.7 Urethra is cut with 270°

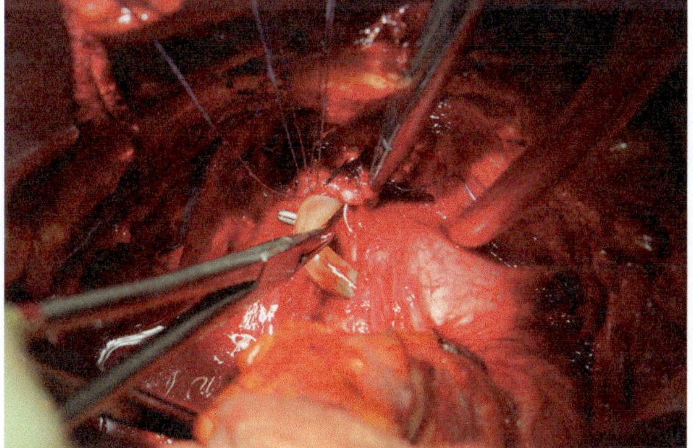

Fig. 13.8 Urethra sutures

vesicles emerge. First, the vas deferens is separated, clipped, and cut. The fibrous adhesions between the distal part of the vas deferens and the seminal vesicles are separated so they are clearly revealed. After this point, the end of the seminal vesicles is reached with blunt and sharp dissection. Here, the seminal vesicle artery is clearly displayed and clipped, which allows mobilization of the seminal vesicle (Fig. 13.10).

Later, the dissection is directed toward the bladder neck in the posterior plane (Fig. 13.11). After finding the bladder neck, separation of the prostate will continue anteriorly (Fig. 13.12). After observing the orifices, the posterior part of

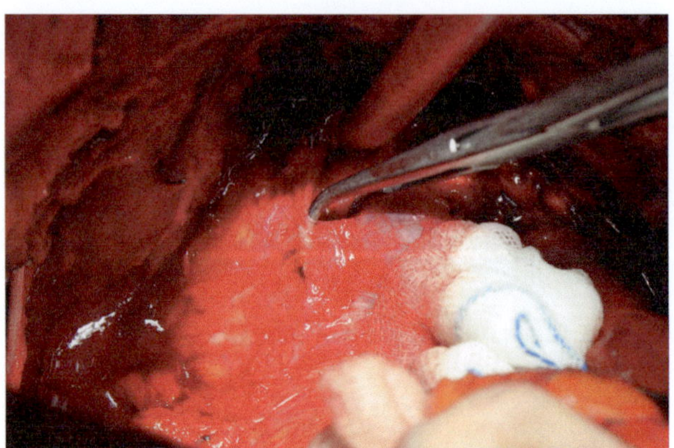

Fig. 13.9 Pararectal fatty tissue

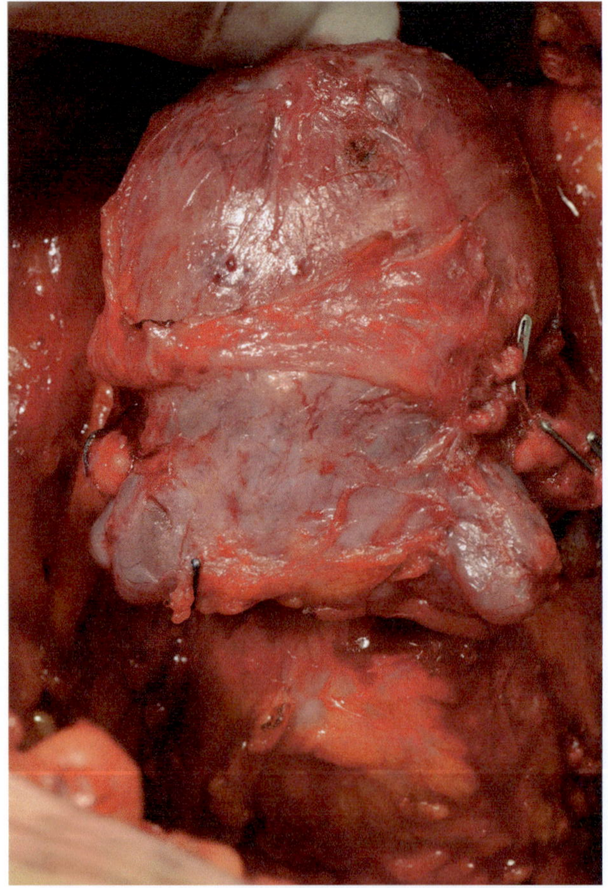

Fig. 13.10 Seminal vesicles mobilized

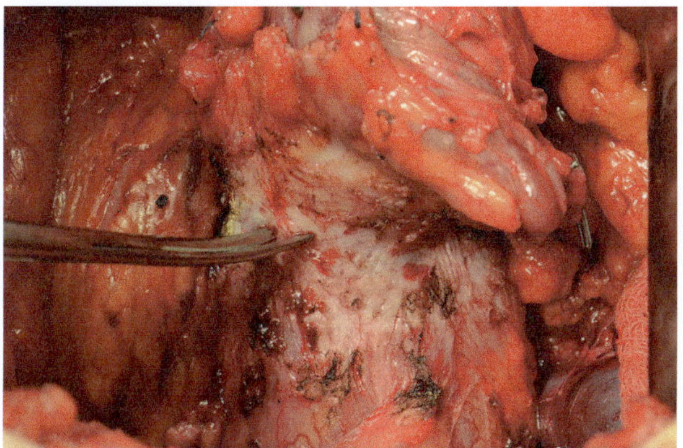

Fig. 13.11 Bladder neck is dissected

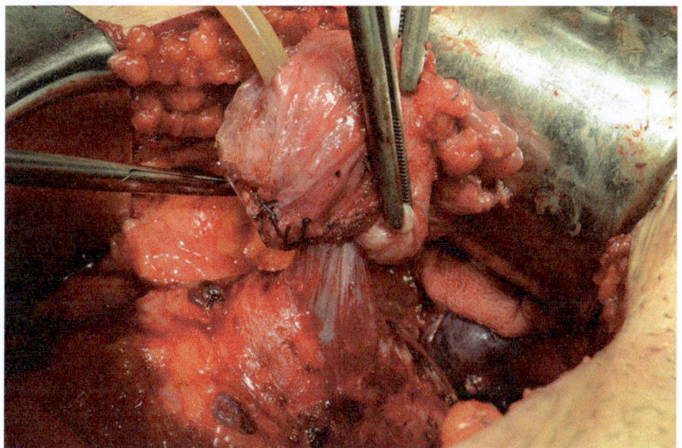

Fig. 13.12 Anterior dissection of prostate

the bladder neck is cut with scissors and taken out. At this point the catheter will be removed with the specimen (Fig. 13.13). The bladder neck is closed posteriorly in a tennis racquet fashion. The mucosa is everted with fine 3.0 Vicryl sutures (Fig. 13.14). When adequate hemostasis has been achieved, 20 F Foley catheter will be advanced into the bladder and inflated with 10–15 cc sterile water. The six sutures placed in the urethra are passed through the appropriate points on the bladder neck—from inside to outside. The catheter is placed on traction to bring the bladder neck down to the urethra, slack is taken out of the sutures, and the bladder is gently retracted with the anastomotic sutures tied in an anterior-to-posterior fashion. A sump drain is then placed through the anterior abdominal wall through a separate stab incision, and then the fascia and skin will be closed.

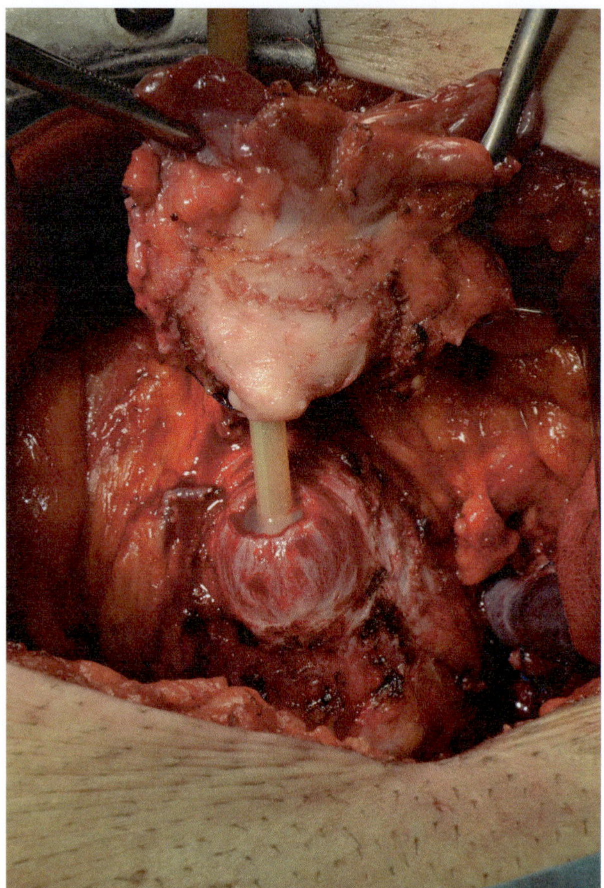

Fig. 13.13 Prostate is removed

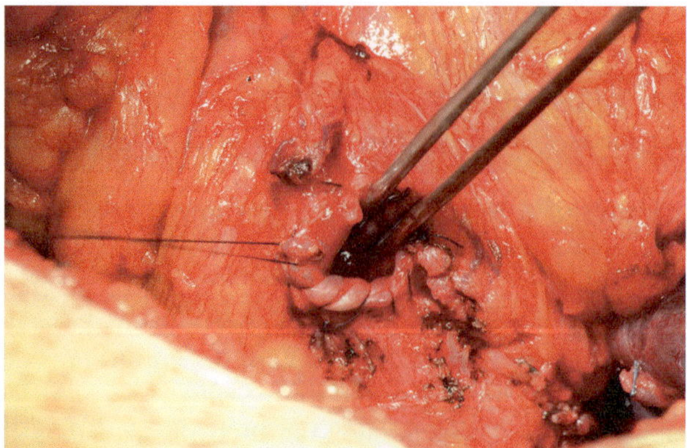

Fig. 13.14 Bladder neck mucosa is everted

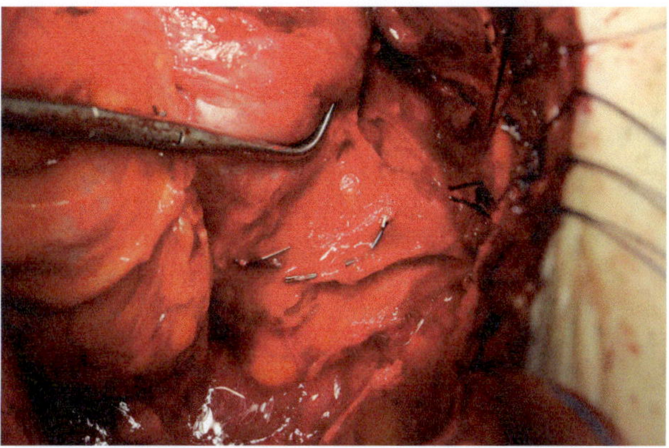

Fig. 13.15 Nerve-sparing technique

13.5 Nerve-Sparing Technique

To preserve nerves, cautery usage should be avoided. Instead, crossing vessels passing to the prostate should be ligated with clips [28] (Fig. 13.15). As cavernous nerves pass between the prostatic and levator fascia, the prostatic fascia should not be harmed. The levator fascia should be opened as much as cranially from the bladder neck level from the thickened part. This approach is preferred, since it will also help to mobilize the prostate. If you start to spare nerves gently from prostatic apex and continue caudally, the rest of procedure will be much easier.

13.6 Complications

Several factors may complicate the surgery in short or long term. Those are mainly the surgeon's experience, patient age, comorbidities, prostate and tumor volume, pelvic anatomy, and neoadjuvant hormone or radiotherapy. In other words, patient selection is the key point here. RP was not so popular for many years mainly because of excessive bleeding [29]. Understanding the anatomy has significantly decreased both the amount of bleeding and transfusion rates. An old study has shown a mean blood loss of 1100 (800–1600) cc during RP [30]. A recent meta-analysis with 167.184 open RP patients reported a median blood loss to be 750 cc [31]. Dorsal vein complex is the main cause of bleeding and so it should be sutured carefully. Nerve-sparing approach may also increase bleeding.

Rectal injury is a rarely reported complication and is directly related to surgical experience and technique [31, 32]. Most surgeons do routine preoperative mechanical bowel preparation besides antibiotics. So they can easily close defect primarily in case of rectal injury. A meta-analysis including 35.099 RP patients reported 0.43% rectal injury rate [33]. Of those with rectal injury, 48% received preoperative mechanical preparation. Infection, delayed colostomy, and length of stay rates were not statistically different between mechanical and nonmechanical bowel preparation groups.

Lymphocele is a relatively common complication for patients who underwent lymphadenectomy. When lymphatics are well controlled by cautery, clips, or sutures, the risk will be minimal. The rate of symptomatic lymphocele requiring intervention was reported to be 1.1–9.1% [34]. However, this rate increases to 27–61% when asymptomatic lymphoceles are also included [35]. Conservative management is the best option for asymptomatic patients. In case of pain or fever, USG or CT-guided drainage and antibiotics are required.

Postoperative infection is very rare and when it occurs is mostly wound infection. Postoperative antibiotics are not required if there are no symptoms. Single-dose second-generation cephalosporin is preferred for prophylaxis at anesthesia induction. Nevertheless, antibiotics could be beneficial when excessive intraoperative bleeding or long-standing postoperative drainage has occurred especially for obese and diabetic patients.

Deep vein thrombosis (DVT) is undoubtedly the most important etiology of 1% mortality observed in RP. Catalona reported 1.3% thromboembolic complication rate [36]. DVT can be prevented by shortening duration of surgery to less than 2 h and early postoperative mobilization and using air compression socks [37]. Low-molecular-weight heparin derivatives such as enoxaparin sodium may be given for high-risk patients.

13.6.1 Erectile Dysfunction

There are several studies related to this subject in limitation. Although there are many valid surveys, there is variable data related to ED. This is related to the patient group heterogeneity and the different erection reporting by the physician and the patients. While physicians always have good results, the situation may be different on the patients' side. This shows that erectile function is a concept assessed and rated relatively not through yes-or-no questions.

Diabetes, hypertension, and drugs used for these reasons may cause adverse effects on the patient's erectile function in the preoperative period and also may cause poor outcome after RP. Another important subject is the preoperative erectile function. It is considered one of the most important factors predicting erection recovery [38].

In his series Catalona followed up 3477 patients treated with RP for 18 months [36]. Erections sufficient for intercourse occurred in 76% of preoperatively potent men treated with bilateral nerve sparing and 53% of men treated with unilateral or partial nerve sparing surgery. Younger age and bilateral nerve sparing were significant factors for erection recovery. Huland et al. followed up patients for more than 12 months and reported erection recovery rate of 70% in patients younger than 55 years old with bilateral NS. They also found that this rate decreases to 37% in patients older than 65 with unilateral NS [39].

Another important factor affecting postoperative potency is the accessory pudendal artery. A study of 2399 patients who underwent bilateral NSRRP showed that accessory pudendal artery preservation provides a twofold advantage in preserving potency and leads to potency recovery sooner [40].

In a prospective, randomized controlled study, the postoperative 12-month potency status of 778 RRP and 1847 robot-assisted laparoscopic radical prostatectomy (RALP) patients with age < 75, PSA < 20, and T < 4 was compared using questionnaire forms [41]. ED was reported to be 74 and 70.1% in both RALP and RRP, respectively. However, it should be noticed that more lymph node dissections were performed with less nerve preservation in RRP group. The first results of a randomized controlled trial of 47 RRP and 22 RRP were published, and the potency rate in the RRP arm at the 12th postoperative month was 26%, and the same rate was found as 55% in the RALP arm [42]. In the study, a questionnaire form was used, and there was no difference between patients' preoperative potency status and tumor characteristics. Krambeck et al. retrospectively studied the results of 403 RRP and 203 RALP after a 1-year follow-up [43]. NS approach was applied less in RRP group. There was no difference in the tumor characteristics between two groups. After 1 year they assessed erectile function by using questionnaire form, and no difference was found between the two groups' potency status (RRP 63%, RALP 70%). The 12-month results of phase 3 study in which 163 RRP and 163 RALP were randomized were published [44]. There was no difference between the 12-month questionnaire form scores between the patients.

13.6.2 Incontinence

The most feared and most devastating complication after PR is urinary incontinence. Fortunately, excellent results are reported in experienced hands. Catalona et al. reported that recovery of urinary continence occurred in 93% of all men and was associated only with younger age [36]. In Walsh's series of more than 1200 patient data, it was reported that at the end of 1 year, 93% of the patients did not use any pads and 98% did not have a serious urinary problem [45]. The complete continence rate of 91% at 12 months reached 95% at 24 months. On multivariable analysis increased patient age, lack of protection of the neurovascular bundle, and development of anastomotic sheath obstruction were the factors that predict and cause postoperative incontinence.

There are some problems in assessing incontinence. Differences in the definition of continence, in the patient population, and in the postoperative evaluation time are important variables that hamper standardization. The most important point is how the physician and the patient interpret the continence. In a study from Japan, continence and its related problems were asked to patients by using "University of California-Los Angeles Prostate Cancer Index" (UCLA-PCI) survey. In this study, patients were not able to understand the 0–100 score scale in the survey, and it was argued that "absolutely no urine leakage" was the best description of continence

[46]. While 97% of patients who said they didn't have any urine leakage didn't use any pads, only 63 and 75% of them reported full continence and full urination control, respectively. This demonstrates that as pad use can change from person to person, it can't define continence in a sufficiently objective way. In prospective studies comparing RARP to RRP, patient-reported urinary incontinence was reported to be 3–12% and 12–20%, respectively [41, 47].

13.7 Surgical Margin Status

The main issue in oncological surgery is appropriate patient selection and complete tumor resection with negative surgical margins. Positive surgical margin (PSM) rates in Catalona's series were reported to decrease to 9.8% after 2000 [36]. Even it was reported to be 1.3% in localized disease [48]. This excellent rate is definitely related to the surgeon's experience and his better understanding of anatomy.

Many studies focused on the effect of PSM on biochemical recurrence-free survival. Schroder et al. found that PSM is a significant risk factor for biochemical relapse [49]. Nevertheless, Soloway et al. found that only 25–50% of patients with PSM had biochemical relapse [50]. A study including about 6000 patients with a 2-year median follow-up was published in 2005 [51]. PSM was observed in 26% of patients. Biochemical recurrence-free survival for patients with and without PSM was 70 and 36%, respectively. Multivariable analysis demonstrated that patients with PSM had 3.66 times increased relapse rate. Another study with 7160 patients reported PSM of 21% [52]. A PSM was significantly associated with biochemical recurrence. Patients with multiple and extensive PSM had an increased risk of biochemical recurrence on multivariable analysis. Al-Ahmadie et al. studied 2150 patients and reported 10% PSMs, 71% of them were in the apex [53]. The linear extension of a PSM was found to be related to lower biochemical recurrence-free survival.

13.8 Cancer Control

In his series of 3478 patients, Catalona et al. reported 5- and 10-year biochemical progression-free survival rate to be 80 and 68%, respectively [54]. They found that actuarial 10-year biochemical progression-free probabilities were 91% (95% CI 83–95) for PSA less than 2.6 ng/mL and 49% (95% CI 44–54) for PSA greater than 10.0 ng/mL. Actuarial 10-year biochemical progression-free survival probabilities were 79% (95% CI 76–82) for organ-confined disease, 62% (95% CI 51–72) for disease with ECE without PSMs, and 53% (95% CI 47–59) for disease with ECE and PSMs. The results of 4478 men who underwent anatomical radical retropubic prostatectomy, as performed by a single surgeon (PCW), at the Johns Hopkins Medical Institutions with a median follow-up of 10 years were published in 2012 [55]. The 10-, 15-, 20-, and 25-year actuarial probabilities of PFS were 82, 78, 74, and 68%, respectively. Increasing age and earlier year of surgery as well as increasing PSA, biopsy Gleason score, and clinical stage were all significant preoperative risk factors associated with lower PFS. Postoperative significant predictors of PFS included prostatectomy Gleason score, pathological stage, and surgical margin status. According to these results, in case of organ-confined disease, RRP offers an excellent 20-year PFS.

Park et al. retrospectively analyzed prospectively collected longitudinal data of 277 RRP and 730 RALP cases over a 5-year period [56]. The pT2 PSM and biochemical recurrence-free rates showed no significant difference between the RRP and RALP series throughout the study period. Although the pT3 PSM rates of the 1st and 2nd RALP series (1st 500 patients) were higher than that of the RRP series, the 3rd RALP series had a comparable rate. The 3-year biochemical-free survival rates of the RRP and RALP series were similar at each pathological stage. The RALP group was significantly associated with a younger age, lower body mass index, lower Gleason score, and lower clinical stage than the RRP group. Punnen et al. in their retrospective study found that recurrence-free survival was similar at 2 years (84 and 79%) and 4 years (68 and 66%) after open RRP and RALP, respectively [57]. In the aforementioned studies, follow-up periods and patient numbers are considered limited [58].

13.9 Hospital and Surgeon Workload

Hu et al. analyzed Medicare data and found that high-volume surgeons had half the complication risk compared with low-volume surgeons [59]. Ellison et al. reported that patients treated at lower-volume institutions are at increased risk of initiation of subsequent adjuvant therapy with radiation therapy, medical hormone ablation, or orchiectomy [60]. It was reported that postoperative mortality, hospitalization time, transfusion rate, surgical margin, and disease recurrence were also associated with hospital volume [61]. In a population-based study of 25,346 men who underwent RP, it was demonstrated that factors predicting surgery for incontinence were patient age at radical prostatectomy, radiotherapy after surgery, and surgeon volume [62]. As a result, among surgeons with high case volume, there are differences that can significantly change the patient's quality of life.

Conclusions

The most desired three outcomes following RP which are full continence, potency, and absence of biochemical recurrence represent "trifecta." Bianco et al. studied 1746 intervention-naïve, newly diagnosed, and clinically localized prostate cancer patients who underwent RP with curative intent beginning in 1983. He has found, at 24 months, 60% of patients were potent, continent, and free of cancer [63]. Saranchuk et al. reported the results of 647 patients who underwent RP between 1998 and 2003. Mean patient age and pretreatment PSA were 58 years and 6.9 ng/mL, respectively [64]. In another study including 831 patients, trifecta rate at 2 and 5 years was 64 and 61%, respectively [65]. A similar study with 1577 patients reported 64% trifecta rate in 2 years.

When analyzing these results, the figures are a little bit below than expectations basically because of erection recovery problem. Although good oncological and continence outcomes are reported from many centers, the trifecta rate is low because of potency problems. So, patients should be counseled about outcomes of the center before curative treatment in order to prevent long-term dissatisfaction.

References

1. Walsh PC, Lepor H, Eggleston JC. Radical prostatectomy with preservation of sexual function: anatomical and pathological considerations. Prostate. 1983;4(5):473–85.
2. Walsh PC. Radical prostatectomy for localized prostate cancer provides durable cancer control with excellent quality of life: a structured debate. J Urol. 2000;163(6):1802–7.
3. Nielsen ME, Schaeffer EM, Marschke P, Walsh PC. High anterior release of the levator fascia improves sexual function following open radical retropubic prostatectomy. J Urol. 2008;180(6):2557–64; discussion 64.
4. Bill-Axelson A, Holmberg L, Ruutu M, Garmo H, Stark JR, Busch C, et al. Radical prostatectomy versus watchful waiting in early prostate cancer. N Engl J Med. 2011;364(18):1708–17.
5. Bill-Axelson A, Holmberg L, Filen F, Ruutu M, Garmo H, Busch C, et al. Radical prostatectomy versus watchful waiting in localized prostate cancer: the Scandinavian prostate cancer group-4 randomized trial. J Natl Cancer Inst. 2008;100(16):1144–54.
6. Draisma G, Boer R, Otto SJ, van der Cruijsen IW, Damhuis RA, Schroder FH, et al. Lead times and overdetection due to prostate-specific antigen screening: estimates from the European randomized study of screening for prostate cancer. J Natl Cancer Inst. 2003;95(12):868–78.
7. Draisma G, Etzioni R, Tsodikov A, Mariotto A, Wever E, Gulati R, et al. Lead time and overdiagnosis in prostate-specific antigen screening: importance of methods and context. J Natl Cancer Inst. 2009;101(6):374–83.
8. Pelzer AE, Bektic J, Akkad T, Ongarello S, Schaefer G, Schwentner C, et al. Under diagnosis and over diagnosis of prostate cancer in a screening population with serum PSA 2 to 10 ng/ml. J Urol. 2007;178(1):93–7; discussion 7.
9. Graif T, Loeb S, Roehl KA, Gashti SN, Griffin C, Yu X, et al. Under diagnosis and over diagnosis of prostate cancer. J Urol. 2007;178(1):88–92.
10. Ohori M, Egawa S, Shinohara K, Wheeler TM, Scardino PT. Detection of microscopic extracapsular extension prior to radical prostatectomy for clinically localized prostate cancer. Br J Urol. 1994;74(1):72–9.
11. Lotan Y, Shariat SF, Khoddami SM, Saboorian H, Koeneman KS, Cadeddu JA, et al. The percent of biopsy cores positive for cancer is a predictor of advanced pathological stage and poor clinical outcomes in patients treated with radical prostatectomy. J Urol. 2004;171(6 Pt 1):2209–14.
12. Balaji KC, Wheeler T, Scardino PT. Poorly differentiated prostate cancer detected by PSA are more likely to be organ confined than those detected by digital rectal examination. Proc Am Soc Clin Oncol. 1999;18:318.
13. Kumar V, Toussi H, Marr C, Hough C, Javle P. The benefits of radical prostatectomy beyond cancer control in symptomatic men with prostate cancer. BJU Int. 2004;93(4):507–9.
14. Walsh PC, Donker PJ. Impotence following radical prostatectomy: insight into etiology and prevention. J Urol. 1982;128(3):492–7.
15. Gontero P, Kirby RS. Nerve-sparing radical retropubic prostatectomy: techniques and clinical considerations. Prostate Cancer Prostatic Dis. 2005;8(2):133–9.
16. Steuber T, Graefen M, Haese A, Erbersdobler A, Chun FK, Schlom T, et al. Validation of a nomogram for prediction of side specific extracapsular extension at radical prostatectomy. J Urol. 2006;175(3 Pt 1):939–44; discussion 44.

17. Zorn KC, Gallina A, Hutterer GC, Walz J, Shalhav AL, Zagaja GP, et al. External validation of a nomogram for prediction of side-specific extracapsular extension at robotic radical prostatectomy. J Endourol. 2007;21(11):1345–51.
18. Ohori M, Kattan MW, Koh H, Maru N, Slawin KM, Shariat S, et al. Predicting the presence and side of extracapsular extension: a nomogram for staging prostate cancer. J Urol. 2004;171(5):1844–9; discussion 9.
19. Palisaar RJ, Noldus J, Graefen M, Erbersdobler A, Haese A, Huland H. Influence of nerve-sparing (NS) procedure during radical prostatectomy (RP) on margin status and biochemical failure. Eur Urol. 2005;47(2):176–84.
20. Masterson TA, Touijer K. The role of endorectal coil MRI in preoperative staging and decision-making for the treatment of clinically localized prostate cancer. MAGMA. 2008;21(6):371–7.
21. Roethke MC, Lichy MP, Kniess M, Werner MK, Claussen CD, Stenzl A, et al. Accuracy of preoperative endorectal MRI in predicting extracapsular extension and influence on neurovascular bundle sparing in radical prostatectomy. World J Urol. 2013;31(5):1111–6.
22. Panebianco V, Salciccia S, Cattarino S, Minisola F, Gentilucci A, Alfarone A, et al. Use of multiparametric MR with neurovascular bundle evaluation to optimize the oncological and functional management of patients considered for nerve-sparing radical prostatectomy. J Sex Med. 2012;9(8):2157–66.
23. de Rooij M, Hamoen EH, Witjes JA, Barentsz JO, Rovers MM. Accuracy of magnetic resonance imaging for local staging of prostate cancer: a diagnostic meta-analysis. Eur Urol. 2016;70(2):233–45.
24. Jager GJ, Barentsz JO, Oosterhof GO, Witjes JA, Ruijs SJ. Pelvic adenopathy in prostatic and urinary bladder carcinoma: MR imaging with a three-dimensional TI-weighted magnetization-prepared-rapid gradient-echo sequence. AJR Am J Roentgenol. 1996;167(6):1503–7.
25. Wang L, Mullerad M, Chen HN, Eberhardt SC, Kattan MW, Scardino PT, et al. Prostate cancer: incremental value of endorectal MR imaging findings for prediction of extracapsular extension. Radiology. 2004;232(1):133–9.
26. D'Amico AV, Whittington R, Malkowicz B, Schnall M, Schultz D, Cote K, et al. Endorectal magnetic resonance imaging as a predictor of biochemical outcome after radical prostatectomy in men with clinically localized prostate cancer. J Urol. 2000;164(3 Pt 1):759–63.
27. Hernandez DJ, Epstein JI, Trock BJ, Tsuzuki T, Carter HB, Walsh PC. Radical retropubic prostatectomy. How often do experienced surgeons have positive surgical margins when there is extraprostatic extension in the region of the neurovascular bundle? J Urol. 2005;173(2): 446–9.
28. Ong AM, Su LM, Varkarakis I, Inagaki T, Link RE, Bhayani SB, et al. Nerve sparing radical prostatectomy: effects of hemostatic energy sources on the recovery of cavernous nerve function in a canine model. J Urol. 2004;172(4 Pt 1):1318–22.
29. Eastham JA, Scardino PT. Radical prostatectomy for clinical stage T1 and T2 prostate cancer. In: Vogelzang NJ, Scardino PT, Shipley WU, Debruyne FMJ, Linehan WM, eds. Comprehensive Text- book of Genitourinary Oncology. 3rd ed. Philadelphia, PA: Lippincott Williams and Wilkins; 2006:166–89.
30. Rabbani F, Yunis LH, Pinochet R, Nogueira L, Vora KC, Eastham JA, et al. Comprehensive standardized report of complications of retropubic and laparoscopic radical prostatectomy. Eur Urol. 2010;57(3):371–86.
31. Tewari A, Sooriakumaran P, Bloch DA, Seshadri-Kreaden U, Hebert AE, Wiklund P. Positive surgical margin and perioperative complication rates of primary surgical treatments for prostate cancer: a systematic review and meta-analysis comparing retropubic, laparoscopic, and robotic prostatectomy. Eur Urol. 2012;62(1):1–15.
32. Schmitges J, Trinh QD, Sun M, Abdollah F, Bianchi M, Budaus L, et al. Annual prostatectomy volume is related to rectal laceration rate after radical prostatectomy. Urology. 2012;79(4):796–803.
33. Sugihara T, Yasunaga H, Horiguchi H, Matsuda S, Fushimi K, Kattan MW, et al. Does mechanical bowel preparation ameliorate damage from rectal injury in radical prostatectomy? Analysis of 151 rectal injury cases. Int J Urol. 2014;21(6):566–70.

34. Anheuser P, Treiyer A, Stark E, Haben B, Steffens JA. Lymphoceles after radical retropubic prostatectomy. A treatment algorithm. Der Urologe Ausg A. 2010;49(7):832–6.
35. Harbin AC, Eun DD. The role of extended pelvic lymphadenectomy with radical prostatectomy for high-risk prostate cancer. Urol Oncol. 2015;33(5):208–16.
36. Kundu SD, Roehl KA, Eggener SE, Antenor JA, Han M, Catalona WJ. Potency, continence and complications in 3,477 consecutive radical retropubic prostatectomies. J Urol. 2004;172(6 Pt 1):2227–31.
37. Lepor H, Nieder AM, Ferrandino MN. Intraoperative and postoperative complications of radical retropubic prostatectomy in a consecutive series of 1,000 cases. J Urol. 2001;166(5):1729–33.
38. Rabbani F, Stapleton AM, Kattan MW, Wheeler TM, Scardino PT. Factors predicting recovery of erections after radical prostatectomy. J Urol. 2000;164(6):1929–34.
39. Graefen M, Walz J, Huland H. Open retropubic nerve-sparing radical prostatectomy. Eur Urol. 2006;49(1):38–48.
40. Rogers CG, Trock BP, Walsh PC. Preservation of accessory pudendal arteries during radical retropubic prostatectomy: surgical technique and results. Urology. 2004;64(1):148–51.
41. Haglind E, Carlsson S, Stranne J, Wallerstedt A, Wilderang U, Thorsteinsdottir T, et al. Urinary incontinence and erectile dysfunction after robotic versus open radical prostatectomy: a prospective, controlled, nonrandomised trial. Eur Urol. 2015;68(2):216–25.
42. Di Pierro GB, Baumeister P, Stucki P, Beatrice J, Danuser H, Mattei A. A prospective trial comparing consecutive series of open retropubic and robot-assisted laparoscopic radical prostatectomy in a centre with a limited caseload. Eur Urol. 2011;59(1):1–6.
43. Krambeck AE, DiMarco DS, Rangel LJ, Bergstralh EJ, Myers RP, Blute ML, et al. Radical prostatectomy for prostatic adenocarcinoma: a matched comparison of open retropubic and robot-assisted techniques. BJU Int. 2009;103(4):448–53.
44. Yaxley JW, Coughlin GD, Chambers SK, Occhipinti S, Samaratunga H, Zajdlewicz L, et al. Robot-assisted laparoscopic prostatectomy versus open radical retropubic prostatectomy: early outcomes from a randomised controlled phase 3 study. Lancet. 2016;388(10049):1057–66.
45. Walsh PC, Marschke P, Ricker D, Burnett AL. Patient-reported urinary continence and sexual function after anatomic radical prostatectomy. Urology. 2000;55(1):58–61.
46. Namiki S, Kuwahara M, Ioritani N, Akito T, Arai Y. An evaluation of urinary function after radical prostatectomy in Japanese men: concordance with definitions of urinary continence. BJU Int. 2005;95(4):530–3.
47. Ficarra V, Novara G, Fracalanza S, D'Elia C, Secco S, Iafrate M, et al. A prospective, non-randomized trial comparing robot-assisted laparoscopic and retropubic radical prostatectomy in one European institution. BJU Int. 2009;104(4):534–9.
48. Chuang AY, Nielsen ME, Hernandez DJ, Walsh PC, Epstein JI. The significance of positive surgical margin in areas of capsular incision in otherwise organ confined disease at radical prostatectomy. J Urol. 2007;178(4 Pt 1):1306–10.
49. Vis AN, Schroder FH, van der Kwast TH. The actual value of the surgical margin status as a predictor of disease progression in men with early prostate cancer. Eur Urol. 2006;50(2):258–65.
50. Simon MA, Kim S, Soloway MS. Prostate specific antigen recurrence rates are low after radical retropubic prostatectomy and positive margins. J Urol. 2006;175(1):140–4; discussion 4–5.
51. Karakiewicz PI, Eastham JA, Graefen M, Cagiannos I, Stricker PD, Klein E, et al. Prognostic impact of positive surgical margins in surgically treated prostate cancer: multi-institutional assessment of 5831 patients. Urology. 2005;66(6):1245–50.
52. Stephenson AJ, Wood DP, Kattan MW, Klein EA, Scardino PT, Eastham JA, et al. Location, extent and number of positive surgical margins do not improve accuracy of predicting prostate cancer recurrence after radical prostatectomy. J Urol. 2009;182(4):1357–63.
53. Udo K, Cronin AM, Carlino LJ, Savage CJ, Maschino AC, Al-Ahmadie HA, et al. Prognostic impact of subclassification of radical prostatectomy positive margins by linear extent and Gleason grade. J Urol. 2013;189(4):1302–7.
54. Roehl KA, Han M, Ramos CG, Antenor JA, Catalona WJ. Cancer progression and survival rates following anatomical radical retropubic prostatectomy in 3,478 consecutive patients: long-term results. J Urol. 2004;172(3):910–4.

55. Mullins JK, Feng Z, Trock BJ, Epstein JI, Walsh PC, Loeb S. The impact of anatomical radical retropubic prostatectomy on cancer control: the 30-year anniversary. J Urol. 2012;188(6):2219–24.
56. Park J, Yoo DS, Song C, Park S, Park S, Kim SC, et al. Comparison of oncological outcomes between retropubic radical prostatectomy and robot-assisted radical prostatectomy: an analysis stratified by surgical experience. World J Urol. 2014;32(1):193–9.
57. Punnen S, Meng MV, Cooperberg MR, Greene KL, Cowan JE, Carroll PR. How does robot-assisted radical prostatectomy (RARP) compare with open surgery in men with high-risk prostate cancer? BJU Int. 2013;112(4):E314–20.
58. Novara G, Ficarra V, Mocellin S, Ahlering TE, Carroll PR, Graefen M, et al. Systematic review and meta-analysis of studies reporting oncologic outcome after robot-assisted radical prostatectomy. Eur Urol. 2012;62(3):382–404.
59. Hu JC, Gold KF, Pashos CL, Mehta SS, Litwin MS. Role of surgeon volume in radical prostatectomy outcomes. J Clin Oncol. 2003;21(3):401–5.
60. Ellison LM, Trock BJ, Poe NR, Partin AW. The effect of hospital volume on cancer control after radical prostatectomy. J Urol. 2005;173(6):2094–8.
61. Trinh QD, Bjartell A, Freedland SJ, Hollenbeck BK, Hu JC, Shariat SF, et al. A systematic review of the volume-outcome relationship for radical prostatectomy. Eur Urol. 2013;64(5):786–98.
62. Nam RK, Herschorn S, Loblaw DA, Liu Y, Klotz LH, Carr LK, et al. Population based study of long-term rates of surgery for urinary incontinence after radical prostatectomy for prostate cancer. J Urol. 2012;188(2):502–6.
63. Bianco FJ Jr, Scardino PT, Eastham JA. Radical prostatectomy: long-term cancer control and recovery of sexual and urinary function ("trifecta"). Urology. 2005;66(5 Suppl):83–94.
64. Saranchuk JW, Kattan MW, Elkin E, Touijer AK, Scardino PT, Eastham JA. Achieving optimal outcomes after radical prostatectomy. J Clin Oncol. 2005;23(18):4146–51.
65. Antebi E, Eldefrawy A, Katkoori D, Soloway CT, Manoharan M, Soloway MS. Oncological and functional outcomes following open radical prostatectomy: how patients may achieve the "trifecta"? Int Braz J Urol. 2011;37(3):320–7; discussion 7.

Guidelines for the Delineation of Primary Tumor Target Volume in Prostate Cancer

14

Gozde Yazici, Sezin Yuce Sari, Pervin Hurmuz, Melis Gultekin, Fadıl Akyol, and Gokhan Ozyigit

Abstract

In recent years, the use of intensity-modulated RT (IMRT) and image-guided RT (IGRT) has increased worldwide. These techniques are highly conformal and the target should be more precise. Therefore, target determination and delineation is crucial in the management of prostate cancer with modern radiotherapy techniques. In this chapter, we will briefly explain the current guidelines for the delineation of primary target volume in prostate cancer.

14.1 Anatomy

The prostate gland is composed of fibrous, glandular, and muscular components, and it has a thin, fibrous capsule continuous with its stroma. The prostate is located in the pelvis, in close vicinity to the rectum and bladder. It is separated from the rectum by the rectovesical septum (Denonvilliers' fascia) posteriorly which decreases the risk of invasion of prostate cancer to the rectum. The prostate is also adjacent to periprostatic and dorsal venous complexes, pelvic plexus, and cavernous nerves. The gland passes through the genitourinary diaphragm (GUD) after it surrounds the prostatic urethra.

The prostate gland has an ovoid shape; the apex is located at the inferior above the GUD which surrounds the membranous sphincter. The puboprostatic ligaments lie between the anterior surface of the prostate and pubic symphysis. The periprostatic fascia covers the anterior surface of the prostate and the lateral pelvic floor. The endopelvic fascia covers the anterolateral surfaces of the prostate gland, and it

G. Yazici, M.D. • S.Y. Sari, M.D. • P. Hurmuz, M.D. • M. Gultekin, M.D. (✉) • F. Akyol, M.D.
G. Ozyigit, M.D.
Department of Radiation Oncology, Hacettepe University, Ankara, Turkey
e-mail: melisgultekin@hacettepe.edu.tr

G. Ozyigit, U. Selek (eds.), *Principles and Practice of Urooncology*,
DOI 10.1007/978-3-319-56114-1_14

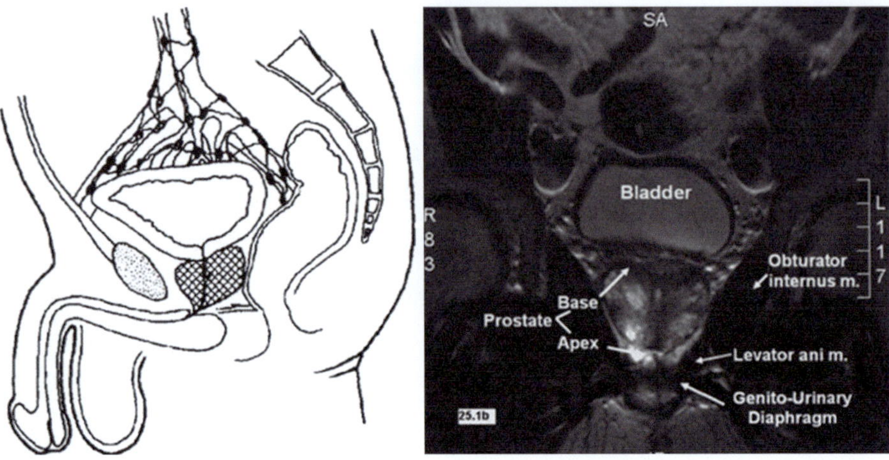

Fig. 14.1 Anatomy of prostate gland (With permission: Levitt SH, Purdy JA, Perez CA (2006) Technical basis of radiation therapy, 4th revised edition, Springer, Berlin)

contains the neurovascular structures such as the dorsal vein complex (venous plexus of Santorini) which is the primary drainage for the penis.

The prostate has four zones histologically: peripheral, transition, central, and anterior fibromuscular stroma zones. The peripheral zone is the posterior part of the gland which can be palpated on digital rectal examination. This is also where prostate cancer usually originates. On the other hand, benign prostate hypertrophy arises from the transition zone. The central zone surrounds the ejaculatory ducts. The fibromuscular tissue in the anterior fibromuscular zone continues with the bladder muscle and external sphincter (Fig. 14.1).

A pair of seminal vesicles (SV) are located posterosuperiorly to the prostate gland. Seminal fluid which protects and nourishes the sperm after ejaculation is mainly secreted from SV as well as the testicles and bulbourethral glands and poured into bilateral ductus deferens which then forms the ejaculatory ducts to finally join the urethra at the verumontanum. This point is where the urethra bends 30–40° to the anterior. A slight percentage of the seminal fluid is also secreted from the prostate gland. This fluid contains enzymes such as acid phosphatase and prostate-specific antigen (PSA) which is a serine protease that functions in the liquefaction of the semen.

14.2 Target Volume Delineation

In recent years, the use of intensity-modulated RT (IMRT) and image-guided RT (IGRT) has increased worldwide. These techniques are highly conformal and the target should be more precise. Fiducial markers should be inserted into the prostate via transrectal ultrasound guidance before IGRT administration. In the study of the Mayo Clinic, the inter- and intra-fractional prostate movements were found a mean

2.5 mm (up to 9.1 mm) at the superior-inferior, 3.7 mm (up to 16.3 mm) at the anterior-posterior, and 1.9 mm (up to 15.2 mm) at the right-left planes [1]. Without localization of the fiducials, the clinical target volume (CTV) received 95% of the prescribed dose with 5.1, 7.3, and 5 mm margins on the superoinferior, anteroposterior, and lateral aspects. The respective margins were decreased to 2.7, 2.9, and 2.8 mm with fiducial visualization. Bony structures should not be trusted while delineating the prostate because the movement of these structures is between 2.8 and 4.4 mm, while the prostate can move between 5.6 and 4.4 mm. Crook et al. found a displacement of gold markers of 0.1–0.5 cm in the lateral and 0.5–1 cm in the inferior aspect of the prostate gland [2]. The displacement in the posterior was >1 cm in 30% of the patients. Zelefsky et al. reported the mean motion of the prostate to be 1.2, 0.6, and 0.5 cm in the anteroposterior, lateral, and superoinferior directions [3]. They also recommended adding wider margins for the planning target volume (PTV) in patients with large rectal and bladder volumes in order to adequately cover the CTV.

After the fiducials are located, approximately 1 week should be awaited for the planning computerized tomography (CT). That is because of the time for fibrosis to happen around the fiducials so that they cannot move and the target would not change during simulation and between fractions. Intravenous contrast injection is not necessary for the CT simulation unless the pelvic LNs would be irradiated. However, the patient should undergo planning CT with a urinary catheter in order to empty the urinary bladder. The catheter can also be used in every treatment fraction, or patients with good cooperation can be told to undergo treatment after voiding the bladder. The patient is then immobilized with a Kneefix and Feetfix in the supine position in which the prostate gland moves less compared to the prone position. This position also helps to remove the small intestines out of the treatment field [4]. The arms should be on the chest in order to keep them away from the treatment area. To define the isocenter, three radiopaque pellet markers are placed: one at the anterior midline and two at right and left lateral points, respectively, on the skin. The CT scan is then acquired in ≤5 mm (ideally ≤3 mm, particularly for stereotactic body RT [SBRT] planning) slices from the superior level of the iliac bones to the inferior of minor trochanters of the femurs or the perineum [5, 6]. The gross tumor volume (GTV), CTV, PTV, and organs at risk (OAR) should be delineated separately in each slice based on the recommendations in International Commission on Radiation Units and Measurements (ICRU) reports 50 and 62 [7, 8].

14.3 Gross Tumor Volume (GTV)

The GTV is the primary tumor in the prostate gland and extraprostatic tissue, if existent. However, delineating a GTV in prostate cancer is not practical because the total dose is prescribed to the CTV and generally no boost dose to the GTV is applied. On the other hand, institutions using simultaneous integrated boost to a malignant nodule determined via MR fusion should delineate entire nodule as boost volume or GTV.

14.4 Clinical Target Volume (CTV)

The prostatic apex is the structure which is the guide for the delineation of the target because of the fact that it can be visualized easily on CT. However, because the apex is not covered with a capsule, the level of the GUD may vary causing a difficulty in discriminating the prostate from the GUD. In this case, magnetic resonance imaging (MRI) can be helpful on which the GUD can also be easily detected. Roach et al. observed a 32% increase in prostate volume when defined by non-contrast CT scan compared to contrast CT and MRI scans [9]. This discrepancy is mainly the result of misinterpretation of the posterior, apical, and posteroinferoapical aspects of the prostate as well as the neurovascular bundles. MRI was found significantly superior in defining the apex and base of the prostate, neurovascular bundle, and anterior wall of the rectum while delineating based on fused CT and MRI images [10]. Rasch et al. reported that the volumes of the prostate and SVs were 40% larger when determined on CT compared to MRI [11]. The most apparent difference was at the base of the SVs and prostatic apex which concluded in an additional 8 and 6-mm delineation, respectively. MRI also has a higher resolution for soft tissues which more clearly defines the organ-confined disease, SV involvement, and capsular and extracapsular extension. Based on these data CT and MRI should be used together while delineating the prostate.

The CTV is defined as the whole prostate gland and bilateral SVs. Prostate cancer is typically multifocal. It was reported that only 17–24% of prostate cancers arise from a solitary focus [12, 13]. The capsule of the gland is invaded in 8–57% of the patients with prostate cancer [14, 15]. Therefore, the whole prostate gland and its capsule should be delineated in all patients independent of the clinical stage and risk group. However, the extent of the delineation of the SVs depends on the risk group. In low-risk and intermediate-risk disease, the delineation of proximal SVs is sufficient, whereas in high-risk disease whole bilateral SVs should be contoured.

There is a wide range of variability among radiation oncologists for prostate contouring. It is crucial to master in prostate and pelvic anatomy for delineating the target and OARs correctly. In 2009, McLaughlin et al. published a study on the common contouring errors while delineating the apex, mid-gland, and base of the prostate on CT images [16]. They reported that the GUD, rectum, and anterior fascia are overestimated at the level of the prostatic apex. The overestimation continued in the anterior and lateral fasciae at the mid-gland and the bladder and anterior fascia at the base. The reason for common errors was claimed to be the transition zone hypertrophy and bladder neck variability at the superior base and the variability in the relationship between the prostate and SVs at the posterior base. They recommended to inspect the lateral view of prostate contours and to improve recognition of certain anatomic structures on CT images, concluding that most errors can be improved without the direct help of MRI.

The delineation the SVs can also be challenging. The risk of involvement of SVs is 15–20% in intermediate- and high-risk prostate cancer [17]. The median length of SV involvement was found to be 1 cm, whereas the rate of ≥2 cm involvement decreased to <4% even in high-risk disease [18]. Therefore, the CTV should encompass at least the proximal SVs. However, the definition of proximal SV varies according to different guidelines. The European Organization for Research and Treatment of Cancer (EORTC) recommends adding the proximal 2 cm SV into the CTV in high-risk disease and the proximal 1 cm in intermediate-risk disease [19]. In the ongoing Radiation Therapy Oncology Group (RTOG) 0815 trial, the proximal 1 cm of SV is recommended to be delineated in both intermediate- and high-risk patients. Qi et al. compared these two recommendations and found that both recommendations failed to encompass the SV under risk, and a 1.4 and 2.2 cm SV should be contoured in intermediate- and high-risk patients, respectively, in order to adequately include the proximal SVs [20].

CTV delineation for a prostate cancer patient treated with definitive IGRT is depicted in Fig. 14.2.

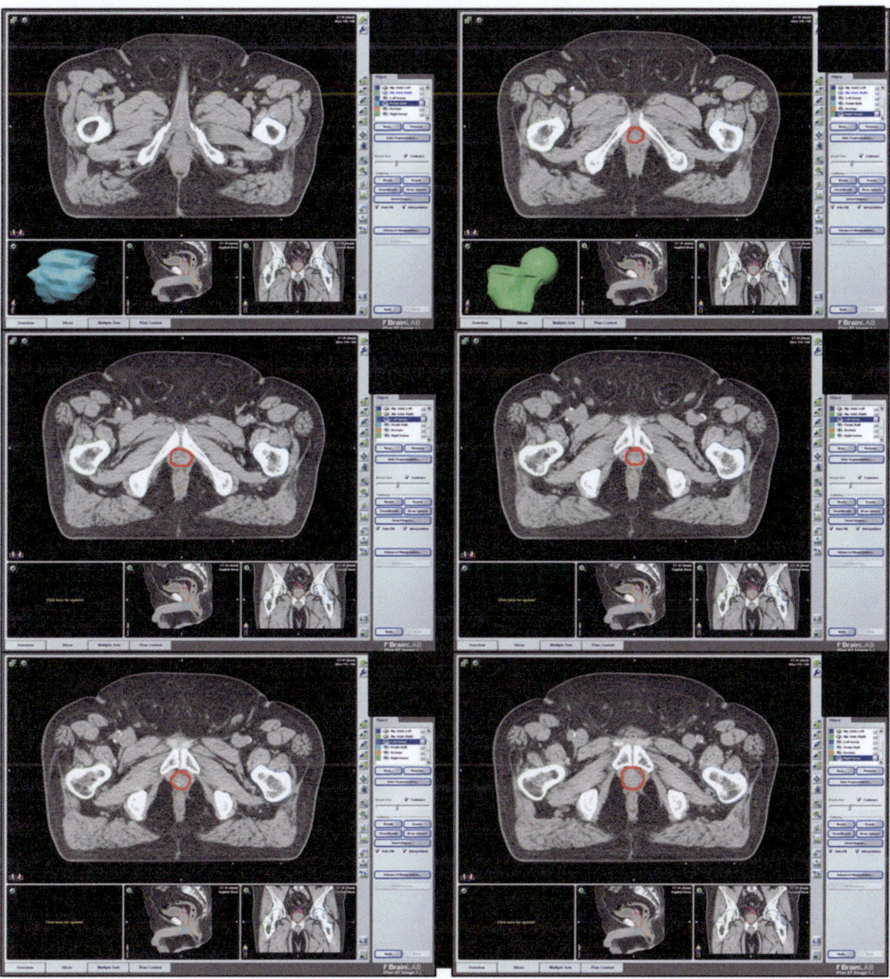

Fig. 14.2 CTV delineation for a prostate cancer patient treated with definitive IGRT (Slices were contoured in the direction of inferior to superior, Red: Prostate, Magenta: Seminal vesicles)

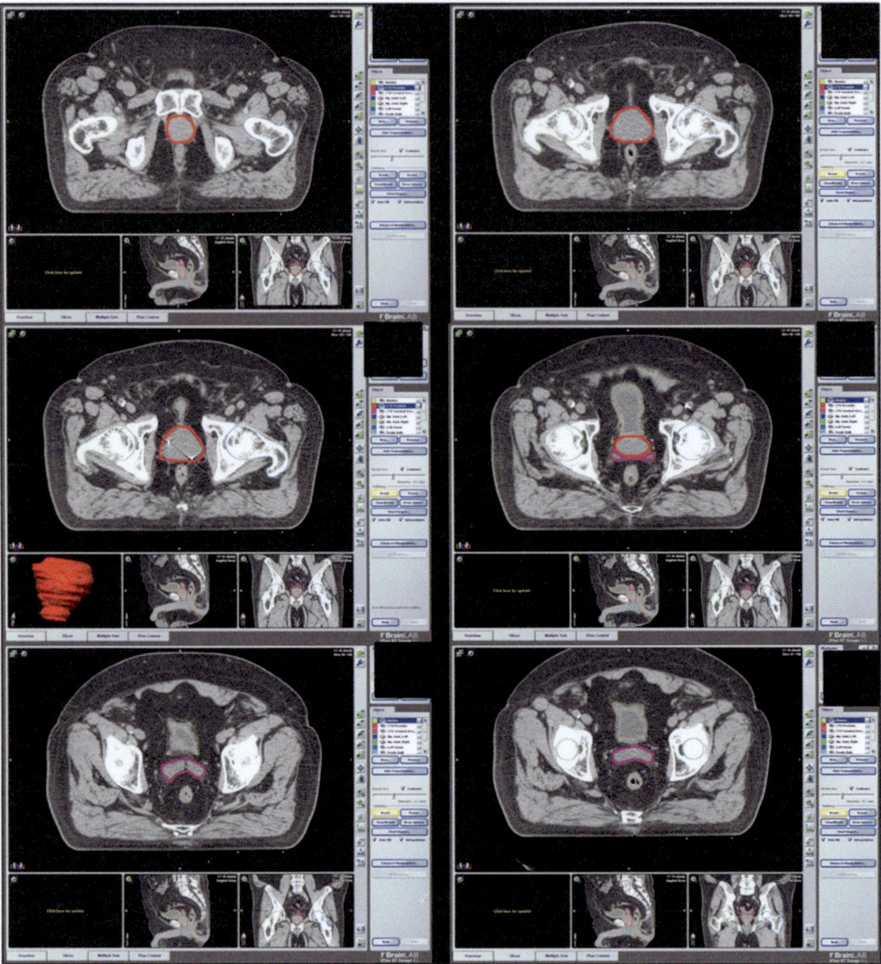

Fig. 14.2 (continued)

14.5 Planning Target Volume (PTV)

There are various recommendations for the constitution of the PTV. Memorial Sloan Kettering Cancer Center (MSKCC) proposes a 1 cm margin to the CTV to form the PTV in all directions but to diminish it to 0.6 cm at the posterior [3]. Fox Chase Cancer Center recommends an 8 mm margin in all directions which should be minimized to 5 mm posteriorly [21]. In SBRT and other IGRT techniques, some centers recommend a 0.6 cm margin in all directions, whereas in MSKCC

0.5 mm is recommended in all but 0.3 mm in the posterior direction [22]. In addition, the central 1 cm diameter portion of the prostate encompassing the prostatic urethra is defined for dosimetric consideration and evaluation during high-dose IMRT planning.

14.6 Target Volume Determination in Adjuvant or Salvage Radiotherapy

In the EORTC-22911 trial, 5-year progression-free survival (PFS) and locoregional control rates were significantly higher in patients with positive SM, extracapsular extension (ECE), and SV involvement after radical prostatectomy (RP) [23]. However, in the subgroup analysis of this study, the only group that benefited from adjuvant RT was the patients with positive surgical margins (SM) [24]. In the South Western Oncology Group (SWOG)-8794 trial, patients with pT3 tumors and/or positive SM had significantly better outcomes with adjuvant RT [25]. Similarly, a German study reported better results with adjuvant RT in patients with T3 tumors and positive SM [26]. According to Grossfeld et al., 24% of patients with clinically organ-confined disease are found to have locally advanced disease and/or lymph node (LN) positivity after RP [27]. Based on the previous studies, adjuvant RT to the prostate is indicated in patients with T3–T4 tumor and positive SM. In the presence of LN positivity and ECE, lymphatic irradiation should also be performed. Delineation of lymphatic regions is discussed in Chap. 9. The following contouring recommendations can also be used for patients that will undergo salvage RT for biochemical failure after RP.

No GTV is present in the adjuvant setting. Four guidelines have been published for the delineation of CTV in postoperative prostate cancer. The first guideline was reported by the EORTC in 2007 [28]. They stated that the most risky areas for recurrence were the vesicourethral anastomosis (VUA) in the central, the bladder neck at the superior, the vicinity of the outer rectal wall and most posterior portion of the bladder neck at the posterior, the prostatic apex at the caudal, the neurovascular bundles at the lateral, and the anastomosis and the urethral axis at the anterior aspects, respectively. After delineating these structures, they recommend a 5 mm margin in all directions excluding the rectal wall, an additional 5 mm margin in the posterolateral aspect in patients with ECE except the rectal wall (as this is where the recurrence mostly occurs), and an additional 5 mm margin in the direction of positive SM. The base of the SV should be included in all patients. If the SVs are involved, they recommend contouring their original location and/or the remnants without an additional margin and irradiating them with a lower dose.

In the second guideline published in 2007 by Princess Margaret Hospital, the inferior border of the CTV was recommended to be 8 mm below the VUA or superior to the penile bulb, whichever is most superior [29]. The superior border was just above the most superior surgical clip, if present, or 5 mm above the inferior border of the vas deferens, anterior border was posterior to the symphysis pubis caudally and posterior 1.5 cm of the urinary bladder cranially, posterior border was anterior to the rectal wall and levator ani muscle caudally and the mesorectal fascia cranially, and lateral border was the medial border of the levator ani and obturator internus muscles caudally and the sacrorectogenitopubic fascia cranially. In case of salvage RT, 1 cm margin was added to the gross disease and surgical clips for the CTV.

The Australian and New Zealand Radiation Oncology Genito-Urinary Group published another guideline in 2008 [30]. They recommend the inferior border of the CTV 5–6 mm below the VUA including all surgical clips. The VUA is just below the last slice with urine or one slice above the penile bulb. The anterior border is the posterior aspect of the symphysis pubis cranially and encompasses the posterior 1.5 cm of the bladder caudally, posterior border is the posterior rectal wall caudally and the anterior mesorectal fascia cranially, lateral border is the medial border of the levator ani or obturator internus muscle, and the superior border should include whole SV bed and the distal portion of the vas deferens. For the PTV, they recommend a 1 cm margin but claim that this can be lowered to 0.5 cm according to the rectal dose.

In 2010, RTOG published the last consensus guideline [6]. They recommend that the CTV should begin from the level of the cut end of the vas deferens and end at >8–12 mm inferior to the VUA. In case the vas deferens is retracted postoperatively, the superior end can start 3–4 cm above the top of the symphysis pubis. In addition, the inferior border may be extended if the apical SM is positive. The VUA can be visualized in one slice below the most inferior urine-containing image in the retropubic region on a CT scan and can be more clearly seen as a hypertensive signal on T2 images of MRI. The VUA can be better visualized if the urinary bladder is full, and the sagittal images can help the identification of the VUA. If the VUA cannot be visualized, the inferior border of the CTV can extend to the last slice above the penile bulb. If pathologically involved, both SV remnants should be included in the CTV. Other borders for the CTV vary according to its location in the pelvis. Above the superior edge of the symphysis pubis, the anterior border of the CTV encompasses the posterior 1–2 cm of the bladder wall, the posterior border is the mesorectal fascia, and lateral borders extend to the sacrorectogenitopubic fascia but may extend to obturator internus muscles if there is extraprostatic disease at the base of the gland. Below the superior edge of the symphysis pubis, the anterior border is the posterior edge of the pubic bone, the posterior border is the anterior rectal wall (the CTV may need to be curved at the level of the VUA), and lateral borders are medial to the levator ani and obturator internus muscles. The RTOG recommends including all surgical clips in the prostate and SV bed into the

CTV. However, the clips above the level of SV can be excluded because they are generally left by the surgeon to control the bleeding, not to mark the sites of the disease.

Finally in 2011, Malone et al. compared these four guidelines and showed that the CTV was significantly different between them, mainly due to the differences at the superior portion [31]. They reported that the recommendations from the Princess Margaret Hospital and RTOG guidelines were similar, their CTVs were larger than the other two, and the CTV of the EORTC trial was the smallest.

CTV delineation in a prostate cancer patient treated with postoperative adjuvant IGRT is depicted in Fig. 14.3.

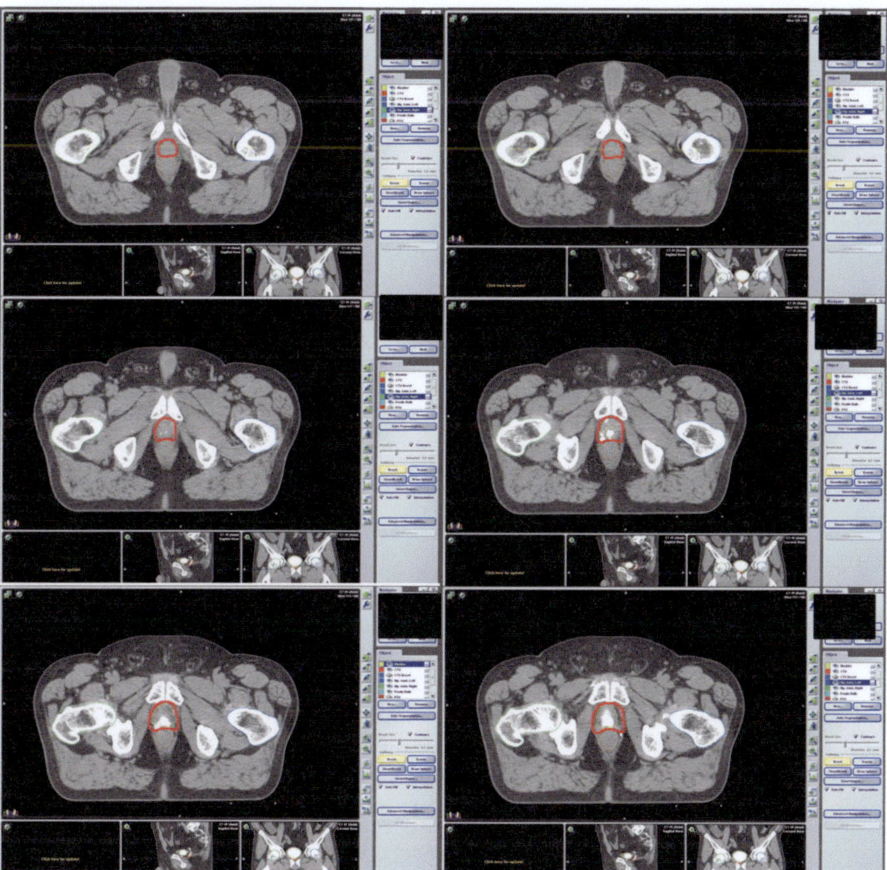

Fig. 14.3 CTV delineation in a prostate cancer patient treated with postoperative adjuvant IGRT (Slices were contoured in the direction of inferior to superior, Red: CTV for surgical bed)

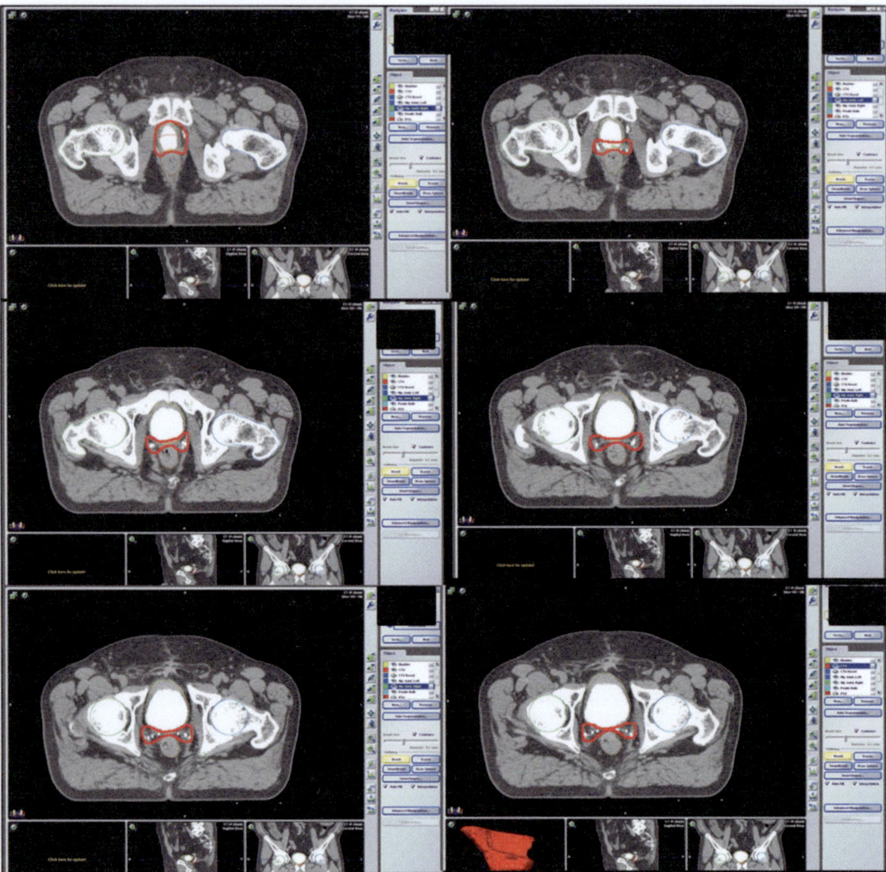

Fig. 14.3 (continued)

Conclusion

Patient-based treatment planning is the standard in prostate cancer. Innovative techniques such as IMRT and IGRT provide better target coverage and decreased toxicity rates compared to conventional RT. Recommended simulation and delineation techniques are summarized in this chapter. If these recommendations are applied in clinical practice, the variations in the treatment techniques between institutions can be minimized.

References

1. Schallenkamp JM, Herman MG, Kruse JJ, Pisansky TM. Prostate position relative to pelvic bony anatomy based on intraprostatic gold markers and electronic portal imaging. Int J Radiat Oncol Biol Phys. 2005;63(3):800–11.
2. Crook JM, Raymond Y, Salhani D, Yang H, Esche B. Prostate motion during standard radiotherapy as assessed by fiducial markers. Radiother Oncol. 1995;37(1):35–42.

3. Zelefsky MJ, Crean D, Mageras GS, Lyass O, Happersett L, Ling CC, et al. Quantification and predictors of prostate position variability in 50 patients evaluated with multiple CT scans during conformal radiotherapy. Radiother Oncol. 1999;50(2):225–34.
4. Malone S, Crook JM, Kendal WS, Szanto J. Respiratory-induced prostate motion: quantification and characterization. Int J Radiat Oncol Biol Phys. 2000;48(1):105–9.
5. Benedict SH, Yenice KM, Followill D, Galvin JM, Hinson W, Kavanagh B, et al. Stereotactic body radiation therapy: the report of AAPM task group 101. Med Phys. 2010;37(8): 4078–101.
6. Michalski JM, Lawton C, El Naqa I, Ritter M, O'Meara E, Seider MJ, et al. Development of RTOG consensus guidelines for the definition of the clinical target volume for postoperative conformal radiation therapy for prostate cancer. Int J Radiat Oncol Biol Phys. 2010;76(2):361–8.
7. Measurements. ICoRUa. ICRU report 50: prescribing, recording and reporting photon beam therapy. Bethesda, Maryland, USA; 1993.
8. Measurements. ICoRUa. ICRU Report 62: prescribing, recording and reporting photon beam therapy (supplement to ICRU report 50). Bethesda, Maryland, USA; 1999.
9. Roach M 3rd, Faillace-Akazawa P, Malfatti C, Holland J, Hricak H. Prostate volumes defined by magnetic resonance imaging and computerized tomographic scans for three-dimensional conformal radiotherapy. Int J Radiat Oncol Biol Phys. 1996;35(5):1011–8.
10. Kagawa K, Lee WR, Schultheiss TE, Hunt MA, Shaer AH, Hanks GE. Initial clinical assessment of CT-MRI image fusion software in localization of the prostate for 3D conformal radiation therapy. Int J Radiat Oncol Biol Phys. 1997;38(2):319–25.
11. Rasch C, Barillot I, Remeijer P, Touw A, van Herk M, Lebesque JV. Definition of the prostate in CT and MRI: a multi-observer study. Int J Radiat Oncol Biol Phys. 1999;43(1):57–66.
12. Jewett HJ. The present status of radical prostatectomy for stages A and B prostatic cancer. Urol Clin North Am. 1975;2(1):105–24.
13. Wise AM, Stamey TA, McNeal JE, Clayton JL. Morphologic and clinical significance of multifocal prostate cancers in radical prostatectomy specimens. Urology. 2002;60(2):264–9.
14. Catalona WJ, Richie JP, Ahmann FR, Hudson MA, Scardino PT, Flanigan RC, et al. Comparison of digital rectal examination and serum prostate specific antigen in the early detection of prostate cancer: results of a multicenter clinical trial of 6,630 men. J Urol. 1994;151(5):1283–90.
15. Villers AA, McNeal JE, Freiha FS, Stamey TA. Development of prostatic carcinoma. Morphometric and pathologic features of early stages. Acta Oncol. 1991;30(2):145–51.
16. McLaughlin PW, Evans C, Feng M, Narayana V. Radiographic and anatomic basis for prostate contouring errors and methods to improve prostate contouring accuracy. Int J Radiat Oncol Biol Phys. 2010;76(2):369–78.
17. Eifler JB, Feng Z, Lin BM, Partin MT, Humphreys EB, Han M, et al. An updated prostate cancer staging nomogram (Partin tables) based on cases from 2006 to 2011. BJU Int. 2013;111(1):22–9.
18. Kestin L, Goldstein N, Vicini F, Yan D, Korman H, Martinez A. Treatment of prostate cancer with radiotherapy: should the entire seminal vesicles be included in the clinical target volume? Int J Radiat Oncol Biol Phys. 2002;54(3):686–97.
19. Boehmer D, Maingon P, Poortmans P, Baron MH, Miralbell R, Remouchamps V, et al. Guidelines for primary radiotherapy of patients with prostate cancer. Radiother Oncol. 2006;79(3):259–69.
20. Qi X, Gao XS, Asaumi J, Zhang M, Li HZ, Ma MW, et al. Optimal contouring of seminal vesicle for definitive radiotherapy of localized prostate cancer: comparison between EORTC prostate cancer radiotherapy guideline, RTOG0815 protocol and actual anatomy. Radiat Oncol. 2014;9:288.
21. Buyyounouski MK, Horwitz EM, Price RA Jr, Feigenberg SJ, Pollack A. Prostate IMRT. In: Bortfeld T, Schmidt-Ullrich, R, De Neve W, Wazer DE, editor Image-guided IMRT Germany: Springer-Verlag Berlin Heidelberg; 2006. p. 391–410.
22. Desai NZM. Prostate adenocarcinoma. In: Lee NY, Lu JJ, editors. Target volume delineation and field setup, a practical guide for conformal and intensity-modulated radiation therapy. Berlin Heidelberg: Springer-Verlag; 2013. p. 213–26.

23. Bolla M, van Poppel H, Collette L, van Cangh P, Vekemans K, Da Pozzo L, et al. Postoperative radiotherapy after radical prostatectomy: a randomised controlled trial (EORTC trial 22911). Lancet. 2005;366(9485):572–8.
24. Van der Kwast TH, Bolla M, Van Poppel H, Van Cangh P, Vekemans K, Da Pozzo L, et al. Identification of patients with prostate cancer who benefit from immediate postoperative radiotherapy: EORTC 22911. J Clin Oncol. 2007;25(27):4178–86.
25. Swanson GPTI, Tangen C. Phase III randomized study of adjuvant radiation therapy versus observation in patients with patohologic T3 prostate cancer (SWOG 8794). Int J Radiat Oncol Biol Phys. 2005;63:S1.
26. Wiegel T, Bottke D, Willich N, et al. Phase III results of adjuvant radiotherapy (RT) versus 'wait and see' (WS) in patients with pT3 prostate cancer following radical prostatectomy (RP) (ARO 96-02/AUO AP 09/95). J Clin Oncol. (Meeting Abstracts) 2005;23(4513).
27. Grossfeld GD, Chang JJ, Broering JM, Li YP, Lubeck DP, Flanders SC, et al. Under staging and under grading in a contemporary series of patients undergoing radical prostatectomy: results from the cancer of the prostate strategic urologic research endeavor database. J Urol. 2001;165(3):851–6.
28. Poortmans P, Bossi A, Vandeputte K, Bosset M, Miralbell R, Maingon P, et al. Guidelines for target volume definition in post-operative radiotherapy for prostate cancer, on behalf of the EORTC radiation oncology group. Radiother Oncol. 2007;84(2):121–7.
29. Wiltshire KL, Brock KK, Haider MA, Zwahlen D, Kong V, Chan E, et al. Anatomic boundaries of the clinical target volume (prostate bed) after radical prostatectomy. Int J Radiat Oncol Biol Phys. 2007;69(4):1090–9.
30. Sidhom MA, Kneebone AB, Lehman M, Wiltshire KL, Millar JL, Mukherjee RK, et al. Post-prostatectomy radiation therapy: consensus guidelines of the Australian and New Zealand radiation oncology genito-urinary group. Radiother Oncol. 2008;88(1):10–9.
31. Malone S, Croke J, Roustan-Delatour N, Belanger E, Avruch L, Malone C, et al. Postoperative radiotherapy for prostate cancer: a comparison of four consensus guidelines and dosimetric evaluation of 3D-CRT versus tomotherapy IMRT. Int J Radiat Oncol Biol Phys. 2012;84(3):725–32.

Guidelines for the Delineation of Lymphatic Target Volumes in Prostate Cancer

15

Gokhan Ozyigit, Gozde Yazici, Sezin Yuce Sari, Melis Gultekin, Pervin Hurmuz, and Fadil Akyol

Abstract

The incidence of regional lymph node (LN) involvement in patients with prostate cancer depends on several factors like the tumor size and the Gleason score (GS). The risk of LN involvement is <10% in low-risk disease. A number of models were developed in order to predict the risk of LN involvement which helps the physicians to decide whether to perform a staging lymphadenectomy or LN irradiation. In this chapter, we will review the current guidelines for the delineation of lymphatic target volumes in prostate cancer.

15.1 Introduction

The incidence of regional lymph node (LN) involvement in patients with prostate cancer depends on the tumor size and degree of differentiation which is represented by the Gleason score (GS) [1, 2]. Partin et al. reported that clinical stage, preoperative prostate-specific antigen (PSA) level, and GS can be used to predict the risk of LN involvement [3]. With this model, the negative predictive value was found 99% in a total of 703 patients. In other prediction models, up to 63% of patients with clinically organ-confined disease would have been spared pelvic lymphadenectomy with 2–10% rate of missed LN metastasis [4, 5].

Stock et al. reported that the incidence of positive LNs correlated with pretreatment PSA level, GS, and clinical stage as well as seminal vesicle (SV) involvement [6]. No patients with GS $\leq$ 4 in this study had pathologically positive LNs, independent of the PSA level. However, in patients with GS > 4 the incidence of LN

G. Ozyigit, M.D. • G. Yazici, M.D. • S.Y. Sari, M.D. • M. Gultekin, M.D. • P. Hurmuz, M.D. (✉)
F. Akyol, M.D.
Department of Radiation Oncology, Hacettepe University, Ankara, Turkey
e-mail: pervin.hurmuz@hacettepe.edu.tr

G. Ozyigit, U. Selek (eds.), *Principles and Practice of Urooncology*,
DOI 10.1007/978-3-319-56114-1_15

metastasis significantly increased with PSA level of >20 ng/mL. Rees et al. observed 2.2% LN metastasis rate in patients with PSA level of ≤5 ng/mL, GS of ≤5, or PSA level of <25 ng/mL together with GS of ≤7 [7].

A formula was proposed by Roach to predict the probability of LN metastasis based on pretreatment PSA level and GS [8]:

Probability of pelvic LN metastasis = 2/3 PSA + (GS − 6) × 10.

The presence of LN metastasis significantly increases the 10-year rate of distant metastasis (DM) development (>85 vs. <20%) and increases the risk of death [9, 10]. However, patients with a single LN metastasis have a similar prognosis compared to patients without LN involvement [11, 12].

15.2 Role of Elective Nodal Irradiation in Prostate Cancer

For a staging lymphadenectomy to be adequate, the TNM classification recommends at least eight LNs to be resected in order to stage a patient as pN0, but there is no exact requirement [13]. Elective nodal irradiation is not required in a patient with pN0 tumor because of the increased rate of toxicity and the lack of a prospective study that shows the benefit of this treatment. Similarly, elective nodal irradiation has no rationale in patients with cN0 disease [14].

There are three prospective randomized trials questioning the role of elective nodal irradiation in prostate cancer. The first study was Radiation Therapy Oncology Group (RTOG) 77-06 trial which resulted in no benefit from prostatic bed and nodal irradiation compared to prostatic bed irradiation only [15]. However, patients that had undergone lymphadenectomy had significantly better outcomes than the patients that did not.

The second trial was the first report of RTOG 9413 which found that whole pelvis RT (WPRT) with short-term neoadjuvant hormonotherapy (HT) increased the rate of progression-free survival (PFS) in 1275 prostate cancer patients without positive LNs but with a risk of LN involvement >15% [16]. However, this study was criticized because of the bias in the duration of HT in different groups. Eventually, in the update of this study, WPRT had no significant benefit over prostate-only RT (PORT) in addition to an increased rate of late gastrointestinal toxicity [17].

The third study was the Groupe d'étude des tumeurs urogénitales (GETUG)-01 trial which similarly found no benefit of pelvic irradiation even in patients with a higher risk of LN involvement [18]. In 2016, the update of this study was published with a median follow-up of 11.4 years [19]. The 10-year overall survival (OS) and event-free survival (EFS) rates were similar in patients that did and did not undergo pelvic irradiation.

In the light of these data, elective nodal irradiation in patients without nodal involvement is not recommended. However, Murthy et al. analyzed the incidental dose received by the pelvic LNs and found an interesting result [20]. When they compared the dose from two-dimensional conventional RT (2D CRT), three-dimensional conformal RT (3D CRT), and intensity-modulated RT (IMRT), they found that the obturator nodes received 44, 29, and 22 Gy from 2D CRT, 3D CRT, and IMRT, respectively, and each was significantly different from the others. On the other hand, the doses to other lymphatic regions were low and not clinically relevant. The authors concluded that in patients that will undergo IMRT, elective pelvic irradiation can be considered.

15.3 Target Volume Delineation

Pelvic organs do not have a hilum so they are supplied and drained into both sides of the pelvis. Major groups of LNs in the pelvis include the sacral, internal, external, and common iliac LNs. There are a few minor groups of LNs such as pararectal LNs in the connective tissue along the branches of internal iliac vessels. Pelvic LNs receive afferent from pelvic, peripheral, visceral, and parietal structures and send efferents to proximal group of LNs. The pelvic LNs are generally named after the arteries they are clustered around.

15.3.1 Common Iliac Lymph Nodes

The common iliac LNs are located along the common iliac vessels, caudal to the aortic bifurcation and cranial to the common iliac bifurcation. They can be subdivided into three groups as lateral (to the common iliac vessels), medial (to the common iliac vessels), and middle (located in the lumbosacral fossa). Common iliac LNs are not local drainage for the prostate and not delineated for RT planning.

15.3.2 External Iliac Lymph Nodes

The external iliac LNs are found along the external iliac vessels, in the lateral pelvis, caudal to the common iliac bifurcation and cranial to the inguinal ligament. They can also be subdivided into lateral, medial, and medium parts. Obturator nodes are generally considered to be a part of the medial external iliac node group by some experts. The external iliac LNs drain lymph from the leg and buttocks (via superficial and deep inguinal nodes), the superior aspect of the urinary bladder, the prostate in men, and superior parts of the uterus in women. These nodes drain into common iliac nodes.

15.3.3 Internal Iliac Lymph Nodes

The internal iliac LNs are found along the internal iliac vessels and its branches. They are more posterior in the pelvis than are the external iliac LNs. Obturator LNs are an important cluster of internal iliac LNs. They are generally found along the obturator artery and continue into the obturator foramen. Internal iliac LNs also include the lateral sacral and presacral LNs. Some authors use the term "hypogastric" for the most superior internal iliac LNs, whereas others use it for the entire internal iliac group [21, 22]. Internal iliac nodes drain lymph from all pelvic structures but they are not the only drainage way. The deep parts of the buttock may drain via the gluteal vessels into internal iliac nodes, and the upper part of the anal canal drains into internal iliac nodes. Internal iliac nodes also drain into common iliac nodes.

15.3.4 Presacral Nodes

The presacral LNs are found in the mesorectum, immediately anterior to the sacrum and posterior to the mesorectal fascia. They drain lymph from the rectum and anal canal, the prostate in men. These nodes may drain into common iliac, lumbar, or inferior mesenteric LNs.

The lymphatic drainage of the prostate is mainly into four stations; first, it drains into the pudendal axis and obturator fossa, then into the internal and lateral external iliacs, continuing with superior external iliacs, and, finally, to the perirectal and presacral area [23]. The posterior part of the prostate mainly drains into the obturator and external iliac and partially into the internal iliac LNs. The apex drains into the internal iliac, common iliac, and presacral lymphatics. The anterior part of the gland mainly drains into the pudendal and internal iliac LNs.

During the era of 2D CRT, a four-field box technique was administered to patients with prostate cancer according to the bony landmarks in the pelvic area. The superior border was at the L4–L5 or L5–S1 interspace, and the inferior border was inferior to the ischial tuberosities. The lateral border was 1.5–2 cm lateral to the pelvic brim on anterior/posterior portals, and anterior border was the anterior aspect of the pubic symphysis, and posterior border was at the S2–S3 interspace on lateral portals. In order to limit the dose to the small bowel and femoral heads, corner blocks were used at all four corners.

With the developing techniques of RT, planning CT is used for patient-based treatment. Unless there is a contraindication, intravenous contrast is administered during simulation to better visualize the nodal disease. The Royal College of Radiologists defined pathologic LNs as having a short axis of >9 mm for common iliac, >10 mm for external iliac, >7 mm for internal iliac, and >8 mm for obturator LNs on imaging techniques [24]. Delineation guidelines for the lymphatic region have been proposed for conformal RT techniques. RTOG published a guideline for delineating pelvic LNs in high-risk prostate cancer in 2009 [25]. The recommendations of this guideline were based on previously published studies of prostatic lymphography which revealed the prostate drains mainly into the internal iliac and presacral and then into the external iliac and common iliac LNs [9, 10]. Prostate cancer usually drains into multiple LNs and drainage is not contiguous [11–15]. The authors defined three main lymphatic drainage areas which are internal iliacs on the superior, external iliacs on the lateral, and subaortic aspect of the S1–S3 presacrals on the posterior [19, 20]. Based on these data and historical 2D CRT portal, they had five final recommendations:

1. Start delineating the LN clinical target volume (CTV) at the L5–S1 interspace in order to include distal common iliac and proximal presacral LNs.
2. Give a margin of 7 mm around the external and internal iliac vessels without including organs at risk (OAR) such as the small bowel, urinary bladder, and bones. They also recommended giving an additional 10 mm margin to the external iliacs anterolaterally along iliopsoas muscle to include lateral external nodes and extending lateral borders of internal iliacs to the pelvic sidewall.
3. Delineate the subaortic portion of presacral LNs between S1 and S3. The posterior border is the anterior sacrum, and give an additional 1 cm margin for the anterior border without including OARs.
4. Stop delineating external iliac LNs when you see the femoral heads on the superior which is the bony landmark for the inguinal ligament, and connect them to internal iliacs on each slice.
5. Stop delineating obturator LNs when you see the pubic symphysis on the superior.
6. Boundaries and recommended margins for pelvic LNs are summarized in Table 15.1.

The ongoing Prostate and pelvIs Versus prOsTate Alone treatment for Locally advanced prostate cancer (PIVOTAL) study uses different delineation techniques than RTOG in certain points. For instance, they do not describe the superior border as “L5–S1 interspace” but as “inferior to L5 vertebra” because they claim that the interspace is not a straight line, and the latter definition is more consistent. Secondly, they recommend the inferior border not the “top of” but “1 cm above the top of the pubic symphysis” in order to eliminate the anatomical variations of individual patients. They add the term “bowel expansion volume (BEV)” which is bowel + 3 mm margin, and they switch it with “bowel” and add the rectum and muscle as critical organs that should not be included in the LN-CTV. They recommend giving a 12 mm margin anterior to the sacrum for presacral LNs. Finally, they claim that internal and external iliac volumes should be connected with an 18 mm strip, intravenous contrast should be used to help identification of vessels, an 18 mm strip should be given from the inner surface of bony pelvic sidewall in order to constitute obturator lymphatic region, and all small white dots which may be representing small blood vessels and associated LNs should be included.

Despite the recommendations of the RTOG guideline, there are studies claiming that these nodal regions do not entirely cover the areas under recurrence risk. Meijer et al. studied the distribution of LN metastases on magnetic resonance (MR) lymphography and found that more than half of the patients had ≥1 LN in areas which are not included in the RTOG guideline [26]. They showed that an important percentage of patients have metastases in the para-aortic, proximal common iliac, perirectal lymphatics, and even in the perivesical and inguinal regions.

They also stated that the risk of perirectal and proximal common iliac LN involvement was associated with GS and PSA level, respectively, concluding that the respective lymphatic areas should be included in the LN-CTV in patients with these high risk factors.

A recent study revealed that in approximately half of the patients, the superior border of the RTOG guideline does not cover the lymphatic area that shows

Table 15.1 Boundaries and recommended margins for the pelvic lymph node levels

LN levels	Boundaries of LN levels						Recommended margins
	Superior	Inferior	Medial	Lateral	Anterior	Posterior	
Internal iliac	Bifurcation of the CI (usually the L5–S1 interspace)	Superior portion of the coccygeal muscle	Bladder, mesocolon, and mesorectum	IIV, iliac bone, sacroiliac joint, and psoas muscle (cranially) Internal obturator and piriform muscles (caudally)	Bladder	Sacral wing (cranially) Piriform muscle (caudally)	7 mm around vessels extend lateral borders to the pelvic sidewall
External iliac	Bifurcation of the CI (usually the L5–S1 interspace)	Femoral ring (when you do not see the lateral muscles of the abdominal wall anymore and the artery gets lateral)	Ureter (cranially) Bladder (caudally)	Iliac muscle (cranially) Iliac bone, iliopsoas muscle, and EIV (caudally)	Fat of small bowel, ductus deference	EIV (cranially) Pubic bone (caudally)	7 mm around vessels extend anterior border by an additional 10 mm anterolaterally along iliopsoas muscle to include lateral external iliac nodes
Obturator	Superior portion of the obturator muscle	Superior border of the inferior branch of the pubic bone	Bladder	Acetabulum (cranially) Internal obturator muscle (caudally)	EIV	Internal obturator muscle	Join external and internal iliac regions with 18-mm-wide strip along pelvic sidewall
Presacral	Aortic bifurcation	Superior portion of the coccygeal bone	Suprapubic fat	Piriform muscle	Posterior wall of the rectum	Anterior surface of the sacrum	10 mm strip over anterior sacrum

LN lymph node, *CI* common iliac, *IIV* internal iliac vein, *EIV* external iliac vein

recurrence [27]. The authors concluded that extending the field can cover these areas or adding androgen deprivation therapy can minimize the risk of more superior LN recurrence in high-risk patients. On the other hand, a study from the Massachusetts General Hospital reported that 95% of the LNs are in 1.5 cm proximity from large vessels and iliac vessels under high-risk of respective LN involvement should be given a radial margin of 2 cm for adequate coverage of the subclinical disease that cannot be shown by imaging techniques [28]. They recommended delineating the distal 2.5 cm portion of common iliac, proximal 9 cm portion of external iliac, and proximal 8.5 cm of internal iliac vessels starting from the iliac bifurcation. Based on these findings, the currently ongoing RTOG 0924 trial is evaluating the benefit of extending the superior border of RT portals.

Pelvic lymphatic delineation in a prostate cancer treated with definitive IGRT is depicted in Fig. 15.1.

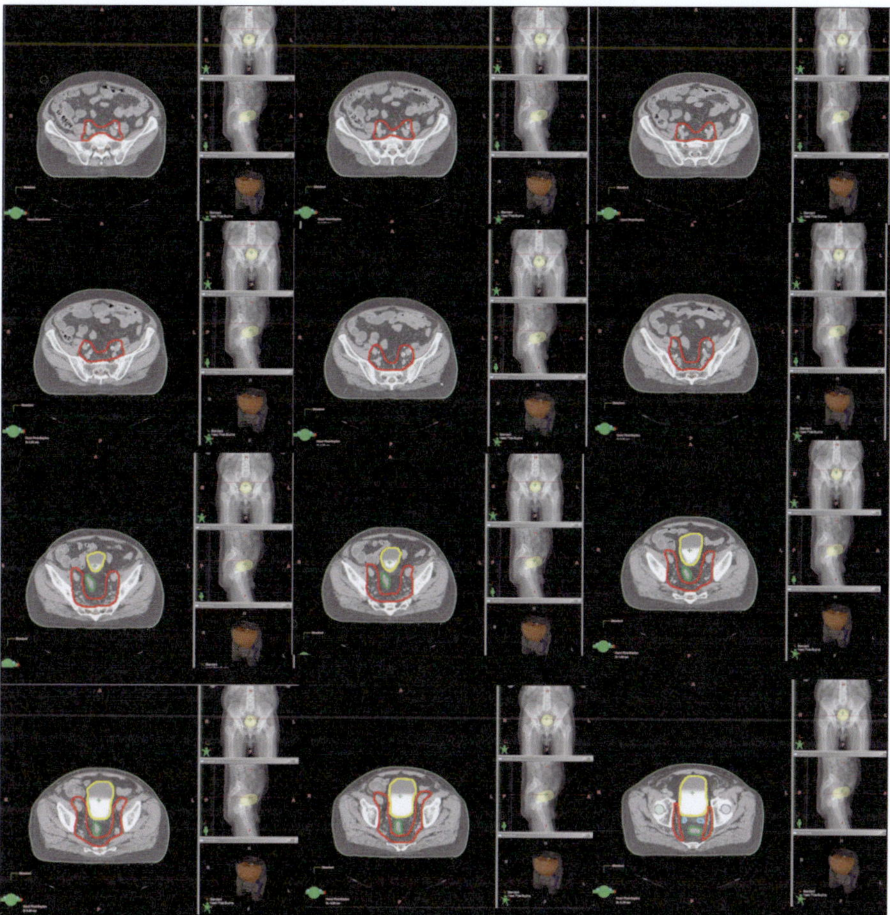

Fig. 15.1 Pelvic lymphatic delineation in a prostate cancer treated with definitive IGRT

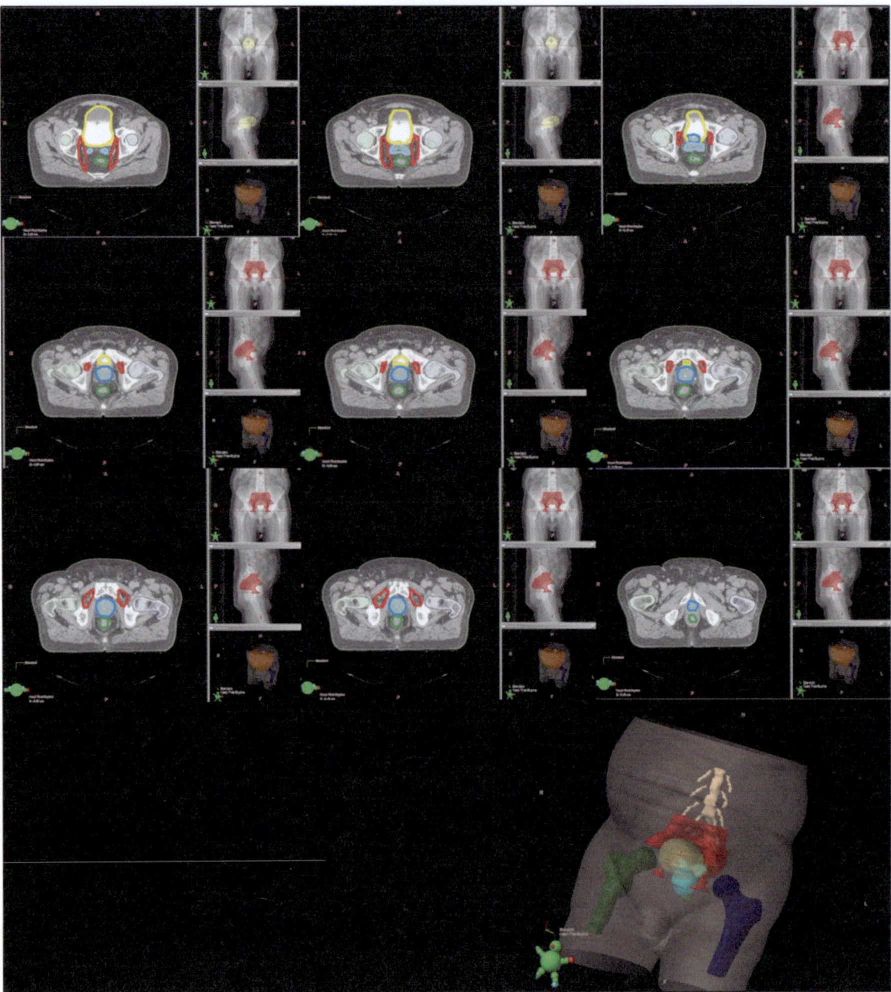

Fig. 15.1 (continued)

Conclusion

Elective nodal irradiation is not a standard procedure in patients with N0 prostate cancer that undergo RT. However, irradiation of pelvic LNs can be performed in patients with a high risk of or that already have LN metastasis. The recommended delineation guideline of the pelvic LNs is given in detail in this chapter. Although there are studies reporting the insufficiency of the available guideline, the variations in contouring the LNs between the institutions can be minimized if these recommendations are applied in clinical practice.

References

1. Fowler JE Jr, Whitmore WF Jr. The incidence and extent of pelvic lymph node metastases in apparently localized prostatic cancer. Cancer. 1981;47(12):2941–5.
2. Pisansky TM, Zincke H, Suman VJ, Bostwick DG, Earle JD, Oesterling JE. Correlation of pretherapy prostate cancer characteristics with histologic findings from pelvic lymphadenectomy specimens. Int J Radiat Oncol Biol Phys. 1996;34(1):33–9.
3. Partin AW, Yoo J, Carter HB, Pearson JD, Chan DW, Epstein JI, et al. The use of prostate specific antigen, clinical stage and Gleason score to predict pathological stage in men with localized prostate cancer. J Urol. 1993;150(1):110–4.
4. Bishoff JT, Reyes A, Thompson IM, Harris MJ, St Clair SR, Gomella L, et al. Pelvic lymphadenectomy can be omitted in selected patients with carcinoma of the prostate: development of a system of patient selection. Urology. 1995;45(2):270–4.
5. Link RE, Morton RA. Indications for pelvic lymphadenectomy in prostate cancer. Urol Clin North Am. 2001;28(3):491–8.
6. Stock RG, Stone NN, Ianuzzi C, Unger P. Seminal vesicle biopsy and laparoscopic pelvic lymph node dissection: implications for patient selection in the radiotherapeutic management of prostate cancer. Int J Radiat Oncol Biol Phys. 1995;33(4):815–21.
7. Rees MA, Campbell S, Kleian EA, et al. Validation of a model for predicting metastatic disease in the pelvic lymph nodes of patients with clinically localized prostate cancer. J Urol. 1996;155:487. (abst).
8. Roach M. Equations for predicting the pathologic state of men with localized prostate cancer using the preoperative prostate specific antigen. J Urol. 1993;150:1923–4.
9. Gervasi LA, Mata J, Easley JD, Wilbanks JH, Seale-Hawkins C, Carlton CE Jr, et al. Prognostic significance of lymph nodal metastases in prostate cancer. J Urol. 1989;142(2 Pt 1):332–6.
10. Cheng L, Zincke H, Blute ML, Bergstralh EJ, Scherer B, Bostwick DG. Risk of prostate carcinoma death in patients with lymph node metastasis. Cancer. 2001;91(1):66–73.
11. Prout GR Jr, Heaney JA, Griffin PP, Daly JJ, Shipley WU. Nodal involvement as a prognostic indicator in patients with prostatic carcinoma. J Urol. 1980;124(2):226–31.
12. Golimbu M, Provet J, Al-Askari S, Morales P. Radical prostatectomy for stage D1 prostate cancer. Prognostic variables and results of treatment. Urology. 1987;30(5):427–35.
13. UICC. TNM supplement. 3rd ed. 2003.
14. Dirix P, Haustermans K, Junius S, Withers R, Oyen R, Van Poppel H. The role of whole pelvic radiotherapy in locally advanced prostate cancer. Radiother Oncol. 2006;79(1):1–14.
15. Asbell SO, Martz KL, Shin KH, Sause WT, Doggett RL, Perez CA, et al. Impact of surgical staging in evaluating the radiotherapeutic outcome in RTOG #77-06, a phase III study for T1BN0M0 (A2) and T2N0M0 (B) prostate carcinoma. Int J Radiat Oncol Biol Phys. 1998;40(4):769–82.
16. Roach M 3rd, DeSilvio M, Lawton C, Uhl V, Machtay M, Seider MJ, et al. Phase III trial comparing whole-pelvic versus prostate-only radiotherapy and neoadjuvant versus adjuvant combined androgen suppression: Radiation Therapy Oncology Group 9413. J Clin Oncol. 2003;21(10):1904–11.
17. Roach M, Yan Y, Lawton CA, Hsu IJ, Lustig RA, Jones CU, et al. Radiation Therapy Oncology Group (RTOG) 9413: randomized trial comparing whole pelvic radiotherapy (WPRT) to prostate only (PORT) and neoadjuvant hormone therapy (NHT) to adjuvant hormone therapy (AHT). J Clin Oncol. 2012;30(suppl 5):96.
18. Pommier P, Chabaud S, Lagrange JL, Richaud P, Lesaunier F, Le Prise E, et al. Is there a role for pelvic irradiation in localized prostate adenocarcinoma? Preliminary results of GETUG-01. J Clin Oncol. 2007;25(34):5366–73.
19. Pommier P, Chabaud S, Lagrange JL, Richaud P, Le Prise E, Wagner JP, et al. Is there a role for pelvic irradiation in localized prostate adenocarcinoma? Update of the long-term survival results of the GETUG-01 randomized study. Int J Radiat Oncol Biol Phys. 2016;96(4):759–69.

20. Murthy V, Lewis S, Sawant M, Paul SN, Mahantshetty U, Shrivastava SK. Incidental dose to pelvic nodal regions in prostate-only radiotherapy. Technol Cancer Res Treat. 2017;16(2):211–7.
21. Saksena MA, Kim JY, Harisinghani MG. Nodal staging in genitourinary cancers. Abdom Imaging. 2006;31(6):644–51.
22. Koh DM, Hughes M, Husband JE. Cross-sectional imaging of nodal metastases in the abdomen and pelvis. Abdom Imaging. 2006;31(6):632–43.
23. Chapet O, Enachescu C, Lorchel F. Pelvic irradiation in prostate cancer: what place for what volumes? Cancer Radiother. 2013;17(5–6):562–5.
24. Padhani AR. Lymph Nodes. In: Nicholson T, editor. Recommendations for cross-sectional imaging in cancer management. London: The Royal College of Radiologists; 2014.
25. Lawton CA, Michalski J, El-Naqa I, Buyyounouski MK, Lee WR, Menard C, et al. RTOG GU radiation oncology specialists reach consensus on pelvic lymph node volumes for high-risk prostate cancer. Int J Radiat Oncol Biol Phys. 2009;74(2):383–7.
26. Meijer HJ, Fortuin AS, van Lin EN, Debats OA, Alfred Witjes J, Kaanders JH, et al. Geographical distribution of lymph node metastases on MR lymphography in prostate cancer patients. Radiother Oncol. 2013;106(1):59–63.
27. Spratt DE, Vargas HA, Zumsteg ZS, Golia Pernicka JS, Osborne JR, Pei X, et al. Patterns of lymph node failure after dose-escalated radiotherapy: implications for extended pelvic lymph node coverage. Eur Urol. 2017;71(1):37–43.
28. Shih HA, Harisinghani M, Zietman AL, Wolfgang JA, Saksena M, Weissleder R. Mapping of nodal disease in locally advanced prostate cancer: rethinking the clinical target volume for pelvic nodal irradiation based on vascular rather than bony anatomy. Int J Radiat Oncol Biol Phys. 2005;63(4):1262–9.

Advanced Radiotherapy Techniques in Prostate Cancer

16

Cem Onal and Ozan Cem Guler

Abstract

Prostate cancer (PC) is the most common tumor in males. Treatment options for localized prostate cancer include radical prostatectomy and radiation therapy (RT), which is delivered either as external beam radiation therapy (EBRT) or brachytherapy (BRT). According to "European Association of Urology" guidelines, although radical prostatectomy is the gold standard treatment option in localized PC, definitive RT could be an alternative treatment option in medically inoperable patients or who refused surgery. Treatment of PC has been evolving since the last decades with the innovation in technology. More precise radiotherapy (RT) techniques provides sharper isodoses while sparing organs at risk (OAR). It is also important that setup margins could be reduced with image guidance. Hence, precisely defining targets and considering organ movement are gaining much more importance. As a consequence of sharper isodoses and image guidance, dose escalation comes into question. It is well known that there is a positive correlation between RT dose and biochemical progression-free survival (BPFS) but not overall survival (OS) rates, with dose escalated conventionally fractionated up to 76–80 Gy in 2 Gy fractions, which is a biologically equivalent dose ($BED_{1.5}$) of 180–200 Gy, assuming an α/β of 1.5. A recent meta-analysis clearly demonstrated an increased disease

C. Onal, M.D. (✉)
Department of Radiation Oncology, Adana Dr Turgut Noyan Research and Treatment Center, Başkent University, Adana, Turkey
e-mail: hcemonal@hotmail.com

O.C. Guler, M.D.
Department of Radiation Oncology, Karadeniz Technical University, Trabzon, Turkey

G. Ozyigit, U. Selek (eds.), *Principles and Practice of Urooncology*,
DOI 10.1007/978-3-319-56114-1_16

control with a $BED_{1.5}$ to 200 Gy, with no additional clinical benefit with doses above 200 Gy. In order to deliver higher doses to the prostate without increasing surrounding organs at risk, it is essential to delineate target volumes properly, deliver RT with high-technology devices, immobilize patient, and track prostate during RT. The aim of this chapter is to review recent advances in prostate RT.

16.1 Advances in Imaging and Tumor Delineation

Major advances in diagnostic imaging dramatically improved the ability to accurately target the prostate with smaller treatment volumes. This, in turn, led to better toxicity profiles, safe dose escalation, and improved disease control [2, 3, 4–6]. More recently, onboard imaging devices (cone beam computed tomography [CBCT]) used to image the prostate during treatment have led to further increase in dose delivered per treatment and an associated decrease in total treatment duration. Trends toward earlier diagnosis during the PSA screening era have led to detection of more focal and smaller volume disease within the prostate. In an effort to intensify treatment and avoid adverse effects in these patients, focal ablative techniques have been used to target only intraprostatic lesions (IPL) as opposed to traditional treatment of the whole gland or dose escalation to IPL lesion with simultaneous integrated boost (SIB) technique.

With increasing technology in radiological imaging, functional and metabolic imaging is taking the place of conventional modalities in oncology. Additionally, functional imaging modalities, such as positron emission tomography (PET-CT), diffusion-weighted magnetic resonance imaging (DW-MRI), or MR spectroscopy, may be potentially used to define the tumor biology. It is important to clearly define the tumor biology during RT because there may be discordance between clinical and pathological staging and Gleason scores of biopsy and prostatectomy specimens. For this reason, a thorough evaluation of the entire prostate is essential before performing definitive RT, in which histopathological evaluation is based on prostate biopsy only, and staging is performed with clinical and radiological findings. Noninvasive methods to evaluate the entire prostate and the tumor biology before performing RT may be a promising alternative. Moreover, this approach would allow optimized treatment delivery to adequately stratified patient risk groups.

The best method of imaging prostate cancer is endorectal T2-weighted MRI, which has 60–82% sensitivity and 55–70% specificity for detecting cancer [7, 8]. Additionally, recent studies have aimed to determine the value of MR correlates of cellular density, metabolite concentration, and tumor vascularization for predicting tumor

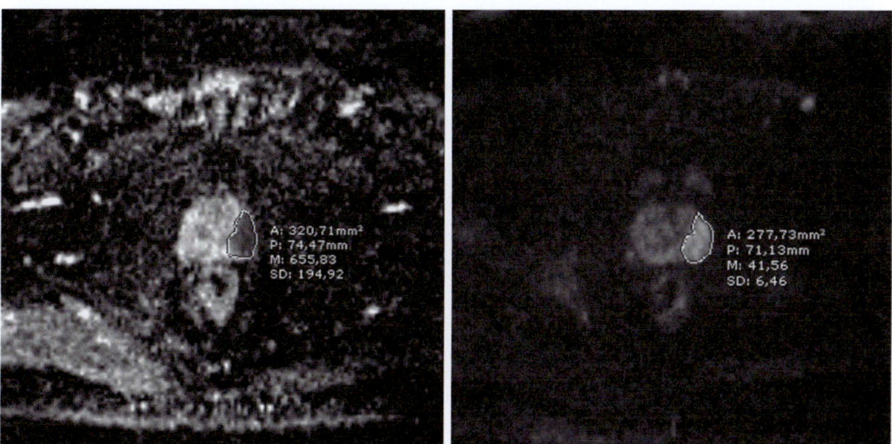

Fig. 16.1 Axial apparent diffusion coefficient map of a corresponding patient demonstrating prostate tumor at left peripheral zone

aggressiveness [9, 10]. The DW-MRI is advantageous in tumor localization [11, 12], and it may also provide qualitative information regarding the pathophysiological character of prostate cancer [13, 14] (Fig. 16.1).The DW-MRI is sensitive to the microscopic motion of water molecules and allows biological characterization of tissues based on their water-diffusion properties. The degree of diffusion is quantified as the apparent diffusion coefficient (ADC).

Conventional 18-fluorodeoxyglucose (FDG) PET-CT has been widely used for various tumors [15–19]; however, its role in prostate cancer is limited. Choline PET and 18F-fluciclovine PET are other nuclear imaging modalities for prostate cancer [20]. The use of choline PET remains unclear for its value in initial staging. In the restaging phase, the detection rate of choline PET varies between 21% and 82%, which is dependent on site of recurrence and PSA levels [21]. A systematic review showed that the sensitivity and specificity of 18F-fluciclovine PET for prostate cancer was 87% and 66% [20]. There is an increasing investigation about specific markers related to prostate cancer. Prostate-specific membrane antigen (PSMA) is overexpressed in prostate cancer cell membranes [22]. The PSMA-PET is a highly selective imaging tool for detecting the primary, involved lymph nodes and distant metastasis in prostate cancer patients (Fig. 16.2). Also the importance of PSMA PET in identification of both local and distant recurrences was shown in many trials with a detection rate for recurrent disease of approximately 85–90% [23, 24]. The detection rate is correlated with PSA value and decreasing to 58% between PSA values of 0.2–0.5 ng/ml [24]. Furthermore, PSMA-PET is useful in demonstrating IPL, for further dose escalation during prostate RT (Fig. 16.3).

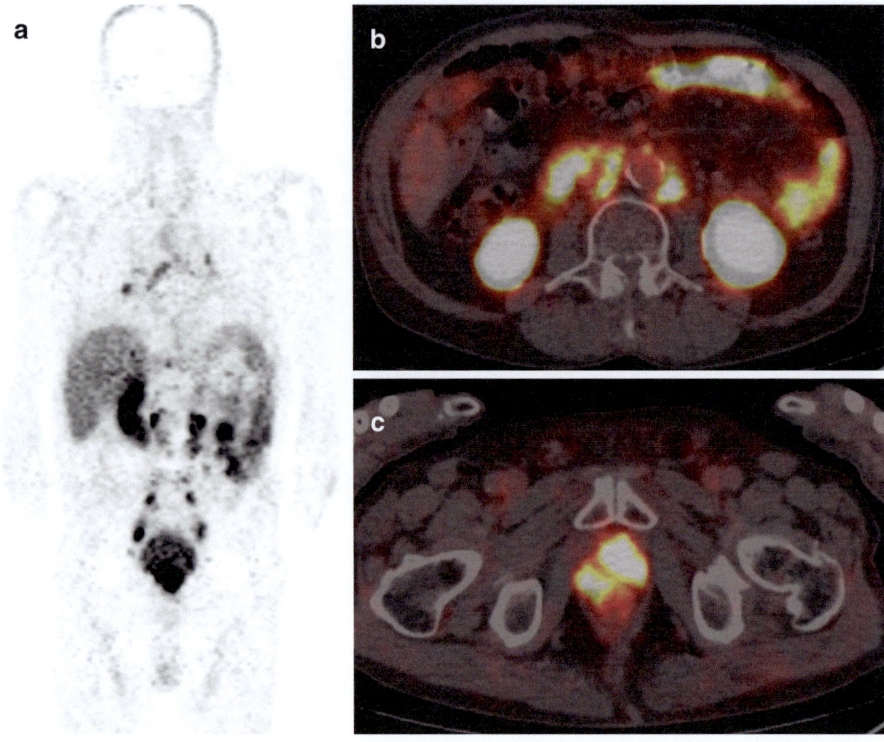

Fig. 16.2 68 Ga-PSMA ligand positron emission tomography/computed tomography images of a representative prostate cancer patient. (**a**) PSMA-PET-CT image, demonstrating increased uptake in the pelvic and para-aortic lymphatics (arrows). (**b**) The co-registered images of PET and CT, demonstrating increased Ga-PSMA uptake in the para-aortic lymphatics and (**c**) in the prostate

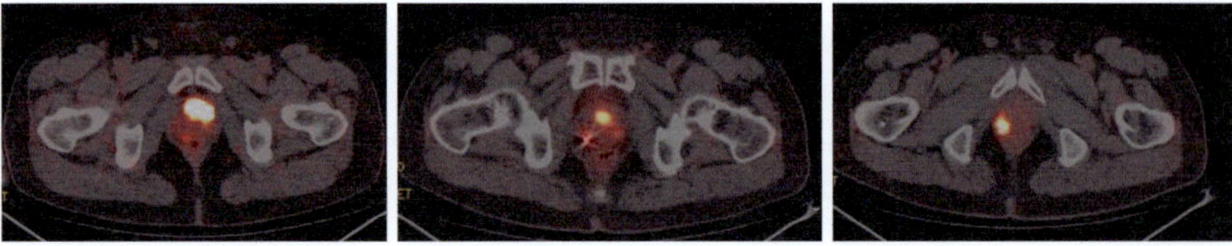

Fig. 16.3 68 Ga-PSMA ligand positron emission tomography/computed tomography images demonstrating intraprostatic lesion (*light yellow area*) in three different representative prostate cancer patients

16.2 New Radiotherapy Delivery Approaches

Historically, the prostate was treated with four static radiation fields designed based on anatomic landmarks. However, with this technique, it is difficult to get idea about the target volume doses and also surrounding organs. As a consequence, geographic misses may be seen more than expected, and it is difficult to know

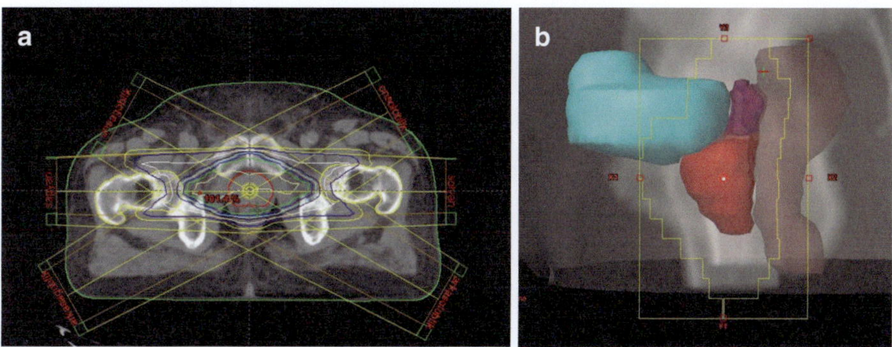

Fig. 16.4 (**a**) Dose distributions of a seven-field coplanar three-dimensional conformal radiotherapy plan. (**b**) Beam's eye view of lateral irradiation field demonstrating prostate and seminal vesicles (*red*), rectum (*brown*), and bladder (*magenta*)

about the toxicities. With the use of a 3D conformal RT (3DCRT) technique, the dose escalation above 70 Gy resulted in a modest increase in rectal and bladder toxicity. With advancements in imaging, more focal three-dimensional treatment plans were developed to target the prostate and seminal vesicles only (Fig. 16.4). Further advances in radiation delivery techniques such as IMRT and volumetric modulated arc therapy (VMAT) led to greater sparing of adjacent normal tissue to reduce toxicity. Techniques such as VMAT and IMRT are able to generate conformal isodoses, which significantly reduce the OAR doses and normal tissue toxicity [25]. Although IMRT is a commonly used method to treat prostate cancer, the potential downsides of IMRT include increased RT delivery time, resulting in a greater integral body dose, which might increase the risk of secondary cancer development [26].

VMAT is an innovative form of IMRT optimization that allows the radiation dose to be efficiently delivered using a dynamic modulated arc. The VMAT simultaneously coordinates gantry rotation, multi-leaf collimator (MLC) motion, and dose-rate modulation, facilitating highly conformal treatment with better normal tissue sparing [27]. Compared with IMRT, the potential advantages of VMAT include a large reduction in monitor units (MU) required to deliver a given fraction size and a concomitant reduction in treatment time (Figs. 16.5 and 16.6). Helical tomotherapy (HT) is an arc-based application of IMRT that uses a fan beam of radiation in conjunction with binary MLC. The gantry rotates at a constant speed, while the binary MLC leaves open 51 times per rotation and close entirely between projections. This rotational treatment modality can establish target dose conformity and OAR dose reduction (Fig. 16.7). Several recent studies have evaluated the use of VMAT delivery methods in prostate cancer (Table 16.1) [28–38].

Image guidance is essential for delivering the high radiation doses to the prostate accurately. The prostate is a mobile organ influenced by bladder and rectal filling. The position of these structures as defined on the planning CT can vary during and between fractions. Delivery of highly conformal treatments

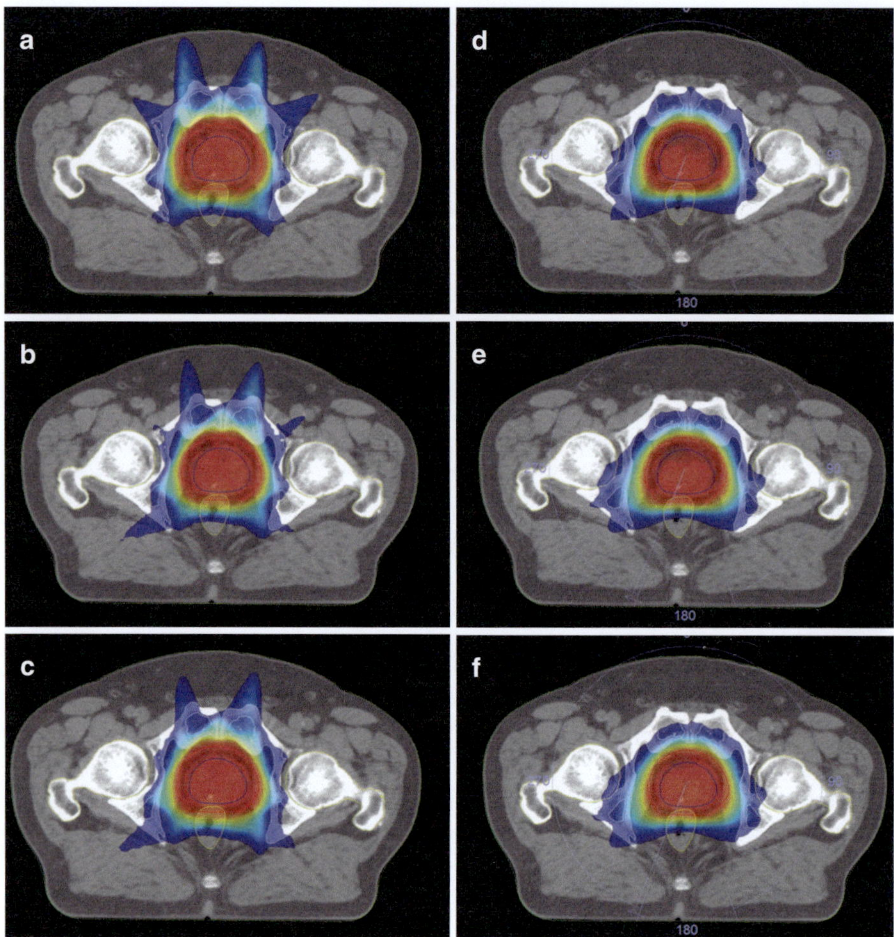

Fig. 16.5 Representative axial computed tomography slices showing 50% of prescribed dose distributions for (**a**) 6 MV, (**b**) 10 MV, and (**c**) 15 MV energy IMRT plans and (**d**) 6 MV, (**e**) 10 MV, and (**f**) 15 MV energy VMAT plans. *Blue* area represents 50%, *red* area represents 95%, and *yellow-orange* area represents 50–95% of prescribed dose

with steep dose gradients demands confidence in localization of the target because motion can lead to geographic miss, underdosing of the tumor, and/or unwanted overdosing of organs at risk. Dedicated CBCT equipment can acquire a 3D CT image in real time in the treatment position just before treatment (Fig. 16.8). Resolution is not of diagnostic quality but enables visualization of soft tissues (prostate, bladder, and rectum) so that table shifts can be made if needed. CBCT can be used in conjunction with fiducial seeds. However, the implantation of fiducial markers is an invasive procedure with the potential for

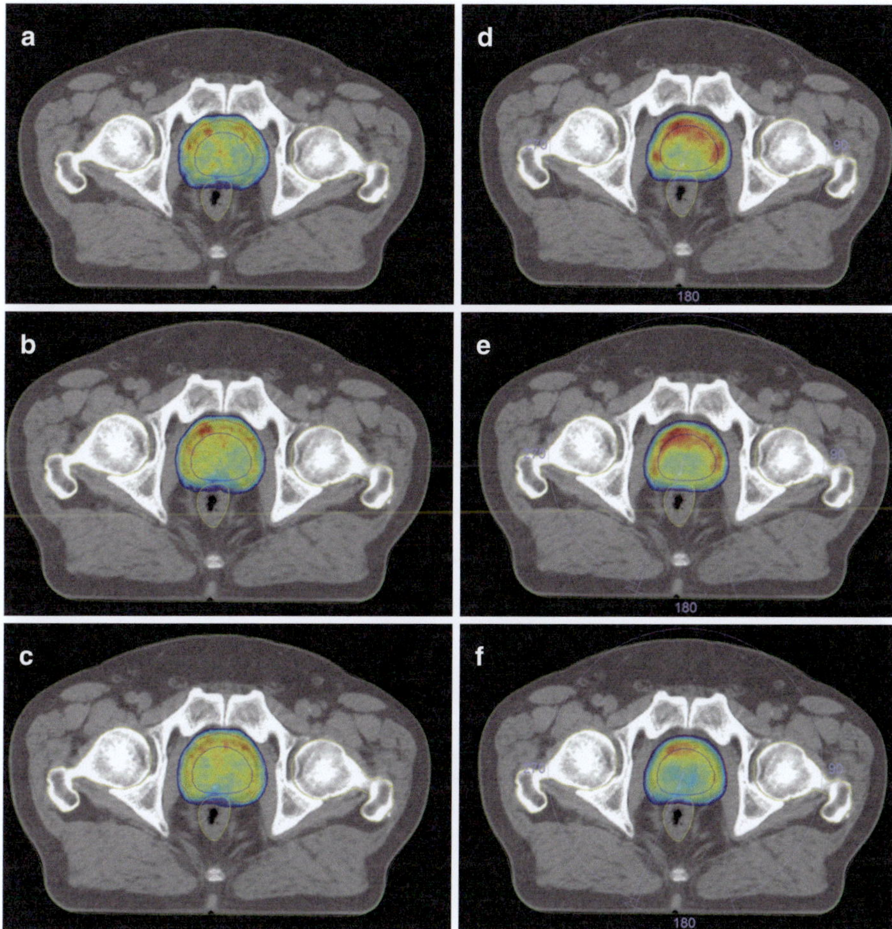

Fig. 16.6 Representative axial computed tomography slices showing 90% of prescribed dose distributions for (**a**) 6 MV, (**b**) 10 MV, and (**c**) 15 MV energy IMRT plans and (**d**) 6 MV, (**e**) 10 MV, and (**f**) 15 MV energy VMAT plans. *Yellow* area represents 95%, and *red* area represents hot spots within the target volume

discomfort, bleeding, and infection. Furthermore, fiducial markers provide little information on deformation of the target, localization of the seminal vesicles, or alteration in the neighboring normal tissue and may cause deformation of the prostate gland after implantation. Although fiducial marker implantation for image-guided RT in prostate cancer allows the localization of the prostate during treatment, this application may cause some complications and dosimetric uncertainties. Therefore, alternative noninvasive methods of CBCT should be considered for IGRT of prostate cancer patients [39].

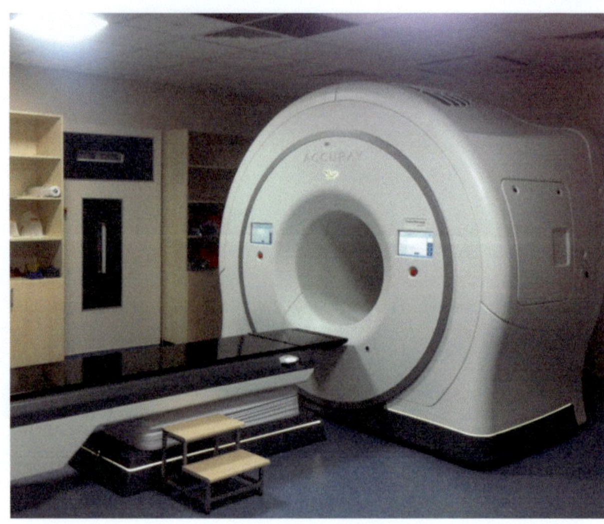

Fig. 16.7 Helical tomotherapy version HDA used for external beam radiotherapy

Table 16.1 Published studies comparing VMAT and IMRT plans for prostate ± seminal vesicle irradiation

Author (year)	Patient no	TPS	RT dose (Gy)	IMRT beam no	VMAT arc no	IMRT MU/VMAT MU
Palma et al. (2008)	10	Eclipse/Eclipse	2/74	5	1/358°	1.73
Wolff et al. (2009)	9	Hyperion/ERGO++	2/76	7	1/360° 1/360° + 2/100°	1.41 1.47
Zhang et al. (2010)	11	MSKCC/MSKCC	1.8/86.4	5	1/360°	2.22
Rao et al. (2010)	6	Pinnacle/Pinnacle SmartArc	2/78	7	1/356°	1.16
Sale et al. (2011)	8	Eclipse/Eclipse	1.8/75.6	5	1/360° 2/360°	
Tsai et al. (2011)	12	Pinnacle/ERGO++	2/78	5	1/360°	1.08
Hardcastle et al. (2011)	10	Pinnacle/Pinnacle SmartArc	2/78	7	1/360°	1.23
Sze et al. (2012)	14	Eclipse/Eclipse	2/76	7	1/360° 2/360°	1.48 1.23
Fontenot et al. (2012)	5	Pinnacle/Pinnacle SmartArc		7	1/350°	1.25
Onal et al. (2014)	12	Monaco/Monaco	2/78	7	1/360°	1.10

Abbreviations: *TPS* treatment planning system, *IMRT* intensity-modulated radiotherapy, *VMAT* volumetric modulated arc therapy, *MU* monitor units, *MSKCC* Memorial Sloan Kettering Cancer Center

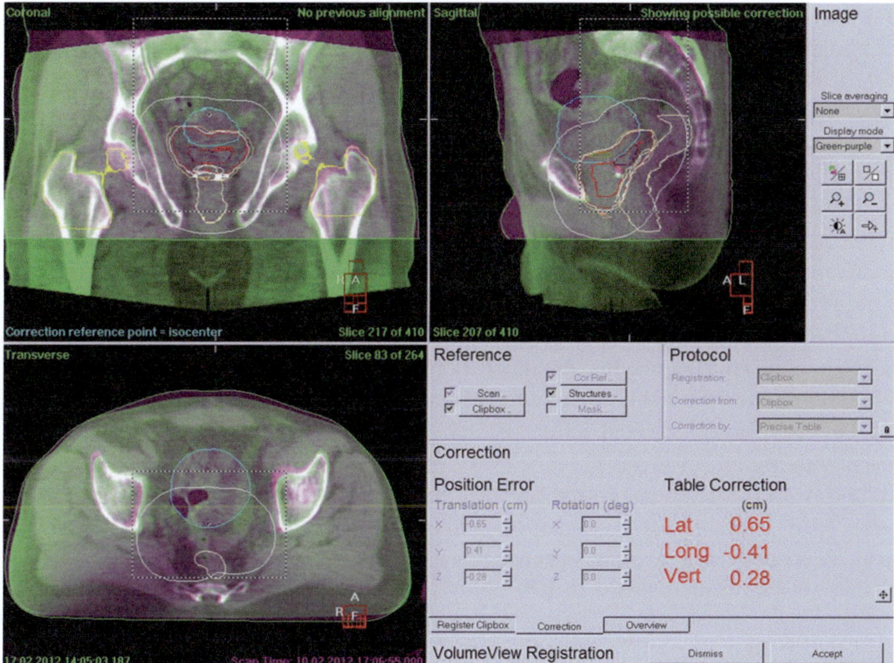

Fig. 16.8 Registration of cone beam CT images and reference CT images. After corrections according to prostate at lateral, superoinferior, and anteroposterior directions, the treatment was delivered with less setup errors

16.3 Radiotherapy Dose Escalation

External beam radiotherapy (EBRT) focusing on intensity-modulated RT (IMRT) and image-guided RT (IMRT), hypofractionation and stereotactic body RT (SBRT), high-dose rate (HDR) brachytherapy, proton beam RT (PBRT), and ablative therapies such as cryoablation, high-intensity focused ultrasound (HIFU), and radiofrequency ablation (RFA) are therapeutic modalities that have been investigated in patients with PC in an attempt to reduce toxicity while improving cancer control. These treatment modalities could be used as monotherapy, whole prostate, or IPL boost.

A 3 mm thickness planning CT should cover the whole pelvis for RT planning. Patients need to be asked to have a comfortably full bladder and an empty rectum [40]. If MRI or PET fusion is planned to fuse with planning CT, these imaging modalities should be obtained in closest possible condition. In addition to that, in patients planning to receive androgen blockade, imaging should be preferred before the initiation of hormonal therapy [31]. Gross tumor volume (GTV), clinical tumor volume (CTV), and planning tumor volume (PTV) are basically defined in the

International Commission of Radiation Units and Measurements (ICRU) [41]. CTV is based on clinical or pathological staging, while appropriate PTV margin is based on the RT technique and image guidance in the oncological center. The rectum, sigmoid colon, small bowels, bladder, and femoral heads are recommended to delineate as OAR. The rectum needs to be delineated from the anal verge to the rectosigmoidal junction. Femoral heads need to be delineated to the level of ischial tuberosities.

Dose escalation for prostate cancer causes improved biochemical control and reduced distant metastasis [2]. However, local failure still occurs in one-third of patients after 78 Gy ERT, and the original IPL is the most frequent location of relapse [42]. Therefore, selectively boosting radiation to these lesions to a very high dose has been hypothesized to be a more effective method to improve the therapeutic ratio than a homogeneous, but more modest, dose escalation to the entire prostate [43]. Randomized trials have shown a gain in BPFS using dose escalation for PC [1, 2]. However, isolated local failure is still reported in nearly one-third of patients, even with higher RT doses [2]. Local recurrence is of clinical importance because a relationship has been suggested between local control, distant metastasis, and survival [44]. Also, it has been demonstrated that local failure mainly originates at IPL. This could be a result of intrinsic resistance of radioresistant tumor clones [42]. So, delivering higher doses to IPL using SIB technique may potentially increase local control and treatment outcomes. The SIB technique can be safely performed by static IMRT, VMAT, or HT (Fig. 16.9). With VMAT plan (Fig. 16.10) and HT plan (Fig. 16.11), a homogeneous dose distribution was observed in target volumes with better sparing of the surrounding organs.

There are several studies investigating SIB boost to IPL/whole gland in treatment of PC [12, 32, 45–47] (Table 16.2). A boost to the IPL has been found to be effective and safe [48]. The reported BRFS and DFS rates were 78–92% and 90–100%, respectively [48]. Although SIB to IPL is not a standard approach, several ongoing studies will evaluate whether this approach is effective in local tumor control or not.

The investigate the benefit of a focal lesion ablative microboost in prostate cancer (FLAME) trial (ClinicalTrials.gov identifier NCT01168479) is a phase III study evaluating an EBRT boost to the DIL [49]. The tumor TARGET PC trial is a nonrandomized phase II study (ClinicalTrials.gov identifier, NCT01802242) comparing a combination of a boost to the DIL with high-dose-rate brachytherapy and a moderate dose of volumetric modulated arc therapy (VMAT) for the rest of the prostate, with VMAT as monotherapy for the whole prostate.

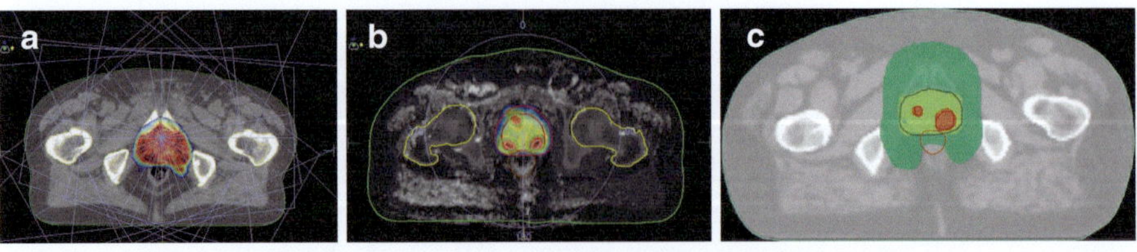

Fig. 16.9 The dose distributions of prostate irradiation and simultaneous integrated boost to intraprostatic lesion in (**a**) static IMRT plan, (**b**) VMAT plan, and (**c**) helical tomotherapy plan

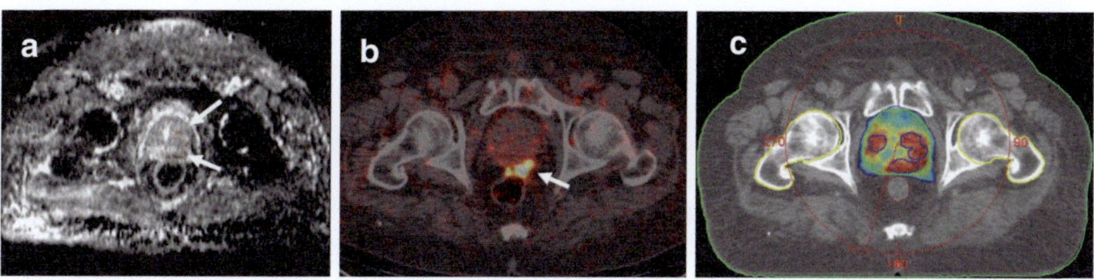

Fig. 16.10 The intraprostatic lesion demonstrated in (**a**) diffusion-weighted MRI and (**b**) 68 Ga-PSMA-PET/CT. (**c**) The dose distribution of prostate (*green-yellow area*) and intraprostatic lesions (*red area*) obtained from VMAT plan

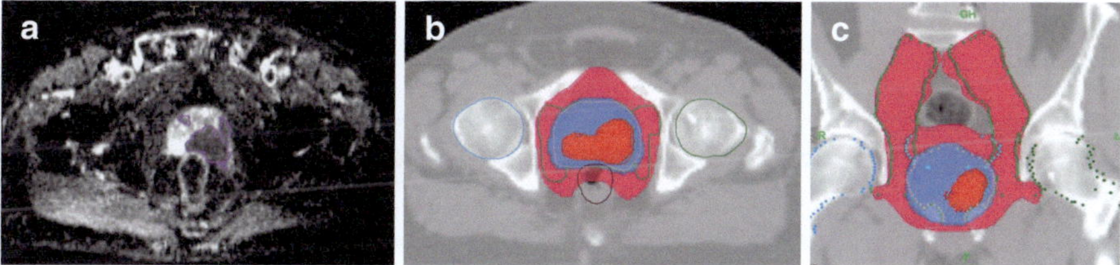

Fig. 16.11 The intraprostatic lesion demonstrated in (**a**) diffusion-weighted MRI. (**b–c**) The dose distribution of prostate (*blue area*) and intraprostatic lesions (*red area*) together with pelvic lymphatics (*pink area*) obtained from helical tomotherapy plan

Table 16.2 Published studies demonstrating the feasibility of simultaneous integrated boost intraprostatic lesion during prostate radiotherapy

Author (year)	Patient no	Imaging	RT technique/dose	Toxicity
De Meerleer et al. (2005)	15	MRI	Step-shoot IMRT Prostate + 7–10 mm 74 Gy IPL + 0 mm 80 Gy	Acute GI Gr II 3/15 Acute GU Gr III 1/15 Acute GU Gr II 6/15
Singh et al. (2007)	3	MRI + fiducial	Step-shoot IMRT Prostate + 7–10 mm 75.6 Gy IPL + 3 mm 94.5 Gy	Acute Gr I 1/3 Acute GU 2/3
Fonteyne et al. (2008)	118 (boost) 112 (no boost)	MRI	Step-shoot IMRT Prostate + 8 mm 78 Gy IPL + 4 mm 80 Gy	No increase in toxicity with SIB plan
Miralbell et al. (2010)	50	MRI	Prostate 64–64.4 Gy Hypofractionated boost 5–8 Gy	Late GI Gr II 10% Late GI Gr III 10% Late GU Gr II 12%
Ippolito et al. (2012)	40	MRI	Step-shoot IMRT Prostate + 10 mm 72 Gy IPL + 5 mm 80 Gy	Late GI Gr II 5% Late GI Gr III 2.5% Late GU Gr II 5%

(continued)

Table 16.2 (continued)

Author (year)	Patient no	Imaging	RT technique/dose	Toxicity
Wong et al. (2011)	Total 71 SIB 14	Indium-111-capromad	Step-shoot IMRT Prostate + 4–8 mm 76 Gy IPL + 4 mm 80 Gy	Late GI Gr II 21% Late GU Gr II 39% Late GU Gr III 4%
Pinkawa et al. (2012)	Total 67 SIB 46	18F-choline PET	Step-shoot IMRT Prostate + 6 mm 75.6 Gy IPL + 0 mm 80 Gy	No increase in toxicity with SIB plan
Aluwini et al. (2013)	50 14 IPL (+)	MRI + fiducial	Prostate + 3 mm 38Gy/4 fx (daily) IPL 44Gy/4fx	Late GI Gr II 3% Late GU Gr II 10% Late GU Gr III 6%
Onal et al. (2016)	173	MRI	Dynamic IMRT/VMAT Prostate + 5–8 mm 78 Gy IPL + 4 mm 86 Gy	Late GI Gr II 4% Late GU Gr II 3%

16.4 Hypofractionation/Stereotactic Body Radiotherapy

Larger fraction per treatment is hypothesized with better radiobiological effect in the treatment of PC [50]. In addition to that, the potentially low alpha/beta ratio of PC is hypothesized as the rationale of hypofractionation and SBRT [51–53]. In moderate hypofractionation, 2.2–4 Gy per fraction is generally delivered with linear accelerators, while doses above 5 Gy are used in SBRT. SBRT uses more intensive immobilization and tracking systems to safely deliver high doses of radiation compared to IMRT.

SBRT and hypofractionation studies generally investigated low-risk and intermediate-risk patients. Because high-risk disease requires more comprehensive approach due to risk of regional spread, SBRT is generally used as boost in such patients. Also, greater likelihood of local recurrence and resistance of conventional RT dose makes high-risk patients a candidate for dose escalation with larger RT fraction [54].

Summaries of hypofractionation and SBRT studies are depicted in Table 16.3. Briefly, SBRT and hypofractionated RT could be used as monotherapy, whole-gland boost therapy, or focal boost of IPL. There are various RT schemes for monotherapy of PC, but the optimal fractionation has not been determined. Most of the studies investigated the BPFS, quality of life (QoL), and toxicity. In general, hypofractionation or SBRT is well tolerated with acceptable results without any serious increase in toxicity.

Radiofrequency tracking or implanted markers such as fiducial can be used for delivering SBRT. Prostate movement can be minimized with careful bladder and rectal/small bowel preparation [55]. If standard cone beam computerized tomography (CBCT) is used instead of tracking systems, it is recommended to perform before and after treatment. Rectal protection is the one of the major issues in PC SBRT. Care should be taken to ensure the rectum receives less than the prescribed radiation dose. The use of an inflatable rectal balloon for rectal distension or

Table 16.3 Published studies of stereotactic radiotherapy and hypofractionation in prostate cancer treatment

Author	Year	n	Design	Risk group	Fractionation	Therapy	Follow-up	Outcome	Toxicity
Arcangeli et al.	2011	168	Randomized	HR	Conv. vs 3.1 Gy × 20 fr	Monotherapy	70 months	5y BPFS 79–85% No difference	Late Grd 2 ≥ 11–17% No difference
Pollack et al.	2013	303	Randomized	HR	Conv. vs 2.7 Gy × 26 fr	Monotherapy	68 months	5y BPFS 81–85% No difference	Late Grd 2 ≥ 13–23% No difference
Hoffman et al.	–	204	Randomized Phase III	LR, IR, HR	Conv. vs 2.4 Gy × 30 fr	Monotherapy	57 months	–	Late Grd 2 ≥ 5.1–16.5%
Norkus et al.	2013	124	Randomized	HR	Conv. vs 3.15 Gy × 20 fr	Monotherapy		–	Acute tx No difference
Wilkins et al. (CHHiP trial)	2015	2054	Randomized Phase III	LR, IR, HR	Conv. vs 3 Gy × 19–20 fr	Monotherapy	50 months	No difference	No difference
Aluvini et al. (HYPRO trial)	2016		Randomized Phase III	IR, HR	Conv. vs 3.4 Gy × 19 fr	Monotherapy			Hypofractionation is more toxic
King et al.	2013	1100	Prospective Phase II	LR, IR, HR	7 Gy × 5 fr 8 Gy × 5 fr	Monotherapy		5y BPFS 81%	
Kang et al.	2011	44	Retrospective	LR, IR, HR	8 Gy × 4 fr 9 Gy × 4 fr	Monotherapy	40 months	5y BPFS 90.8%	Late Grd 2 ≥ 6.8–11.4%
Anwar et al.	2016	48	Prospective	IR, HR	9.5–10.5 Gy × 2 fr	Prostate boost	43 months	5y BPFS 90%	Late Grd 3 ≥ 2.1%
Kim et al.	2016			IR, HR		Prostate boost			
Oermann et al.	2010	45		IR, HR		Prostate boost		5y BPFS 83%	Late Grd 3 ≥ 2.2%
Aluwini et al.	2013	50	Prospective	LR, IR	9.5 Gy × 4 fr SIB: 11 Gy × 4 fr	IPL boost	23 months		Late Grd 3 ≥ 8%
Kotecha et al.	2016	24		IR, HR	7.25 Gy × 5 fr SIB: 10 Gy × 5 fr	IPL boost	25 months	2y BPFS 95.8%	Late Grd 2 ≥ 8%

rectoprostatic injectable hydrogel can be used for organ motion. Another issue about PC SBRT is homogeneity. Ideally care should be taken with maximal dose inhomogeneity of less than 107% of the prescription dose within the prostate to prevent ureteral complications. Caution and care must be taken for appropriate education, immobilization, and RT delivery.

16.5 Brachytherapy

High-dose rate (HDR) BRT delivers radiation at a dose rate of >12 Gy/h. Iridium-192 is the most commonly used isotope in BRT. The use of BRT allows for a degree of conformality and dose distribution that is difficult to achieve with EBRT.

BRT is recommended in patients with cT1-2a, PSA $\leq$ 10, GS $\leq$ 7, and prostate volume $\leq$ 50 cc [56].

16.6 Proton Beam Radiation Therapy

PBRT aims to deliver radiation to the prostate while taking advantage of the physical property of protons to minimize dose to surrounding tissue and OAR [57]. Researchers mainly focus on low-risk PC [58, 59], but it is possible to use PBRT in combination with photon energies as a boost treatment [60, 61].

Mendenhall et al. conducted a prospective study investigating the role of PBRT in 40 high-risk PC patients. Patients were given weekly concomitant docetaxel chemotherapy followed by hormonotherapy for 6 months. Five-year BPFS was 76% and grade III toxicities for GIS and GUS were 0.5% and 1%, respectively [57]. Bryant et al. retrospectively analyzed 229 high-risk PC patients treated with PBRT. They reported 5 year BPFS of 76, and grade III or higher toxicities for GIS and GUS were 0.6% and 2.9%, respectively [62]. Unlike these authors, Slater et al. reported a relatively poor 5 year BPFS of 48–50% in the 133 high-risk patients in retrospective analysis [59]. Caution should be taken when interpreting these findings because of small sample sizes and lack of the number of studies.

16.7 Ablative Focal Therapies

Alternative focal treatment methods to RT and RP continue to be investigated for the treatment of PC. There are various focal treatments but cryoablation, high-intensity focused ultrasound (HIFU), and radiofrequency ablation (RFA) are the most studied approaches. These technologies aim to deliver focal ablation with minimally or noninvasive methods. Although most investigations are about low-risk PC, it is unclear for high-risk patients [63].

16.7.1 Cryoablation

Cryoablation is based on focal areas of freezing (minus 30 °C) and cell death. Because it is not possible for this technique to use it for the whole gland, studies focused on partial or targeted treatments. Bahn et al. investigated hemiablation in 73 low- and intermediate-risk patients. The authors reported that potency sparing is about 86–100% [64]. Also, cryoablation is investigated as salvage therapy after recurrence of postradiation treatment [65].

16.7.2 High-Intensity Focused Ultrasound (HIFU)

HIFU is based on coagulation necrosis by thermal energy and cell death. It has been investigated for mostly low-risk PC. Generally the treatment is considered as more toxic and potentially less efficacious than modern RT treatments [66, 67]. Also, rectourethral fistula after HIFU had been reported [68]. Therefore, the role of HIFU against RT is limited by only experimental studies.

16.7.3 Radiofrequency Ablation (RFA)

RFA uses thermal damage to cause death. RFA has two major differences from HIFU. Firstly, RFA is an invasive technique with interstitial electrodes. Secondly, RFA uses electric energy instead of ultrasonography. Nevertheless, the lack of data concerning RFA and its role in PC still remain controversial.

Conclusion

The evidence in PC treatment continues to increase. Sharper dose gradients can be obtained, and OAR doses can be reduced with new technologies, but care must be taken to organ motion and targeting. The use of SBRT, BRT, and PBRT is promising. Clinical data supports the use of SBRT in selected patients with low-risk and intermediate-risk, while it is still controversial in high-risk PC. Focal ablation therapies are not recommended in routine clinical practice unless in clinical trial.

References

1. Viani GA, Stefano EJ, Afonso SL. Higher-than-conventional radiation doses in localized prostate cancer treatment: a meta-analysis of randomized, controlled trials. Int J Radiat Oncol Biol Phys. 2009;74(5):1405–18. doi:10.1016/j.ijrobp.2008.10.091.
2. Zietman AL, DeSilvio ML, Slater JD, Rossi CJ Jr, Miller DW, Adams JA, et al. Comparison of conventional-dose vs high-dose conformal radiation therapy in clinically localized adenocarcinoma of the prostate: a randomized controlled trial. JAMA. 2005;294(10):1233–9. doi:10.1001/jama.294.10.1233.

3. Kuban DA, Tucker SL, Dong L, Starkschall G, Huang EH, Cheung MR, et al. Long-term results of the M. D. Anderson randomized dose-escalation trial for prostate cancer. Int J Radiat Oncol Biol Phys. 2008;70(1):67–74. doi:10.1016/j.ijrobp.2007.06.054.
4. Beckendorf V, Guerif S, Le Prise E, Cosset JM, Bougnoux A, Chauvet B, et al. 70Gy versus 80 Gy in localized prostate cancer: 5-year results of GETUG 06 randomized trial. Int J Radiat Oncol Biol Phys. 2011;80(4):1056–63. doi:10.1016/j.ijrobp.2010.03.049.
5. Pawlowski JM, Yang ES, Malcolm AW, Coffey CW, Ding GX. Reduction of dose delivered to organs at risk in prostate cancer patients via image-guided radiation therapy. Int J Radiat Oncol Biol Phys. 2010;76(3):924–34. doi:10.1016/j.ijrobp.2009.06.068.
6. Heemsbergen WD, Al-Mamgani A, Slot A, Dielwart MF, Lebesque JV. Long-term results of the Dutch randomized prostate cancer trial: impact of dose-escalation on local, biochemical, clinical failure, and survival. Radiother Oncol. 2014;110(1):104–9. doi:10.1016/j.radonc.2013.09.026.
7. Tilak G, Tuncali K, Song SE, Tokuda J, Olubiyi O, Fennessy F, et al. 3T MR-guided in-bore transperineal prostate biopsy: a comparison of robotic and manual needle-guidance templates. J Magn Reson Imaging. 2015;42(1):63–71. doi:10.1002/jmri.24770.
8. Le JD, Tan N, Shkolyar E, Lu DY, Kwan L, Marks LS, et al. Multifocality and prostate cancer detection by multiparametric magnetic resonance imaging: correlation with whole-mount histopathology. Eur Urol. 2015;67(3):569–76. doi:10.1016/j.eururo.2014.08.079.
9. Kobus T, Hambrock T, Hulsbergen-van de Kaa CA, Wright AJ, Barentsz JO, Heerschap A, et al. In vivo assessment of prostate cancer aggressiveness using magnetic resonance spectroscopic imaging at 3 T with an endorectal coil. Eur Urol. 2011;60(5):1074–80. doi:10.1016/j.eururo.2011.03.002.
10. Watanabe Y, Nagayama M, Araki T, Terai A, Okumura A, Amoh Y, et al. Targeted biopsy based on ADC map in the detection and localization of prostate cancer: a feasibility study. J Magn Reson Imaging. 2013;37(5):1168–77. doi:10.1002/jmri.23908.
11. Quentin M, Schimmoller L, Arsov C, Rabenalt R, Antoch G, Albers P, et al. Increased signal intensity of prostate lesions on high b-value diffusion-weighted images as a predictive sign of malignancy. Eur Radiol. 2014;24(1):209–13. doi:10.1007/s00330-013-2999-3.
12. Onal C, Sonmez S, Erbay G, Guler OC, Arslan G. Simultaneous integrated boost to intraprostatic lesions using different energy levels of intensity-modulated radiotherapy and volumetric-arc therapy. Br J Radiol. 2014;87(1034):20130617. doi:10.1259/bjr.20130617.
13. Wu LM, Xu JR, Ye YQ, Lu Q, Hu JN. The clinical value of diffusion-weighted imaging in combination with T2-weighted imaging in diagnosing prostate carcinoma: a systematic review and meta-analysis. AJR Am J Roentgenol. 2012;199(1):103–10. doi:10.2214/AJR.11.7634.
14. Thormer G, Otto J, Horn LC, Garnov N, Do M, Franz T, et al. Non-invasive estimation of prostate cancer aggressiveness using diffusion-weighted MRI and 3D proton MR spectroscopy at 3.0 T. Acta Radiol. 2015;56(1):121–8. doi:10.1177/0284185113520311.
15. Onal C, Guler OC, Reyhan M, Yapar AF. Prognostic value of 18F-fluorodeoxyglucose uptake in pelvic lymph nodes in patients with cervical cancer treated with definitive chemoradiotherapy. Gynecol Oncol. 2015;137(1):40–6. doi:10.1016/j.ygyno.2015.01.542.
16. Madsen PH, Holdgaard PC, Christensen JB, Hoilund-Carlsen PF. Clinical utility of F-18 FDG PET-CT in the initial evaluation of lung cancer. Eur J Nucl Med Mol Imaging. 2016;43(11):2084–97. doi:10.1007/s00259-016-3407-4.
17. Engert A, Raemaekers J. Treatment of early-stage Hodgkin lymphoma. Semin Hematol. 2016;53(3):165–70. doi:10.1053/j.seminhematol.2016.05.004.
18. Onal C, Torun N, Guler OC, Yildirim BA. Prognostic value of metabolic response measured by 18F-FDG-PET in oesophageal cancer patients treated with definitive chemoradiotherapy. Nucl Med Commun. 2016;37(12):1282–9. doi:10.1097/MNM.0000000000000594.
19. Onal C, Reyhan M, Parlak C, Guler OC, Oymak E. Prognostic value of pretreatment 18F-fluorodeoxyglucose uptake in patients with cervical cancer treated with definitive chemoradiotherapy. Int J Gynecol Cancer. 2013;23(6):1104–10. doi:10.1097/IGC.0b013e3182989483.
20. Evangelista L, Briganti A, Fanti S, Joniau S, Reske S, Schiavina R, et al. New clinical indications for (18)F/(11)C-choline, new tracers for positron emission tomography and a promising

hybrid device for prostate cancer staging: a systematic review of the literature. Eur Urol. 2016;70(1):161–75. doi:10.1016/j.eururo.2016.01.029.

21. Mamede M, Ceci F, Castellucci P, Schiavina R, Fuccio C, Nanni C, et al. The role of 11C-choline PET imaging in the early detection of recurrence in surgically treated prostate cancer patients with very low PSA level <0.5 ng/mL. Clin Nucl Med. 2013;38(9):e342–5. doi:10.1097/RLU.0b013e31829af913.
22. Mease RC, Foss CA, Pomper MG. PET imaging in prostate cancer: focus on prostate-specific membrane antigen. Curr Top Med Chem. 2013;13(8):951–62.
23. Afshar-Oromieh A, Avtzi E, Giesel FL, Holland-Letz T, Linhart HG, Eder M, et al. The diagnostic value of PET/CT imaging with the (68)Ga-labelled PSMA ligand HBED-CC in the diagnosis of recurrent prostate cancer. Eur J Nucl Med Mol Imaging. 2015;42(2):197–209. doi:10.1007/s00259-014-2949-6.
24. Eiber M, Maurer T, Souvatzoglou M, Beer AJ, Ruffani A, Haller B, et al. Evaluation of hybrid (6)(8)Ga-PSMA ligand PET/CT in 248 patients with biochemical recurrence after radical prostatectomy. J Nucl Med. 2015;56(5):668–74. doi:10.2967/jnumed.115.154153.
25. Palma D, Vollans E, James K, Nakano S, Moiseenko V, Shaffer R, et al. Volumetric modulated arc therapy for delivery of prostate radiotherapy: comparison with intensity-modulated radiotherapy and three-dimensional conformal radiotherapy. Int J Radiat Oncol Biol Phys. 2008;72(4):996–1001. doi:10.1016/j.ijrobp.2008.02.047.
26. Hall EJ, Wuu CS. Radiation-induced second cancers: the impact of 3D-CRT and IMRT. Int J Radiat Oncol Biol Phys. 2003;56(1):83–8.
27. Pardo-Montero J, Fenwick JD. An approach to multiobjective optimization of rotational therapy. Med Phys. 2009;36(7):3292–303. doi:10.1118/1.3151806.
28. Onal C, Arslan G, Parlak C, Sonmez S. Comparison of IMRT and VMAT plans with different energy levels using Monte-Carlo algorithm for prostate cancer. Jpn J Radiol. 2014;32(4):224–32. doi:10.1007/s11604-014-0291-3.
29. Wolff D, Stieler F, Welzel G, Lorenz F, Abo-Madyan Y, Mai S, et al. Volumetric modulated arc therapy (VMAT) vs. serial tomotherapy, step-and-shoot IMRT and 3D-conformal RT for treatment of prostate cancer. Radiother Oncol. 2009;93(2):226–33. doi:10.1016/j.radonc.2009.08.011.
30. Tsai CL, Wu JK, Chao HL, Tsai YC, Cheng JC. Treatment and dosimetric advantages between VMAT, IMRT, and helical tomotherapy in prostate cancer. Med Dosim. 2011;36(3):264–71. doi:10.1016/j.meddos.2010.05.001.
31. Chen M, Hricak H, Kalbhen CL, Kurhanewicz J, Vigneron DB, Weiss JM, et al. Hormonal ablation of prostatic cancer: effects on prostate morphology, tumor detection, and staging by endorectal coil MR imaging. AJR Am J Roentgenol. 1996;166(5):1157–63. doi:10.2214/ajr.166.5.8615261.
32. Fonteyne V, Villeirs G, Speleers B, De Neve W, De Wagter C, Lumen N, et al. Intensity-modulated radiotherapy as primary therapy for prostate cancer: report on acute toxicity after dose escalation with simultaneous integrated boost to intraprostatic lesion. Int J Radiat Oncol Biol Phys. 2008;72(3):799–807. doi:10.1016/j.ijrobp.2008.01.040.
33. Sale C, Moloney P. Dose comparisons for conformal, IMRT and VMAT prostate plans. J Med Imaging Radiat Oncol. 2011;55(6):611–21. doi:10.1111/j.1754-9485.2011.02310.x.
34. Zhang P, Happersett L, Hunt M, Jackson A, Zelefsky M, Mageras G. Volumetric modulated arc therapy: planning and evaluation for prostate cancer cases. Int J Radiat Oncol Biol Phys. 2010;76(5):1456–62. doi:10.1016/j.ijrobp.2009.03.033.
35. Rao M, Yang W, Chen F, Sheng K, Ye J, Mehta V, et al. Comparison of Elekta VMAT with helical tomotherapy and fixed field IMRT: plan quality, delivery efficiency and accuracy. Med Phys. 2010;37(3):1350–9. doi:10.1118/1.3326965.
36. Hardcastle N, Tome WA, Foo K, Miller A, Carolan M, Metcalfe P. Comparison of prostate IMRT and VMAT biologically optimised treatment plans. Med Dosim. 2011;36(3):292–8. doi:10.1016/j.meddos.2010.06.001.
37. Sze HC, Lee MC, Hung WM, Yau TK, Lee AW. RapidArc radiotherapy planning for prostate cancer: single-arc and double-arc techniques vs. intensity-modulated radiotherapy. Med Dosim. 2012;37(1):87–91. doi:10.1016/j.meddos.2011.01.005.

38. Fontenot JD, King ML, Johnson SA, Wood CG, Price MJ, Lo KK. Single-arc volumetric-modulated arc therapy can provide dose distributions equivalent to fixed-beam intensity-modulated radiation therapy for prostatic irradiation with seminal vesicle and/or lymph node involvement. Br J Radiol. 2012;85(1011):231–6. doi:10.1259/bjr/94843998.
39. Yildirim BA, Onal C, Dolek Y. Is it essential to use fiducial markers during cone-beam CT-based radiotherapy for prostate cancer patients? Jpn J Radiol. 2017;35(1):3–9. doi:10.1007/s11604-016-0590-y.
40. Onal C, Topkan E, Efe E, Yavuz M, Arslan G, Yavuz A. The effect of concurrent androgen deprivation and 3D conformal radiotherapy on prostate volume and clinical organ doses during treatment for prostate cancer. Br J Radiol. 2009;82(984):1019–26. doi:10.1259/bjr/65939531.
41. Gregoire V, Mackie TR. State of the art on dose prescription, reporting and recording in intensity-modulated radiation therapy (ICRU report no. 83). Cancer Radiother. 2011;15(6–7):555–9. doi:10.1016/j.canrad.2011.04.003.
42. Cellini N, Morganti AG, Mattiucci GC, Valentini V, Leone M, Luzi S, et al. Analysis of intraprostatic failures in patients treated with hormonal therapy and radiotherapy: implications for conformal therapy planning. Int J Radiat Oncol Biol Phys. 2002;53(3):595–9.
43. Geier M, Astner ST, Duma MN, Jacob V, Nieder C, Putzhammer J, et al. Dose-escalated simultaneous integrated-boost treatment of prostate cancer patients via helical tomotherapy. Strahlenther Onkol. 2012;188(5):410–6. doi:10.1007/s00066-012-0081-8.
44. Morgan PB, Hanlon AL, Horwitz EM, Buyyounouski MK, Uzzo RG, Pollack A. Radiation dose and late failures in prostate cancer. Int J Radiat Oncol Biol Phys. 2007;67(4):1074–81. doi:10.1016/j.ijrobp.2006.10.023.
45. Ishii K, Ogino R, Okada W, Nakahara R, Kawamorita R, Nakajima T. A dosimetric comparison of RapidArc and IMRT with hypofractionated simultaneous integrated boost to the prostate for treatment of prostate cancer. Br J Radiol. 2013;86(1030):20130199. doi:10.1259/bjr.20130199.
46. Ost P, Speleers B, De Meerleer G, De Neve W, Fonteyne V, Villeirs G, et al. Volumetric arc therapy and intensity-modulated radiotherapy for primary prostate radiotherapy with simultaneous integrated boost to intraprostatic lesion with 6 and 18 MV: a planning comparison study. Int J Radiat Oncol Biol Phys. 2011;79(3):920–6. doi:10.1016/j.ijrobp.2010.04.025.
47. Pinkawa M, Attieh C, Piroth MD, Holy R, Nussen S, Klotz J, et al. Dose-escalation using intensity-modulated radiotherapy for prostate cancer—evaluation of the dose distribution with and without 18F-choline PET-CT detected simultaneous integrated boost. Radiother Oncol. 2009;93(2):213–9. doi:10.1016/j.radonc.2009.07.014.
48. von Eyben FE, Kiljunen T, Kangasmaki A, Kairemo K, von Eyben R, Joensuu T. Radiotherapy boost for the dominant intraprostatic cancer lesion-a systematic review and meta-analysis. Clin Genitourin Cancer. 2016;14(3):189–97. doi:10.1016/j.clgc.2015.12.005.
49. Lips IM, van der Heide UA, Haustermans K, van Lin EN, Pos F, Franken SP, et al. Single blind randomized phase III trial to investigate the benefit of a focal lesion ablative microboost in prostate cancer (FLAME-trial): study protocol for a randomized controlled trial. Trials. 2011;12:255. doi:10.1186/1745-6215-12-255.
50. Fowler JF, Ritter MA, Chappell RJ, Brenner DJ. What hypofractionated protocols should be tested for prostate cancer? Int J Radiat Oncol Biol Phys. 2003;56(4):1093–104.
51. Lee WR. Extreme hypofractionation for prostate cancer. Expert Rev Anticancer Ther. 2009;9(1):61–5. doi:10.1586/14737140.9.1.61.
52. Magnuson WJ, Mahal A, Yu JB. Emerging technologies and techniques in radiation therapy. Semin Radiat Oncol. 2017;27(1):34–42. doi:10.1016/j.semradonc.2016.08.004.
53. Pollack A, Walker G, Horwitz EM, Price R, Feigenberg S, Konski AA, et al. Randomized trial of hypofractionated external-beam radiotherapy for prostate cancer. J Clin Oncol. 2013;31(31):3860–8. doi:10.1200/JCO.2013.51.1972.
54. Zumsteg ZS, Spratt DE, Romesser PB, Pei X, Zhang Z, Kollmeier M, et al. Anatomical patterns of recurrence following biochemical relapse in the dose escalation era of external beam radiotherapy for prostate cancer. J Urol. 2015;194(6):1624–30. doi:10.1016/j.juro.2015.06.100.

55. QJ W, Li T, Yuan L, Yin FF, Lee WR. Single institution's dosimetry and IGRT analysis of prostate SBRT. Radiat Oncol. 2013;8:215. doi:10.1186/1748-717X-8-215.
56. Heidenreich A, Bastian PJ, Bellmunt J, Bolla M, Joniau S, van der Kwast T, et al. EAU guidelines on prostate cancer. Part 1: screening, diagnosis, and local treatment with curative intent-update 2013. Eur Urol. 2014;65(1):124–37. doi:10.1016/j.eururo.2013.09.046.
57. Mendenhall NP, Hoppe BS, Nichols RC, Mendenhall WM, Morris CG, Li Z, et al. Five-year outcomes from 3 prospective trials of image-guided proton therapy for prostate cancer. Int J Radiat Oncol Biol Phys. 2014;88(3):596–602. doi:10.1016/j.ijrobp.2013.11.007.
58. Grimm P, Billiet I, Bostwick D, Dicker AP, Frank S, Immerzeel J, et al. Comparative analysis of prostate-specific antigen free survival outcomes for patients with low, intermediate and high risk prostate cancer treatment by radical therapy. Results from the prostate cancer results study group. BJU Int. 2012;109(Suppl 1):22–9. doi:10.1111/j.1464-410X.2011.10827.x.
59. Slater JD, Rossi CJ Jr, Yonemoto LT, Bush DA, Jabola BR, Levy RP, et al. Proton therapy for prostate cancer: the initial Loma Linda University experience. Int J Radiat Oncol Biol Phys. 2004;59(2):348–52. doi:10.1016/j.ijrobp.2003.10.011.
60. Shipley WU, Verhey LJ, Munzenrider JE, Suit HD, Urie MM, McManus PL, et al. Advanced prostate cancer: the results of a randomized comparative trial of high dose irradiation boosting with conformal protons compared with conventional dose irradiation using photons alone. Int J Radiat Oncol Biol Phys. 1995;32(1):3–12. doi:10.1016/0360-3016(95)00063-5.
61. Yonemoto LT, Slater JD, Rossi CJ Jr, Antoine JE, Loredo L, Archambeau JO, et al. Combined proton and photon conformal radiation therapy for locally advanced carcinoma of the prostate: preliminary results of a phase I/II study. Int J Radiat Oncol Biol Phys. 1997;37(1):21–9.
62. Bryant C, Smith TL, Henderson RH, Hoppe BS, Mendenhall WM, Nichols RC, et al. Five-year biochemical results, toxicity, and patient-reported quality of life after delivery of dose-escalated image guided proton therapy for prostate cancer. Int J Radiat Oncol Biol Phys. 2016;95(1):422–34. doi:10.1016/j.ijrobp.2016.02.038.
63. Giannarini G, Gandaglia G, Montorsi F, Briganti A. Will focal therapy remain only an attractive illusion for the primary treatment of prostate cancer? J Clin Oncol. 2014;32(13):1299–301. doi:10.1200/JCO.2013.54.8214.
64. Bahn D, de Castro Abreu AL, Gill IS, Hung AJ, Silverman P, Gross ME, et al. Focal cryotherapy for clinically unilateral, low-intermediate risk prostate cancer in 73 men with a median follow-up of 3.7 years. Eur Urol. 2012;62(1):55–63. doi:10.1016/j.eururo.2012.03.006.
65. Duijzentkunst DA, Peters M, van der Voort van Zyp JR, Moerland MA, van Vulpen M. Focal salvage therapy for local prostate cancer recurrences after primary radiotherapy: a comprehensive review. World J Urol. 2016;34(11):1521–31. doi:10.1007/s00345-016-1811-9.
66. Chin JL. Editorial comment. J Urol. 2013;190(2):710. doi:10.1016/j.juro.2013.02.3238.
67. Gardner TA. Editorial comment. J Urol. 2013;190(2):710. doi:10.1016/j.juro.2013.02.3239.
68. Koch MO, Gardner T, Cheng L, Fedewa RJ, Seip R, Sanghvi NT. Phase I/II trial of high intensity focused ultrasound for the treatment of previously untreated localized prostate cancer. J Urol. 2007;178(6):2366–70; discussion 70–1. doi:10.1016/j.juro.2007.08.014.

Adjuvant or Salvage Radiotherapy in Postoperative Prostate Cancer

17

Ugur Selek, Yasemin Bolukbasi, and Deborah A. Kuban

Abstract

Prostate-specific antigen (PSA) screening increased the diagnosis of prostate cancer at a localized stage to be treated with a curative intent; approximately half of them undergo radical prostatectomy, and roughly one third of surgically treated patients are expected to experience a recurrence in 10 years' follow-up. Once PSA failure occurs, many develop distant metastases at a median of 8 years and afterward followed by cancer-related death at a median of 5 years. Biochemical failure risk after radical prostatectomy is mainly expected mostly in men with any of the following features: detectable postoperative PSA, positive surgical margins, extraprostatic extension of tumor (T3a), seminal vesicle invasion (T3b), and Gleason score ≥ 8. The radiotherapy in the undetectable PSA environment (<0.01 ng/mL) within 4 months after prostatectomy is termed as "adjuvant," while radiotherapy in rising PSA within any time after prostatectomy is defined as "salvage."

17.1 Introduction

Prostate cancer is the most frequent malignancy in males and a major cause of cancer-related mortality [1, 2]. Prostate-specific antigen (PSA) screening increased the diagnosis of prostate cancer at a localized stage and, therefore, treatment with a

U. Selek, M.D. • Y. Bolukbasi, M.D.
Department of Radiation Oncology, Koc University, Istanbul, Turkey

Department of Radiation Oncology, The University of Texas, MD Anderson Cancer Center, Houston, TX, USA

D.A. Kuban, M.D., F.A.C.R., F.A.S.T.R.O. (✉)
Department of Radiation Oncology, The University of Texas, MD Anderson Cancer Center, Houston, TX, USA
e-mail: dakuban@mdanderson.org

G. Ozyigit, U. Selek (eds.), *Principles and Practice of Urooncology*,
DOI 10.1007/978-3-319-56114-1_17

curative intent. Approximately half of the men with localized disease undergo radical prostatectomy, and roughly one third of these are expected to experience a recurrence within 10 years' time [3, 4]. Once PSA failure occurs, the median time to distant metastasis is 8 years followed by prostate cancer-related death at a median of 5 years [5]. Biochemical failure risk after radical prostatectomy increases with the following features: detectable postoperative PSA, positive surgical margins, extraprostatic extension of tumor (T3a), seminal vesicle invasion (T3b), and Gleason score ≥ 8 [3, 6, 7]. Postoperative radiotherapy with undetectable PSA (<0.1 ng/mL) within 4 months of surgery is defined as "adjuvant," while radiotherapy for rising PSA at any point after prostatectomy is referred to as "salvage."

There have been ongoing arguments as to whether patients with unfavorable disease features benefit from adjuvant therapy and as to when the window of opportunity for salvage treatment is greatest. The American Society of Clinical Oncology Clinical Practice Guideline Endorsement in 2014 sought to clarify the confusion on four fundamentals: patient counseling, adjuvant versus salvage radiotherapy settings, an acceptable definition of biochemical recurrence, and the restaging evaluation [8].

The preference for salvage radiotherapy is based on allowing enough time for post-prostatectomy urinary and erectile function recovery, avoiding potentially unnecessary radiotherapy in a large group of patients and avoiding radiotherapy-related toxicity. Accumulation of retrospective knowledge from prostatectomy series has provided patterns of relapse and valuable information by which to define patients at high risk of recurrence in order to rationalize therapeutic measures [5, 9, 10]. A recent update of the Stephenson nomogram by Tendulkar et al. has been published on multi-institutional outcomes for salvage radiotherapy (SRT) derived from 2460 node-negative patients with a detectable post-RP PSA treated with SRT with or without concurrent androgen-deprivation therapy (ADT) with a median follow-up of 5 years [11]. Overall, the pathologic features of positive surgical margins (58%), extraprostatic tumor extension (T3a, 56%), seminal vesicle invasion (T3b, 18%), Gleason score (76%: 7, 56%; 8, 10%; 9–10, 9%), and pre-radiation PSA levels were significantly associated with biochemical failure-free survival at 5 years after treatment.

Most of the biopsy-proven biochemical failures occur in the prostate or seminal vesicle bed [12, 13]. Connolly et al. analyzed the characteristics of local recurrence after radical prostatectomy in 114 patients with an elevated PSA and a negative bone scan using ultrasound-guided prostate fossa biopsies. The authors concluded that the majority of the recurrences were at the anastomosis (66%), the bladder neck (16%), and posterior to the trigone (13%) [12]. Furthermore, the examination of pathological details demonstrated that local recurrences are associated with organ-confined disease just 20% of the time but with positive surgical margins in 66% of patients. (Leventis et al. also evaluated the accuracy of transrectal ultrasonography-guided prostatic fossa biopsy in the detection of local recurrence in their 99 patients with biochemical recurrence after radical prostatectomy [13]; they revealed positive biopsies in more than half of the suspected lesions at the urethrovesical anastomotic area and bladder neck in addition to rare lesions in the retrovesical space.) Instead of this reference which basically says that + bx is 50/50, you may want to quote the reference from MDA—Jingya Wang—Practical Radiation Oncology which looks at the location of bx-proven local recurrences on MRI and creates a map. This would go along with the Connolly reference above.

In the Johns Hopkins Hospital radical prostatectomy series of 1997 patients operated on between 1982 and 1997, 15% of the cohort recurred mainly in the first 5 years after prostatectomy and 34% with metastatic disease [5]. Three key pathologic and clinical factors delineated those likely to develop metastases: Gleason scores of 8–10, ≤2 years' time to PSA recurrence, and ≤10 months PSA doubling time (PSADT). This study led to the clinical question as to whether a therapeutic salvage intervention might decrease the risk of metastases in these patients [9, 10]. Stephenson et al. retrospectively reviewed 501 salvage radiotherapy patients treated between 1987 and 2002 at five US academic centers and concluded that in multivariate analysis, poor response after salvage radiotherapy was directly related to these prognostic predictors of progression: Gleason score (8–10, hazard ratio [HR], 2.6), pre-radiotherapy PSA level (>2.0 ng/mL,HR, 2.3), surgical margins (negative margins, HR, 1.9), PSADT (10 months or less, HR, 1.7), and seminal vesicle invasion (HR, 1.4) [9]. Progression-free probability (PFP) of patients without adverse features was 77% at 4 years, treatment of early recurrence (PSA level ≤ 2.0 ng/mL) documented PFP of 64% for positive surgical margins and of 22% for negative margins in patients with Gleason scores ≤7 and a rapid PSADT, and PFP of 81% for longer PSADT and of 37% for shorter PSADT in patients with Gleason scores of ≥8 and positive margins [9].

Trock et al. retrospectively studied a cohort of 635 biochemically recurrent patients who had radical prostatectomy between 1982 and 2004; 397 patients had no salvage treatment, 160 were treated with radiotherapy alone, and 78 had radiotherapy plus hormonal therapy [10]. Salvage radiotherapy alone was shown to improve cancer-specific survival (PCSS) threefold (HR, 0.32) in comparison to no salvage treatment, while no benefit for adding hormonal therapy to radiotherapy was detected. The patients with improved PCSS after salvage radiotherapy had PSADT <6 months which remained significant in multivariate analysis. Delayed salvage radiotherapy, more than 2 years after recurrence, did not provide any benefit in PCSS in this cohort. Likewise, patients whose PSA did not become undetectable after salvage radiotherapy had no survival gain. In Duke cohort of 519 patients with biochemical failure after prostatectomy analyzed by Cotter et al., salvage radiotherapy was significantly associated with longer overall survival both in PSADT of <6 months and ≥6 months [14].

Since retrospective data points to the frequent need for salvage radiation in patients with high-risk features, prospective data would be helpful in determining who would benefit most from adjuvant radiotherapy. Three prospective randomized clinical trials, Southwest Oncology Group (SWOG) 8794, European Organization for Research and Treatment of Cancer (EORTC) 22,911, and Arbeitsgemeinschaft Radiologische Onkologie (ARO) 9602, have been published comparing adjuvant postoperative RT versus observation in radical prostatectomy patients who had adverse pathologic features: positive margins, extracapsular extension, or seminal vesicular invasion [15–21]. These publications led to the joint guidelines of both the American Society for Radiation Oncology (ASTRO) and the American Urological Association (AUA) which encourage consideration of adjuvant radiotherapy in case of these adverse pathologic findings and also salvage radiotherapy in patients with post-prostatectomy PSA recurrence or local recurrence without distant metastasis [3, 22].

17.2 Randomized Adjuvant Radiotherapy Trials

All three adjuvant radiotherapy randomized trials treated intermediate or high-risk disease patients delivering radiotherapy to the prostatic fossa encompassing the vesicourethral anastomosis, the bladder neck, and the area posterior to the trigone, with 60 Gy in 30 fractions (64 Gy allowed in SWOG 8794). Primary end points varied: metastasis-free survival in SWOG, local control, and clinical progression-free survival in EORTC 22911 and progression-free survival in ARO. All now have long-term follow-up, >9 years. The most recent trial, ARO 9602 (307 patients), did not allow accrual of patients with detectable PSA at the time of postoperative RT as did SWOG 8794 (425 patients) and EORTC 22911 (1005 patients) [15–18]. Approximately one third of patients in SWOG 8794 and one out of eight to ten patients in EORTC 22911 had a pre-radiation PSA ≥ 0.2 ng/mL, while ARO 9602 only included patients with "undetectable PSA" values <0.1 ng/mL [19–21]. The treatment technique was conventional RT with three or four fields in SWOG 8794 (between 1988 and 1997) and EORTC 22911 (between 1992 and 2001), while 3D-CRT planning was done in ARO 9602 (between 1997 and 2004).

Thompson et al. reported on SWOG 8794 [15, 16] with a median follow-up of more than 12 years in the most recent publication showing a significant improvement at 10 years with postoperative radiotherapy in comparison to observation alone in overall survival (74% vs. 66%; HR 0.72; $p = 0.023$) and in metastasis-free survival (71% vs. 61%; HR 0.71; $p = 0.016$). Freedom from biochemical failure (absence of a rise in PSA to >0.4 ng/mL) at 5 years was also improved significantly with postoperative radiotherapy (70% vs. 45%). Salvage hormonal therapy was given to 21% of patients in the observation arm and to only 10% in the radiotherapy arm, whereas salvage radiotherapy was applied after failure to 33% of patients in the observation arm such that some say this was actually a comparison of early versus late radiation. The reported toxicity in the SWOG trial was 11.9% in the observation arm (urethral strictures, 9.5%; total urinary incontinence, 2.8%) and 23.8% in the treatment arm (rectal, 3.3%; urethral strictures, 17.8%, RR 1.9, $p = 0.02$; total urinary incontinence, 6.5%, RR 2.3, $p = 0.11$).

Bolla et al. published EORTC 22911 [17, 18] noting a significant improvement at 10 years in biochemical progression-free survival (absence of a rise in PSA of >0.2 ng/mL over post-radiotherapy nadir), 60.6% vs. 41.1%, HR 0.49; $p < 0.0001$, in locoregional control (cumulative relapse rate, 7.3% vs. 16.6%, HR 0.45; $p < 0.0001$), and in distant metastases-free survival (cumulative metastasis rate, 10.1% vs. 11.0%, HR 0.99; $p = 0.94$). No significant difference in 10 year in OS was seen (76.9% vs. 80.7%, HR 1.18; $p = 0.2024$), and there was no difference in prostate cancer-specific mortality rates (3.9% vs. 5.4%, HR 0.78; $p = 0.3407$). One third of the patients in observation arm were salvaged with radiotherapy, while salvage hormonal therapy rates at 5 years were 10.1% in the radiotherapy arm and 15.5% in observation arm. Toxicity in the EORTC trial was higher as expected in postoperative RT arm (cumulative any-grade toxicity, 70.8% vs. 59.7%, $p = 0.001$). Most toxicities were grades 1–2, and none were grade 4. Grade 3 toxicity at 10 years with postoperative radiotherapy was 5.3% in comparison to 2.5% in the observation arm ($p = 0.052$).

ARO 9602 [19–21] showed a significant improvement for adjuvant radiation in 10 year progression-free survival (progression defined as two consecutive PSA rises), 56% vs. 35%, $p < 0.0001$, but no significant difference in metastasis-free or overall survival as SWOG 8794 did. There was a third reported arm in the ARO study which was excluded from randomization: 74 patients with persistent PSA (median 0.6, range 0.05–5.6 ng/mL) after prostatectomy. These patients received 66 Gy to the prostate bed at a median of 86 days after surgery [20]. In comparison to patients with an undetectable PSA, this group had significantly worse outcomes with a poorer 10 year metastasis-free survival (67% vs. 83%) and overall survival (68% vs. 84%). For the randomized patients, multivariate Cox regression analysis defined risk factors for progression as Gleason score ≥ 8 (HR 2.8), pT ≥ 3c (HR 2.4), and extraprostatic extension ≥2 mm (HR 3.6). ARO 9602 reported that there was no grade 4 acute toxicity and very low grade 3 acute toxicity associated with radiotherapy (single event bladder toxicity, 1/148 0.7%) and higher but acceptable late grade 1–2 toxicity with radiotherapy (late grade 1–2 genitourinary toxicity: 15.5% vs. 2.5%; late grade 1–2 gastrointestinal toxicity: 10.8% vs. 3.1%).

In summary, the SWOG trial asserted that adjuvant radiation reduced metastases and improved overall survival, although the other two trials, EORTC and ARO, with roughly 10 years of follow-up, revealed no such benefit in either end point. The SWOG study critics make the argument that a significant number of patients in the observation arm received later, salvage radiotherapy when the median PSA was >1 ng/mL and that this may have served to decrease the survival difference between the two randomized groups. Ongoing trials will answer the question whether early radiation for rising PSA is equivalent to adjuvant radiation: RADICALS (radiotherapy and androgen deprivation in combination after local surgery) [23], RAVES (radiotherapy–adjuvant versus early salvage) [24, 25], and GETUG-17 (Groupe d' Étude des Tumeurs Uro-Génitales) [26].

17.3 Nomograms and Systematic Reviews

Stephenson et al. retrospectively studied the outcomes with salvage radiotherapy in a multi-institutional cohort of 501 patients from five US academic centers [9]. In patients treated between 1987 and 2003 for detectable and rising PSA with a median follow-up of 45 months, the 4 year progression-free probability (PFP) was 77% if no adverse features were present in comparison to 45% for the entire cohort. Multivariable analysis defined the following predictors of progression as after radiation: Gleason score of ≥8 (HR, 2.6, $p < 0.001$), pre-radiotherapy PSA ≥2.0 ng/mL (HR, 2.3, $p < 0.001$), negative surgical margins (HR, 1.9, $p < 0.001$), PSA doubling time (PSADT) ≤10 months (HR, 1.7, $p = 0.001$), and seminal vesicle invasion (HR, 1.4, $p = 0.02$). Earlier salvage radiation in patients with PSA ≤2.0 ng/mL, Gleason score ≤ 7, and a rapid PSADT provided better PFP at 4 years, 64%, if surgical margins were positive as compared to negative, 22%. Earlier salvage radiation in patients with PSA ≤2.0 ng/mL, Gleason scores ≥8, and positive margins produced better PFP outcome at 4 years, 81%, if PSADT was >10 months as compared to ≤10 months, 37%.

Stephenson et al. updated their analysis in a multi-institutional cohort of 1540 patients using multivariable Cox regression analysis to construct a model to predict the disease progression probability after salvage radiation [27]. The resultant nomogram produced the following significant variables: PSA level before salvage radiation($p < 0.001$), prostatectomy Gleason score ($p < 0.001$), PSADT ($p < 0.001$), surgical margins ($p < 0.001$), androgen ablation before or during salvage radiotherapy ($p < 0.001$), and nodal disease ($p = 0.019$); the concordance index was 0.69. Salvage radiotherapy administered at the earliest sign of PSA recurrence seemed to provide a long-term PSA response in nearly half of the patients, while higher PSA levels at the time of salvage radiotherapy were found to be detrimental, and in fact PSA levels of ≥1.25 ng/mL carried a high risk of pathologic nodal metastasis [27].

King et al. also studied the timing of salvage radiotherapy in their systematic review of 41 studies containing 5597 patients in order to define the factors associated with relapse-free survival (RFS) [28]. Importantly, PSA level before salvage radiotherapy ($p < 0.0001$) as well as radiotherapy dose ($p = 0.0052$) was found to be significantly and independently associated with RFS with an average 2.6% loss in RFS for each incremental 0.1 ng/mL PSA increase prior to salvage radiotherapy. The authors noted that a PSA level of ≤0.2 ng/mL would ensure RFS of approximately 64%. Additionally, although less robust on sensitivity analysis, the salvage radiotherapy dose was important and defined by a sigmoidal dose-response curve which showed a 2% per Gy incremental improvement in RFS such that the RFS was 54% with a dose of 70 Gy but 34% with a dose of 60 Gy. This publication encouraged initiating salvage radiotherapy at the lowest possible PSA level leading to the question of early salvage radiation being equivalent to adjuvant therapy [28]. Tendulkar et al. recently published a contemporary update of the Stephenson nomogram which included 2460 node-negative patients with a median follow-up of 5 years treated with salvage radiotherapy at ten academic institutions. This work also concluded that early salvage radiotherapy at low PSA levels, especially ≤0.2 ng/mL, was significantly associated with improved freedom from biochemical failure and distant metastasis [11].

Fossati et al. recently published a retrospective review of a multi-institutional cohort of 716 node-negative patients with undetectable PSA after radical prostatectomy who subsequently experienced a PSA rise and were salvaged with early radiotherapy to the prostate and seminal vesicle bed while the PSA was still ≤0.5 ng/mL [29]. Biochemical relapse-free survival at 5 years was 82%, and in multivariable Cox regression analysis, the pre-salvage radiotherapy PSA level was very significantly associated with biochemical relapse after salvage (HR: 4.89; $p < 0.0001$). When stratified according to the following three pathological risk factors, ≥pT3b, Gleason score ≥ 8, and negative surgical margins, each incremental 0.1 ng/mL of PSA rise increased the risk of PSA recurrence. At 5 years after treatment, patients with ≥2 risk factors had a PSA recurrence risk of 10% as compared to only 1.5% in patients with 0–1 factor. Salvage radiotherapy at the earliest PSA rise conferred better biochemical control in patients with more adverse pathologic features although the benefit of very early salvage radiotherapy was less evident with favorable disease at radical prostatectomy.

Another study emphasizing the importance of early salvage radiotherapy at low PSA levels by Mir et al. attempted to define the optimal definition of biochemical recurrence after radical prostatectomy in order to identify early salvage radiotherapy candidates [30]. 2348 patients with a detectable PSA of ≥0.03 ng/mL at least 6 weeks after radical prostatectomy were used to test 14 biochemical recurrence definitions: six standard and eight requiring one or more successive PSA rises ≤0.1 ng/mL [30]. The optimal PSA failure definitions were as follows based on discrimination and calibration analysis: a single PSA ≥0.05 ng/mL with two or more rising PSAs ≥0.05 ng/mL, PSA ≥0.2 ng/mL and rising, or PSA ≥0.4 ng/mL and rising associated with progression-free probability at 5 years of <50%, 50–75%, 76–90%, and >90%, respectively [30].

17.4 Genomic Classification

There is an ongoing search to identify candidates who would benefit most from adjuvant radiation therapy [31, 32], based on the development of metastatic disease after adjuvant versus salvage treatment [33, 34]. A genomic classifier (GC) which would provide predictive insight to aid in identifying patients who would have lower rates of developing systemic disease when treated adjuvantly was proposed by Den et al. [31]. GC scores calculated from 188 pT3 or margin-positive prostate cancer patients who received post-radical prostatectomy radiotherapy were analyzed with the primary end point of clinical metastasis. Patients with low GC scores (<0.4) demonstrated no difference in metastatic rate whether they received adjuvant or salvage radiotherapy; however, cumulative incidence of metastasis at 5 years was 6% with adjuvant RT versus 23% with salvage RT ($p < 0.01$) in patients with higher GC scores (≥0.4). The other important finding was the correlation of the PSA level with the incidence of metastasis in high GC score patients who were treated with salvage radiotherapy; there were no metastases in patients with a PSA level < 0.1 ng/mL at the time of treatment [31].

17.5 Androgen Deprivation in Adjuvant/Salvage Radiotherapy

Overall, single-institutional reports of post-radical prostatectomy radiotherapy have shown a significant improvement in biochemical and clinical relapse-free rates with the addition of androgen deprivation [35–39].

Ost et al. reported on 225 node-negative patients who received high-dose (>69 Gy) adjuvant radiotherapy to the prostate and seminal vesicle bed and were shown in multivariate analysis to benefit from the addition of androgen deprivation [39].

RTOG 9601 (NCT00002874) was designed as a phase III, randomized (antiandrogen therapy, AAT, $n = 387$ vs. placebo, $n = 383$), double-blinded study, to address the use of daily bicalutamide 150 mg with salvage radiotherapy to the prostate bed (64.8 Gy, 1.8 Gy/fraction) in patients who had radical prostatectomy with pT3 pN0 or pT2 pN0 with positive margins and subsequent PSA elevation to a level of

0.2–4.0 ng/mL [40]. Two years of bicalutamide daily during and after radiotherapy was shown to significantly improve freedom from biochemical progression and to reduce the incidence of metastatic disease [41]. Shipley et al. demonstrated a significant OS advantage at 10 years, 82% when AAT was added to radiation vs. 78% with placebo ($p = 0.036$). There was also significant benefit in freedom from PSA failure with AAT, 46% vs. 30% ($p < 0.001$), and significantly lower prostate cancer mortality and development of metastatic disease at 12 years. The problem with bicalutamide was the high rate of gynecomastia, 70%.

The other randomized trial which added hormonal therapy to salvage radiotherapy (66 Gy, 2 Gy/fraction to prostatic fossa, ± pelvic nodal radiotherapy) was Groupe d'Etudes des Tumeurs Uro-Génitales (GETUG)-16 trial (NCT00423475) which enrolled 369 patients with and 374 patients without hormonal therapy consisting of 6 months of goserelin [42]. The addition of goserelin improved progression-free survival (79.6% vs. 62.1%, $p < 0.0001$) at 5 years without significant overall survival benefit (96.2% vs. 94.8%, $p = 0.18$) and without difference in grade 3 acute and late toxicities.

RTOG 0534 (NCT00567580) was designed to address the use of androgen deprivation therapy with salvage postoperative radiotherapy (64.8–70.2 Gy, 1.8 Gy/fraction/day to the prostate/seminal vesicle bed ± flutamide t.i.d or bicalutamide q.d. plus a luteinizing hormone-releasing hormone (LHRH) agonist starting 2 months prior to radiotherapy for a total of 4–6 months). In 2015, the trial completed the enrollment of 1792 patients with pT2–3N0M0 R0 or R1 after prostatectomy and a PSA of 0.1–2.0 ng/mL at least 6 weeks after surgery. RTOG 0534 also enrolled patients to a third arm of whole pelvis radiotherapy (45 Gy, 1.8 Gy/fraction/day) with cone-down radiotherapy to the prostate bed (total of 64.8–70.2 Gy) in combination with the antiandrogen.

The RADICALS trial (radiotherapy and androgen deprivation in combination after local surgery, initiated in 2007; NCT00541047; Medical Research Council MRC PR10) is enrolling patients with at least one of the four adverse features of pT3/4, Gleason score 7–10, preoperative PSA ≥10 ng/mL, or R1 resection aiming to investigate the role of androgen deprivation (none, 6 months short-term GnRH agonist, or 24 months long-term GnRH agonist; 3 weeks antiandrogen initiated a week prior to GnRH agonist) and the timing of radiotherapy (early or deferred; 66 Gy, 2 Gy/fraction/day, or 52.5 Gy, 2.625 Gy/fraction/day; pelvic nodes at the discretion of the treating physician) [23]. The radiotherapy timing portion of RADICALS trial is ongoing (target enrollment, 2500), while the hormonal therapy accrual has been completed. A very similar study initiated by EORTC (EORTC 22043–30,041; NCT00949962) for adjuvant versus early salvage radiotherapy with or without hormonal therapy had poor accrual and was closed early. A phase III randomized controlled trial, RAVES 08–03, initiated and led by the Trans Tasman Radiation Oncology Group (TROG) is enrolling post-prostatectomy patients with pT3 (extraprostatic extension +/− seminal vesicle involvement) and/or positive surgical margins and will be analyzing biochemical failure with observation with early salvage radiotherapy, triggered by a PSA level > 0.20 ng/mL, versus adjuvant radiotherapy immediately after surgery [24, 25].

17.6 Postoperative Radiation Target and Dose

RTOG has generated an expert consensus guideline atlas for delineation of the clinical target volume (CTV) for postoperative radiotherapy in the adjuvant or salvage setting [43, 44]. It is recommended that the CTV encompasses the caudal vas deferens remnant superiorly which is estimated to extend 3 or 4 cm above the top of the pubic symphysis, at least 8–12 mm below the vesicourethral anastomosis inferiorly, the pubic symphysis anteriorly, 1–2 cm of the bladder wall above the pubic symphysis, and the anterior rectal wall posteriorly. The lateral borders are bounded by the anatomic barriers of the bilateral levator ani and obturator internus muscles inferiorly and the sacrorectogenitopubic fascia superiorly [43]. The RTOG template is important for standardization, while patient-specific individualization also plays an important role in tailoring treatment to the patients' pathologic findings and imaging.

Croke et al. proposed guidelines to delineate post-prostatectomy target volumes based upon the patient's co-registered preoperative MRI and concluded that using MRI may improve coverage of the individual's prostate bed by sparing more anterior lower bladder wall and ensuring better coverage of the superior lateral bladder walls in comparison to basic RTOG guidelines without significant increase in the PTV size or dose to the bladder/rectum [45]. Wang et al. delineated the common areas of recurrence post-prostatectomy on individual MRI images which were then mapped onto a "template" MRI image which served to demonstrate the areas which should be carefully contoured in postoperative patients undergoing adjuvant or salvage radiation [46]. The authors noted that target volumes using RTOG consensus could result in marginal coverage on posterolateral recurrences near the rectum and mesorectal fascia and also in inadequate coverage on recurrences very inferiorly located at the posterior urogenital diaphragm [46]. Current diagnostic evolution with MRI along with newer techniques with 68 Ga-prostate-specific membranous antigen (PSMA), NA Fl, and choline PET-CT is demonstrating higher detection rates of prostate cancer recurrence outside the prostatic fossa in some patients [47]. This will likely aid in the selection of the best candidates for postoperative radiation.

It has been concluded from several studies that postoperative radiotherapy is more effective at lower as compared to higher PSA levels and likely most effective at the earliest PSA rise or in the adjuvant setting. This of course is thought to relate the PSA level to disease burden [9, 11, 36, 48, 49]. Ohri et al. pointed out that the therapeutic ratio for postoperative radiotherapy seems to be improved by initiating treatment at low PSA levels and by applying appropriately high doses [48]. The dose response of salvage radiotherapy has also been noted in the previous and latest reports by King et al. (28) [50]. Although the randomized adjuvant radiation trials used doses in the 60–64 Gy range with conventional fractionation, subsequent analyses and general consensus in designing current cooperative group trials now accept doses in the range of 64–66 Gy for adjuvant and 70 Gy for salvage radiation as standard levels with conventional fractionation [28, 48, 50, 51]. Improvement in radiation techniques has allowed the increase in dose with less or similar toxicity.

Radiation has been shown to modestly add to surgical toxicity, gastrointestinal and genitourinary events, in the postoperative setting [17, 18, 21, 51]. It has been questioned whether earlier radiation therapy is in fact associated with higher morbidity. In this regard, the recent Surveillance, Epidemiology, and End Results (SEER)—Medicare database study by Hegarty et al. identified 6137 patients with one or more adverse pathological features after prostatectomy (prostatectomy alone, 4509; with adjuvant radiotherapy, 894; salvage radiotherapy, 734) and showed that earlier treatment with adjuvant radiotherapy was not associated with increased rates of genitourinary or erectile dysfunction in comparison to delayed salvage radiotherapy in adjusted models [51]. However, SEER data lacked detailed information such as IIEF scoring of erectile function and daily pad usage related to incontinence. In addition, patients who received adjuvant postoperative radiotherapy in the 3–12 months interval after surgery were not included in this dataset. Recently, van Stam et al. evaluated the effect of radiotherapy timing on the quality of life in their cohort of 241 salvage radiotherapy and 1005 radical prostatectomy patients in a prospective database (2004–2015) containing health-related quality of life (HRQoL) assessments up to 2 years after the last treatment [52]. They noted that delaying the start of postoperative radiotherapy may decrease the incidence and duration of urinary and sexual problems; patients with a $\geq$ 7 months interval between prostatectomy and radiotherapy had significantly better urinary function recovery ($p = 0.03$) in addition to better sexual satisfaction ($p = 0.02$). Zaffuto et al. also documented that early postoperative radiotherapy in prostatectomy patients was associated with worse functional outcomes; [53] 3 year erectile function recovery rates (no radiotherapy—35%; salvage radiotherapy—29%; adjuvant radiotherapy—11.6%, $p < 0.001$) were significantly affected by time to radiotherapy (<1 year, 11.7% vs ≥1 year, 34.7%, $p < 0.001$), as well as 3 year urinary continence recovery rates (no radiotherapy—70.7%; salvage radiotherapy—59%; adjuvant radiotherapy,—42.2%, $p < 0.001$), differing by delay of radiotherapy (<1 year, 43.5% vs ≥1 year, 62.7%, $p < 0.001$) [53]. Therefore, the length of the interval between prostatectomy and radiotherapy does seem to play a role in the recovery of erectile function and urinary continence.

17.7 Recommendations

Based on current AUA/ASTRO consensus guidelines along with up-to-date clinical evidence, the benefits and risks of postoperative radiotherapy should be discussed for any patient without evidence of distant metastatic disease but demonstrating ≥1 adverse pathologic features including positive surgical margins, ECE, or SVI in the adjuvant setting or immediately post-op with detectable PSA [3, 22]. Salvage radiotherapy should be delivered early at lower versus higher PSA levels, typically at the first documented and verified rise.

Evidence-based radiotherapy delivery guidelines suggest a dose of 64–66 Gy conventionally fractionated to the prostate fossa ± seminal vesicle bed (at least

50 Gy to the seminal vesical fossa and ideally 64–66 Gy if seminal vesicles are positive) following urinary function maximization 3–6 months post-op in the adjuvant setting. A higher dose or 70 Gy in 35 fractions for detectable or rising PSA in the salvage setting is recommended. Again, 50 Gy to the seminal vesicular fossa can be considered if seminal vesicles are negative and70 Gy if positive; dose escalation to clinical gross disease at the prostate fossa can be boosted to 72–74 Gy. Androgen deprivation can be added in the salvage setting, especially if PSA is ≥0.5 ng/mL. The typical duration of androgen deprivation is at least 6 months for patients without distant and nodal metastasis and is initiated 2–3 months prior to radiation.

Conclusion

While ongoing trials will highlight and clarify the postoperative radiotherapy timing and indications as well as the patients who will possibly benefit from radiotherapy, each institution is encouraged to develop an algorithm agreed upon by urology and radiation oncology to standardize the clinical approach in post-operative prostate cancer patients until there is an enhanced and customized consensus guideline.

References

1. American Cancer Society: Cancer Facts & Figures. http://www.cancer.org/acs/groups/content/@research/documents/document/acspc-047079.pdf
2. Siegel RL, Miller KD, Jemal A. Cancer statistics, 2016. CA Cancer J Clin. 2016;66(1):7–30.
3. Thompson IM, Valicenti RK, Albertsen P, Davis BJ, Goldenberg SL, Hahn C, Klein E, Michalski J, Roach M, Sartor O, et al. Adjuvant and salvage radiotherapy after prostatectomy: AUA/ASTRO guideline. J Urol. 2013;190(2):441–9.
4. Pound CR, Partin AW, Epstein JI, Walsh PC. Prostate-specific antigen after anatomic radical retropubic prostatectomy. Patterns of recurrence and cancer control. Urol Clin North Am. 1997;24(2):395–406.
5. Pound CR, Partin AW, Eisenberger MA, Chan DW, Pearson JD, Walsh PC. Natural history of progression after PSA elevation following radical prostatectomy. JAMA. 1999;281(17):1591–7.
6. Moreira DM, Presti JC Jr, Aronson WJ, Terris MK, Kane CJ, Amling CL, Freedland SJ. Natural history of persistently elevated prostate specific antigen after radical prostatectomy: results from the SEARCH database. J Urol. 2009;182(5):2250–5.
7. Moreira DM, Jayachandran J, Presti JC Jr, Aronson WJ, Terris MK, Kane CJ, Amling CL, Stephenson AJ, Freedland SJ. Validation of a nomogram to predict disease progression following salvage radiotherapy after radical prostatectomy: results from the search database. BJU Int. 2009;104(10):1452–6.
8. Freedland SJ, Rumble RB, Finelli A, Chen RC, Slovin S, Stein MN, Mendelson DS, Wackett C, Sandler HM. Adjuvant and salvage radiotherapy after prostatectomy: American Society of Clinical Oncology clinical practice guideline endorsement. J Clin Oncol Off J Am Soc Clin Oncol. 2014;32(34):3892–8.
9. Stephenson AJ, Shariat SF, Zelefsky MJ, Kattan MW, Butler EB, Teh BS, Klein EA, Kupelian PA, Roehrborn CG, Pistenmaa DA, et al. Salvage radiotherapy for recurrent prostate cancer after radical prostatectomy. JAMA. 2004;291(11):1325–32.
10. Trock BJ, Han M, Freedland SJ, Humphreys EB, DeWeese TL, Partin AW, Walsh PC. Prostate cancer-specific survival following salvage radiotherapy vs observation in men with biochemical recurrence after radical prostatectomy. JAMA. 2008;299(23):2760–9.

11. Tendulkar RD, Agrawal S, Gao T, Efstathiou JA, Pisansky TM, Michalski JM, Koontz BF, Hamstra DA, Feng FY, Liauw SL, et al. Contemporary update of a multi-institutional predictive nomogram for salvage radiotherapy after radical prostatectomy. J Clin Oncol. 2016.
12. Connolly JA, Shinohara K, Presti JC Jr, Carroll PR. Local recurrence after radical prostatectomy: characteristics in size, location, and relationship to prostate-specific antigen and surgical margins. Urology. 1996;47(2):225–31.
13. Leventis AK, Shariat SF, Slawin KM. Local recurrence after radical prostatectomy: correlation of US features with prostatic fossa biopsy findings. Radiology. 2001;219(2):432–9.
14. Cotter SE, Chen MH, Moul JW, Lee WR, Koontz BF, Anscher MS, Robertson CN, Walther PJ, Polascik TJ, D'Amico AV. Salvage radiation in men after prostate-specific antigen failure and the risk of death. Cancer. 2011;117(17):3925–32.
15. Thompson IM Jr, Tangen CM, Paradelo J, Lucia MS, Miller G, Troyer D, Messing E, Forman J, Chin J, Swanson G, et al. Adjuvant radiotherapy for pathologically advanced prostate cancer: a randomized clinical trial. JAMA. 2006;296(19):2329–35.
16. Thompson IM, Tangen CM, Paradelo J, Lucia MS, Miller G, Troyer D, Messing E, Forman J, Chin J, Swanson G, et al. Adjuvant radiotherapy for pathological T3N0M0 prostate cancer significantly reduces risk of metastases and improves survival: long-term followup of a randomized clinical trial. J Urol. 2009;181(3):956–62.
17. Bolla M, van Poppel H, Collette L, van Cangh P, Vekemans K, Da Pozzo L, de Reijke TM, Verbaeys A, Bosset JF, van Velthoven R, et al. Postoperative radiotherapy after radical prostatectomy: a randomised controlled trial (EORTC trial 22911). Lancet. 2005;366(9485):572–8.
18. Bolla M, van Poppel H, Tombal B, Vekemans K, Da Pozzo L, de Reijke TM, Verbaeys A, Bosset JF, van Velthoven R, Colombel M, et al. Postoperative radiotherapy after radical prostatectomy for high-risk prostate cancer: long-term results of a randomised controlled trial (EORTC trial 22911). Lancet. 2012;380(9858):2018–27.
19. Wiegel T, Bartkowiak D, Bottke D, Bronner C, Steiner U, Siegmann A, Golz R, Storkel S, Willich N, Semjonow A, et al. Adjuvant radiotherapy versus wait-and-see after radical prostatectomy: 10-year follow-up of the ARO 96-02/AUO AP 09/95 trial. Eur Urol. 2014;66(2):243–50.
20. Wiegel T, Bartkowiak D, Bottke D, Thamm R, Hinke A, Stockle M, Rube C, Semjonow A, Wirth M, Storkel S, et al. Prostate-specific antigen persistence after radical prostatectomy as a predictive factor of clinical relapse-free survival and overall survival: 10-year data of the ARO 96-02 trial. Int J Radiat Oncol Biol Phys. 2015;91(2):288–94.
21. Wiegel T, Bottke D, Steiner U, Siegmann A, Golz R, Storkel S, Willich N, Semjonow A, Souchon R, Stockle M, et al. Phase III postoperative adjuvant radiotherapy after radical prostatectomy compared with radical prostatectomy alone in pT3 prostate cancer with postoperative undetectable prostate-specific antigen: ARO 96-02/AUO AP 09/95. J Clin Oncol Off J Am Soc Clin Oncol. 2009;27(18):2924–30.
22. Valicenti RK, Thompson I Jr, Albertsen P, Davis BJ, Goldenberg SL, Wolf JS, Sartor O, Klein E, Hahn C, Michalski J, et al. Adjuvant and salvage radiation therapy after prostatectomy: American Society for Radiation Oncology/American Urological Association guidelines. Int J Radiat Oncol Biol Phys. 2013;86(5):822–8.
23. Parker C, Sydes MR, Catton C, Kynaston H, Logue J, Murphy C, Morgan RC, Mellon K, Morash C, Parulekar W, et al. Radiotherapy and androgen deprivation in combination after local surgery (RADICALS): a new Medical Research Council/National Cancer Institute of Canada phase III trial of adjuvant treatment after radical prostatectomy. BJU Int. 2007;99(6):1376–9.
24. Taneja SS. Re: a phase III trial to investigate the timing of radiotherapy for prostate cancer with high-risk features: background and rationale of the Radiotherapy-Adjuvant Versus Early Salvage (RAVES) trial. J Urol. 2015;193(2):539.
25. Pearse M, Fraser-Browne C, Davis ID, Duchesne GM, Fisher R, Frydenberg M, Haworth A, Jose C, Joseph DJ, Lim TS, et al. A phase III trial to investigate the timing of radiotherapy for prostate cancer with high-risk features: background and rationale of the Radiotherapy—Adjuvant Versus Early Salvage (RAVES) trial. BJU Int. 2014;113(Suppl 2):7–12.
26. Nguyen PL. Value of extra-early initiation of salvage radiation for increasing prostate-specific antigen after prostatectomy. J Clin Oncol Off J Am Soc Clin Oncol. 2016.

27. Stephenson AJ, Scardino PT, Kattan MW, Pisansky TM, Slawin KM, Klein EA, Anscher MS, Michalski JM, Sandler HM, Lin DW, et al. Predicting the outcome of salvage radiation therapy for recurrent prostate cancer after radical prostatectomy. J Clin Oncol Off J Am Soc Clin Oncol. 2007;25(15):2035–41.
28. King CR. The timing of salvage radiotherapy after radical prostatectomy: a systematic review. Int J Radiat Oncol Biol Phys. 2012;84(1):104–11.
29. Fossati N, Karnes RJ, Cozzarini C, Fiorino C, Gandaglia G, Joniau S, Boorjian SA, Goldner G, Hinkelbein W, Haustermans K, et al. Assessing the optimal timing for early salvage radiation therapy in patients with prostate-specific antigen rise after radical prostatectomy. Eur Urol. 2016;69(4):728–33.
30. Mir MC, Li J, Klink JC, Kattan MW, Klein EA, Stephenson AJ. Optimal definition of biochemical recurrence after radical prostatectomy depends on pathologic risk factors: identifying candidates for early salvage therapy. Eur Urol. 2014;66(2):204–10.
31. Den RB, Yousefi K, Trabulsi EJ, Abdollah F, Choeurng V, Feng FY, Dicker AP, Lallas CD, Gomella LG, Davicioni E, et al. Genomic classifier identifies men with adverse pathology after radical prostatectomy who benefit from adjuvant radiation therapy. J Clin Oncol Off J Am Soc Clin Oncol. 2015;33(8):944–51.
32. Perrapato SD, Gore J, du Plessis M, Santiago-Jimenez M, Yousefi K, Thompson D, Chen D, Clark W, Franks M, Karsh L, et al. A genomic classifier impacts adjuvant treatment decision making among patients with high-risk pathology at radical prostatectomy: results from the multicenter prospective PRO-IMPACT study. Int J Radiat Oncol Biol Phys. 2016;96(2S):S104.
33. Klein EA, Yousefi K, Haddad Z, Choeurng V, Buerki C, Stephenson AJ, Li J, Kattan MW, Magi-Galluzzi C, Davicioni E. A genomic classifier improves prediction of metastatic disease within 5 years after surgery in node-negative high-risk prostate cancer patients managed by radical prostatectomy without adjuvant therapy. Eur Urol. 2015;67(4):778–86.
34. Freedland SJ, Choeurng V, Howard L, De Hoedt A, du Plessis M, Yousefi K, Lam LL, Buerki C, Ra S, Robbins B, et al. Utilization of a genomic classifier for prediction of metastasis following salvage radiation therapy after radical prostatectomy. Eur Urol. 2016.
35. King CR. Adjuvant radiotherapy after prostatectomy: does waiting for a detectable prostate-specific antigen level make sense? Int J Radiat Oncol Biol Phys. 2011;80(1):1–3.
36. Cheung R, Kamat AM, de Crevoisier R, Allen PK, Lee AK, Tucker SL, Pisters L, Babaian RJ, Kuban D. Outcome of salvage radiotherapy for biochemical failure after radical prostatectomy with or without hormonal therapy. Int J Radiat Oncol Biol Phys. 2005;63(1):134–40.
37. Kurokawa K, Ito K, Suzuki K, Ono Y, Yamamoto T, Akimoto T, Yamanaka H. Salvage external beam radiotherapy for local recurrence without systemic progression or prostate specific antigen recurrence of prostate cancer after initial hormonal therapy: is it possible to identify patients likely to have good treatment outcomes? Jpn J Clin Oncol. 2002;32(11):466–71.
38. Spiotto MT, Hancock SL, King CR. Radiotherapy after prostatectomy: improved biochemical relapse-free survival with whole pelvic compared with prostate bed only for high-risk patients. Int J Radiat Oncol Biol Phys. 2007;69(1):54–61.
39. Ost P, Cozzarini C, De Meerleer G, Fiorino C, De Potter B, Briganti A, Nagler EV, Montorsi F, Fonteyne V, Di Muzio N. High-dose adjuvant radiotherapy after radical prostatectomy with or without androgen deprivation therapy. Int J Radiat Oncol Biol Phys. 2012;83(3):960–5.
40. Shipley WU, Hunt D, Lukka HR, Major P, Heney NM, Grignon D, Patel M, Bahary J, Lawton CA, Sandler HM. Initial report of RTOG 9601, a phase III trial in prostate cancer: effect of anti-androgen therapy (AAT) with bicalutamide during and after radiation therapy (RT) on freedom from progression and incidence of metastatic disease in patients following radical prostatectomy (RP) with pT2-3,N0 disease and elevated PSA levels. J Clin Oncol Off J Am Soc Clin Oncol. 2011;29(7_suppl):1.
41. Shipley WU, Hunt D, Lukka HR, Major P, Heney NM, Grignon D, Patel M, Bahary J, Lawton CA, Sandler HM. Report of NRG Oncology/RTOG 9601, a phase III trial in prostate cancer: anti-androgen therapy (AAT) with bicalutamide during and after radiation therapy (RT) in patients following radical prostatectomy (RP) with pT2–3pN0 disease and an elevated

PSA. Presented at the 2015 Annual Meeting of the American Society for Radiation Oncology, San Antonio, TX (Late Breaking Abstract 5). 2015.
42. Carrie C, Hasbini A, de Laroche G, Richaud P, Guerif S, Latorzeff I, Supiot S, Bosset M, Lagrange JL, Beckendorf V, et al. Salvage radiotherapy with or without short-term hormone therapy for rising prostate-specific antigen concentration after radical prostatectomy (GETUG-AFU 16): a randomised, multicentre, open-label phase 3 trial. Lancet Oncol. 2016;17(6):747–56.
43. Prostate Post-Op RTOG Atlas. https://www.rtog.org/CoreLab/ContouringAtlases/ProstatePostOp.aspx
44. Michalski JM, Lawton C, El Naqa I, Ritter M, O'Meara E, Seider MJ, Lee WR, Rosenthal SA, Pisansky T, Catton C, et al. Development of RTOG consensus guidelines for the definition of the clinical target volume for postoperative conformal radiation therapy for prostate cancer. Int J Radiat Oncol Biol Phys. 2010;76(2):361–8.
45. Croke J, Maclean J, Nyiri B, Li Y, Malone K, Avruch L, Kayser C, Malone S. Proposal of a post-prostatectomy clinical target volume based on pre-operative MRI: volumetric and dosimetric comparison to the RTOG guidelines. Radiat Oncol. 2014;9:303.
46. Wang J, Kudchadker R, Choi S, Pettaway CA, Choi H, Hobbs BD, Occena MC, McGuire SE, Pugh TJ, Hoffman K, et al. Local recurrence map to guide target volume delineation after radical prostatectomy. Pract Radiat Oncol. 2014;4(6):e239–46.
47. van Leeuwen PJ, Stricker P, Hruby G, Kneebone A, Ting F, Thompson B, Nguyen Q, Ho B, Emmett L. (68) Ga-PSMA has a high detection rate of prostate cancer recurrence outside the prostatic fossa in patients being considered for salvage radiation treatment. BJU Int. 2016;117(5):732–9.
48. Ohri N, Dicker AP, Trabulsi EJ, Showalter TN. Can early implementation of salvage radiotherapy for prostate cancer improve the therapeutic ratio? A systematic review and regression meta-analysis with radiobiological modelling. Eur J Cancer. 2012;48(6):837–44.
49. Swanson GP, Hussey MA, Tangen CM, Chin J, Messing E, Canby-Hagino E, Forman JD, Thompson IM, Crawford ED. Predominant treatment failure in postprostatectomy patients is local: analysis of patterns of treatment failure in SWOG 8794. J Clin Oncol Off J Am Soc Clin Oncol. 2007;25(16):2225–9.
50. King CR. The dose-response of salvage radiation therapy following radical prostatectomy: a systematic review and meta-analysis. Int J Radiat Oncol Biol Phys. 2016;96(2S):S101–2.
51. Hegarty SE, Hyslop T, Dicker AP, Showalter TN. Radiation therapy after radical prostatectomy for prostate cancer: evaluation of complications and influence of radiation timing on outcomes in a large, population-based cohort. PLoS One. 2015;10(2):e0118430.
52. van Stam MA, Aaronson NK, Pos FJ, Bosch JL, Kieffer JM, Tillier CN, van der Poel HG. The effect of salvage radiotherapy and its timing on the health-related quality of life of prostate cancer patients. Eur Urol. 2016;70(5):751–7.
53. Zaffuto E, Gandaglia G, Fossati N, Dell'Oglio P, Moschini M, Cucchiara V, Suardi N, Mirone V, Bandini M, Shariat SF, et al. Early postoperative radiotherapy is associated with worse functional outcomes in patients with prostate cancer. J Urol. 2016;197(3 Pt 1):669–75.

Stereotactic Body Radiotherapy for Prostate Cancer

18

Fadil Akyol, Gozde Yazici, Melis Gultekin, Pervin Hurmuz, Sezin Yuce Sari, and Gokhan Ozyigit

Abstract

The term stereotactic implies that the target is localized relative to a fixed three-dimensional spatial coordinate system. Stereotactic body radiation therapy (SBRT) is defined as giving a high dose of radiation per fraction, in up to five fractions, using sophisticated image guidance to deliver a potent ablative dose to cancerous tissues while minimizing the risk to normal structures. The alpha-beta ratios for the rectum and bladder, both of which are late-responding tissues, are 2.5–5 Gy and 3–7 Gy, respectively. This unique biologic nature of prostate cancer explains the therapeutic gain with hypofractionation. These radiobiologic assumptions were supported by prospective randomized trials that used 2.5–3.1 Gy per fraction.

18.1 The Rationale for High Dose per Fraction

The concept of conventional radiation fractionation (1,8–2 Gy/fraction) dates back to observations in 1932 when Coutard reported successful treatment results with fractionated radiotherapy in deep-seated tumors with moderate toxicity [1]. With the advances in radiobiology, the advantages of fractionation were better understood. The therapeutic index of radiotherapy increases as the fractionation dose decreases due to differences in DNA repair between tumor and normal tissues, and the decrease in the dose of fractions preferentially spares normal structures [2]. However, this generalization is not true for every tumor type. The alpha-beta ratio describes the fractionation sensitivity of a specific cell type. The linear quadratic

F. Akyol, M.D. (✉) • G. Yazici, M.D. • M. Gultekin, M.D. • P. Hurmuz, M.D. • S.Y. Sari, M.D.
G. Ozyigit, M.D.
Department of radiation Oncology, Hacettepe University, Ankara, Turkey
e-mail: hakyol@hacettepe.edu.tr

G. Ozyigit, U. Selek (eds.), *Principles and Practice of Urooncology*,
DOI 10.1007/978-3-319-56114-1_18

model described by Fowler formulates the response of cells to radiation according to their specific alpha-beta ratios [3]. The alpha-beta ratio is generally high (≥10 Gy) for early-responding tissues (skin, mucosa, and most tumors). In contrast, it is low (<5 Gy) for late-responding tissues (connective tissues and muscles). When the alpha-beta ratio of the tumor is high and the alpha-beta ratio of the late responding tissues around the tumor is low, fractionation provides sparing of the normal tissues. In cases where the alpha-beta ratio of the tumor is lower than the alpha-beta ratio of the surrounding normal tissues, fractionation causes decreased tumoricidal effect.

Haustermans et al.'s observation back in 1997 was a pioneering study that proposed a low alpha-beta ratio for prostate cancer [4]. Later in 1999, Brenner and Hall showed that the clinical data also supported Haustermans's findings [5]. The same biochemical control of prostate cancer either by external beam treatment with a 2 Gy per fraction to 70 Gy or by permanent iodine-125 low-dose-rate irradiation to 145 Gy was their starting point, and they calculated an alpha-beta ratio of 1.5 Gy for prostate cancer. The consensus for the alpha-beta ratio for prostate cancer is within the limits of 1–4 Gy [4–8]. In prostate cancer treatment, the critical structures at risk are the bladder, rectum, and small bowel. The alpha-beta ratios for the rectum and bladder, both of which are late-responding tissues, are 2.5–5 Gy and 3–7 Gy, respectively. This unique biologic nature of prostate cancer explains the therapeutic gain with hypofractionation. These radiobiologic assumptions were supported by prospective randomized trials that used 2.5–3.1 Gy per fraction [9–11].

18.2 Technical Aspects of SBRT

The term stereotactic implies that the target is localized relative to a fixed three-dimensional spatial coordinate system [12]. For prostate cancer treatments, these coordinate systems are marked with internal fiducial markers (bony landmarks or implanted markers). Many contemporary linear accelerators are now integrated with SBRT treatment delivery systems that include image guidance technology. These systems allow the use of considerably smaller fields compared with conventional radiation therapy. The SBRT treatment planning is a multistep process that starts with patient immobilization. Motion assessment and management, planning computed tomography (CT), target delineation, patient-specific quality assurance testing, and patient setup are examples of other steps in treatment planning which are beyond the scope of this chapter. However, for practical issues, we need to know some of the technical properties of linear accelerators or target localization systems currently used for SBRT. The minimum requirement for SBRT is target localization prior to daily treatments. This can be performed using X-ray imaging of implanted fiducials or onboard CT imaging. However there is also variation that occurs during the treatment, and this is referred as the intra-fractional motion. If this intra-fractional motion is not followed by image guidance during the treatment, we need to define at least a 5 mm margin around the target to deliver the prescribed dose to the prostate effectively. If the target can be localized during treatment, then smaller PTV expansions can be employed. Xie et al. showed that with proper monitoring and intervention during the treatment, a submillimeter accuracy can be achieved [13]. They used a stereoscopic X-ray system to obtain the position of the prostate target through the monitoring of implanted gold fiducial markers, and they found that a sampling rate of every 40 s during the treatment was ideal.

18.3 Dosimetric Studies of SBRT

King et al. evaluated the SBRT plan of CyberKnife (CK; Accuray Inc., Sunnyvale, CA), a robotic arm-driven linear accelerator, for a localized prostate cancer [14]. Conformal isodose curves and dose volume histograms (DVH) were used to compare with an optimized intensity-modulated radiotherapy (IMRT) plan delivered to the patient. The SBRT plan produced better sparing of the rectum and bladder and superior target coverage compared with IMRT.

Fuller et al. hypothesized that CK may be used to deliver high-dose-rate (HDR) brachytherapy like dosimetry to the prostate noninvasively, and they created HDR plans using common contour sets and simulated HDR catheters for ten low-intermediate-risk prostate cancer patients that were treated with CK [15]. They found that the planning target volume coverage by the prescription dose was similar for CK SBRT and HDR plans, and the urethra dose comparisons were lower for CK SBRT in nine of ten cases. Bladder maximum point doses were higher with HDR, and the maximum rectal wall doses were similar. Fukuda et al. reported a similar study, but they performed SBRT plans on six patients who were treated with HDR [16]. In this dosimetric study, they found that the CK SBRT plans' dosimetric profiles were better for PTV coverage of the prostate, and the maximum dose in the rectum was lower. However, the HDR plan provided a sharper dose falloff around the PTV. SBRT was significantly superior in most of the dosimetric profiles for the bladder and urethra.

18.4 Clinical Results of SBRT

There are accumulating data on the use of SBRT for prostate cancer; however the published literature consists phase I or II trials and retrospective studies. In the previous chapter, Chap. 16, selected series are summarized in Table 16.3. The vast majority of the patients included in these trials are low-intermediate-risk prostate cancers.

A phase I/II dose escalation study from 45 to 50 Gy in five fractions in low- to intermediate-risk prostate cancer patients showed a 10% ≥ grade 3 rectal toxicity rate in the 50 Gy arm, demonstrating that SBRT with 50 Gy in five fractions is unsafe [17]. This study had a multi-institutional design, and patients were enrolled from five different institutions. Fiducial markers consisting of gold seeds (Calypso beacons were permitted) were placed within the prostate, and the prostate was expanded uniformly by 2–3 mm to create the planning target volume (PTV) based on institutional PTV guidelines. SBRT was delivered via ring gantry helical accelerator (Tomotherapy; TomoTherapy Inc., Madison, WI, USA) or on a linear accelerator with image guidance (Trilogy; Varian Medical Systems, Palo Alto, CA, USA and Synergy; Elekta AB, Stockholm, Sweden) with energies of 6–15 MV.

Madsen et al. reported their results of SBRT in 40 patients with a dose of 33.5 Gy in five fractions [18]. They calculated this dose to be biologically equivalent to 78 Gy in 2 Gy fractions. They used noncoplanar conformal fields and daily stereotactic localization of implanted fiducials. However they used a 4–5 mm margin from the prostate to the block edge. Acute GU grade 1–2 toxicity rate was 48.5% (GU), and this value for GI toxicity was 39%. Late grade 1–2 toxicity for GU and GI was 45% and 37%, respectively. No late grade 3 or higher toxicity was reported. The actuarial 48 month biochemical freedom from relapse was 90% according to the nadir 2 ng/mL failure definition.

Loblaw et al. performed phase I/II SBRT study in patients with low-risk localized prostate cancer [19]. They prescribed 35 Gy in five fractions, and the treatment was given once weekly. To account for intra-fractional motion, they defined a 4 mm margin for PTV. They achieved 98% biochemical control in 5 years with only 1% of late grade 3 GI and GU toxicity.

Katz et al. reported the results of 477 patients treated with CK SBRT [20]. Three hundred twenty-four patients were low risk (PSA <10 ng/mL and Gleason <7), and 153 were intermediate risk (PSA 10–20 ng/mL or Gleason = 7). One hundred fifty-four patients received 35 Gy delivered in five daily fractions; the rest received 36.25 Gy in five daily fractions. They reported an actuarial 7 year freedom from biochemical failure as 95.6% and 89.6% for low- and intermediate-risk groups, respectively. They reported that the biochemical control rate did not differ between doses of 35 and 36.25 Gy. They did not observe any grade 3–4 acute GI or GU toxicity. Late grade 3 GU toxicity rate was 1.7%, and all occurred in the 36.25 Gy cohorts.

For patients with low- or intermediate-risk prostate cancer, the largest published study is a pooled analysis of multiple phase II trials across eight institutions [21]. This analysis included 1100 patients. Fifty eight percent of patients had a low-risk disease, 30% had intermediate risk, and 11% had high-risk disease. The radiotherapy dose was 36.25 Gy (range 35–40 Gy) in median over five fractions (given daily among >95% of patients, every other day for the remainder). The vast majority of the patients (89%) received a dose of 35–36.25 Gy in five fractions. The 5 year biochemical relapse-free survival rate was 95%, 84%, and 81% for low-, intermediate-, and high-risk patients, respectively. For 135 patients with a minimum of 5 years follow-up, the 5 year biochemical relapse-free survival rate was

99% for low-risk patients and was 99% for intermediate-risk group. Patient-reported quality of life data from 864 patients in this pooled analysis showed a transient decline in GU and GI domains within the first 3 months after SBRT, which returned to baseline or better within 6 months and remained so through 5 years of follow-up [22].

We evaluated the long-term results of two different fractionation schemes in our patients treated with robotic SBRT (CyberKnife™) [23]. D'Amico risk classification system was used to group patients. In the low-risk (LR) group (n = 54), 20 patients received androgen blockade (AB). In the intermediate-risk (IR) group (n = 52), 42 patients received neoadjuvant/adjuvant AB. SBRT was delivered in five fractions to a total dose of 36.5 Gy either sequentially (n = 58) or every other day (n = 48). Five year BRFS rate was 89% in patients with PSA bounce phenomenon compared to 94.2% in patients without bounce (p = 0.9). There was no difference in the incidence of late toxicities for two different SBRT schemes.

18.5 Robotic Radiosurgery with CyberKnife at Hacettepe University

18.5.1 Patient Selection

We recommend robotic SBRT (rSBRT) with CyberKnife® in low-intermediate-risk patients (PSA < 20 ng/mL, Gleason score < 8, T1-T2N0M0) (Fig. 18.1). If a patient has a very large prostate volume (>50 cc), it might be worthwhile to consider having the patient undergo hormonal therapy for volume reduction rSBRT.

We do not recommend rSBRT in patients with collagen vascular disease and inflammatory bowel disease. We can treat patients with metal in the pelvis, which consists of artificial hips, since the delivery of multiple small beamlets can find appropriate alternative pathways.

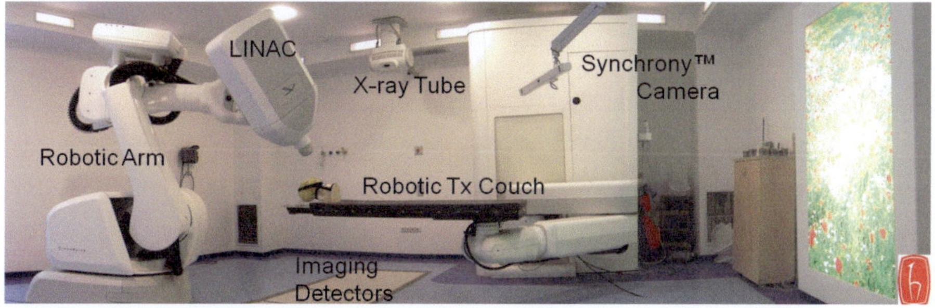

Fig. 18.1 Robotic stereotactic body radiotherapy unit (Courtesy of Hacettepe University)

18.5.2 Fiducial Placement

Once the patient is a candidate for rSBRT, the patient is scheduled for his fiducial placement and simulation. We used specific four golden fiducials manufactured to be used with CyberKnife® (Fig. 18.2). Prophylactic antibiotic and urinary antiseptics are given prior to procedure.

At our institution, the fiducials are inserted transrectally under ultrasound guidance by the urologist under local anesthesia (Fig. 18.3). We also try to place the fiducials in certain regions of the prostate gland due to the fact that all fiducials should be in certain geometry accordingly with the imaging X-ray tubes (Fig. 18.4). Once the fiducials have been placed, there should be 7–10 days before the simulation is done.

18.5.3 Simulation

For the simulation, we place the patient in a supine position and place a 14 Gauge Foley catheter into the bladder to visualize prostatic urethra (Fig. 18.5). We then inflate its balloon with 6 cc of water. Once the Foley is placed, a non-contrast planning CT with less than 1 mm slice thickness is performed to the entire pelvis.

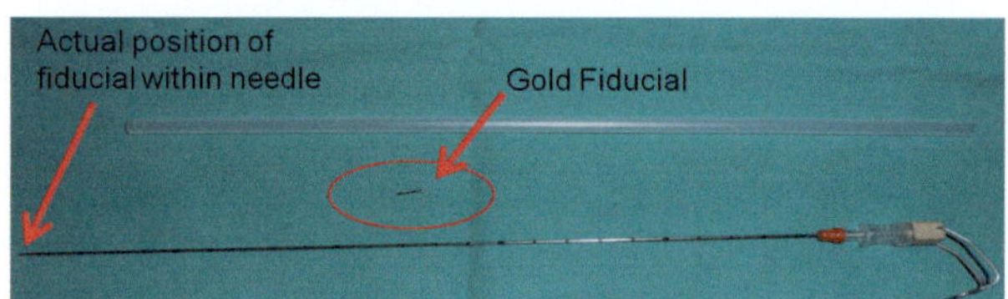

Fig. 18.2 Golden fiducials for CyberKnife

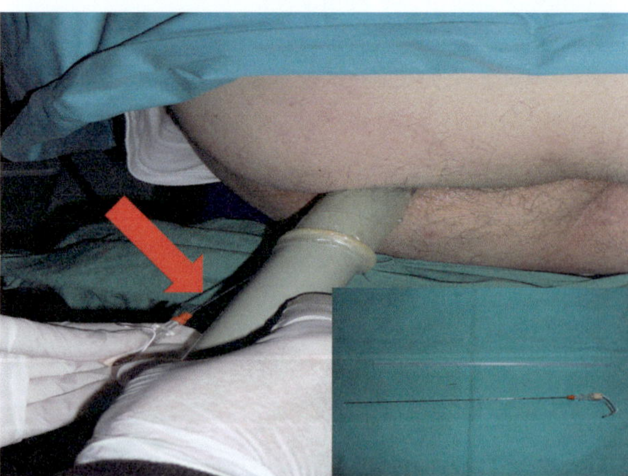

Fig. 18.3 Transrectal fiducial placement for rSBRT

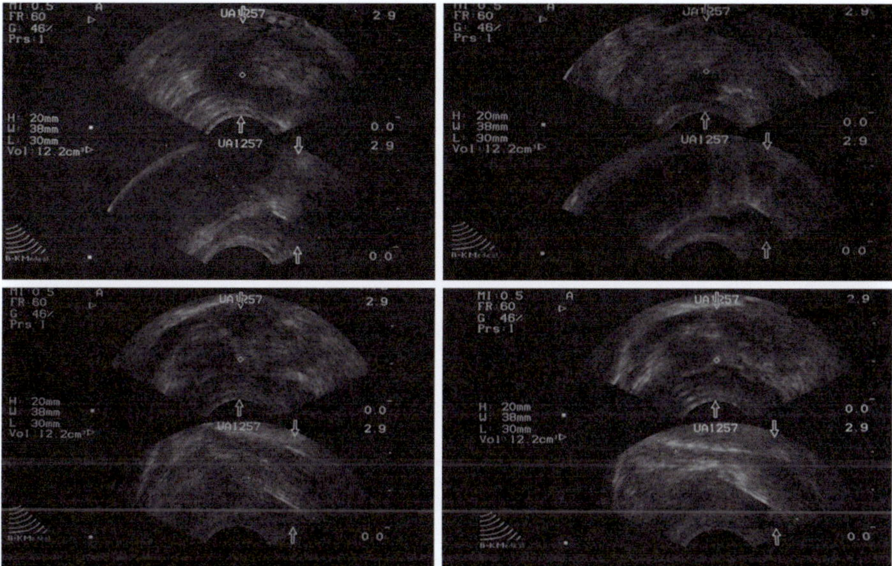

Fig. 18.4 Locations for the fiducial placement within the prostate gland

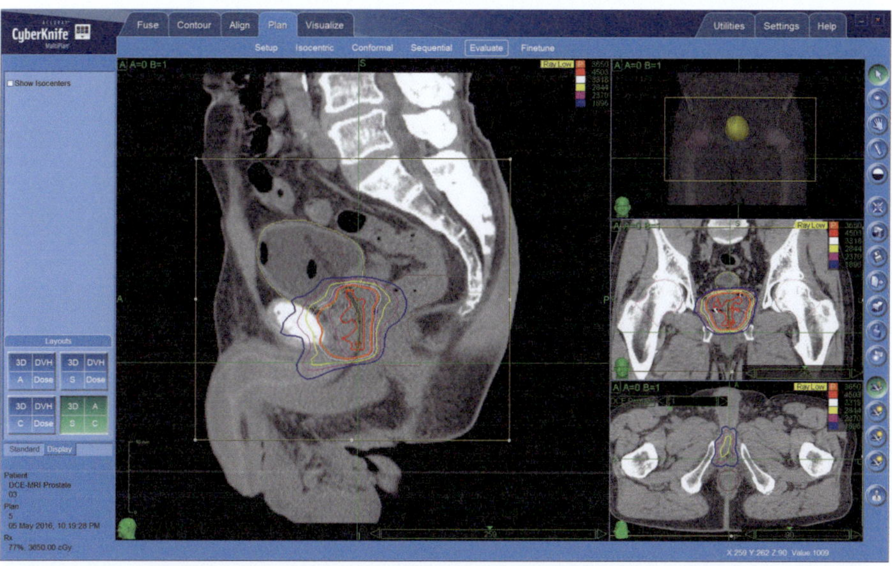

Fig. 18.5 14 G Foley catheter visualized within the prostatic urethra. Sample plan is showing hot points within the urethra that is not acceptable

18.5.4 Contouring

At our institution, the CTV for definitive prostate cancer patients is as per the following: prostate only for low risk; prostate proximal seminal vesicles (SV) for intermediate risk. Proximal is defined as the proximal 1 cm of the SV.

18.5.5 Dosing

The standard dose is 36.5 Gy in 7.3 Gy daily fractions either in consecutive (Monday–Friday) or every-other-day regimen (2 weeks regimen) (Fig. 18.6).

18.5.6 Plan Evaluation

Our rSBRT treatment plan acceptance criteria are summarized as following:

PTV

- PTV prescribed dose: 7.3 Gy in five fractions with a total dose of 36.5 Gy.
- Inhomogeneities. 110–130% high-dose region within CTV if possible within GTV.

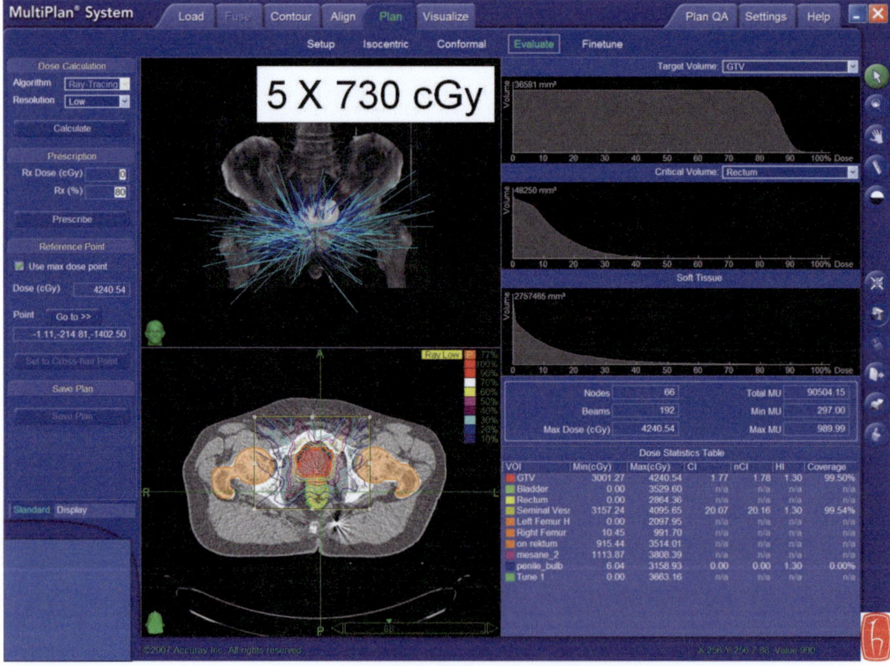

Fig. 18.6 Treatment plan of a patient receiving rSBRT with every-other-day protocol

- Maximum dose < 45.5 Gy.
- Ninety-five percent volume of PTV should receive 36.25 Gy.
- Minimum PTV dose 34.4 Gy.

Rectum
- V33.5 Gy < 1 cc.
- Minor variation: V33.5 Gy ≥ 1 cc but <3 cc.
- Major variation: V33.5 Gy ≥ 3 cc.
- Max dose (0.03 cc) ≤ 38.06 Gy.
- Less than 3 cc volume may receive 34.4 Gy.
- V32.6 Gy ≤ 90% rectum.
- V29 Gy ≤ 80% rectum.
- V18.125 Gy ≤ 50% rectum.

Bladder
- V35 Gy < 5 cc
- Minor variation: V35Gy ≥ 5 cc but <10 cc
- Major variation: V35 Gy ≥ 10 cc
- Max point dose (0.03 cc) ≤ 38.06 Gy
- V32.625 Gy ≤ 90% bladder
- V18.125 Gy ≤ 50% bladder

Urethra
- V45.5 Gy < 10%
- Minor variation: V45.5 Gy ≥ 10% but <20%
- Major variation: V45.5 Gy ≥ 20%
- Max Doz < 38.78 Gy

Penile Bulb
- V27.5 Gy ≤ 50%.
- Minor variation: V27.5 Gy ≥ 50% ama <70%.
- Major variation: V27.5 Gy ≥ 70%.
- Max dose does not exceed the prescribed dose.
- V20 Gy < 3 cc.

Femur
- V20 Gy < 10 cc

18.5.7 Image Guidance

Daily image-guided radiation therapy (IGRT) is achieved using real-time daily kV imaging with fiducials (Fig. 18.7).

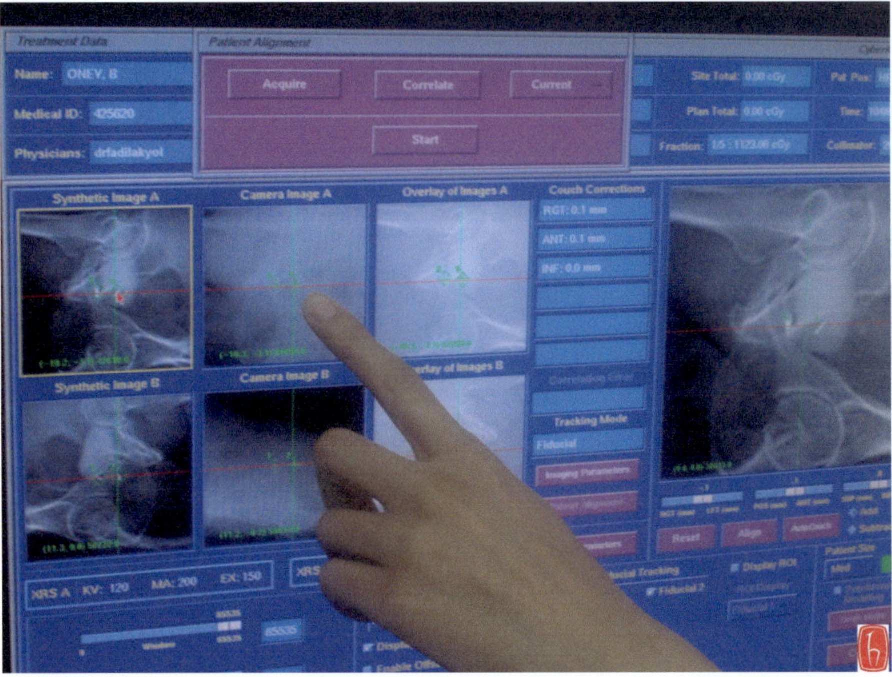

Fig. 18.7 Daily kV imaging of gold fiducials for rSBRT

Conclusion

Based on these currently available data, the American Society for Radiation Oncology has included SBRT as "an appropriate alternative for select patients with low to intermediate-risk disease." Meanwhile, multiple randomized trials are ongoing directly comparing SBRT with conventionally fractionated RT for prostate cancer (NCT01839994, NCT01794403, ISRCTN45905321, and CRUKE/12/025).

References

1. Coutard H. Roentgentherapy of epitheliomas of the tonsillar region, hypopharynx, and larynx from 1920 to 1926. Am J Roentgenol. 1932;28:313–31.
2. Withers HR. Biologic basis for altered fractionation schemes. Cancer. 1985;55:2086–95.
3. Fowler JF. The linear-quadratic formula and progress in fractionated radiotherapy. Br J Radiol. 1989;62:679–94.
4. Haustermans KM, Hofland I, Van Poppel H, et al. Cell kinetic measurements in prostate cancer. Int J Radiat Oncol Biol Phys. 1997;37:1067–70.
5. Brenner DJ, Hall EJ. Fractionation and protraction for radiotherapy of prostate carcinoma. Int J Radiat Oncol Biol Phys. 1999;43:1095–101.
6. Fowler JFCR, Ritter MA. Is a/b for prostate tumors really low? Int J Radiat Oncol Biol Phys. 2001;50:1021–31.

7. Brenner DJ, Martinez AA, Edmundson GK, et al. Direct evidence that prostate tumors show high sensitivity to fractionation (low alpha/beta ratio), similar to late-responding normal tissue. Int J Radiat Oncol Biol Phys. 2002;52:6–13.
8. Wang JZ, Guerrero M, Li XA. How low is the alpha/beta ratio for prostate cancer? Int J Radiat Oncol Biol Phys. 2003;55:194–203.
9. Kupelian PA, Willoughby TR, Reddy CA, et al. Hypofractionated intensity-modulated radiotherapy (70 Gy at 2.5 Gy per fraction) for localized prostate cancer: Cleveland Clinic experience. Int J Radiat Oncol Biol Phys. 2007;68:1424–30.
10. Yeoh EE, Botten RJ, Butters J, et al. Hypofractionated versus conventionally fractionated radiotherapy for prostate carcinoma: final results of phase III randomized trial. Int J Radiat Oncol Biol Phys. 2011;81:1271–8.
11. Arcangeli S, Strigari L, Gomellini S, et al. Updated results and patterns of failure in a randomized hypofractionation trial for high-risk prostate cancer. Int J Radiat Oncol Biol Phys. 2012;84:1172–8.
12. Solberg TD, Balter JM, Benedict SH, et al. Quality and safety considerations in stereotactic radiosurgery and stereotactic body radiation therapy: executive summary. Pract Radiat Oncol. 2012;2:2–9.
13. Xie Y, Djajaputra D, King CR, et al. Intrafractional motion of the prostate during hypofractionated radiotherapy. Int J Radiat Oncol Biol Phys. 2008;72:236–46.
14. King CR, Lehmann J, Adler JR, Hai J. CyberKnife radiotherapy for localized prostate cancer: rationale and technical feasibility. Technol Cancer Res Treat. 2003;2:25–30.
15. Fuller DB, Naitoh J, Lee C, et al. Virtual HDR CyberKnife treatment for localized prostatic carcinoma: dosimetry comparison with HDR brachytherapy and preliminary clinical observations. Int J Radiat Oncol Biol Phys. 2008;70:1588–97.
16. Fukuda S, Seo Y, Shiomi H, et al. Dosimetry analyses comparing high-dose-rate brachytherapy, administered as monotherapy for localized prostate cancer, with stereotactic body radiation therapy simulated using CyberKnife. J Radiat Res. 2014;55:1114–21.
17. Kim DW, Straka C, Cho LC, Timmerman RD. Stereotactic body radiation therapy for prostate cancer: review of experience of a multicenter phase I/II dose-escalation study. Front Oncol. 2014;4:319.
18. Madsen BL, Hsi RA, Pham HT, et al. Stereotactic hypofractionated accurate radiotherapy of the prostate (SHARP), 33.5 Gy in five fractions for localized disease: first clinical trial results. Int J Radiat Oncol Biol Phys. 2007;67:1099–105.
19. Loblaw A, Cheung P, D'Alimonte L, et al. Prostate stereotactic ablative body radiotherapy using a standard linear accelerator: toxicity, biochemical, and pathological outcomes. Radiother Oncol. 2013;107:153–8.
20. Katz AJ, Kang J. Stereotactic body radiotherapy as treatment for organ confined low and intermediate-risk prostate carcinoma, a 7-year study. Front Oncol. 2014;4:240.
21. King CR, Freeman D, Kaplan I, et al. Stereotactic body radiotherapy for localized prostate cancer: pooled analysis from a multi-institutional consortium of prospective phase II trials. Radiother Oncol. 2013;109:217–21.
22. King CR, Collins S, Fuller D, et al. Health-related quality of life after stereotactic body radiation therapy for localized prostate cancer: results from a multi-institutional consortium of prospective trials. Int J Radiat Oncol Biol Phys. 2013;87:939–45.
23. Ozyigit G, Hurmuz P, Akyol F. Comparison of two fractionation schemes in prostate cancer patients treated with robotic SBRT. Proceedings of ESTRO 36, Vienna, Austria, 5–9 May 2017.

Proton Therapy for the Treatment of Prostate Cancer

19

Seungtaek Choi

Abstract

Treatment using proton beam has advantages over X-rays due to its physical characteristics, which allow for dose escalation of the tumor with less scatter radiation dose to the surrounding tissues. There have been multiple published reports showing excellent clinical outcomes after treatment with proton therapy for prostate cancer. However, there continues to be significant controversy regarding the clinical advantage of proton therapy over using X-rays with intensity-modulated radiation therapy (IMRT) as there have been no randomized trials comparing the two treatments reported. This chapter will summarize the physics of the proton therapy and the recent technical advances in the delivery of the proton beam, review the clinical results, and describe the treatment protocol used at our institution for the use of proton therapy in the treatment of prostate cancer patients.

19.1 Introduction

The use of proton therapy for the treatment of cancer was first proposed by Robert Wilson in 1946 [1]. The physical characteristics of proton therapy make it especially attractive for cancer treatment. Proton therapy gives most of its dose at a fixed depth into tissue called the Bragg peak with almost no dose given beyond that depth. Therefore, there is an improved ability to deliver high doses of radiation therapy with decreased scattered dose to the nearby critical structures. Because of this perceived advantages of the proton beam over X-ray therapy, radiation therapy centers offering proton therapy for treatment of cancer have opened throughout the world.

S. Choi, M.D.
Department of Radiation Oncology, The University of Texas, MD Anderson Cancer Center, Houston, TX, USA
e-mail: stchoi@mdanderson.org

G. Ozyigit, U. Selek (eds.), *Principles and Practice of Urooncology*,
DOI 10.1007/978-3-319-56114-1_19

Currently there are 61 centers which are in operation in the world, with 24 of them located in the United States [2].

Several studies have shown the importance of dose escalation in the treatment of prostate cancer. These studies have shown that a higher radiation dose to the prostate leads to improved biochemical relapse-free survival and freedom from clinical failure rate [3–5]. However, the higher dose often comes at the cost of higher risk of side effects. Therefore, it is crucial to minimize the dose to the normal tissues with dose escalation to minimize the risk of side effects. As mentioned earlier, the physical characteristics of the proton beam therapy allow for such dose escalation of the tumor with less scatter and exit dose to the surrounding normal tissues.

This chapter will summarize the physics of proton therapy and the recent technical advances in the delivery of the proton beam, review the clinical results, and describe the treatment protocol used at our institution in the treatment of prostate cancer patients.

19.2 Physics of Proton Beam Radiation Therapy

The proton is a positively charged particle. A beam made of protons deposits most of its energy at a fixed depth known as the Bragg peak with very little dose deposited beyond that depth (Fig. 19.1). In contrast, an X-ray beam deposits its maximum dose just inside the patient's body and then continues to travel through the body

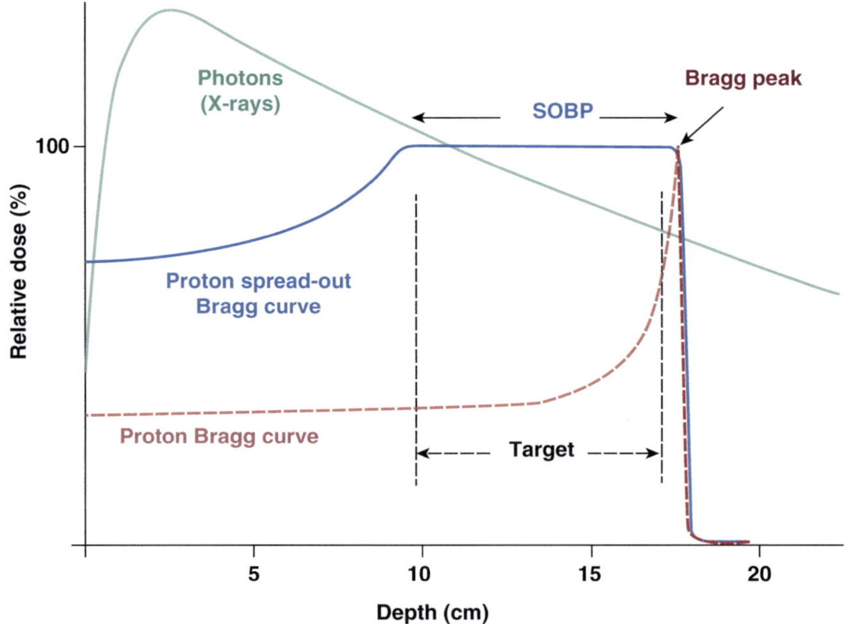

Fig. 19.1 Dose deposition characteristics of protons vs. X-rays

depositing dose until it exits the body. The depth of the Bragg peak is based on the energy of the proton beam. Normally, the Bragg peak is too narrow to treat the entire tumor. Therefore, the width of the Bragg peak is spread out to cover the entire target volume with margin (spread out Bragg peak, also known as SOBP).

Because of the absence of an exit dose, proton therapy can be used to treat cancer patients with less scatter radiation dose compared to X-rays. For prostate cancer patients treated with protons, the most common beam arrangement used for treatment is two beams coming in from the right lateral and left lateral directions. In contrast, X-rays with intensity-modulated radiation therapy (IMRT) use multiple angles or arcs to be able to concentrate the radiation dose around the prostate. This means that there is low-dose scatter to the rest of the pelvis, including to the bladder and rectum.

19.3 Modes of Proton Delivery

Currently there are two types of proton therapy delivery: passively scattered proton therapy and pencil beam proton therapy. Passively scattered proton therapy consists of a monoenergetic beam of protons, which is scattered by a snout to a square-shaped beam. As mentioned before, the Bragg peak is usually spread out to cover the entire tumor with margin in the direction of the beam using a range modulator wheel. This beam is shaped by a custom aperture (usually made of brass) and a custom tissue compensator (usually made of acrylic or wax), unique to the patient's anatomy. The aperture determines the shape of the radiation field (akin to multileaf collimators for X-rays), and the compensator shapes the distal edge of the proton beam dose to the shape of the target volume (Fig. 19.2).

Pencil beam proton therapy (also known as actively scanned proton therapy or spot-scanning proton therapy) uses a small proton beam ("pencil beam") to deliver dose by sequentially layering multiple pristine Bragg peaks (or "spots"). An electromagnetic field is used in the pencil beam to scan the protons in both directions perpendicular to the beam direction (i.e., X and Y axes) without the need for a scattering device [6–8]. Dose delivery in the distal and proximal directions (i.e., Z axis) is achieved by changing the energy of the pencil beam and delivering multiple layers of

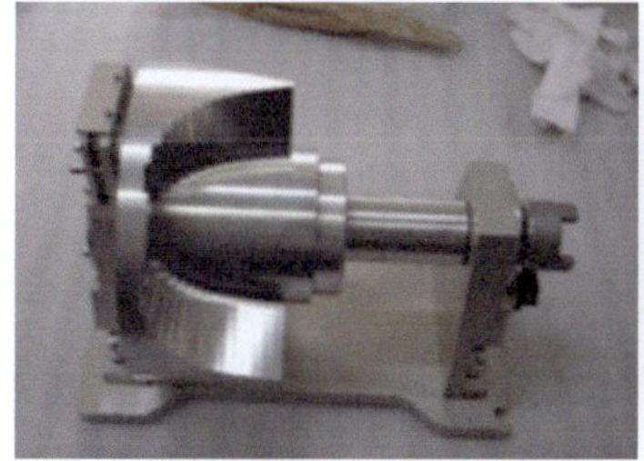
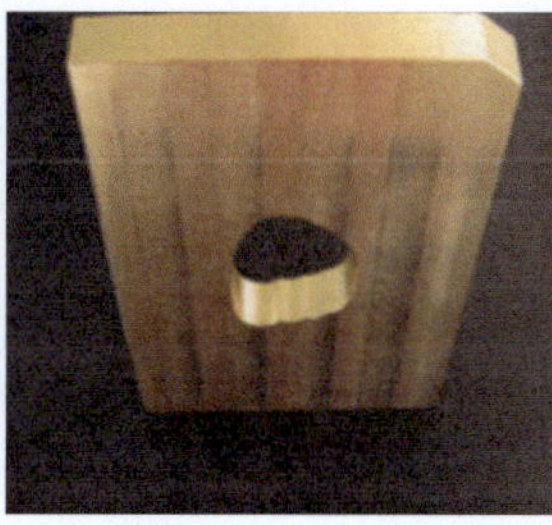
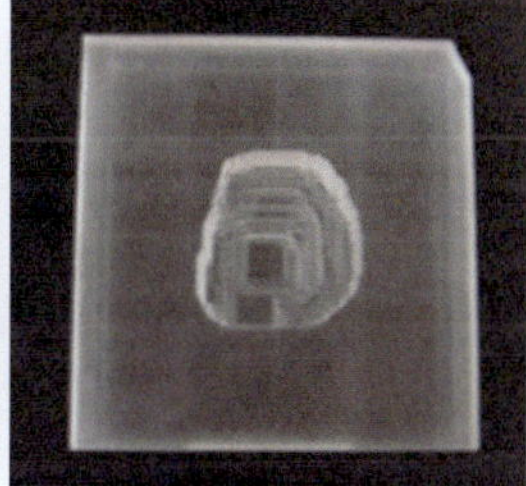

Fig. 19.2 Hardware used for passively scattered protons (from *left*, range moderator wheel, aperture, tissue compensator)

dose, instead of using a range-modulator wheel. Because this layering of dose allows for better conformity of the proximal edge of the target volume compared to passively scattered proton therapy, there is improved normal tissue sparing.

Pencil beam proton therapy has several advantages over passively scattered proton beam therapy. Pencil beam allows for improved conformality of the proton dose with improved tumor coverage and normal tissue sparing, especially around curved structures. The pencil beam does not require the use of brass apertures and acrylic compensators, which saves time and effort normally needed to make such hardware. It also makes it easier and faster for radiation therapists to treat the patient, as they no longer need to mount the hardware on the treatment machine. Because each beam angle with the passively scattered proton therapy needs its own set of aperture and compensator, the number of beam angles that can be used per patient is limited. With the pencil beam, there is less of a limit on how many angles can be used for the treatment. Furthermore, the hardware in the pathway of the passively scattered proton therapy (which includes the range-modulator wheel, aperture, and tissue compensator) leads to increased neutron production. Therefore, the pencil beam proton therapy also has the advantage of decreased neutron dose, which should decrease the risk of affecting implanted medical devices and the risk of secondary cancers. Finally, the pencil beam is required for intensity-modulated proton therapy (IMPT) using multifield optimization. IMPT allows for further improvements in dose conformality and simultaneous integrated boosts (SIB) of the gross tumor. However, the pencil beam plans require more rigorous quality assurance to make sure that the dose delivery matches the treatment plan.

The main difference between a pencil beam plan and a passively scattered plan for treatment of a prostate cancer patient is that the radiation dose lateral and posterior to the prostate is much more conformal with the pencil beam. Most of the proton therapy centers now have pencil beam available for treatment. In fact, the newest proton therapy centers are being built with only pencil beam capability (and will no longer have passively scattered proton beam). Figure 19.3 shows the difference between plans using passively scattered and pencil beam proton therapy.

19.4 Clinical Outcomes

Several studies have shown the benefit of dose escalation in the treatment of prostate cancer. Kuban et al. randomized 301 patients with stage T1b–T3 prostate cancer to either 70 or 78 Gy using X-ray therapy. At a median follow-up of 8.7 years, the patients who received 78 Gy had an improved freedom from biochemical or clinical failure of 78% compared to 59% in patients who received 70 Gy ($p = 0.004$) [4]. There was also improvement in the clinical failure-free survival in the 78 Gy arm (93% vs. 85%, $p = 0.014$), but there was no overall survival benefit. Unfortunately, the 78 Gy arm was also associated with higher toxicity, with the rate of RTOG grade 2 or higher gastrointestinal (GI) toxicity being 26% vs. 13% ($p = 0.013$). There was no significant difference in the RTOG grade 2 or higher genitourinary (GU) toxicity (13% vs. 8%).

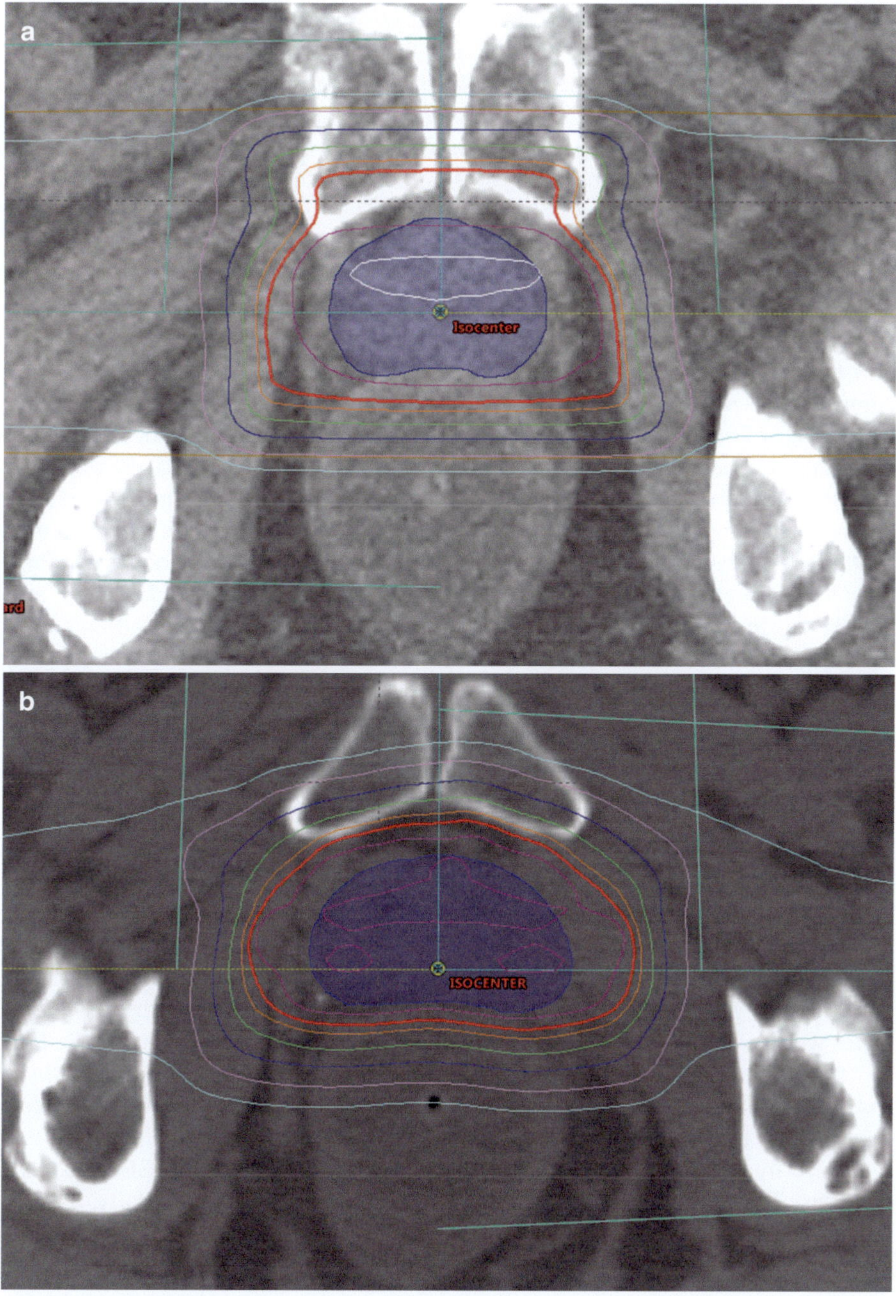

Fig. 19.3 Difference between treatment plans using passively scattered (**a**) and pencil beam (**b**) proton therapy

The Dutch Multicenter Trial randomized 669 patients with localized prostate cancer to either 68 or 78 Gy using X-ray therapy. After a median follow-up of 70 months, the 7 year freedom from failure was improved in the 78 Gy arm compared to 68 Gy (54% vs. 47%, $p = 0.04$) [9]. Once again, there was an increased late grade 2 or higher GI toxicity seen in the 78 Gy arm compared to the 68 Gy arm (35% vs. 25%, $p = 0.04$). There was no significant difference in the late grade 2 or higher GU toxicity (40% vs. 41%, $p = 0.6$).

The Proton Radiation Oncology Group (PROG) 95–09 study randomized a total of 393 patients with stage T1b–T2b with PSA <15 ng/mL at either Loma Linda University Medical Center (LLUMC) or Massachusetts General Hospital (MGH). All patients received 3D conformal X-ray therapy to the prostate and seminal vesicles to a dose of 50.4 Gy, followed by either a proton boost of 28.8 cobalt Gy equivalent (CGE) or 19.8 CGE. Therefore, the patients were randomized to either 79.2 CGE or 70.2 CGE. At LLUMC, < patients were treated in the supine position using opposed lateral 250 MeV proton beams. At the MGH, patients were treated in the lithotomy position using a single transperineal 160 MeV proton beam. At a median follow-up of 8.9 years, patients who received the 79.2 CGE were significantly less likely to have local failure with a hazard ratio of 0.57. The 10 year biochemical failure rate using the ASTRO definition was 16.7% for the 79.2 CGE arm and 32.4% for the 70.2 CGE arm (p = <0.0001). The patient reported outcomes using the prostate cancer symptom indices (PCSI) were published in a separate publication. At a median of 9.4 years, there was no difference in urinary obstruction/irritation ($p = 0.36$), urinary incontinence ($p = 0.99$), bowel problems ($p = 0.70$), or sexual dysfunction ($p = 0.65$) [10]. Unfortunately, the PROG 95–09 was not a randomized study comparing protons to X-rays; all of the patients received a combination of photons and X-rays. However, it is interesting to note that there is no increased GI toxicity seen with dose escalation in this study where proton therapy was used.

Several single-institution reports on the outcomes of prostate cancer patients after proton therapy have been published. Slater et al. published the LLUMC experience of 1255 patients treated between October 1991 and December 1997. Patients with 15% or greater risk of having pelvic lymph node metastasis by the Partin tables were treated with a conformal "boost" using protons to a dose of 30 CGE in 15 fractions which was given to the prostate and seminal vesicles, followed by a conformal treatment using X-rays to a dose of 45 Gy to the prostate, seminal vesicles, and the first- and second-echelon lymphatics. Patients who did not have this risk were treated with proton therapy only to a total dose of 74 CGE in 2 CGE fractions. These patients were treated with a rectal balloon placed daily, usually with one field per day. With a median follow-up of 62 months, the overall biochemical disease-free survival was 73% [11]. In patients with initial PSAs $\leq$ 4.0, it was 90% and in patients with posttreatment PSA $\leq$0.5, 87%. The actuarial 5 year and 10 year rates for freedom from grades 3 and 4 GI toxicity were both 99%. The actuarial 5 year and 10 year rates for freedom from grades 3 and 4 GU toxicity were also both 99%.

Bryant et al. published the outcomes of 1327 patients treated between 2006 and 2010. With a median follow-up of 5.5 years, the 5 year freedom from biochemical progression was 99%, 94%, and 74% in low-risk, intermediate-risk, and high-risk patients, respectively [12]. The actuarial 5-year rates of late grade ≥ 3 Common Terminology Criteria for Adverse Events, version 4.0 (CTCAE 4.0), GI and GU toxicities were 0.6% and 2.9%, respectively. There was no significant change in median and mean expanded prostate cancer index (EPIC) summary scores for the bowel, urinary irritative/obstructive, and urinary incontinence domains. Only the sexual function summary scores in patients who did not get hormone ablation therapy significantly declined from baseline to 5 years.

Pugh et al. reported the patient-reported outcomes of 291 patients after proton therapy from the MD Anderson Cancer Center (MDACC) who had a minimum follow-up of 2 years. All patients were treated with opposed lateral beams to a total dose of 76 CGE in 2 CGE fractions. Interestingly, 226 patients were treated with passively scattered proton therapy, and 65 patients were treated with pencil beam proton therapy. Cumulative grade ≥ 2 GU and GI toxicities at 24 months were 13.4% and 9.6%, respectively [13]. There was 1 grade 3 GI toxicity, but no grade ≥ 3 GU toxicity. There was slight higher incidence of argon plasma coagulation application in the passively scattered proton therapy compared to pencil beam proton therapy, but it was not statistically significant (4.4% vs. 1.5%, $p = 0.21$).

There have been several retrospective comparisons between protons and IMRT. A Surveillance, Epidemiology, and End Results (SEER)-Medicare analysis by Sheets et al. showed a lower rate of GI morbidity (RR 0.66) with IMRT compared to protons in a propensity score-matched comparison. However, this analysis was severely limited as any GI procedure after the treatment was coded as a morbidity. Hoppe et al. performed a comparison of patients undergoing either proton therapy or IMRT using prospectively collected quality of life (QoL) data using the EPIC. There were 1243 proton patients treated with 76–82 CGE and 204 IMRT patients treated with 75.6–79.4 Gy. There was no difference seen between the two groups for the bowel, urinary incontinence, urinary irritative/obstructive, and sexual domains [14]. However, more patients in the IMRT group reported moderate/big problems with rectal urgency ($p = 0.02$) and frequent bowel movements ($p = 0.05$) compared to patients in the proton therapy group. Fang et al. compared 181 proton therapy patients and 213 IMRT patients treated between 2010 and 2012 using maximum acute and late GI/GU CTCAE-graded toxicities. On multivariate analysis, there were no statistically significant differences in the acute/late grade ≥ 2 GU and GI toxicities between the two groups [15]. Yu et al. performed an analysis using the Medicare database of 27,647 men. In this analysis, patients who received proton therapy had significant less GU toxicity at 6 months compared to IMRT (5.9% vs. 9.5%, $p = 0.03$); however, the difference disappeared by 12 months (18.8% vs. 17.5%, $p = 0.66$) [16]. There was no difference in GI or other toxicities at 6 or 12 months.

Proton therapy may also reduce the risk of secondary cancer when compared to IMRT. Several analyses have predicted that IMRT would increase the risk of secondary cancer over conventional 3D conformal radiation therapy due to the increased scattered dose, while proton therapy would decrease the risk [16–19]. A retrospective matched cohort analysis of 558 proton patients and 558 X-ray patients matched using the SEER registry published by Chung et al. showed that there is a significant reduction of secondary cancer risk (RR 0.52, $p = 0.009$) in patients treated with proton therapy compared to X-ray therapy. However, due to the limitation of this retrospective study, the authors stated that these results should only be considered as hypothesis generating.

These results show that proton therapy is an effective and safe method for the treatment of prostate cancer. However, as there has been no randomized trial comparing proton therapy to IMRT, it is difficult to know if protons are superior to IMRT in terms of efficacy and/or risk of side effects. There is one randomized trial currently ongoing called the Proton Therapy vs. IMRT for Low or Intermediate Risk Prostate Cancer (PARTIQoL). However, we will need to wait several years until the results of that trial are available.

19.5 Proton Treatment at MD Anderson Cancer Center

19.5.1 Patient Selection

Although the results of the PARTIQoL trial are not yet available, there are probably several specific instances where proton therapy may be especially beneficial. For instance, we recommend proton therapy in younger patients (although the definition of "younger" can vary significantly among clinicians) and patients with larger prostates, especially with a large median lobe. Trying to cover a large median lobe using IMRT usually leads to giving radiation dose to a much larger area of the bladder. However, if a patient has a very large median lobe, it might be worthwhile to consider having the patient undergo a transurethral resection of the prostate (TURP) or greenlight laser enucleation of the median lobe before the radiation therapy. If a patient were to undergo such a procedure, we recommend waiting 2–3 months before the start of the radiation therapy to allow for adequate healing to minimize the risk of urinary incontinence after the radiation therapy.

Just like with IMRT, we do not recommend proton therapy in patients with certain collagen vascular disease (such as Lupus and scleroderma) and inflammatory bowel disease (i.e., Crohn's disease and ulcerative colitis). We also do not treat patients with metal in the pelvis in the pathway of the proton therapy, which most often consists of artificial hips. There are two reasons why we avoid treating patients with metal in the pelvis. The first reason is that the proton therapy can be significantly blocked by the metal in the pathway, which could decrease the dose delivered to the prostate. The second reason is that the artifact from the metal makes the treatment planning less accurate due to increased uncertainty in tissue density calculation from the planning CT. We also tend to discourage patients who are pacemaker dependent from undergoing proton therapy due to the neutron dose from the proton therapy. When we do treat patients with pacemakers (or any other implanted electronics), we treat these patients with the pencil beam to try to decrease the neutron dose as low as possible.

19.5.2 Fiducial Placement

Once the patient is deemed to be a candidate for proton therapy, the patient is scheduled for his fiducial placement and simulation.

At our institution, the fiducials are inserted transrectally under ultrasound guidance by the radiation oncologist. However at other institutions, either urology or interventional radiology may be the ones placing these fiducials. Unlike with IMRT, fiducial placement may be more important as there can be shadowing of the proton dose from the fiducials. Tables 19.1 and 19.2 show the actual amount of dose attenuation from various types of fiducials. Of the three types of fiducials listed, gold

Table 19.1 Gold fiducial dose attenuation [20]

Marker	Orientation	Z_c(cm)	ΔD_{max}(%)	Z_s(cm)
Small gold	Perpendicular	19.5	−15	>0.93
Small gold	Perpendicular	23.5	−17	0.58
Small gold	Perpendicular	26.5	−24	Fluctuates
Small gold	Perpendicular	27.5	−46	0.46
Small gold	Parallel	19.5	−37	0.35
Small gold	Parallel	23.5	−41	0.35
Small gold	Parallel	26.5	−67	0.00
Small gold	Parallel	27.5	−86	0.00
Large gold	Perpendicular	19.5	−21	>0.93
Large gold	Perpendicular	23.5	−25	0.93
Large gold	Perpendicular	26.5	−42	1.04
Large gold	Perpendicular	27.5	−69	0.46
Large gold	Parallel	19.5	−43	0.69
Large gold	Parallel	23.5	−48	0.46
Large gold	Parallel	26.5	−83	0.00
Large gold	Parallel	27.5	−91	0.00

Table 19.2 Carbon and PEEK fiducial dose attenuation [20]

Marker	Orientation	Z_c(cm)	ΔD_{max}(%)	Z_s(cm)
C/ZrO_2	Perpendicular	19.5	–	–
C/ZrO_2	Perpendicular	23.5	−8	0.35
C/ZrO_2	Perpendicular	26.5	−7	Fluctuates
C/ZrO_2	Perpendicular	27.5	−18	0.58
C/ZrO_2	Parallel	19.5	−10	0.58
C/ZrO_2	Parallel	23.5	−15	0.35
C/ZrO_2	Parallel	26.5	−21	0.12
C/ZrO_2	Parallel	27.5	−38	0.23
PEEK/stainless steel	Perpendicular	19.5	–	–
PEEK/stainless steel	Perpendicular	23.5	–	–
PEEK/stainless steel	Perpendicular	26.5	−2	Fluctuates
PEEK/stainless steel	Parallel	19.5	−7	0.58
PEEK/stainless steel	Parallel	23.5	−8	0.58
PEEK/stainless steel	Parallel	26.5	−12	0.35

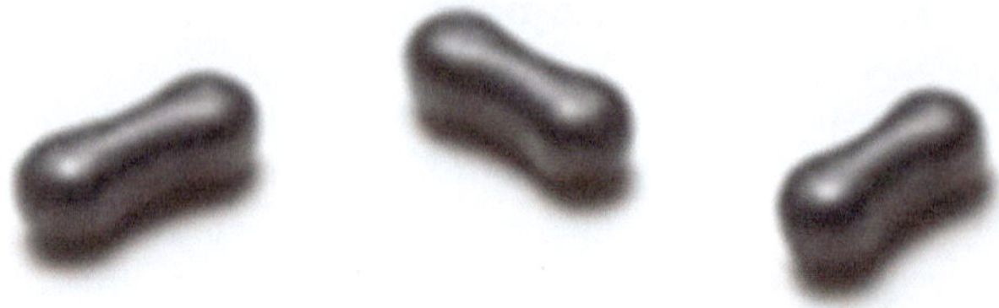

Fig. 19.4 Carbon-coated zirconium dioxide fiducials

fiducials have the highest proton attenuation. Therefore we use the carbon/ZrO2 fiducial at our institution (Fig. 19.4). We also usually place two fiducials in the prostate (as opposed to 3 for IMRT) to minimize the risk of the shadowing of the dose to areas of the tumor. We also try to place the fiducials in areas where there is no or minimal cancer.

Once the fiducials have been placed, there should ideally be 7 days before the simulation is done. However, as many of our patients are out of town, we often perform the simulation on the same day as the fiducial placement. There is no fiducial placement for postoperative patients undergoing radiation therapy.

19.5.3 Simulation

For the simulation, we place the patient in a supine position and place the endorectal balloon in the rectum. We then inflate the balloon with 60–80 cc of warm water based on the size of the balloon that is used (either "short" or "long"). Once the balloon is placed, we immobilize the patient's legs in a foot–knee indexed cradle. After ensuring that the patient is straight and not rotated, a non-contrast planning CT is performed to the pelvis. There has been some concern of the effect of patient rotation on the daily treatment using protons. Sejpal et al. and Meyer et al. showed that patient rotational setup errors up to 5° on either side do not significantly change the dose to the target volume or critical structures using passively scattered proton therapy and pencil beam proton therapy, respectively [21, 22].

The rectal balloon is used to immobilize the prostate in the pelvis. Having a consistent tissue path that the protons have to travel to reach the prostate is important as change in this path length can affect the dose deposition of the proton beam. The rectal balloon can also push the posterior aspect of the rectum, as well as the sigmoid colon and small bowel away from the prostate, which likely decreases the risk of toxicity to these structures. However, at the same time, the anterior wall of the rectum is often placed next to the prostate more consistently by the rectal balloon, which may negate some of the benefit of pushing the rest of the rectum away.

For postoperative patients, rectal balloon use is determined on an individual basis as there is no prostate to immobilize. In some patients, the balloon can help push the sigmoid and bowel away, while in others, it can lead to more rectum getting radiation dose due to the balloon pushing the prostate fossa more posteriorly and laterally around the rectum.

19.5.4 Contouring

At our institution, the CTV for definitive prostate cancer patients is based on the National Cancer Center Network (NCCN) risk classification for prostate cancer as per the following: prostate only for low risk, prostate proximal seminal vesicles (SV) for intermediate risk, and prostate and entire SV for high risk. Proximal is defined as the proximal 1.5 cm of the SV. Pelvic lymph nodes are generally not treated even for high-risk prostate cancer at our institution. However, when the pelvic lymph nodes are treated, proton therapy offers significant bowel sparing compared to IMRT (Fig. 19.5).

19.5.5 Dosing

The standard dose is 78 CGE in two CGE daily fractions. We do consider using a slower fractionation scheme (i.e., 77.4 or 79.2 CGE in 1.8 CGE daily fractions) in patients with previous treatments to the prostate (i.e., cryotherapy, HIFU) to minimize the risk of urethral toxicity.

We also have a protocol evaluating a hypofractionation regimen of 55.5 CGE in 3.7 CGE fractions given three times per week (for a total of 15 fractions given over 5 weeks).

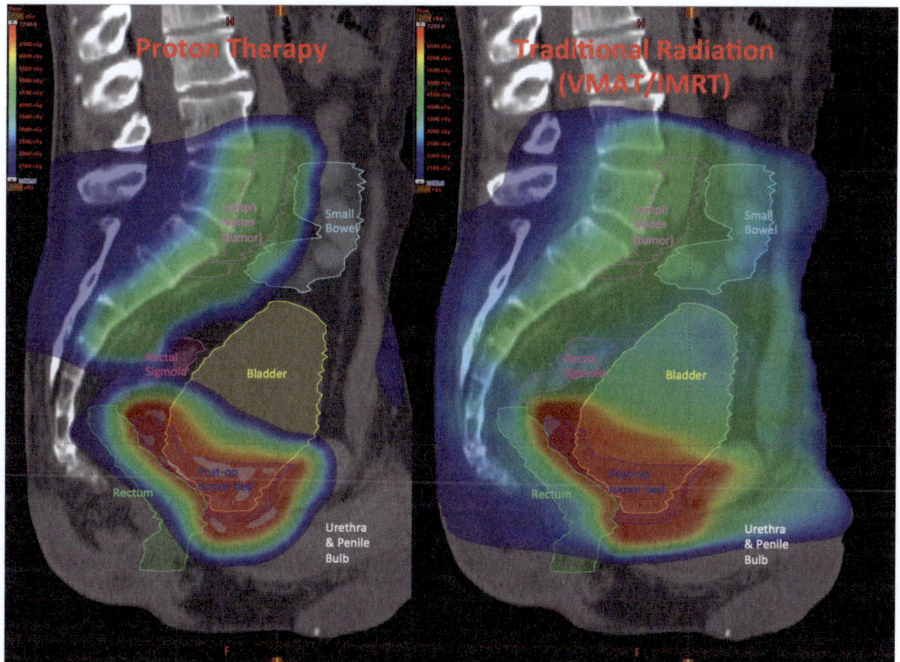

Fig. 19.5 Proton therapy offers significant bowel sparing compared to IMRT when the pelvic lymph nodes are treated

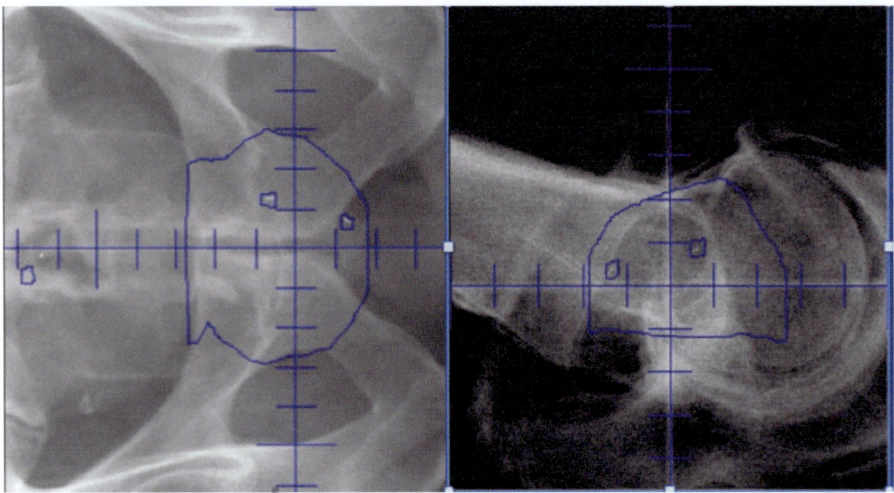

Fig. 19.6 Daily kV imaging of carbon fiducials for proton therapy

19.5.6 Image Guidance

Daily image-guided radiation therapy (IGRT) is achieved using daily kV imaging with fiducials (Fig. 19.6). For the postoperative patients, we use daily kV imaging of the pelvic bony anatomy.

Conclusions

Proton therapy is an effective and safe treatment modality for the treatment of prostate cancer. Pencil beam proton therapy and the advent of IMPT have allowed further improvements in the planning and dose delivery.

In the future, we aim to incorporate more MRI imaging into the planning with an MRI simulator which, when combined with IMPT, will allow us to target dominant lesions. We will also likely move more toward hypofractionated proton therapy and even start treating patients with stereotactic body proton therapy (SBPT) to the prostate.

References

1. Wilson RR. Radiological use of fast protons. Radiology. 1946;45(7):487–91.
2. Particle Therapy Co-Operative Group (PTCOG) website.
3. Pollack A, Zagars GK, Starkschall G, et al. Prostate cancer radiation dose response: results of the M.D. Anderson phase III randomized trial. Int J Radiat Oncol Biol Phys. 2002;53(5):1097–105.
4. Kuban DA, Tucker SL, Dong L, et al. Long-term results of the M.D. Anderson randomized dose-escalation trial for prostate cancer. Int J Radiat Oncol Biol Phys. 2008;70(1):67–74.
5. Zietman AL, Bae K, Slater JD, et al. Randomized trial comparing conventional-dose with high-dose conformal radiation therapy in early stage adenocarcinoma of the prostate: long-term

results from proton radiation oncology group/American college of radiology 95–09″. JCO. 2010;28(7):1106–11.

6. Zhu XR, Sahoo N, Zhang X, et al. Intensity modulated proton therapy treatment planning using single-field optimization: the impact of monitor unit constraints on plan quality. Med Phys. 2010;37(3):1210–9.
7. Pedroni E, Bacher R, Blattmann H, et al. The 200-MeV proton therapy project at the Paul Scherrer Institute: conceptual design and practical realization. Med Phys. 1995;22(1):37–53.
8. Haberer T, Becher W, Schardt D, et al. Magnetic scanning system for heavy ion therapy. Nucl Instrum Methods Phys Res A. 1993;330:296–305.
9. Al-Mamgani A, van Putten WL, Heemsbergen WD, et al. Update of Dutch multicenter dose-escalation trial for radiotherapy for localized prostate cancer. Int J Radiat Biol Phys. 2008;72(4):980–8.
10. Talcott JA, Rossi C, Shipley WU, et al. Patient-reported long-term outcomes after conventional and high-dose combined proton and photon radiation for early prostate cancer. JAMA. 2010;303(11):1046–53.
11. Slater JD, Rossi CJ, Yonemoto LT, et al. Proton therapy for prostate cancer: the initial Loma Linda University experience. Int J Radiat Oncol Biol Phys. 2004;59(2):348–52.
12. Bryant C, Smith TL, Henderson RH, et al. Five-year biochemical results, toxicity, and patient-reported quality of life after delivery of dose-escalated image guided proton therapy for prostate cancer. Int J Radiat Oncol Biol Phys. 2016;95(1):422–34.
13. Pugh TJ, Munsell MF, Choi S, et al. Quality of life and toxicity from passively scattered and spot-scanning proton beam therapy for localized prostate cancer. Int J Radiat Oncol Biol Phys. 2013;87(5):946–53.
14. Hoppe BS, Michalski JM, Mendenhall NP, et al. Comparative effectiveness study of patient-reported outcomes after proton therapy or intensity-modulated radiotherapy for prostate cancer. Cancer. 2014;120(7):1076–82.
15. Fang P, Mick R, Deville C, et al. A case-matched study of toxicity outcomes after proton therapy and intensity-modulated radiation therapy for prostate cancer. Cancer. 2015;121(7):1118–27.
16. Yu JB, Soulos PR, Herrin J, et al. Proton versus intensity-modulated radiotherapy for prostate cancer: patterns of care and early toxicity. J Natl Cancer Inst. 2013;105(1):25–32.
17. Hall EJ, Wuu CS. Radiation-induced second cancers: the impact of 3D-CRT and IMRT. Int J Radiat Oncol Biol Phys. 2003;56(1):83–8.
18. Hall EJ. Intensity-modulated radiation therapy, protons, and the risk of second cancers. Int J Radiat Oncol Biol Phys. 2006;65(1):1–7.
19. Fontenot JD, Lee AK, Newhauser WD. Int J Radiat Oncol Biol Phys. 2009;74(2):616–22.
20. Cheung J, Kudchadker RJ, Zhu XR, et al. Dose perturbations and image artifacts caused by carbon-coated ceramic and stainless steel fiducials used in proton therapy for prostate cancer. Phys Med Biol. 2010;55(23):7135–47.
21. Sejpal SV, Amos RA, Bluett JB, et al. Dosimetric changes resulting from patient rotational setup errors in proton therapy prostate plans. Int J Radiat Oncol Biol Phys. 2009;75(1):40–8.
22. Meyer J, Bluett JB, Amos RA, et al. Spot scanning proton beam therapy for prostate cancer: treatment planning technique and analysis of consequences of rotational and translational alignment error. Int J Radiat Oncol Biol Phys. 2010;78(2):428–34.

The Role of Hormonal Treatment in Prostate Cancer

20

Pervin Hurmuz, Fadıl Akyol, Melis Gultekin, Gozde Yazici, Sezin Yuce Sari, and Gokhan Ozyigit

Abstract

Androgens are endocrine secretions produced mainly by the testes under stimulation of the pituitary gland. They are also synthesized from the adrenal glands in both sexes and from ovaries in females. Luteinizing hormone (LH) produced by the anterior pituitary gland regulates the secretion of androgens from the Leydig cells in the testes. LH secretion is controlled by the hypothalamus via gonadotropin-releasing hormone (GnRH). Androgens play a major role in the development and maintenance of male sex characteristics. The primary and most well-known androgen is testosterone that is rapidly and irreversibly converted to dihydrotestosterone (DHT) in prostate by types 1 and 2 5α-reductase. Androgens stimulate the growth of both normal and cancerous prostate cells by binding to and activating the androgen receptor (AR), a protein that is expressed in prostate cells. Then, AR stimulates the expression of specific genes that cause prostate cells to grow. The role of androgens in prostate cancer was first established in 1941 by Huggins and Hodges. Since then androgen deprivation therapy (ADT) has become the standard of care for patients with advanced prostate cancer. In this chapter ADT and its use in prostate cancer will be discussed.

P. Hurmuz, M.D. • F. Akyol, M.D. • M. Gultekin, M.D. • G. Yazici, M.D. (✉)
S.Y. Sari, M.D. • G. Ozyigit, M.D.
Department of Radiation Oncology, Hacettepe University, Ankara, Turkey
e-mail: yazicig@hacettepe.edu.tr

G. Ozyigit, U. Selek (eds.), *Principles and Practice of Urooncology*,
DOI 10.1007/978-3-319-56114-1_20

20.1 Androgen Deprivation Therapy

ADT aims to reduce the serum testosterone to castrate level. The castrate level was defined as testosterone being less than 50 ng/dL (1.7 nmol/L), many years ago. However contemporary laboratory testing methods showed that the mean value after surgical castration is 15 ng/dL [1]. Thus, recently the level is defined as being less than 20 ng/dL (1 nmol/L). Recent definition is associated with better outcomes compared to the previous one [2–4]. However, current guidelines from the National Comprehensive Cancer Network (NCCN) recommend testosterone level of <50 ng/dL (1.7 nmol/L) as the castration level [5].

ADT can be used as adjuvant or neoadjuvant therapy in conjunction with initial treatment of patients with intermediate- or high-risk prostate cancer, patients with rising PSA after curative treatment, or patients with metastatic disease at diagnosis. It can either be used before radiotherapy in patients with large prostate to decrease the tumor volume.

ADT can be accomplished either by surgical or medical orchiectomy. The decision between two treatment options is based upon factors like the preference of the patient, cost, and availability. Combined androgen blockade (CAB) refers to the combination of any ADT with an antiandrogen.

20.2 Surgical Castration

Bilateral orchiectomy is a simple and a cheap procedure which results in rapid decrease in serum testosterone to castration levels and improvement in disease-related symptoms. Although less frequently used in North America and Europe, it is a widely used method in many countries where availability and cost of medical castration are an issue. This type of castration is permanent and irreversible; thus the psychological impact of the treatment should be discussed with the patient. Subcapsular orchiectomy is another method in which the tunica albuginea and epididymis remain intact.

20.3 Medical Castration

There are several methods of medical castration. Measuring serum PSA levels is a way to monitor patient's response to treatment.

20.3.1 Estrogens

Estrogens inhibit the release of GnRH from the hypothalamus resulting in reduction in testicular production of testosterone via suppressed LHRH secretion from the pituitary. Historically, diethylstilbestrol (DES) was used as an alternative to surgical orchiectomy. However it was shown that DES significantly increased the risk of dying from heart disease and stroke without any survival benefit [6–7]. Due to severe side effects related to DES, estrogens are not considered as a first-line treatment.

20.3.2 Gonadotropin-Releasing Hormone Agonists

Gonadotropin-releasing hormone (GnRH) agonists bind to GnRH receptors on pituitary gland resulting in initial release of luteinizing hormone (LH) and follicle-stimulating hormone (FSH). This causes a subsequent increase in testosterone production from testes. However, this is a transient rise that is followed by a down-regulation of the GnRH receptors on gonadotropin-producing cells in a week. Decline in serum LH and FSH decreases testosterone levels within 3–4 weeks. Transient rise in LH 2–3 days after first injection leads to a surge in serum testosterone that lasts about a week and results in increase in the tumor growth. This is called "flare-up" phenomenon and is associated with increase in bone pain, acute bladder outlet obstruction, or other disease-related symptoms. Thus, initial treatment with GnRH is contraindicated in patients with severe urinary tract obstruction, painful bone metastases, or spinal cord compression. This can be prevented by antiandrogen treatment at least 1 week before GnRH application.

Approved GnRH analogs are leuprolide, goserelin, triptorelin, and histrelin. GnRH agonists are delivered as depot injections on a one-, two-, three-,or six-monthly periods. A castration level is usually obtained within 2–4 weeks and is reversible upon cessation of GnRH analog [8]. Klotz et al. showed that low nadir serum testosterone (<0.7 mmol/L) within the first year of ADT correlates with improved cause-specific survival (CSS) and duration of response to treatment in men being treated for biochemical failure undergoing continuous ADT [9].

20.3.3 Gonadotropin Hormone-Releasing Hormone Antagonists

GnRH antagonists immediately and reversibly bind to GnRH receptors of the anterior pituitary leading to a rapid decrease in LH, FSH, and testosterone levels without any flare. Currently approved GnRH antagonists are degarelix, abarelix, ganirelix, and cetrorelix. They are administered in parental way. They are used in the treatment where fast control of disease is needed. They do not have a long-acting depot formulation. Early GnRH antagonists leaded to histamine release and resulted in anaphylactic reactions [10–12].

Degarelix is the most extensively studied and widely available new GnRH antagonist with a monthly subcutaneous formulation. The standard dosage is 240 mg in the first month, followed by monthly injections of 80 mg. Most patients achieve a castrate level at the third day. An extended follow-up has been published, suggesting a better PFS compared to monthly leuprorelin [13]. Compared with GnRH agonists, degarelix is associated with faster decline in serum testosterone and PSA levels [8]. Its definitive superiority over the LHRH analogues remains to be proven.

20.3.4 Antiandrogens

Antiandrogens (AAs) are oral compounds that competitively inhibit the binding of androgens to the androgen receptor. They can be either steroidal (e.g., cyproterone acetate (CPA), megestrol acetate, and medroxyprogesterone acetate) or nonsteroidal (e.g., bicalutamide, flutamide, and nilutamide). Nonsteroidal AAs competitively inhibit the binding of androgens to the androgen receptor. Thus serum testosterone levels are not suppressed and may even be elevated by nonsteroidal AAs. However steroidal AAs have additional progestational and antigonadotropic properties. Its application via a feedback suppression of pituitary LHRH release thus leads to a reduction of serum testosterone levels.

20.3.4.1 Steroidal AAs

They are synthetic derivatives of hydroxyprogesterone. Their main side effects are suppression of libido and erectile dysfunction. Cardiovascular toxicity and hepatotoxicity may also be seen. Cyproterone acetate (CPA), megestrol acetate, and medroxyprogesterone acetate are examples of steroidal AAs. CPA has no overall survival (OS) advantage compared to LHRH analogues [14]. Another study comparing CPA with flutamide in M1b disease did not show any difference in disease specific- and OS at a median follow-up of 8.6 years [15].

20.3.4.2 Nonsteroidal AAs

Bicalutamide is the most widely used form of nonsteroidal AAs. The licensed dosages are 50 mg or 150 mg. Bicalutamide monotherapy seems to be a tolerable regimen for patients with biochemical failure following 3D-CRT and TAD and may be effective in patients with low PSA levels at biochemical failure [16]. Its main side effects are gynecomastia and breast pain that occur in 70–80% of patients [17–19]. However it was shown that bicalutamide monotherapy increases bone mineral density, lessens fat accumulation, and has fewer bothersome side effects than treatment with a gonadotropin-releasing hormone agonist [20].

Nilutamide and flutamide are the other forms of nonsteroidal AAs. All of them have potential liver hepatotoxicity; thus liver enzymes should be regularly monitored during treatment. Nilutamide is not licensed for monotherapy. Its side effects are visual disturbances, alcohol intolerance, nausea, and specifically severe interstitial pneumonitis. Flutamide has been studied as monotherapy. The half-life of the active metabolite of flutamide is 5–6 h; thus it should be used three times daily. Its frequent side effect is diarrhea.

Castration resistance may occur during the course of the disease. Castration-resistant prostate cancer (CRPC) is considered to be mediated through two mechanisms: either androgen-receptor (AR)- dependent or AR-independent ways. Abiraterone acetate is a CYP17 inhibitor. It significantly decreases the intracellular testosterone level by suppressing its synthesis at the adrenal level and inside the tumor cells. It must be used together with prednisone/prednisolone (2 × 5 mg) to prevent drug-induced hyperaldosteronism.

Enzalutamide is another AA with a higher affinity for the androgen receptor. Nonsteroidal AAs allow transfer of ARs to the nucleus, but enzalutamide additionally blocks AR transfer leading to suppression of any possible agonist-like activity.

20.4 Combined Androgen Blockade with Antiandrogens

CAB is defined as the combination of an AA with orchiectomy or medical castration. It blocks the effect of both testicular and adrenal androgens. AAs are not indicated as monotherapy for treatment naïve patients. However it is used in conjunction with medical castration to block the side effects associated with the flare phenomenon at the initiation of ADT. Given 7–10 days before the initiation of GnRH analogue, GnRH receptors are downregulated at the hypophysis. This results in decline of LH and FSH secretion leading to decrease in testosterone to castrate level within 3–4 weeks after the start of treatment.

The decrease in testosterone production is generally reversible. However depending on the duration of ADT and patient-related other factors, it may not return to baseline levels after treatment cessation. Murthy et al. showed that after LHRHa treatment and radiotherapy, the testosterone levels of most men had recovered to normal by 18–24 weeks after the last injection [21]. D'Amico et al. showed that time to testosterone recovery was associated with a lower risk of death in men with no or minimal comorbidity [22].

Studies of short-term and long-term neoadjuvant ADT all have used CAB. To date, there are no trials comparing the use of initial CAB with AA monotherapy in nonmetastatic prostate cancer patients. Safety and Efficacy Study of Enzalutamide Plus Leuprolide in Patients with Nonmetastatic Prostate Cancer (EMBARK) trial is an ongoing trial that randomizes patients to enzalutamide plus leuprolide, enzalutamide monotherapy, or leuprolide monotherapy after radical prostatectomy (RP) or radiotherapy [23].

There are two studies comparing CAB with AA monotherapy in metastatic prostatic cancer. Intergroup trial INT 0036 is a randomized, double-blind trial that compared leuprolide in combination with either placebo or flutamide in 603 patients with disseminated, previously untreated prostate cancer. Patients who received leuprolide and flutamide had a longer progression-free survival (16.5 vs. 13.9 months; $p = 0.039$) and an increase in the median length of survival (35.6 vs. 28.3 months; $p = 0.035$) with symptom control [24]. Intergroup trial INT 0105 enrolled 1387 patients with metastatic prostate cancer to orchiectomy and either flutamide or placebo. The addition of flutamide to orchiectomy does not result in a clinically significant improvement in survival. Patients who received flutamide had more toxicity compared to placebo group [25].

20.5 Intermittent Androgen Deprivation

ADT has several side effects including loss of libido, hot flashes, night sweats, psychological stress, osteoporosis, anemia, fatigue, loss of muscle mass, glucose intolerance, and changes in lipid profile. Prolonged ADT may also lead to progression of androgen independence. The aim of intermittent androgen deprivation (IAD) is to minimize the adverse effects of continuous ADT and to delay progression of castration resistance. IAD is delivered for a period of time or until a maximal response is achieved based on PSA levels. Then ADT is withdrawn and patient is followed with PSA. ADT is initiated in case of recurrence or disease progression based on PSA levels.

20.5.1 Metastatic Disease

The intergroup trial INT 0162 was designed to assess whether intermittent therapy was noninferior to continuous therapy with respect to survival in patients with metastatic, hormone-sensitive prostate cancer. Patients with PSA level of ≥5 ng/mL received aN LHRH analogue and an AA agent for 7 months. Patients in whom the PSA level fell to ≤4 ng/mL were randomly assigned to continuous or IAD [26]. ADT was reinitiated in the IAD group when the PSA level rose to 20 ng per milliliter (or returned to baseline in the case of patients who had PSA levels of <20 ng/mL before enrollment). A total of 3040 patients were enrolled, of whom 1535 were included in the analysis. The median follow-up period was 9.8 years. Median survival was 5.8 years in the continuous-therapy group and 5.1 years in the IAD group (hazard ratio for death with intermittent therapy, 1.10; 90% confidence interval, 0.99–1.23). Intermittent therapy was associated with better erectile function and mental health ($p < 0.001$ and $p = 0.003$, respectively) at month 3 but not thereafter. There were no significant differences between the groups in the number of treatment-related high-grade adverse events. Based on these results, continuous ADT remains the standard of care in patients with metastatic prostate cancer.

20.5.2 Rising PSA

Crook et al. evaluated the noninferiority of IAD compared to continuous ADT in terms of overall survival. Patients with PSA level greater than 3 ng/mL more than 1 year after primary or salvage radiotherapy for localized prostate cancer were included. All of the 1386 enrolled patients did not have detectable metastases. Intermittent treatment was provided in 8 month cycles, with nontreatment periods determined according to the PSA level. Median follow-up was 6.9 years. Median OS was 8.8 years in the IAD group versus 9.1 years in the continuous-therapy group (hazard ratio for death, 1.02; 95% confidence interval, 0.86–1.21). There were no significant differences in adverse events. IAD provided potential benefits with respect to physical function, fatigue, and hormonal, urinary, and erectile function. This study showed that IAD was noninferior to continuous therapy with respect to OS and some quality-of-life factors improved with intermittent therapy [27].

Table 20.1 Randomized studies of radiotherapy and androgen blockade in patients with prostate cancer

Study	No of patients	Randomization	Results
RTOG 85-31 [31]	977	RT vs. RT + LHRHa (continuous)	Combined arm is better in all end points
RTOG 86-10 [32]	456	RT vs. RT + 4 month CAB	No significant difference in OS GS 2–6 patients have better OS
RTOG 92-02 [33]	1554	RT + 4 month LHRHa vs. RT + 2 year LHRHa	Long-term arm is better in all end points except OS GS 8–10 patients have better OS with long-term LHRHa
EORTC 22863 [34]	415	RT vs. RT + 3 year LHRHa	Combined arm is better in all end points

RT radiotherapy, *LHRH* luteinizing hormone-releasing hormone, *CAB* complete androgen blockade, *GS* Gleason score, *OS* overall survival

20.6 Timing of Hormonal Therapy

ADT was shown to improve OS and PFS in patients with locally advanced disease [28–30]. Table 20.1 represents the results of ADT combined with RT.

ADT was shown to be the most cost-effective therapy if started at the time that the patient developed symptomatic metastases [35] Thus ADT should be started immediately in case of symptomatic metastases in order to palliate symptoms and prevent complications; however, controversy still exists regarding asymptomatic metastatic patients because of the lack of high-quality studies.

20.7 Hormonal Treatment Combined with Chemotherapy

Three large RCTs compared ADT alone as the standard of care with ADT combined with immediate docetaxel (75 mg/m^2 every 3 weeks; within 3 months of ADT initiation) in terms of OS [36–38].

In the GETUG-15 trial [36], all patients had newly diagnosed M1 prostate cancer, either primary or after a primary treatment. After a median follow-up of 83.9 months, updated results of GETUG-15 trial were published [37]. Median OS was 62.1 months and 48.6 months for ADT plus docetaxel and ADT arms, respectively (hazard ratio [HR]: 0.88 [95% CI, 0.68–1.14]; $p = 0.3$). Median OS in ADT plus docetaxel and ADT arms, respectively, was for high-volume disease (HVD) patients 39.8 months versus 35.1 months (HR: 0.78 [95% CI, 0.56–1.09]; $p = 0.14$) for low-volume disease (LVD) patients; median was not reached and 83.4 months (HR: 1.02 [95% CI, 0.67–1.55]; $p = 0.9$). For up-front metastatic patients, OS was 52.6 months and 41.5 months, respectively (HR: 0.93 [95% CI, 0.69–1.25]; $p = 0.6$). The bPFS (HR: 0.73 [95% CI, 0.56–0.94]; $p = 0.014$) and rPFS (HR: 0.75 [95% CI,

0.58–0.97]; $p = 0.030$) were significantly longer in the ADT plus D arm. Docetaxel should not be used as part of first-line treatment for patients with non-castrate metastatic prostate cancer.

In the CHAARTED trial [38], the same inclusion criteria applied. High-volume disease was defined as either presence of visceral metastases or four or more bone metastases, with at least one outside the spine and pelvis. After a median follow-up of 28.9 months, the median overall survival was 13.6 months longer with ADT plus docetaxel than with ADT alone (57.6 months vs. 44.0 months; $p < 0.001$). The median time to progression was 20.2 months in the combination group, as compared with 11.7 months in the ADT-alone group ($p < 0.001$). The rate of a prostate-specific antigen level of less than 0.2 ng/mL at 12 months was 27.7% in the combination group versus 16.8% in the ADT-alone group ($p < 0.001$). In the combination group, the rate of grade 3 or 4 febrile neutropenia was 6.2%, the rate of grade 3 or 4 infection with neutropenia was 2.3%, and the rate of grade 3 sensory neuropathy and of grade 3 motor neuropathy was 0.5%. It was concluded that ADT plus docetaxel for metastatic prostate cancer resulted in significantly longer overall survival than that with ADT alone.

STAMPEDE [39] was a multiarm, multistage trial including high-risk, locally advanced, metastatic, or recurrent prostate cancer who is starting first-line long-term hormone therapy. The standard of care (SOC) arm was ADT ($n = 1184$). The experimental arms were ADT combined with docetaxel ($n = 593$) and ADT combined with zoledronic acid ($n = 593$), and another was ADT combined with docetaxel and zoledronic acid ($n = 593$). Median follow-up was 43 months. Median overall survival was 71 months for SOC only, not reached for SOC + ZA ($p = 0.450$), 81 months for SOC + docetaxel ($p = 0.006$), and 76 months for SOC + ZA + docetaxel ($p = 0.022$). Grade 3–5 adverse events were reported for 399 (32%) patients receiving SOC, 197 (32%) receiving SOC + ZA, 288 (52%) receiving SOC + docetaxel, and 269 (52%) receiving SOC + ZA + docetaxel. Zoledronic acid showed no evidence of survival improvement, but docetaxel chemotherapy, given at the time of long-term hormone therapy initiation, showed evidence of improved survival accompanied by an increase in adverse events. Thus it was concluded that docetaxel treatment should become part of standard of care for adequately fit men commencing long-term hormone therapy. Table 20.2 summarizes the results of those four important trials.

Table 20.2 Hormonal treatment combined with chemotherapy in patients with metastatic disease

Study	No of patients	Median FU, months	Median OS, months (ADT + D vs. ADT)	*p* value
Gravis et al. [36]	385	50	58.9 vs. 54.2	0.955
Gravis et al. [37]	385	82.9	60.9 vs. 46.5	0.44
Sweeney et al. [38]	790	28.9	57.6 vs. 44	<0.001
STAMPEDE trial [39]	SOC 1184	43	81 vs. 71	0.006
	D 593		76 vs. NR	0.022
	D + ZA 593		60 vs. 45	0.005

ADT androgen deprivation therapy, *D* docetaxel, *FU* follow-up, *NR* not reported, *ZA* zoledronic acid, *OS* overall survival

20.8 Side Effects of Hormonal Treatment

ADT has been shown to improve survival when used with radiation for patients with intermediate- and high-risk disease and locally advanced and node-positive disease. However it may cause side effects on bone, metabolic, cardiovascular, sexual, and cognitive health as well as body composition that negatively affect quality of life of patients.

20.8.1 Osteoporosis and Bone Fractures

ADT decreases bone mineral density (BMD). It was shown that ADT significantly increases risk for any clinical fracture, hip fractures, and vertebral fractures in men with prostate cancer, and the duration of treatment affects the onset of complications [40, 41]. Calcium (1000–1200 mg daily from diet and supplements) and vitamin D (800–1000 IU daily) are recommended to reduce the ADT side effects [42]) Osteoclast inhibition with either bisphosphonates or denosumab is recommended for men with bone metastases. Osteoclast inhibition can decrease bone turnover and increase bone mineral density in men receiving ADT [43].

20.8.2 Cardiovascular Events

The first report identifying a possible CV risk with LHRH agonists was by Keating et al., who analyzed the Surveillance, Epidemiology, and End Results (SEER) Medicare data of 73,196 men with locoregional prostate cancer [44]. A significantly increased risk of coronary heart disease, myocardial infarction, and sudden cardiac death was reported for men receiving an LHRH agonist compared with those not undergoing ADT. Prospective clinical trials have demonstrated that ADT may increase cardiovascular disease risk by increasing body weight, reducing insulin sensitivity, and/or resulting in dyslipidemia. In a prospective 12-month study of 40 men with prostate cancer, ADT increased serum total cholesterol, low-density lipoprotein cholesterol, high-density lipoprotein cholesterol, and triglycerides by 9%, 7%, 11%, and 27%, respectively [45].

It is advisable that patients in whom ADT is initiated be on periodic follow-up that includes assessment of blood pressure, lipid profile, and glucose level. Some of the effects of ADT occur within the first 3 months of treatment; thus it may be reasonable for an initial follow-up evaluation to occur within 3–6 months after initiation of therapy. There are no data to guide at what intervals periodic further follow-up should occur, and this is left to the discretion of the physician initiating ADT and to the patient's primary care physician. Prudence and good medical care dictate that patients with cardiac disease receive appropriate secondary preventive measures as recommended by the American Heart Association and other expert organizations, including, when appropriate, lipid-lowering therapy, antihypertensive therapy, glucose-lowering therapy, and antiplatelet therapy [46].

20.8.3 Sexual Dysfunction

Since the incidence of prostate cancer is higher among older patients, at least one-third of men have sexual problems at diagnosis. However, most of the patients receiving continuous ADT who are potent prior to therapy develop sexual dysfunction. Loss of libido in patients receiving LHRH agonists usually develops within the first months followed by erectile dysfunction [47]. Erections do not recover in about one-half of men, even if ADT is discontinued. Although intermittent ADT allows some recovery of sexual function, serum testosterone requires 9–12 months off ADT to recover [48].

20.8.4 Vasomotor Symptoms

The most common symptom associated with ADT is hot flashes. Hot flashes are usually described as an intense sensation of warmth in the face and upper part of the body which seems similar to postmenopausal symptoms in women. The treatment should be decided depending on the degree of symptoms and potential side effects of the treatment. Megestrol and estrogen appear substantially more effective than venlafaxine. However, estrogen is associated with breast symptoms, megestrol is associated with increased appetite and weight, and venlafaxine is associated with dry mouth. It is recommended to start with a selective serotonin reuptake inhibitor and reserve hormonal treatment (estrogen, megestrol) for refractory cases.

20.8.5 Body Composition and Metabolism

A prospective study of 32 men receiving 12 months of GnRH agonists found a 2.4% weight gain, 9.4% increase in body fat percentage, and 2.7% decrease in lean body mass at 12 months [49]. Another prospective study of 25 patients without diabetes found that 12 weeks of combined androgen blockade resulted in a 12.8% decrease in insulin sensitivity and a 25.9% increase in fasting plasma insulin [50]. Basaria et al. conducted a cross-sectional study among 53 men, including 18 men with PCa who received ADT for at least 12 months prior to the onset of the study (the ADT group), 17 age-matched men with nonmetastatic PCa who had undergone prostatectomy and/or received radiotherapy and who were not receiving ADT (the non-ADT group), and 18 age-matched controls (the control group). It was shown that men on long-term ADT had significantly higher fasting glucose (131 vs. 103; $p < 0.01$) and greater insulin resistance (17 vs. 6; $p < 0.01$) and that 44% of the men on ADT had fasting glucose in the diabetic range (>126 mg/dL) compared with 11–12% for the controls [51].

Per the Adult Treatment Panel III (ATP III) guidelines, the diagnosis of metabolic syndrome requires the presence of three of the following five criteria: (1) serum triglycerides ≥150 mg/dL, (2) high-density lipoprotein (HDL) < 40 mg/dL, (3) fasting serum glucose >110 mg/dL, (4) waist circumference ≥ 40 inches, and (5) blood pressure ≥ 130/85 [52]. As noted earlier, patients receiving ADT are at risk for higher fasting serum glucose and increased waist size due to central weight gain. Triglycerides have also been reported to rise by 26.5% (±10%; $p = 0.01$) with 1 year of ADT [49]. There are currently no specific recommendations regarding the management of insulin resistance and lipid increases for men on ADT.

20.8.6 Gynecomastia

Gynecomastia and breast pain may be seen in patients on ADT. The incidence of gynecomastia was reported to be as high as 85% in patients receiving high-dose 150 mg daily bicalutamide antiandrogen monotherapy [53]. However, the incidence is lower (13–22%) in men receiving combined androgen blockade [54]. Di Lorenzo et al. investigated the role of tamoxifen and radiotherapy for the prevention and treatment of gynecomastia and breast pain during adjuvant bicalutamide monotherapy after RP in patients with prostate cancer [55]. It was shown that gynecomastia and breast pain induced by bicalutamide monotherapy after RP can be prevented and treated. Tamoxifen has been shown to be more effective and safe than RT (12 Gy) in this setting, and QOL and sexual function are not negatively influenced by these two treatment options. Ozen et al. investigated the efficacy of prophylactic radiotherapy for gynecomastia/breast pain induced by 150 mg bicalutamide in a prospective, randomized, multi-institutional trial [56]. After definitive treatment for localized prostate cancer, 125 patients were randomized to 12 Gy radiotherapy before bicalutamide as prophylactic radiotherapy or bicalutamide only for nonprophylactic radiotherapy. With a follow-up of 12 months, the gynecomastia rate was 15.8% in the prophylactic group and 50.8% in the nonprophylactic group ($p < 0.001$). Although prophylactic breast irradiation seemed to decrease the gynecomastia rate in patients on 150 mg bicalutamide, not all patients need prophylaxis since only 52% were significantly bothered by gynecomastia. Thus, it was recommended to select patients who need prophylactic radiation based on individual assessment.

20.8.7 Other

Fatigue is another side effect of ADT. The main strategy to reduce fatigue is exercise. Anemia and reduction in penile and testis size may be seen. Hypogonadism has been linked to cognitive declines in patients on ADT [57].

20.9 Follow-Up During Hormonal Treatment

EAU-ESTRO recommends follow-up of 3–6 month intervals. As a minimum, tests should include serum PSA measurement, physical examination, serum testosterone, and careful evaluation of symptoms to assess the treatment response and side effects. Patients should be warned about the signs of metastatic situations like occult cord compression, urinary tract complications/obstruction signs, and bone pain. Routine imaging is not indicated asymptomatic in patients. However, new-onset bone pain requires a bone scan, as does PSA progression suggesting CRPC status, if a treatment modification is considered [43].

The measurement of serum testosterone levels should be a part of follow-up of patients on LHRH therapy. Although timing of measurements is not clearly defined, a 3–6 month assessment of the testosterone level might be performed to evaluate the effectiveness of treatment and to ensure that the castration level is being maintained. If it is not achieved, switching to another type of treatment modality can be attempted. In patients with rising PSA and/or clinical progression, serum testosterone must be evaluated in all cases to confirm a castrate-resistant state.

Long-term ADT reduces bone mineral density (BMD) and increases the risk of fractures [58]. In the absence of associated risk factors, it is recommended that BMD and serum vitamin D and calcium levels should be measured every 2 years [59]. Patients should be screened for the development of alterations in lipid profiles and decreased insulin sensitivity [60]. ADT may increase the risk of diabetes and cardiovascular disease [61]. Patients should be given advice on modifying their lifestyle (e.g., diet, exercise, smoking cessation) and should be treated for any existing conditions, such as diabetes, hyperlipidemia, and/or hypertension. Furthermore, the risk–benefit ratio of ADT must be considered for patients with a higher risk of cardiovascular complications, especially if it is possible to delay starting ADT.

20.10 Castration-Resistant Prostate Cancer

CRPC is defined as castrate serum testosterone <50 ng/dl plus either biochemical or radiological progression. Biochemical progression is defined as three consecutive rises in PSA 1 week apart, resulting in two 50% increases over the nadir, and PSA >2 ng/mL. Radiological progression is defined as the appearance of new lesions, either two or more new bone lesions on bone scan or a soft tissue lesion using the Response Evaluation Criteria in Solid Tumors.

20.10.1 First-Line Treatment in Metastatic Castration-Resistant Prostate Cancer

Abiraterone was evaluated in 1088 chemonaïve metastatic CRPC patients in the phase 3 trial. Patients were randomized to abiraterone acetate or placebo, both combined with prednisone [62]. After a median follow-up of 22.2 months, there was significant improvement of radiographic PFS (median: 16.5 vs. 8.2 months; HR: 0.52; $p < 0.001$). At the final analysis, with a median follow-up of 49.2 months, the OS end point was significantly improved (34.7 vs. 30.3 months; HR: 0.81; 95% CI, 0.70–0.93; $p = 0.0033$) [63].

PREVAIL is a randomized phase 3 trial that included a similar patient population and compared enzalutamide with placebo. It was conducted in 1717 chemonaïve mCRPC patients and showed significant improvement in both radiographic PFS (HR: 0.186; 95% CI, 0.15–0.23; $p < 0.0001$) and OS (HR: 0.706; 95% CI, 0.6–0.84; $p < 0.001$). The most common clinically relevant AEs were fatigue and hypertension. The results showed that enzalutamide significantly decreased the risk of radiographic progression and death and delayed the initiation of chemotherapy in men with metastatic prostate cancer [64].

In a phase 2 randomized controlled trial of a Poxviral-based PSA-targeted immunotherapy in metastatic CRPC, 125 patients were randomly assigned in a multicenter trial of vaccination series. After a median follow-up of 34 months, median survival was 25.8 months in the sipuleucel-T group compared with 21.7 months in the placebo group ($p = 0.03$). PFS was similar in both groups and treatment tolerance was very good [65].

Tannock et al. compared docetaxel plus prednisone with mitoxantrone plus prednisone in 1006 men with metastatic hormone-refractory prostate cancer. The median survival was 16.5 months in the mitoxantrone group, 18.9 months in the group given docetaxel every 3 weeks, and 17.4 months in the group given weekly docetaxel. Among these three groups, 32%, 45%, and 48% of men, respectively, had at least a 50% decrease in the serum PSA level ($p < 0.001$ for both comparisons with mitoxantrone); 22%, 35% ($p = 0.01$), and 31% ($p = 0.08$) had predefined reductions in pain; and 13%, 22% ($p = 0.009$), and 23% ($p = 0.005$) had improvements in the quality of life. Adverse events were also more common in the groups that received docetaxel [66].

ALSYMPCA is a phase 3 trial that enrolled 921 patients with symptomatic mCRPC who failed or were unfit for docetaxel. Patients were randomized to six injections of 50 kBq/kg Ra 223, every 4 weeks. or placebo, plus standard of care. Ra 223, an alpha emitter, significantly improved median OS by 3.6 months (HR: 0.70; $p < 0.001$) [67]. Ra-223 treatment was associated with prolonged time to first skeletal event and improvement in pain scores and QoL. Radium-223 was associated with low myelosuppression rates and fewer adverse events. The updated analysis of ALSYMPCA trial showed that Ra-223 was effective and safe regardless of previous docetaxel use [68].

20.10.2 Second-Line Treatment Options and Beyond in Metastatic Castration-Resistant Prostate Cancer

Cabazitaxel is a form of taxane that has an activity in docetaxel-resistant cancers. TROPIC trial is a large prospective randomized phase 3 trial comparing cabazitaxel plus prednisone versus mitoxantrone plus prednisone in 755 patients with mCRPC who had progressed after or during docetaxel-based chemotherapy [69]. Patients received a maximum of ten cycles of cabazitaxel (25 mg/m^2) or mitoxantrone (12 mg/m^2) plus prednisone (10 mg/dL), respectively. OS was significantly longer with cabazitaxel (median: 15.1 vs. 12.7 months; $p < 0.0001$). Treatment-associated World Health Organization grade 3–4 AEs developed significantly more often in the cabazitaxel arm, particularly hematological toxicity (68.2% vs. 47.3%; $p < 0.0002$)

but also nonhematological toxicity (57.4% vs. 39.8%; $p < 0.0002$). This drug should be administered preferably with prophylactic granulocyte colony-stimulating factor and by physicians with expertise in handling neutropenia and sepsis [70].

AFFIRM is a trial including 1199 mCRPC patients with randomization in a 2:1 fashion to enzalutamide or placebo [71]. The patients had progressed after docetaxel treatment, according to the PCWG2 criteria. After a median follow-up of 14.4 months, median survival in the enzalutamide group was 18.4 months compared with 13.6 months in the placebo arm (HR: 0.63; $p < 0.001$). The benefit was observed regardless of age, baseline pain intensity, and type of progression. All secondary objectives including soft tissue response, QoL response rate, and time to PSA progression or objective progression were in favor of enzalutamide. Rates of fatigue, diarrhea, and hot flashes were higher in the enzalutamide group. Seizures were reported in five patients (0.6%) receiving enzalutamide compared to none in the placebo group.

Conclusion

ADT has become the standard of care for patients with advanced prostate cancer. ADT aims to reduce the serum testosterone to castrate level. The contemporary laboratory testing methods showed that the mean value after surgical castration is 15 ng/dL. Thus, recently the level is defined as being less than 20 ng/dL (1 nmol/L). Recent definition is associated with better outcomes compared to the previous one. ADT can be used as adjuvant or neoadjuvant therapy in conjunction with initial treatment of patients with intermediate or high-risk prostate cancer, patients with rising PSA after curative treatment, or patients with metastatic disease at diagnosis. It can either be used before radiotherapy in patients with large prostate to decrease the tumor volume.

References

1. Oefelein MG, Feng A, Scolieri MJ, et al. Reassessment of the definition of castrate levels of testosterone: implications for clinical decision making. Urology. 2000;56:1021–4.
2. Morote J, Planas J, Salvador C, et al. Individual variations of serum testosterone in patients with prostate cancer receiving androgen deprivation therapy. BJU Int. 2009;103:332–5.
3. Pickles T, Hamm J, Morris WJ, et al. Incomplete testosterone suppression with luteinizing hormone-releasing hormone agonists: does it happen and does it matter? BJU Int. 2012;110:E500–7.
4. Klotz L, O'Callaghan C, Higano T, et al. MP74-01 nadir testosterone on ADT predicts for time to castrate resistant progression: a secondary analysis of the PR-7 intermittent vs continuous ADT trial. J Urol. 2014;191(4):e855–6.
5. https://www.nccn.org/professionals/physician_gls/pdf/prostate.pdf. Accessed Jan 2017.
6. Klotz L, McNeill I, Fleshner N. A phase 1-2 trial of diethylstilbestrol plus low dose warfarin in advanced prostate carcinoma. J Urol. 1999;161:169–72.
7. Farrugia D, Ansell W, Singh M, Philp T, et al. Stilboestrol plus adrenal suppression as salvage treatment for patients failing treatment with luteinizing hormone-releasing hormone analogues and orchiectomy. BJU Int. 2000;85:1069–173.
8. Klotz L, Boccon-Gibod L, Shore ND, et al. The efficacy and safety of degarelix: a 12-month, comparative, randomized, open-label, parallel-group phase III study in patients with prostate cancer. BJU Int. 2008;102:1531–8.

9. Klotz L, O'Callaghan C, Ding K, et al. Nadir testosterone within first year of androgen-deprivation therapy (ADT) predicts for time to castration-resistant progression: a secondary analysis of the PR-7 trial of intermittent versus continuous ADT. J Clin Oncol. 2015;33(10):1151–6.
10. Schmidt F, Sundaram K, Thau RB, Bardin CW. [Ac-D-NAL(2)1,4FD-Phe2,D-Trp3,D-Arg6]-LHRH, a potent antagonist of LHRH, produces transient edema and behavioral changes in rats. Contraception. 1984;29(3):283–9.
11. Hook WA, Karten M, Siraganian RP. Histamine release by structural analogs of LHRH. Fed Am Soc Exp Biol. 1985;44:1323.
12. Broqua P, Riviere P, Conn P, Rivier J, Aubert M, Junien J. Pharmacological profile of a new, potent, and longacting gonadotropin-releasing hormone antagonist: degarelix. J Pharmacol Exp Ther. 2002;301:95–102.
13. Crawford ED, Tombal B, Miller K, et al. A phase III extension trial with a 1-arm crossover from leuprolide to degarelix: comparison of gonadotropin-releasing hormone agonist and antagonist effect on prostate cancer. J Urol. 2011;186:889–97.
14. Moffat LE. Comparison of Zoladex, diethylstilbestrol and cyproterone acetate treatment in advanced prostate cancer. Eur Urol. 1990;18(Suppl 3):26–7.
15. Schroder FH, Whelan P, de Reijke TM, et al. Metastatic prostate cancer treated by flutamide versus cyproterone acetate. Final analysis of the "European Organization for Research and Treatment of Cancer" (EORTC) Protocol 30892. Eur Urol. 2004;45:457–64.
16. Akyol F, Selek U, Ozyigit G, Onal C, Akdogan B, Karabulut E, Ozen H. Preliminary results of bicalutamide monotherapy on biochemical failure of localized prostate cancer. J Natl Med Assoc. 2006;98(7):1058–61.
17. Wirth M, Tyrrell C, Delaere K, et al. Bicalutamide ('Casodex') 150 mg in addition to standard care in patients with nonmetastatic prostate cancer: updated results from a randomised double-blind phase III study (median followup 5.1 y) in the early prostate cancer programme. Prostate Cancer Prostatic Dis. 2005;8:194–200.
18. Abrahamsson PA, Anderson J, Boccon-Gibod L, et al. Risks and benefits of hormonal manipulation as monotherapy or adjuvant treatment in localised prostate cancer. Eur Urol. 2005;48:900–5.
19. Tyrrell CJ, Payne H, See WA, et al. Bicalutamide ('Casodex') 150 mg as adjuvant to radiotherapy in patients with localised or locally advanced prostate cancer: results from the randomised early prostate cancer programme. Radiother Oncol. 2005;76:4–10.
20. Smith MR, Goode M, Zietman AL, et al. Bicalutamide monotherapy versus leuprolide monotherapy for prostate cancer: effects on bone mineral density and body composition. J Clin Oncol. 2004;22:2546–53.
21. Murthy V, Norman AR, Shahidi M, et al. Recovery of serum testosterone after neoadjuvant androgen deprivation therapy and radical radiotherapy in localized prostate cancer. BJU Int. 2006;97(3):476–9.
22. D'Amico AV, Chen MH, Renshaw AA, et al. Interval to testosterone recovery after hormonal therapy for prostate cancer and risk of death. Int J Radiat Oncol Biol Phys. 2009;75(1):10–5.
23. https://clinicaltrials.gov/ct2/show/NCT02319837. Accessed Jan 2017.
24. Crawford ED, Eisenberger MA, McLeod DG, et al. A controlled trial of leuprolide with and without flutamide in prostatic carcinoma. N Engl J Med. 1989;321(7):419–24.
25. Eisenberger MA, Blumenstein BA, Crawford ED, et al. Bilateral orchiectomy with or without flutamide for metastatic prostate cancer. N Engl J Med. 1998;339(15):1036–42.
26. Hussain M, Tangen CM, Berry DL, et al. Intermittent versus continuous androgen deprivation in prostate cancer. N Engl J Med. 2013;368(14):1314–25.
27. Crook JM, O'Callaghan CJ, Duncan G, et al. Intermittent androgen suppression for rising PSA level after radiotherapy. N Engl J Med. 2012;367(10):895–903.
28. Ozyigit G. The role of radiotherapy in the management of prostate cancer. Turkiye Klinikleri J Med Oncol-Special Topics. 2015;8(3):23–30.
29. Ozdemir Y, Akyol F, Ozyigit G, Hurmuz P, Onal C, Selek U, Karabulut E. Three dimensional conformal radiotherapy and androgen deprivation therapy in patients with clinically localized prostate cancer; Hacettepe University experience. UHOD 2015;25(2):107–17.

30. Ozyigit G, Akyol F, Onal C, Sari S, Gurdalli S, Yapici B. Combined hormonotherapy and definitive radiation therapy in localized prostate adenocarcinoma. UHOD 2003;13(4):177–89.
31. Lawton CA, Winter K, Grignon D, Pilepich MV. Androgen suppression plus radiation versus radiation alone for patients with stage D1/pathologic node-positive adenocarcinoma of the prostate: updated results based on national prospective randomized trial radiation therapy oncology group 85-31. J Clin Oncol. 2005;23(4):800–7.
32. Roach M III, Bae K, Speight J, Wolkov HB, Rubin P, Lee RJ, et al. Short-term neoadjuvant androgen deprivation therapy and external-beam radiotherapy for locally advanced prostate cancer: long-term results of RTOG 8610. J Clin Oncol. 2008;26(4):585–91.
33. Horwitz EM, Bae K, Hanks GE, Porter A, Grignon DJ, Brereton HD, et al. Ten-year follow-up of radiation therapy oncology group protocol 92-02: a phase III trial of the duration of elective androgen deprivation in locally advanced prostate cancer. J Clin Oncol. 2008;26(15):2497–504.
34. Bolla M, Van Tienhoven G, Warde P, Dubois JB, Mirimanoff RO, Storme G, et al. External irradiation with or without long-term androgen suppression for prostate cancer with high metastatic risk: 10-year results of an EORTC randomised study. Lancet Oncol. 2010;11(11):1066–73.
35. Bayoumi AM, Brown AD, Garber AM. Cost-effectiveness of androgen suppression therapies in advanced prostate cancer. J Natl Cancer Inst. 2000;92:1731–9.
36. Gravis G, Fizazi K, Joly F, Oudard S, et al. Androgen-deprivation therapy alone or with docetaxel in non-castrate metastatic prostate cancer (GETUG-AFU 15): a randomised, open-label, phase 3 trial. Lancet Oncol. 2013;14:149–58.
37. Gravis G, Boher JM, Joly F, et al. Androgen deprivation therapy (ADT) plus docetaxel versus ADT alone in metastatic non castrate prostate cancer: impact of metastatic burden and long-term survival analysis of the randomized phase 3 GETUG-AFU15 trial. Eur Urol. 2016;70:256–62.
38. Sweeney CJ, Chen YH, Carducci M, et al. Chemohormonal therapy in metastatic hormone-sensitive prostate cancer. N Engl J Med. 2015;373:737–46.
39. James ND, Sydes MR, Clarke NW, et al. Addition of docetaxel, zoledronic acid, or both to first-line long-term hormone therapy in prostate cancer (STAMPEDE): survival results from an adaptive, multiarm, multistage, platform randomised controlled trial. Lancet. 2016;387:1163–77.
40. Smith MR, Lee WC, Brandman J, et al. Gonadotropin-releasing hormone agonists and fracture risk: a claims-based cohort study of men with nonmetastatic prostate cancer. J Clin Oncol. 2005;23(31):7897–903.
41. Krupski TL, Smith MR, Lee WC, et al. Natural history of bone complications in men with prostate carcinoma initiating androgen deprivation therapy. Cancer. 2004;101(3):541–9.
42. http://www.nof.org/files/nof/public/content/file/344/upload/159.pdf. Accessed Jan 2017.
43. Cornford P, Bellmunt J, Bolla M, et al. EAU-ESTRO-SIOG guidelines on prostate cancer. Part II: treatment of relapsing, metastatic, and castration-resistant prostate cancer. Eur Urol. 2016;71(4):630–42.
44. Keating NL, O'Malley AJ, Smith MR. Diabetes and cardiovascular disease during androgen deprivation therapy for prostate cancer. J Clin Oncol. 2006;24(27):4448–56.
45. Smith MR, Finkelstein JS, McGovern FJ, et al. Changes in body composition during androgen deprivation therapy for prostate cancer. J Clin Endocrinol Metab. 2002;87(2):599–603.
46. Levine GN, D'Amico AV, Berger P, et al. Androgen-deprivation therapy in prostate cancer and cardiovascular risk: a science advisory from the American Heart Association, American Cancer Society, and American Urological Association: endorsed by the American Society for Radiation Oncology. CA Cancer J Clin. 2010;60(3):194–201.
47. Wilke DR, Parker C, Andonowski A, et al. Testosterone and erectile function recovery after radiotherapy and long-term androgen deprivation with luteinizing hormone-releasing hormone agonists. BJU Int. 2006;97(5):963–8.
48. Schover LR. Sexual healing in patients with prostate cancer on hormone therapy. Am Soc Clin Oncol Educ Book. 2015:e562–6.
49. Smith MR, Finkelstein JS, McGovern FJ, et al. Changes in body composition during androgen deprivation therapy for prostate cancer. J Clin Endocrinol Metab. 2002;87(2):599–603.

50. Smith MR, Lee H, Nathan DM. Insulin sensitivity during combined androgen blockade for prostate cancer. J Clin Endocrinol Metab. 2006;91(4):1305–8.
51. Basaria S, Muller DC, Carducci MA, et al. Hyperglycemia and insulin resistance in men with prostate carcinoma who receive androgen-deprivation therapy. Cancer. 2006;106(3):581–8.
52. Executive Summary of The Third Report of The National Cholesterol Education Program (NCEP) Expert Panel on Detection, Evaluation, and Treatment of High Blood Cholesterol in Adults (Adult Treatment Panel III). JAMA. 2001;285(19):2486–97.
53. Tyrrell CJ, Payne H, Tammela TL, et al. Prophylactic breast irradiation with a single dose of electron beam radiotherapy (10 Gy) significantly reduces the incidence of bicalutamide-induced gynecomastia. Int J Radiat Oncol Biol Phys. 2004;60(2):476–83.
54. Di Lorenzo G, Autorino R, Perdonà S, De Placido S. Management of gynaecomastia in patients with prostate cancer: a systematic review. Lancet Oncol. 2005;6(12):972–9.
55. Di Lorenzo G, Perdonà S, De Placido S, et al. Gynecomastia and breast pain induced by adjuvant therapy with bicalutamide after radical prostatectomy in patients with prostate cancer: the role of tamoxifen and radiotherapy. J Urol. 2005;174(6):2197–203.
56. Ozen H, Akyol F, Toktas G, Eskicorapci S, Unluer E, Kuyumcuoglu U, Abay E, Cureklibatur I, Sengoz M, Yalcin V, Akpinar H, Zorlu F, Sengor F, Karaman I. Is prophylactic breast radiotherapy necessary in all patients with prostate cancer and gynecomastia and/or breast pain? J Urol. 2010;184(2):519–24.
57. Nguyen PL, Alibhai SM, Basaria S, et al. Adverse effects of androgen deprivation therapy and strategies to mitigate them. Eur Urol. 2015;67(5):825–36.
58. Smith MR, Boyce SP, Moyneur E, et al. Risk of clinical fractures after gonadotropin-releasing hormone agonist therapy for prostate cancer. J Urol. 2006;175(1):136–9.
59. Conde FA, Aronson WJ. Risk factors for male osteoporosis. Urol Oncol. 2003;21(5):380–3.
60. Saylor PJ, Smith MR. Metabolic complications of androgen deprivation therapy for prostate cancer. J Urol. 2008;181(5):1998–2006.
61. Faris JE, Smith MR. Metabolic sequelae associated with androgen deprivation therapy for prostate cancer. Curr Opin Endocrinol Diabetes Obes. 2010;17(3):240–6.
62. Ryan CJ, Smith MR, de Bono JS, et al. Abiraterone in metastatic prostate cancer without previous chemotherapy. N Engl J Med. 2013;368(2):138–48.
63. Ryan CJ, Smith MR, Fizazi K, et al. Abiraterone acetate plus prednisone versus placebo plus prednisone in chemotherapy-naive men with metastatic castration-resistant prostate cancer (COU-AA-302): final overall survival analysis of a randomised, double-blind, placebo-controlled phase 3 study. Lancet Oncol. 2015;16(2):152–60.
64. Beer TM, Armstrong AJ, Rathkopf DE, et al. Enzalutamide in metastatic prostate cancer before chemotherapy. N Engl J Med. 2014;371(5):424–33.
65. Kantoff PW, Schuetz TJ, Blumenstein BA, et al. Overall survival analysis of a phase II randomized controlled trial of a Poxviral-based PSA-targeted immunotherapy in metastatic castration-resistant prostate cancer. J Clin Oncol. 2010;28(7):1099–105.
66. Tannock IF, de Wit R, Berry WR, et al. Docetaxel plus prednisone or mitoxantrone plus prednisone for advanced prostate cancer. N Engl J Med. 2004;351(15):1502–12.
67. Parker C, Nilsson S, Heinrich D, et al. Alpha emitter radium-223 and survival in metastatic prostate cancer. N Engl J Med. 2013;369(3):213–23.
68. Hoskin P, Sartor O, O'Sullivan JM, et al. Efficacy and safety of radium-223 dichloride in patients with castration-resistant prostate cancer and symptomatic bone metastases, with or without previous docetaxel use: a prespecified subgroup analysis from the randomised, double-blind, phase 3 ALSYMPCA trial. Lancet Oncol. 2014;15(12):1397–406.
69. de Bono JS, Oudard S, Ozguroglu M, et al. Prednisone plus cabazitaxel or mitoxantrone for metastatic castration-resistant prostate cancer progressing after docetaxel treatment: a randomised open-label trial. Lancet. 2010;376(9747):1147–54.
70. Resnick MJ, Lacchetti C, Bergman J, et al. Prostate cancer survivorship care guideline: American Society of clinical oncology clinical practice guideline endorsement. J Clin Oncol. 2015;33(9):1078–85.
71. Scher HI, Fizazi K, Saad F, et al. Increased survival with enzalutamide in prostate cancer after chemotherapy. N Engl J Med. 2012;367(13):1187–97.

Chemotherapy in the Management of Prostate Cancer

21

Sevil Bavbek

Abstract

Less than a decade ago, metastatic castration-resistant prostate cancer (mCRPC) was deemed to be a "chemoresistant" disease, with a poor prognosis. The landmark TAX327 trial, published in 2004, showed that a course of chemotherapy based on the taxane docetaxel could extend survival for men with mCRPC. Then, in 2010 it was reported that men with mCRPC who progressed during or after docetaxel could gain a further survival benefit from a second line of chemotherapy, based on another taxane, cabazitaxel.

21.1 Introduction

Less than a decade ago, mCRPC was deemed to be a "chemoresistant" disease, with a poor prognosis. Up until the establishment of mitoxantrone, in combination with prednisone or prednisolone, as a palliative treatment, chemotherapy for prostate cancer remained anecdotal with weekly anthracyclines and estramustine playing the lead roles. The trial reported by Tannock et al. [1], where mitoxantrone with corticosteroids was tested against corticosteroids only, was the first phase III trial reported in castration-resistant prostate cancer (CRPC), and the major effect of the agent mitoxantrone was only palliation of symptoms without improvement in survival. There was a 29% pain response rate for mitoxantrone versus 12% for prednisone alone. This trial clearly showed that chemotherapy with mitoxantrone decreased pain scores and analgesic use in CRPC, and the quality of life (QOL) analysis incorporated into the trial showed better QOL in the chemotherapy arm. Mitoxantrone was well tolerated in this group of elderly and quite sick patient

S. Bavbek, M.D.
Department of Medical Oncology, American Hospital, Istanbul, Turkey
e-mail: sbavbek@yahoo.com

G. Ozyigit, U. Selek (eds.), *Principles and Practice of Urooncology*,
DOI 10.1007/978-3-319-56114-1_21

population. A CCO systematic review reported on three small trials of mitoxantrone plus prednisone or hydrocortisone, which showed modest clinical benefit (including improved pain response, QOL, and/or time to disease progression) but no improvement in OS, and increased risk of harm, compared with treatment with prednisone or hydrocortisone alone [2]. Mitoxantrone is still listed in the ASCO and Ontario Cancer Care guidelines as a palliative agent with QOL benefit [3]. The landmark TAX327 trial, published in 2004, showed that a course of chemotherapy based on the taxane docetaxel could extend survival for men with mCRPC (vs. mitoxantrone-based chemotherapy) [4]. With this trial, prostate cancer entered the chemotherapy age. For several years, docetaxel remained the only chemotherapy to offer a survival benefit in this setting. Then, in 2010 it was reported that men with mCRPC who progressed during or after docetaxel could gain a further survival benefit from a second line of chemotherapy, based on another taxane, cabazitaxel [5]. Once again, the palliative chemotherapy agent mitoxantrone was the comparator. This was followed by reports of different combination chemotherapies for high-grade prostate cancer and the special subtype of neuroendocrine prostate cancer. Finally, chemotherapy was carried up to the hormone-sensitive metastatic phase, changing practice and increasing survival by an even greater fraction than in the CRPC phase.

21.2 First-Line Chemotherapy

In the pivotal trial TAX327, 1006 men with mCRPC were randomized to prednisone 10 mg/day plus weekly or three-weekly docetaxel or three-weekly mitoxantrone [4]. Efficacy and survival were better in the three-weekly docetaxel arm, compared to mitoxantrone. The survival in the weekly docetaxel arm was not statistically improved. Toxicity was different among the treatment arms. The most common grade 3/4 adverse event was neutropenia (three-weekly docetaxel, 32%; weekly docetaxel, 2%; mitoxantrone, 22%), but febrile neutropenia was rare (three-weekly docetaxel, 3%; weekly docetaxel, 0%; mitoxantrone, 2%) [4]. More docetaxel recipients than mitoxantrone recipients experienced at least one serious adverse event (three-weekly docetaxel, 26%; weekly docetaxel, 29%; mitoxantrone, 20%). Based on their findings, the investigators suggested that three-weekly docetaxel plus prednisone improved survival, prostate-specific antigen (PSA) response, pain response, and quality of life versus mitoxantrone plus prednisone.

The SWOG 9916 was a confirmatory trial, although it had a slightly different setup. In the SWOG 9916 trial, 770 men with mCRPC received docetaxel/estramustine and showed improvement in OS compared with a regimen of mitoxantrone/prednisone (median OS 17.5 months vs. 15.6 months, respectively; hazard ratio [HR]: 0.80, 95% confidence interval [CI] 0.67–0.97; $P = 0.02$) [6]. In the phase III TAX327 study, docetaxel/prednisone every 3 weeks prolonged OS by 2.9 months in 1006 men with mCRPC compared with a schedule of mitoxantrone/prednisone (median OS 19.2 months vs. 16.3 months, respectively; HR: 0.79; P ¼ 0.004) [4]. As a regimen of docetaxel/estramustine was associated with greater toxicity and less efficacy compared with docetaxel/prednisone every 3 weeks, the latter was adopted as the preferred standard of care (SOC) in symptomatic patients with metastatic CRCP.

At an updated analysis of the TAX 327, median overall survival was 19.2 months with three-weekly docetaxel, 17.8 months with weekly docetaxel, and 16.3 months with mitoxantrone [7]. The percentages of patients who survived for more than 3 years in the D3P, D1P, and MP arms were 18.6, 16.8, and 13.5%, respectively. Survival among subgroups was expressed in a forest plot within the article; patients above and below age 68, with or without pain/symptoms, with or without visceral disease, with PSA above or below 115, and with perfect or less than perfect performance status, benefited consistently from chemotherapy with docetaxel, although patients with visceral disease, pain, poorer performance status, and high baseline PSA values had shorter survival.

One key question was the patient age, particularly given the elderly demographic range of the disease and the toxicity associated with any cytotoxic treatment course. However, TAX327 showed that the survival benefits of docetaxel applied to older as well as younger men [8]. The International Society of Geriatric Oncology (SIOG) states that chronological age per se should not be a guide to treatment choice for mCRPC [9]. Instead, SIOG recommends individual patient assessment based on the use of established, validated tools. Men with mCRPC who are judged to be healthy (i.e., with controlled comorbidities, independence in daily living, and good nutritional status) should be considered candidates for standard chemotherapy, regardless of their age. Those categorized as vulnerable (i.e., with reversible impairment) may be considered for standard chemotherapy once their comorbidities are taken care of. For the vulnerable patient with no chance of improvement, reports of small trials with weekly or biweekly docetaxel show clinical benefit, although there is no significant survival benefit.

As a result of both randomized trials, docetaxel became the mainstay of chemotherapy in CRPC, the optimal treatment duration was described as 6–12 cycles, and the next question raised was when to start chemotherapy after castration resistance, since it was the only line of survival prolonging effective treatment. The TAX 327 trial included patients with and without symptoms. In general, the chances of prolonging survival with three-weekly docetaxel seemed similar among patients with higher and lower disease burden as indicated by level of serum PSA, the presence or absence of substantial pain, and the QOL or performance score. The trial did not specifically address whether docetaxel should be used in patients with minimal symptoms or whether it is appropriate to defer treatment until more symptoms occur. However, considering the similar benefit among subgroups and the potential for QOL to deteriorate as a result of disease progression, it seemed reasonable to offer treatment to patients with symptoms and to those who are likely to develop symptoms in the near future, based on the burden of disease and the PSA doubling time. Prostate cancer guidelines from the National Comprehensive Cancer Network (NCCN) also state that docetaxel may be considered for asymptomatic men with mCRPC who have signs of rapid progression or soft tissue/visceral metastases [10].

This conservative approach of deferring chemotherapy until symptoms appear was widely accepted until the introduction of many more survival prolonging therapies, whereby initiation and change of treatments became less conservative. Rechallenge with docetaxel initial response and a certain off-treatment period and disease progression also became obsolete with the introduction of new therapies, since rechallenge never had any proof of improved survival [11].

21.3 Second-Line Chemotherapy

Docetaxel set the stage for the standard treatment of metastatic CRPC, creating an arbitrary setting for the testing and licensing of the next generation of drugs. From this time point, all new drugs introduced into metastatic CRPC were either tested in the "post-docetaxel" or the "pre-docetaxel" settings. The terms pre- and post-docetaxel refer to the use of docetaxel in the metastatic CRPC phase.

The first chemotherapy drug showing survival benefit in the post-docetaxel setting as second-line chemotherapy is cabazitaxel [5]. The activity of another taxane came as a pleasant surprise, since cross-resistance would have been a major drawback, and progression on or shortly after docetaxel would be likely to predict resistance to another taxane [12]. Cabazitaxel (XRP6258), a tubulin-binding taxane drug, showed potent antitumor activity comparable with docetaxel in docetaxel-sensitive cell lines and exhibited more potent cytotoxic activity than docetaxel in cancer cell lines with acquired resistance to docetaxel due to P-GP overexpression [13, 14]. Based on these findings, cabazitaxel entered the clinical trial phase and found to have antitumor activity and good tolerability in phase I and II trials.

The groundbreaking phase III clinical data on cabazitaxel emerged from the TROPIC trial, conducted in 26 countries in North and South America, Eastern and Western Europe, and Asia, involving 755 patients with mCRPC in the post-docetaxel setting [5]. About one-third of the patient population had already received two or more lines of chemotherapy and thus were heavily pretreated, and two-thirds had developed progressive disease either during or within 3 months of docetaxel treatment, therefore representing taxane-resistant disease. Visceral metastases were present in 25% of the patients, indicating that the patient population had poor prognostic disease.

The patients were randomized to receive cabazitaxel or mitoxantrone, plus prednisone or prednisolone 10 mg/day. Mitoxantrone was chosen as the comparative arm due to its proven efficacy as a palliative agent in CRPC. Cabazitaxel improved survival over mitoxantrone (15.1 months vs. 12.7 months), meeting the primary endpoint of the trial. It provided a 30% risk reduction of death (hazard ratio: 0.70; 95% confidence interval, 0.59–0.83; $p < 0.0001$). Progression-free survival and safety were the secondary endpoints of the trial. Median progression-free survival was 2.8 months in the cabazitaxel arm and 1.4 months in the mitoxantrone arm. There was also significant improvement in tumor response, time to tumor progression, PSA response rate, and median time to PSA progression in cabazitaxel arm. The PSA response rate was 39.2% ($P = 0.002$), and median time to PSA progression was 6.1 months ($P = 0.001$) with cabazitaxel. However, pain control and time to pain progression were similar among the two treatment arms.

Cabazitaxel benefit was consistent for both the older and younger patient groups (age <65 vs. ≥65 years), for patients with or without pain at baseline. The benefit was evident particularly for those patients who had progressed during or within 3 months following docetaxel therapy. In an updated analysis, 15.9% of the 378 patients in the cabazitaxel group and 8.2% of the 377 patients in the mitoxantrone group survived ≥2 years (odds ratio 2.11; 95% CI 1.33–3.33). Based on the updated Kaplan–Meier curve, the probability of surviving ≥2 years was 27% (95% CI 23–32%) with cabazitaxel versus 16% (95% CI 12–20%) with mitoxantrone [15]. In the multivariate analysis, prognostic factors for survival ≥2 years were rising PSA at baseline, treatment group (cabazitaxel vs. mitoxantrone), baseline pain, and time from last docetaxel dose to randomization in TROPIC (<6 vs. ≥6 months) [15].

The major concern for cabazitaxel in the trial was toxicity. Neutropenia, leukopenia, anemia, febrile neutropenia, and diarrhea were the most common grade 3/4 side effects [5]. Grade 3/4 neutropenia was recorded in 82% of the cabazitaxel and 58% of the mitoxantrone patients, with febrile neutropenia in 8 and 1%, respectively. Diarrhea at any grade occurred in 47% of the cabazitaxel and 11% of the mitoxantrone patients. Eighteen patients died on the cabazitaxel arm within 30 days of the last cycle, compared with nine in the mitoxantrone arm. Neutropenic complications were the most common cause of death associated with cabazitaxel. All of the deaths occurred early in the trial before investigators were allowed the prophylactic use of granulocyte colony-stimulating factor and dose modification in the event of febrile neutropenia. The fact that the management of febrile neutropenia varied grossly over TROPIC centers across the world contributed to this excess death rate. Analysis of the data from the North American centers ($n = 235$) showed that only one patient (<1%) in each treatment group died as a result of treatment side effects [16].

The real-life data from expanded access programs (EAP) of cabazitaxel all over the world proved the efficacy and provided very precious insight into the safety of the drug. The international cabazitaxel early-access program collected data on treatment safety and patients' quality of life [17]. Data from the UK arm of this study showed a 4.9% incidence of febrile neutropenia and 2.4% incidence of diarrhea. In the Canadian arm of the early-access program (33 patients, median age 65 years, >50% received ≥5 cycles), the incidence of grade 3/4 diarrhea was 3%, and no treatment-related deaths were reported [18]. In the Spanish EAP, the most frequent grade ≥3 AEs were neutropenia (16.3%) and asthenia (11.1%). Febrile neutropenia and grade ≥3 diarrhea occurred in 5.2% of the patients each. There were five (3.3%) possibly treatment-related deaths, mainly infection related. Grade ≥3 peripheral neuropathy and nail disorders were rare [19].

The difference in the treatment-related morbidity and mortality between the registration trial TROPIC and the EAP's lies in the use of prophylactic G-CSF in the latter. The dose can be decreased to 20 mg/m^2 if prophylactic G-CSF does not prevent neutropenia and its complications. A randomized trial of 25 versus 20 mg/m^2, PROSELICA has been presented at the American Society of Clinical Oncology meeting in 2016, showing the efficacy of the two doses to be equal [20]. A recent interesting finding was announced after a post hoc analysis of the TROPIC trial [21]. The occurrence of grade ≥3 neutropenia during cabazitaxel therapy was associated with a prolonged OS (median 16.3 vs. 14.0 months, hazard ratio (HR) [95% confidence interval] = 0.65 [0.43 – 0.97], $p = 0.035$), a twice longer PFS (median 5.3 vs. 2.6 months, HR = 0.56 [0.40 – 0.79], $p = 0.001$), and a higher confirmed PSA response ≥50% (49.8% vs. 24.4%, $p = 0.005$), as compared with patients who did not develop grade ≥3 neutropenia. In the subgroup of neutropenic patients, the median OS was 19.7 months in those treated with granulocyte colony-stimulating factor (G-CSF) and 16 months on those without G-CSF support. Primary or secondary prophylactic use of G-CSF had no adverse impact for outcome. If prospectively confirmed, these results would justify maintaining the intended cabazitaxel dose of 25 mg/m^2 whenever possible.

Today, the routine use of G-CSF is the standard of care in cabazitaxel chemotherapy. Aside from neutropenia, cabazitaxel treatment is well tolerated, causing less alopecia, nail changes, neuropathy, and dysgeusia compared with docetaxel [22].

The major question remains as to whom will benefit from cabazitaxel versus further androgen receptor (AR)-targeted therapy in the post-docetaxel setting. Two competing AR-directed therapies, the AR-receptor antagonist enzalutamide and the AR-pathway inhibitor abiraterone, both prolong survival in this clinical situation, and proper sequencing of therapies, as well as choosing the right treatment for the patient, is crucial to provide the best clinical outcome in CRPC. It is well recognized that approximately one-third of patients are primarily resistant to AR-directed therapies. The theoretic tool to recognize resistance would be the measurement of the protein encoded by AR-V7 (AR splice variant 7), since it lacks the ligand-binding domain of the androgen receptor (the direct target of enzalutamide and the indirect target of abiraterone) while remaining constitutively active as a transcription factor in a ligand-independent manner [23–26].

The clinical association AR-V7 with resistance to AR-directed therapy has been evaluated prospectively in 62 patients (31 abiraterone and 31 enzalutamide recipients) [27]. AR-V7 was measured in circulating tumor cells by reverse transcriptase–polymerase chain reaction in patients with metastatic CRPC who were initiating treatment with either enzalutamide or abiraterone. The association of AR-V7 status (positive vs. negative) and PSA response rates (the primary endpoint), PSA progression-free survival, clinical or radiographic progression-free survival, and overall survival were evaluated. In this study, looking at waterfall plots, no AR-V7-positive patient had any appreciable clinical benefit from enzalutamide or abiraterone therapy. The study showed a strong association between the presence of AR-V7 and resistance to enzalutamide and abiraterone, but it failed to provide the mechanism of resistance by AR-V7. It concluded that, after validation in larger trials, AR-V7 could be used as a biomarker to predict resistance to enzalutamide and abiraterone and to facilitate treatment selection.

The same investigators tested whether the presence of AR-V7 affected taxane efficacy [28]. They enrolled taxane-treated patients into the study and pooled the results with their previous group of patients receiving AR-directed therapies. Of the

37 taxane-treated patients enrolled, 17 (46%) had detectable AR-V7 in CTCs. There was no significant difference in PSA response (41% vs. 65%; $P = 0.19$), PSA PFS (hazard ratio [HR], 1.7, 95% CI, 0.6–5.0; $P = 0.32$), and PFS (HR, 2.7, 95% CI, 0.8–8.8; $P = 0.11$) between AR-V7-positive and AR-V7-negative men. A significant interaction was observed between AR-V7 status and treatment type ($P < 0.001$). Clinical outcomes were superior with taxanes compared with enzalutamide or abiraterone therapy in AR-V7-positive men, whereas outcomes did not differ by treatment type in AR-V7-negative men. Investigators have also shown in serial measurements over time in patients receiving chemotherapy and AR-directed treatments that AR-V7 status changes over time with therapy, converting both from negative to positive and from positive to negative status [29]. Interestingly, conversion from positive to negative status only occurred during taxane treatment. Technology for CTC extraction also needs to be developed and standardized before presented for routine use in the clinical setting [30].

21.4 Docetaxel Combination Regimens

Clinical trials and real-life evidence show that only about 50% of patients with CRPC respond to docetaxel and many develop resistance after a certain time of drug exposure. Hypothesis that the microtubulin inhibitor taxanes have additional activity through AR has been proven in studies which have shown that docetaxel causes cytoplasmic AR sequestration ex vivo [31, 32], in circulating tumor cells [33], significant downregulation of the AR and PSA expression, and repression of AR function [34, 35]. These data support that the anticancer activity of docetaxel is partially through the disruption of AR signaling [36]. Resistance to docetaxel seems very complex, such as apoptosis inhibition [37], activation of several survival pathways, and loss of sensitivity of AR leading to continuous signaling, accounting for the activity of further AR-directed therapies after docetaxel in CRPC. The influence of the tumor microenvironment and drug resistance interactions between tumor cells and bone cells may also account for docetaxel resistance [37, 38].

Combinations of docetaxel to other targeted agents have been proposed to overcome resistance. There are many small phase II trials, but ten large negative phase III trials have been completed with negative results.

The MAINSAIL trial tested docetaxel/prednisone with or without the antiangiogenic agent lenalidomide in metastatic CRPC with the primary endpoint of OS [39]. The trial was terminated early based on interim analysis showing no additional benefit. In the SWOG-S0421 trial, docetaxel/prednisone was combined with either the endothelin-A (ET-A) receptor antagonist atrasentan or placebo in 991 eligible patients with mCRPC with bone metastases [40]. This phase III trial reported no differences in OS (median OS 18 months vs. 17 months, respectively; HR: 1.01, 95% CI 0.87–1.18; P ¼ 0.88).

The Cancer and Leukemia Group B (CALGB)/Eastern Cooperative Oncology Group (ECOG)-90401 trial evaluated the combination of bevacizumab with docetaxel/prednisone compared to docetaxel/prednisone alone in men with mCRPC [41].

Despite an improvement in PFS (median PFS 9.9 months vs. 7.5 months, respectively; HR: 0.77, 95% CI 0.68–0.88; P o 0.0001), the trial did not meet its primary endpoint, OS benefit. The VENICE trial evaluated the primary endpoint of OS in patients with mCRPC treated with a regimen of either placebo or aflibercept, an antiangiogenic agent, in combination with docetaxel/prednisone. This trial also did not meet the primary endpoint [42]. The ENTHUSE M1C trial compared a regimen of docetaxel in combination with the ET-A receptor antagonist zibotentan at 10 mg/d versus docetaxel/placebo in patients with mCRPC (NCT00617669) [43]. The primary endpoint, OS, was unmet. The READY trial test the addition of dasatinib to docetaxel/prednisone in a double-blind randomized manner to improve overall survival [44]. Secondary endpoints in the READY trial included comparison of objective response, time to first SRE and PFS, time to PSA progression, reduction of urinary N-telopeptide, pain intensity from baseline between treatment groups, and safety analyses. This trial also was a negative trial, not meeting the OS benefit endpoint. The SYNERGY is an open label, international, randomized trial comparing the addition of custirsen to the standard docetaxel/prednisone in patients with mCRPC. This study follows encouraging results from a phase II trial (n 1⁄4 82) which demonstrated an improvement in survival in patients with mCRPC when custirsen was combined with docetaxel/prednisone relative to SOC docetaxel/prednisone (median OS of 23.8 months vs. 16.9 months, respectively; HR: 0.61, 95% CI 0.36–1.02) [44].

21.5 Neuroendocrine Prostate Cancer (NEPC)

Neuroendocrine prostate cancer (NEPC) is an aggressive subtype of prostate cancer that can arise de novo but much more commonly arises after hormonal therapy for prostate adenocarcinoma (PCA) [1]. NEPC frequently metastasizes to visceral organs and responds only transiently to chemotherapy, and most patients die within 1–2 years of diagnosis [45]. NEPC differs histologically from PCA and is characterized by the presence of small, round, blue neuroendocrine cells, which do not express AR or secrete PSA, but usually express neuroendocrine markers such as chromogranin A, synaptophysin, and neuron-specific enolase (NSE) [46]. Pure localized small cell carcinoma of the prostate gland is rare (<1% of cases); focal neuroendocrine differentiation admixed with adenocarcinoma is more commonly observed in approximately 5–10% of cases, depending on the criteria and biomarkers used [47].

Treatment-related NEPC detected by immunohistochemical staining is found in approximately 20–30% of metastatic castration-resistant tumors [47].The true incidence of NEPC may become even higher with the recent introduction of more potent androgen receptor signaling inhibitors, underdiagnosis as a result of tumor heterogeneity, lack of metastatic site biopsies, lack of a uniform consensus definition based on histology or biomarker expression, and frequent misclassification as high-grade prostate adenocarcinoma, especially in tumors with mixed histologies.

The presence of neuroendocrine differentiation is suggested by a limited response duration to primary ADT (<6 months); high PSA nadir on ADT (>4 ng/mL); visceral metastatic disease, including to the lung, liver, and central nervous system; predominantly lytic bone metastases; low absolute serum PSA in relation to disease burden; elevated serum markers of neuroendocrine differentiation, including chromogranin and neuron-specific enolase; and high levels of lactate dehydrogenase and/or elevated carcinoembryonic antigen (CEA) serum levels [48–50].

One of the hallmarks of NEPC is loss of androgen receptor, and androgen receptor knockdown in an androgen receptor-sensitive cell line correlates with neuroendocrine differentiation [51].

Another study showed overexpression of the AURKA protein in all NEPC tumors and amplification of the *AURKA* gene in four of seven NEPC tumors [52]. Inhibition of AURKA led to a loss of neuroendocrine differentiation, suggesting a link between AURKA signaling and reversible NEPC. Amplification of *MYCN* was found in 40% of NEPC cases compared with only 4% of prostate adenocarcinoma cases [52]. The PI3K/Akt-mTOR pathway has also been shown to be necessary for NEPC formation. Inhibition of PI3K has decreased neuron-specific enolase expression, and transfection of activated Akt led to increased neuron-specific enolase expression, indicating a reversible NEPC activation [53].

21.6 Chemotherapy for NEPC

Advanced small cell prostate cancer and prostate cancer with extensive neuroendocrine differentiation, both highly proliferative subsets of prostate cancer, generally respond rapidly to cytotoxic chemotherapy with minimal (if any) response to androgen deprivation. Pure small cell carcinoma with distant metastases should largely be treated with up-front chemotherapy rather than ADT. In prostate cancer with extensive neuroendocrine differentiation, a trial of ADT in combination with cytotoxic chemotherapy may be reasonable. For small cell cancer, the treatment of choice is platinum plus etoposide combination; for prostatic adenocarcinoma with neuroendocrine differentiation, the choice is docetaxel, or a combination of carboplatin plus docetaxel. Platinum-based treatment should be strongly considered in cases involving more extensive neuroendocrine differentiation and/or small cell features within the tumor biopsy. A retrospective series of 21 patients with metastatic small cell prostate cancer was treated with a combination of platinum plus etoposide, and 62% of patients experienced an objective tumor response. The duration of response was short, and median survival was less than 12 months.

Prospective clinical trials have tested combination chemotherapy. A single-arm phase II study investigated the use of carboplatin plus docetaxel in combination with prednisone in 113 patients with one or more of seven prespecified criteria designed to capture anaplastic or aggressive phenotype prostate cancer: (1) histologic evidence of small cell prostate cancer (pure or mixed); (2) exclusively visceral metastases; (3) predominantly lytic bone metastases; (4) bulky pelvic soft tissue masses greater than 5 cm; (5) low serum PSA level (<10 ng/mL) in combination with high-volume (>20) bone metastases; (6) positive immunohistochemistry staining of chromogranin or synaptophysin A or elevated serum markers of neuroendocrine differentiation plus elevations in lactate dehydrogenase (LDH), CEA, or malignant hypercalcemia; or (7) short-interval (<6 months) response to primary ADT [54]. After disease progression on carboplatin plus docetaxel, patients were treated with cisplatin plus etoposide. Median OS was 16 months (95% CI, 13.6–19.0), and the proportion of patients who were progression-free after four cycles of carboplatin plus docetaxel and subsequent treatment with cisplatin plus etoposide ($N = 71$) was 65.4 and 33.8%, respectively. The trial results suggest that continued platinum-based chemotherapy with the addition of etoposide may be a reasonable second-line therapy in patients with NEPC who experience disease progression on platinum plus taxane combinations. Serum LDH and CEA seemed to have more prognostic value than levels of chromogranin A or immunohistochemical positivity of chromogranin A and synaptophysin, showing that traditional NEPC biomarkers may not be prognostic. More effective targeted therapies are awaited in the future.

21.7 Chemotherapy for Hormone-Naïve Prostate Cancer

The up-front systemic treatment of patients who present with metastatic prostate cancer has long remained androgen deprivation therapy (ADT). The use of intermittent ADT, or the addition of an antiandrogen to ADT, has not improved survival [55, 56]. The addition of chemotherapy, docetaxel, to ADT in newly diagnosed metastatic prostate has been recently tested in three randomized trials [57–59]. A meta-analysis of these three trials has confirmed the benefit of adding chemotherapy to hormonal treatment in this patient population [60].

The CHAARTED trial randomized 790 newly diagnosed metastatic prostate cancer patients between docetaxel + ADT and ADT only [57]. Patients were stratified according to disease volume (high vs. low), age (≥70 vs. <70), ECOG performance status (0–1 vs. 2), ADT ≥ 30 days (yes vs. no), previous adjuvant ADT (>12 months vs. ≤12), bisphosphonates, or denosumab (yes vs. no). High-volume disease was defined as the presence of visceral metastases or ≥4 bone lesions with ≥1 beyond the vertebral bodies and pelvis.

The median overall survival was 13.6 months longer with the addition to ADT of early docetaxel than with ADT alone (57.6 months vs. 44.0 months; HR for death 0.61; 95% CI 0.47–0.80; $P < 0.001$). There were 101 prostate cancer deaths in the combination group and 136 prostate cancer deaths in the ADT-alone group. The benefit at the last analysis was more apparent in the subgroup with high-volume disease than in the overall study population, with a median overall survival that was 17.0 months longer in the combination group than in the ADT-alone group (49.2 months vs. 32.2 months; HR for death, 0.60; 95% CI, 0.45–0.81; $P < 0.001$). The median survival at the time of the analysis had not been reached in the subgroup with low-volume disease in either study group. A benefit of docetaxel treatment was detected in all the subgroups analyzed [57].

Decrease in the PSA level to less than 0.2 ng per milliliter at 12 months was 27.7% in the combination group, compared to 16.8% in the ADT-alone group ($P < 0.001$). The median time to the development of CRPC (biochemical, symptomatic, or radiographic) was 20.2 months with combination therapy, compared to 11.7 months with ADT alone (HR 0.61; 95% CI, 0.51–0.72; $P < 0.001$). The median time to clinical progression was 33.0 months with combination therapy, as compared with 19.8 months with ADT alone (HR 0.61; 95% CI, 0.50–0.75; $P < 0.001$).

In the chemotherapy group, 2% had a grade 3 or 4 allergic reaction; grade 3 fatigue occurred in 4% of the patients, and grade 3 diarrhea, stomatitis, motor neuropathy, and sensory neuropathy each occurred at a rate of 1% or less. Rate of thromboembolic events was 1% in the combination group. One patient died suddenly at home of an unknown cause during the course of docetaxel therapy. Neutropenic fever occurred in 6% of the patients in the combination group; rate of grade 3–4 infection remained at 2%.

The GETUG-15 trial included 385 patients, which were not stratified for disease extent [58]. Based on 176 events, the trial found a similar progression-free survival but no survival difference between chemo-hormonal treatment and ADT alone (HR 1.01; 95% CI 0.76–1.25). The contradictory result may be the consequence of smaller sample size, non-selection of patients according to tumor volume, or the different rate of de novo metastatic disease in these two trials.

STAMPEDE was a multi-arm, multistage trial that included both metastatic and nonmetastatic prostate cancer patients [59]. The current report of the STAMPEDE trial reflects results of four study arms, including standard of care (SOC; ADT ± radiotherapy), SOC plus docetaxel, SOC plus zoledronic acid, and SOC plus docetaxel and zoledronic acid. Docetaxel was administered as six cycles of 75 mg/m^2 every 3 weeks with prednisone 10 mg daily, as opposed to docetaxel alone in the CHAARTED trial. Approximately 61% of patients had metastatic disease at presentation, whereas 15% presented with node-positive disease and 24% with high-risk locally advanced disease (T3/4, PSA >40, or Gleason 8–10). This trial demonstrated that docetaxel in combination with SOC improved OS by 10 months as compared with SOC alone (HR, 0.78; 95% CI, 0.66–0.93; $P = 0.006$). When patients with metastatic disease were analyzed separately, the OS benefit was 15 months for docetaxel plus SOC versus SOC alone (HR, 0.76; 95% CI, 0.62–0.92; $P = 0.005$). These results compared favorably with the results of the CHAARTED trial and confirmed the benefit of the addition of docetaxel to ADT in the treatment of hormone-naïve metastatic prostate cancer.

A meta-analysis, including patients from all three trials, revealed a robust 9% absolute OS benefit at 4 years (HR = 0.77; 95% CI: 0.68–0.87; $p < 0.0001$) by the use of docetaxel plus ADT in men with mHSPC [60].

Many wonder why six cycles of docetaxel in the hormone-naïve setting have such greater benefit than that administered in CRPC. The answer may lie within the early kill of hormone-resistant cell clones or in the different docetaxel pharmacokinetics in these different patient subsets. The difference is evident in the 2.7% rate of neutropenic fever between TAX-327 versus 6–12% in all three hormone-naïve metastatic prostate cancer studies. In the study by Franke et al. [61], the clearance of docetaxel is increased by 100% in castrated men. Steroids may also influence taxane pharmacokinetics. A recent report has suggested a higher incidence of neutropenic fever in patients receiving docetaxel alone as compared to docetaxel with prednisone [62]. The CHAARTED trial used docetaxel without prednisone, and the STAMPEDE coadministered docetaxel with prednisone, producing the same magnitude of benefit. Prednisone alone has shown activity as the control arm in many trials, and the addition of prednisone to docetaxel enhances the efficacy of the regimen. The recommendation today is to coadminister docetaxel with prednisone in all settings.

Conclusion

Chemotherapy in addition to ADT should be offered to all metastatic hormone-naïve prostate cancer patients, who are fit enough for chemotherapy.

References

1. Tannock IF, Osoba D, Stocker MF. Chemotherapy with mitoxantrone plus prednisone or prednisone alone for symptomatic hormone-resistant prostate cancer: a Canadian randomized trial with palliative end points. J Clin Oncol. 1996;14:1756–64.
2. Winquist E, Waldron T, Berry S, et al. Non-hormonal systemic therapy in men with hormone-refractory prostate cancer and metastases: a systematic review from the cancer care Ontario program in evidence-based care's genitourinary cancer disease site group. BMC Cancer. 2006;6:112.
3. Basch EM, Loblaw DA, Oliver TK, et al. Systemic therapy in men with metastatic castration-resistant prostate cancer: American society of clinical oncology and cancer care Ontario clinical practice guideline. J Clin Oncol. 2014;32(30):3436–48.
4. Tannock IF, de Wit R, Berry WR, et al. for the TAX 327 Investigators. Docetaxel plus prednisone or mitoxantrone plus prednisone for advanced prostate cancer. N Engl J Med. 2004;351:1502–12.
5. de Bono JS, Oudard S, Ozguroglu M, et al. TROPIC investigators. Prednisone plus cabazitaxel or mitoxantrone for metastatic castration-resistant prostate cancer progressing after docetaxel treatment: a randomised open-label trial. Lancet. 2010;376:1147–54.
6. Petrylak DP, Tangen CM, Hussain MH, et al. Docetaxel and estramustine compared with mitoxantrone and prednisone for advanced refractory prostate cancer. N Engl J Med. 2004;351:1513–20.
7. Berthold DR, Pond GR, Soban F, et al. Docetaxel plus prednisone or mitoxantrone plus prednisone for advanced prostate cancer: updated survival in the TAX 327 study. J Clin Oncol. 2008;26(2):242–5.
8. Horgan AM, Seruga B, Pond GR, et al. Tolerability and efficacy of docetaxel in older men with metastatic castrate-resistant prostate cancer (mCRPC) in the TAX 327 trial. J Geriatr Oncol. 2014;5(2):119–26.
9. Droz JP, Balducci L, Bolla M, et al. Background for the proposal of SIOG guidelines for the management of prostate cancer in senior adults. Crit Rev Oncol Hematol. 2010;73:68–91.
10. National Comprehensive Cancer Network. NCCN clinical practice guidelines in oncology. Prostate cancer. Version 3.2012. NCCN: Pennsylvania; 2012.
11. Loriot Y, Massard C, Gross-Goupil M, et al. The interval from the last cycle of docetaxel-based chemotherapy to progression is associated with the efficacy of subsequent docetaxel in patients with prostate cancer. Eur J Cancer. 2010;46:1770–2.

12. Shimura T, Kitagawa M, Yamada T, et al. The impact of cross-resistance between paclitaxel and docetaxel for metastatic gastric cancer. Onkologie. 2012;35:176–83.
13. Pivot X, Koralewski P, Hidalgo JL, et al. A multicenter phase II study of XRP6258 administered as a 1-h i.v. infusion every 3 weeks in taxane-resistant metastatic breast cancer patients. Ann Oncol. 2008;19:1547–52.
14. Mita AC, Denis LJ, Rowinsky EK, et al. Phase I and pharmacokinetic study of XRP6258 (RPR116258A), a novel taxane, administered as a 1-hour infusion every 3 weeks in patients with advanced solid tumors. Clin Cancer Res. 2009;15:723–30.
15. Bahl A, Oudard S, Tombal B, et al. Impact of cabazitaxel on 2-year survival and palliation of tumour-related pain in men with metastatic castration-resistant prostate cancer treated in the TROPIC trial. Ann Oncol. 2013;24(9):2402–8.
16. de Bono JS, Oudard S, Ozguroglu M, et al. Cabazitaxel or mitoxantrone with prednisone in patients with metastatic castration-resistant prostate cancer (mCRPC) previously treated with docetaxel: final results of a multinational phase III trial (TROPIC). J Clin Oncol. 2010;(Suppl):abstract 9.
17. Bahl A, Masson S, Malik Z, et al. Cabazitaxel for metastatic castration-resistant prostate cancer (mCRPC): Interim safety and quality-of-life (QOL) data from the U.K. early access program (NCT01254279). J Clin Oncol 2012;30(Suppl):abstract 44.
18. Sridhar SS, Winquist E, Hubay S, et al. Cabazitaxel early access program (EAP)—Canadian interim results: safety, QOL, and utility values in metastatic castration resistant prostate cancer (mCRPC). Ann Oncol. 2012;23(Suppl 9):abstract 960.
19. Castellano D, Aparicio LMA, Esteban E, et al. Cabazitaxel for castration-resistant prostate cancer: safety data from the Spanish expanded access program. J Expert Opin Drug Safety. 2014;13:1165–73.
20. de Bono J, Hardy-Bessard AC, Kim CS, et al. Phase III non-inferiority study of cabazitaxel 20 mg/m^2 versus cabazitaxel 25 mg/m^2 in patients with metastatic castration-resistant prostate cancer previously treated with docetaxel (PROSELICA). Proceedings of the ASCO, 2016.
21. Meisel A, von Felten S, Vogt DR, et al. Severe neutropenia during cabazitaxel treatment is associated with survival benefit in men with metastatic castration-resistant prostate cancer (mCRPC): a post-hoc analysis of the TROPIC phase III trial. Eur J Cancer. 2016;56:93–100.
22. Omlin A, Sartor O, Rothermundt C, et al. Analysis of side effect profile of alopecia, nail changes, peripheral neuropathy, and dysgeusia in prostate cancer patients treated with docetaxel and cabazitaxel. Clin Genitour Cancer. 2015;13:e205–8.
23. Hu R, Dunn TA, Wei S, et al. Ligand-independent androgen receptor variants derived from splicing of cryptic exons signify hormone-refractory prostate cancer. Cancer Res. 2009; 69:16–22.
24. Hu R, Lu C, Mostaghel EA, et al. Distinct transcriptional programs mediated by the ligand-dependent full-length androgen receptor and its splice variants in castration-resistant prostate cancer. Cancer Res. 2012;72:3457–62.
25. Li Y, Chan SC, Brand LJ, Hwang TH, Silverstein KA, Dehm SM. Androgen receptor splice variants mediate enzalutamide resistance in castration-resistant prostate cancer cell lines. Cancer Res. 2013;73:483–9.
26. Guo Z, Yang X, Sun F, et al. A novel androgen receptor splice variant is upregulated during prostate cancer progression and promotes androgen depletion-resistant growth. Cancer Res. 2009;69:2305–13.
27. Antonarakis ES, Lu C, Wang H, et al. ARV7 and resistance to enzalutamide and abiraterone in prostate cancer. N Engl J Med. 2014;371:1028–38.
28. Antonarakis ES, Lu C, Luber B, et al. Androgen receptor splice variant 7 and efficacy of taxane chemotherapy in patients with metastatic castration-resistant prostate cancer. JAMA. 2015;1(5):582–91.
29. Nakazawa M, Lu C, Chen Y, et al. Serial blood-based analysis of AR-V7 in men with advanced prostate cancer. Ann Oncol. 2015;26:1859–65.
30. Zhang T, Armstrong AJ. Clinical utility of circulating tumor cells in advanced prostate cancer. Curr Oncol Rep. 2016;18:3.

31. Jiang J, Huang H. Targeting the androgen receptor by taxol in castration resistant prostate cancer. Mol Cell Pharmacol. 2010;2:1–5.
32. Zhu ML, Horbinski CM, Garzotto M, et al. Tubulin-targeting chemotherapy impairs androgen receptor activity in prostate cancer. Cancer Res. 2010;70:7992–8002.
33. Darshan MS, Loftus MS, Thadani-Mulero M, et al. Taxane-induced blockade to nuclear accumulation of the androgen receptor predicts clinical responses in metastatic prostate cancer. Cancer Res. 2011;71:6019–29.
34. Gan L, Chen S, Wang Y, et al. Inhibition of the androgen receptor as a novel mechanism of taxol chemotherapy in prostate cancer. Cancer Res. 2009;69:8386–94.
35. Kuroda K, Liu H, Kim S, et al. Docetaxel down-regulates the expression of androgen receptor and prostate-specific antigen but not prostate-specific membrane antigen in prostate cancer cell lines: implications for PSA surrogacy. Prostate. 2009;69:1579–85.
36. Mezynski J, Pezaro C, Bianchini D, et al. Antitumour activity of docetaxel following treatment with the CYP17A1 inhibitor abiraterone: clinical evidence for cross-resistance? Ann Oncol 2012. [Epub ahead of print].
37. Seruga B, Tannock IF. Chemotherapy-based treatment for castration- resistant prostate cancer. J Clin Oncol. 2011;29:3686–94.
38. Seruga B, Ocana A, Tannock IF. Drug resistance in metastatic castration-resistant prostate cancer. Nat Rev Clin Oncol. 2011;8:12–23.
39. NCT00988208. Study to evaluate safety and effectiveness of lenalidomide in combination with docetaxel and prednisone for patients with castrate-resistant prostate cancer (Mainsail). Celgene announces discontinue phase III MAINSAIL trial.
40. Quinn DI, Tangen CM, Hussain M, et al. SWOG S0421: phase III study of docetaxel (D) and atrasentan (A) versus docetaxel and placebo (P) for men with advanced castrate resistant prostate cancer (CRPC). J Clin Oncol. 2012;30(Suppl):[abstract 4511].
41. Kelly WK, Halabi S, Carducci MA, et al. A randomized, double- blind, placebo-controlled phase III trial comparing docetaxel, prednisone, and placebo with docetaxel, prednisone, and bevacizumab in men with metastatic castration-resistant prostate cancer (mCRPC): survival results of CALGB 90401. J Clin Oncol. 2010;28(Suppl):344s. [abstract LBA4511].
42. Tannock IF, Fizazi K, Ivanov S, et al. VENICE investigators. Aflibercept versus placebo in combination with docetaxel and prednisone for treatment of men with metastatic castration-resistant prostate cancer (VENICE): a phase 3, double-blind randomised trial. Lancet Oncol. 2013;14(8):760–8.
43. Fizazi K, Higano CS, Nelson JB, et al. Phase III, randomized, placebo-controlled study of docetaxel in combination with zibotentan in patients with metastatic castration-resistant prostate cancer. J Clin Oncol. 2013;31:1740–7.
44. Araujo JC, Trudel GC, Armstrong AJ, et al. Docetaxel and dasatinib or placebo in men with metastatic castration-resistant prostate cancer (READY): a randomised, double-blind phase 3 trial. Lancet Oncol. 2013;14:1307–16.
45. Palmgren JS, Karavadia SS, Wakefield MR. Unusual and underappreciated: small cell carcinoma of the prostate. Semin Oncol. 2007;34:22–9.
46. Wang W, Epstein JI. Small cell carcinoma of the prostate: a morphologic and immunohistochemical study of 95 cases. Am J Surg Pathol. 2008;32:65–71.
47. Mucci NR, Akdas G, Manely S, Rubin MA. Neuroendocrine expression in metastatic prostate cancer: evaluation of high throughput tissue microarrays to detect heterogeneous protein expression. Hum Pathol. 2000;31:406–14.
48. Furtado P, Lima MV, Nogueira C, et al. Review of small cell carcinomas of the prostate. Prostate Cancer. 2011;2011:543272.
49. Isshiki S, Akakura K, Komiya A, et al. Chromogranin a concentration as a serum marker to predict prognosis after endocrine therapy for prostate cancer. J Urol. 2002;167:512–5.
50. Ather MH, Abbas F, Faruqui N, et al. Correlation of three immunohistochemically detected markers of neuroendocrine differentiation with clinical predictors of disease progression in prostate cancer. BMC Urol. 2008;8:21.

51. Rigo DE, McDonnell DP. Differential effects of prostate cancer therapeutics on neuroendocrine transdifferentiation. Mol Cancer Ther. 2008;7:659–69.
52. Beltran H, Rickman DS, Park K, et al. Molecular characterization of neuroendocrine prostate cancer and identification of new drug targets. Cancer Discov. 2011;1:487–95.
53. Wu C, Huang J. Phosphatidylinositol 3-kinase-AKT-mammalian target of rapamycin pathway is essential for neuroendocrine differentiation of prostate cancer. J Biol Chem. 2007;282:3571–83.
54. Aparicio AM, Harzstark AL, Corn PG, et al. Platinum-based chemotherapy for variant castrate-resistant prostate cancer. Clin Cancer Res. 2013;19:3621–30.
55. Hussain M, Tangen CM, Higano CS, et al. Intermittent (IAD) versus continuous androgen deprivation (CAD) in hormone sensitive metastatic prostate cancer (HSM1PC) patients (pts): results of S9346 (INT-0162), an international phase III trial. N Engl J Med. 2013;368:1314–25.
56. Prostate Cancer Trialists' Collaborative Group. Maximum androgen blockade in advanced prostate cancer: an overview of the randomised trials. Lancet. 2000;355:1491–8.
57. Sweeney C, Chen Y-H, Carducci M, et al. Chemohormonal therapy in hormone-sensitive metastatic prostate cancer. N Engl J Med. 2015;373(8):737–46.
58. Gravis G, Fizazi K, Joly F, et al. Androgen-deprivation therapy alone or with docetaxel in non-castrate metastatic prostate cancer (GETUG-AFU 15): a randomised, open-label, phase 3 trial. Lancet Oncol. 2013;14:149–58.
59. James ND, Sydes MR, Mason MD, et al. Addition of docetaxel, zoledronic acid, or both to first-line long-term hormone therapy in prostate cancer (STAMPEDE): survival results from an adaptive, multiarm, multistage, platform randomised controlled trial. Lancer. 2016;387:1163–77.
60. Vale CL, Burdett S, Tierney JF. Addition of docetaxel or bisphosphonates to standard of care in men with localised or metastatic, hormone-sensitive prostate cancer: a systematic review and meta-analyses of aggregate data. Lancet Oncol. 2016;17(2):243–56.
61. Franke RM, Carducci MA, Rudek MA, Baker SD, Sparreboom A. Castration- dependent pharmacokinetics of docetaxel in patients with prostate cancer. J Clin Oncol. 2010;28(30):4562–7.
62. Kongsted P, Svane IM, Lindberg H, Daugaard G, Sengelov L. Low-dose prednisolone in first-line docetaxel for patients with metastatic castration- resistant prostate cancer: is there a clinical benefit? Urol Oncol. 2015;33(11):494.e15–20.

Targeted Therapies and Immunotherapy in Prostate Cancer

22

Sercan Aksoy and Mehmet Ali Nahit Şendur

Abstract

In the era of the molecular medicine, new targets are discovered and testing for clinical benefits in prostate carcinoma. Recent clinical and preclinical studies focused on understanding the molecular landscape of castration-resistant prostate cancer (CRPC) to find out the potential therapeutic targets. Androgen pathway is the main study field. And new-generation androgen pathway targeting agents are testing and new molecular targets also defined. Androgen receptor targeting is demonstrated as overall survival benefit in CRPC. Abiraterone and enzalutamide that targets androgen pathway had survival benefit and had FDA approval in castration-resistant prostate carcinoma (CRPC) patients. Besides the androgen pathway, PARP inhibitors, PI3K/Akt, immune checkpoints, and PD1 and PDL1 inhibitors are drugable targets. This chapter focuses on the targeted therapies and immunotherapies in prostate adenocarcinoma, especially CRPC.

22.1 New Molecules Targeting the Androgen Receptor Pathway

Better understanding of the disease biology comes with next-generation active compounds. Some clinically active androgen receptors and androgen receptor inhibitors are shown in Table 22.1.

S. Aksoy, M.D. (✉)
Department of Medical Oncology, Hacettepe University Cancer Institute, Ankara, Turkey
e-mail: saksoy07@yahoo.com

M.A.N. Şendur, M.D.
Department of Medical Oncology, Ankara Yıldırım Beyazıt University, Ankara, Turkey

G. Ozyigit, U. Selek (eds.), *Principles and Practice of Urooncology*,
DOI 10.1007/978-3-319-56114-1_22

Table 22.1 New molecules that targeting the androgen receptor pathway in prostate carcinoma and related ongoing phase III clinical trials

Androgen inhibitors	
Abiraterone	FDA approval For metastatic CRPC before chemotherapy For metastatic CRPC following docetaxel
Orteronel (TAK-700)	Phase III Maintenance therapy in patients with mCRPC previously treated with novel hormonal agents (NCT02053311) Orteronel Maintenance therapy in patients with metastatic castration-resistant prostate cancer and nonprogressive disease after first-line docetaxel therapy (NCT01707966) Study comparing orteronel plus prednisone in patients with metastatic castration-resistant prostate cancer (NCT01193257) Study comparing orteronel plus prednisone in patients with chemotherapy-naive metastatic castration-resistant prostate cancer (NCT01193244) Phase III ADT + TAK-700 versus ADT + bicalutamide for metastatic prostate cancer (NCT01809691) Hormone therapy, radiation therapy, and steroid 17alpha-monooxygenase TAK-700 in treating patients with high-risk prostate cancer (NCT01546987)
Galeterone	A study of galeterone compared to enzalutamide in men expressing androgen receptor splice variant-7 mRNA (AR-V7) metastatic CRPC (NCT02438007)
ODM-204	Safety and pharmacokinetics of ODM-204 in patients with metastatic castration-resistant prostate cancer (NCT023440179)
Androgen receptor inhibitors	
Bicalutamide	FDA approval for metastatic prostate adenocarcinoma
Enzalutamide	For metastatic CRPC following docetaxel
ODM-201	Efficacy and safety study of BAY1841788 (ODM-201) in men with high-risk nonmetastatic castration-resistant prostate cancer (ARAMIS) (NCT02200614) ODM-201 in addition to standard ADT and docetaxel in metastatic castration sensitive prostate cancer (NCT02799602)
ARN 509	A study of apalutamide (ARN-509) in men with nonmetastatic castration-resistant prostate cancer (NCT01946204) A study of apalutamide (JNJ-56021927, ARN-509) plus androgen deprivation therapy (ADT) versus ADT in participants with mHSPC (NCT02489318) An efficacy and safety study of JNJ-56021927 (ARN-509) in high-risk prostate cancer subjects receiving primary radiation therapy: ATLAS (NCT02531516)
Galeterone	A study of galeterone compared to enzalutamide in men expressing androgen receptor splice variant-7 mRNA (AR-V7) metastatic CRPC (NCT02438007)

Up to date, docetaxel, sipuleucel-T, cabazitaxel, abiraterone acetate, enzalutamide, and radium-223 showed overall survival benefit in CRPC patients.

Cabazitaxel is a new-generation and semisynthetic derivative of a natural taxane. It is formerly known as XRP-6258. It is a microtubule inhibitor. It was tested in a phase III trial with 755 men for the treatment of castration-resistant prostate cancer, median survival was 15.1 months for patients receiving cabazitaxel versus 12.7 months for patients receiving mitoxantrone. Cabazitaxel was associated with more grades 3–4 neutropenia than mitoxantrone. Cabazitaxel in combination with prednisone is a treatment option for hormone-refractory prostate cancer following docetaxel-based treatment [1].

Abiraterone acetate blockade CYP17 inhibits androgen synthesis. Abiraterone was tested in patients received first- or second-line chemotherapy in CRPCP (COU-301) [2]. Abiraterone acetate approved for use with prednisone for metastatic castration-resistant prostate cancer following docetaxel. This phase III study demonstrated a statistically significant improvement in OS in patients receiving abiraterone acetate compared with patients who received the placebo (HR = 0.646; 95% CI: 0.543, 0.768; $P = 0.0001$). The median OS was 14.8 months for patients who received abiraterone acetate compared with 10.9 months OS for patients who received the placebo. An updated OS analysis, conducted after 775 events, demonstrated a median OS of 15.8 months for patients who received abiraterone acetate compared with 11.2 months for patients who received the placebo (HR = 0.740; 95 percent CI: 0.638, 0.859).

Enzalutamide has FDA approval for metastatic CRPC patients. The approval was based on a single randomized placebo-controlled multicenter trial that enrolled 1199 patients with metastatic castration-resistant prostate cancer who had received prior docetaxel. Patients were randomly assigned to receive enzalutamide 160 mg orally once daily ($N = 800$) or placebo ($N = 399$).

A statistically significant improvement in OS [HR 0.63 (95% CI: 0.53, 0.75), $p < 0.0001$, log rank test] was observed in patients in the enzalutamide group compared with patients in the placebo group. The median OS was 18.4 months for patients who received enzalutamide and 13.6 months for patients who received placebo.

Grades 3–4 adverse reactions were reported in 47% of patients treated with enzalutamide and in 53% of those who received placebo. Seizures occurred in 0.9% of patients treated with enzalutamide [3].

Other new-generation drugs targeting the AR are orteronel and ARN-509, ODM-204, and galeterone.

Orteronel (TAK-700) is an investigational, nonsteroidal, reversible, selective 17,20-lyase inhibitor. Orteronel was tested in phase III study in patients with metastatic castration-resistant prostate cancer that progressed after docetaxel therapy (ELM-PC 5). In this study, there was no statistically significant improvement in OS with orteronel-prednisone versus placebo-prednisone. Furthermore, the longer rPFS and higher rate of ≥50% PSA decrease suggest that orteronel may have antitumor activity in mCRPC after docetaxel therapy [4].

ARN-509 (apalutamide) is another nonsteroidal antiandrogen being actively investigated in the nonmetastatic CRPC setting. This compound inhibits binding of androgens to the AR and prevents nuclear translocation and DNA binding of the receptor to androgen response elements. An ongoing phase II trial of ARN-509 that recruited 47 patients between November 2011 and June 2012 is studying this drug in patients with nonmetastatic CRPC. The primary endpoint is PSA response at 12 weeks according to PCWG2 criteria. Inclusion criteria included nonmetastatic

CRPC and high risk for disease progression, based on PSA level ≥8 ng/mL within 3 months of enrollment and/or PSA doubling time of ≤10 months. Patients were given 240 mg of ARN-509 per day and had their PSA level checked every 4 weeks and imaging studies every 16 weeks. The median follow-up was 13.4 months. The PSA response rate at both 12 and 24 weeks was 91%, and the median metastasis-free survival has not been reached. AEs in the metastatic CRPC group included grade 3 or higher fatigue back pain, constipation, musculoskeletal pain, and vomiting.

An ongoing phase III trial is randomly assigning men with nonmetastatic CRPC 2:1 to ARN-509 versus placebo (ClinicalTrials.gov identifier: NCT01946204). Participants must have a PSA doubling time of ≤10 months.

Earlier use of AR pathway targeting drugs have been tested in de novo metastatic patients (latitude study-abiraterone). Abiraterone is also testing in de novo metastatic patients in combination with local radiotherapy (PEACE-1).

There are emerging drugs target in CRPC. PARP inhibitors, PI3K/Akt, immune checkpoints, and PD1 and PDL1 inhibitors are intensively studied and some promising results were published.

22.2 PARP Inhibitors

Metastatic, castration-resistant prostate cancer can have genomic aberrations that interfere with DNA repair. Some of these aberrations have been associated with sensitivity to platinum and poly(adenosine diphosphate [ADP]–ribose) polymerase (PARP) inhibitors, suggesting that treatment with a PARP inhibitor may exploit a synthetic lethal interaction. PARP is involved in multiple aspects of DNA repair, and the PARP inhibitor olaparib (Lynparza, AstraZeneca) has recently been studied in mCRPC for with BRCA1/2 mutations. It is known that BRCA-mutant patients is exquisitely sensitive to PARP inhibition [5]. DNA repair defect is 22.7% and DNA repair defects. 12.7% BRCA2 altered including 5.3% germline [6].

TOPARP trial is an open-label, single-arm, two-part adaptive design phase II trial of olaparib in patients with advanced castration-resistant prostate cancer.

The trial aims to evaluate the antitumor activity of olaparib in metastatic castration-resistant prostate cancer, identify molecular signatures of tumor cells in responding and nonresponding patients, and identify predictive biomarkers of olaparib response. In this study overall response rate is 33%; however, response rate is 88% in the patients with DNA repair defect [7].

There is an ongoing trial that targeting PARP in mCRPC (PROfound Study). PROfound Study is going to evaluate the efficacy and safety of olaparib versus enzalutamide or abiraterone acetate in subjects with metastatic castration-resistant prostate cancer who have failed prior treatment with a new hormonal agent and have homologous recombination repair gene mutations (NCT02987543). Many combination studies with PARP inhibitors + AR-targeted agents are tested in phase I and phase II trials.

22.3 PI3K/Akt Pathway Inhibitors

PI3K/Akt pathway controls key cellular processes including growth, survival, proliferation, and angiogenesis. CRCP patients had 49% PI3K pathway alterations. There is reciprocal regulation between AR and PI3K. This interaction is a strong preclinical rationale for co-targeting [6, 8].

A phase II trial studied the AKT inhibitors ipatasertib in combination with antiandrogen abiraterone in patients with CRPC. There was no statistically rPFS difference between placebo-abiraterone and abiraterone-ipatasertib arms in unselected patients. However when the patients were evaluated according to the PTEN status (PTEN loss and PTEN no loss), abiraterone-ipatasertib combination arm was statistically better rPFS in patients who have PTEN loss group. But there were no statistically difference in patients who have PTEN no-loss group. PTEN loss is a key biomarker for AKT inhibitors in CRPC patients.

There are ongoing studies that targeting PI3K/Akt in mCRPC. A phase III study is going on that compare the abiraterone + ipatasertib versus abiraterone + placebo. There are also new AKT inhibitors (AZD5363 and GSK2636771) in combination with enzalutamide.

Some immunological mechanisms in prostate carcinoma are summarized in Table 22.2. Sipuleucel-T (PROVENGE) consists of autologous peripheral blood mononuclear cells, including antigen-presenting cells (APCs) that are obtained in cell culture with recombinant prostatic acid phosphatase (PAP)-granulocyte-macrophage colony-stimulating factor (GM-CSF) [PA2024]. The final product of sipuleucel-T is autologous APCs and PAP-GM-CSF.

Sipuleucel-T is the first approved vaccine by FDA. This treatment generated patient's own immune cells. Immune cells drawn by leukopheresis ship to central laboratory for processing, and it is exposed to target antigen PAP and GM-CSF for immunization. After this processing, this immune cells get back to hospital, and patients receive this immune cells. Kantoff et al. studied this approaches in minimally symptomatic CRPC patients that compared the placebo. Sipuleucel-T arm had better overall survival in (36 vs 25.8 months; HR = 0.759 (95% CI: 0.606, 0.951). The median overall survival benefit was 4.1 months ($P = 0.017$). Three-year overall survival rate was also better than the placebo arm (32.1% vs 23.0%). However, the technical and processing difficulties is the major concern about the sipuleucel-T [16].

Table 22.2 Some immunological mechanisms in prostate carcinoma [9–15]

1. Antigen–targeted immunotherapy • Prostatic acid phosphatase (PAP) (sipuleucel-T) • PSA (PROSTVAC) • PSMA • Whole-cell vaccine
2. Immunomodulatory immunotherapy • CTLA4 Blockage • PD1 Blockage • OX40 Activation • GITR Activation

DCVAC/PCA is an active autologous cellular immunotherapy consisting of dendritic cells (DCs) produced ex vivo from a patient's monocytes, which are pulsed with tumor cells killed and subsequently activated by a maturation agent. There is phase I/II clinical trial in patients with the biochemical relapse.

Administration of DCVAC/PCa in patients with biochemical relapse of the prostate cancer led to the significant prolongation of PSA doubling time [17].

22.4 Immune Checkpoints

Ipilimumab (trade name Yervoy) is a monoclonal antibody that works to activate the immune system by targeting cytotoxic T lymphocyte associated protein 4 (CTLA-4), a protein receptor that downregulates the immune system. Cytotoxic T lymphocytes (CTLs) can recognize and destroy cancer cells. However, an inhibitory mechanism interrupts this destruction. Ipilimumab turns off this inhibitory mechanism and allows CTLs to function.

A phase III study that compared the ipilimumab versus placebo after radiotherapy in patients with metastatic castration-resistant prostate cancer that had progressed after docetaxel chemotherapy had resulted (CA184-043).

Ipilimumab prolonged the median overall survival marginally (11.2 months (95% CI: 9.5–12.7) versus 10.0 months (95% CI: 8.3–11.0): HR: 0.85 (95% CI: 0.72–1.00; $P = 0.053$) [18].

Another phase III study evaluated treatment with ipilimumab in asymptomatic or minimally symptomatic patients with chemotherapy-naive metastatic castration-resistant prostate cancer without visceral metastases.

Median OS was 28.7 months (95% CI: 24.5–32.5 months) in the ipilimumab arm versus 29.7 months (95% CI: 26.1–34.2 months) in the placebo arm (hazard ratio, 1.11; 95.87% CI: 0.88–1.39; $P = 0.3667$). Median progression-free survival was 5.6 months in the ipilimumab arm versus 3.8 with placebo arm (hazard ratio, 0.67; 95.87% CI: 0.55–0.81). Exploratory analyses showed a higher prostate-specific antigen response rate with ipilimumab (23%) than with placebo (8%). Ipilimumab did not improve OS in patients with metastatic castration-resistant prostate cancer. The observed increases in progression-free survival and prostate-specific antigen response rates suggest antitumor activity in a patient subset [19].

Expression of the programmed death 1 (PD-1) receptor and its ligand, PD-L1, has been reported in CRPC. Pembrolizumab, an anti–PD-1 antibody, blocks the interaction between PD-1 and PD-L1. KEYNOTE-028 (NCT02054806) is a nonrandomized, phase Ib trial to evaluate the safety and efficacy of pembrolizumab in 20 advanced solid tumor cohorts. One of these cohorts is prostate adenocarcinoma. Patients who have advanced adenocarcinoma of the prostate, failure of standard therapy, and PD-L1 expression in ≥1% of tumor or stroma cells by immunohistochemistry were included this cohort. Of the 23 patients enrolled in this cohort. Three patients had a confirmed partial response, for an ORR of 13% (95% CI, 3–34%); median duration of response was 59 weeks (range, 28–62 weeks). Stable disease rate was 39% ($n = 9$; 95% CI: 20–61%). Median OS was 8 months, and the 6-month PFS rate was 39%. In this small cohort, pembrolizumab produced durable responses among heavily pretreated patients with advanced PD-L1–positive prostate cancer with favorable side effect profile. There are many running phase II trials with pembrolizumab and nivolumab in different set of prostate carcinoma patients.

It is important to develop new biomarkers to predict the new targeted therapies and immunotherapies. Newly defined AR genomic aberrations in circulating tumor DNA has been associated with decreased clinical response to abiraterone or enzalutamide.

Prospective trials underway are evaluating the prognostic and predictive utility of AR-V7 and exploring novel agents with potential activity against AR-V-expressing CRPC. Detection of androgen receptor splice variant 7 (AR-V7) in circulating tumor cells (CTCs) from men with castration-resistant prostate cancer (CRPC) was associated with primary resistance to enzalutamide and abiraterone therapy.

Conclusion

In the era of the molecular medicine and immunotherapies, prostate carcinoma will have positive results with these extensive researches. Although the androgen pathway is the main fertile study field, new targets have promising results like PARP inhibitors, PI3K/AKT inhibitors, and immunotherapies. We need more powerful biomarkers to predict the new targeted therapies and immunotherapies.

References

1. de Bono JS, et al. Prednisone plus cabazitaxel or mitoxantrone for metastatic castration-resistant prostate cancer progressing after docetaxel treatment: a randomised open-label trial. Lancet. 2010;376(9747):1147–54.
2. Fizazi K, et al. Abiraterone acetate for treatment of metastatic castration-resistant prostate cancer: final overall survival analysis of the COU-AA-301 randomised, double-blind, placebo-controlled phase 3 study. Lancet Oncol. 2012;13(10):983–92.
3. Scher HI, et al. Increased survival with enzalutamide in prostate cancer after chemotherapy. N Engl J Med. 2012;367(13):1187–97.
4. Fizazi K, et al. Phase III, randomized, double-blind, multicenter trial comparing orteronel (TAK-700) plus prednisone with placebo plus prednisone in patients with metastatic castration-resistant prostate cancer that has progressed during or after docetaxel-based therapy: ELM-PC 5. J Clin Oncol. 2015;33(7):723–31.
5. Lavery A, Gilson C, Chowdhury S. PARP inhibitors and stratified treatment of prostate cancer. Expert Rev Anticancer Ther. 2016;16(12):1213–5.
6. Robinson D, et al. Integrative clinical genomics of advanced prostate cancer. Cell. 2015;161(5):1215–28.
7. Mateo J, et al. DNA-repair defects and olaparib in metastatic prostate cancer. N Engl J Med. 2015;373(18):1697–708.
8. Toren P, et al. Combination AZD5363 with enzalutamide significantly delays enzalutamide-resistant prostate cancer in preclinical models. Eur Urol. 2015;67(6):986–90.
9. Eaton JD, et al. Allogeneic whole-cell vaccine: a phase I/II study in men with hormone-refractory prostate cancer. BJU Int. 2002;89(1):19–26.
10. Kantoff PW, Gulley JL, Pico-Navarro C. Revised overall survival analysis of a phase II, randomized, double-blind, controlled study of PROSTVAC in men with metastatic castration-resistant prostate cancer. J Clin Oncol. 2017;35(1):124–5.

11. Singh P, et al. Development of PROSTVAC immunotherapy in prostate cancer. Future Oncol. 2015;11(15):2137–48.
12. Albisinni S. et al. Clinical impact of 68 Ga-prostate-specific membrane antigen (PSMA) positron emission tomography/computed tomography (PET/CT) in patients with prostate cancer with rising prostate-specific antigen after treatment with curative intent: preliminary analysis of a multidisciplinary approach. BJU Int. 2016. doi:10.1111/bju.13739
13. Linch SN, Redmond WL. Combined OX40 ligation plus CTLA-4 blockade: more than the sum of its parts. Oncoimmunology. 2014;3:e28245.
14. Schaer DA, Murphy JT, Wolchok JD. Modulation of GITR for cancer immunotherapy. Curr Opin Immunol. 2012;24(2):217–24.
15. Knee DA, Hewes B, Brogdon JL. Rationale for anti-GITR cancer immunotherapy. Eur J Cancer. 2016;67:1–10.
16. Kantoff PW, et al. Sipuleucel-T immunotherapy for castration-resistant prostate cancer. N Engl J Med. 2010;363(5):411–22.
17. Podrazil M, et al. Phase I/II clinical trial of dendritic-cell based immunotherapy (DCVAC/PCa) combined with chemotherapy in patients with metastatic, castration-resistant prostate cancer. Oncotarget. 2015;6(20):18192–205.
18. Kwon ED, et al. Ipilimumab versus placebo after radiotherapy in patients with metastatic castration-resistant prostate cancer that had progressed after docetaxel chemotherapy (CA184-043): a multicentre, randomised, double-blind, phase 3 trial. Lancet Oncol. 2014;15(7):700–12.
19. Beer TM, et al. Randomized, double-blind, phase III trial of ipilimumab versus placebo in asymptomatic or minimally symptomatic patients with metastatic chemotherapy-naive castration-resistant prostate cancer. J Clin Oncol. 2017;35(1):40–7.

PSA After Radiotherapy: PSA Bounce and Biochemical Failure

23

Fadil Akyol, Melis Gultekin, Gozde Yazici, Pervin Hurmuz, Sezin Yuce Sari, and Gokhan Ozyigit

Abstract

Prostate cancer is one of the major health problems in the world. Active surveillance (AS), radical prostatectomy (RP) or radiotherapy (RT) options can be selected in patients with localized prostate cancer according to risk groups. RT can be given as external beam therapy (EBT) or as brachytherapy (BRT). EBT can be delivered by three-dimensional conformal RT (3BKRT) or intensity modulated RT (IMRT) with conventional fractionation, hypofractionated RT (HFRT), stereotactic body RT (SBRT) and proton treatment. High-dose rate (HDR) or low-dose rate (LDR) BRT can be used as a sole treatment modality or as a combined treatment modality with EBT. Treatment success after local treatment is often evaluated by "biochemical failure." Approximately one-third of patients undergoing RP and 20–30% of patients treated with EBT and hormonal treatment show local recurrence or biochemical failures.

23.1 Introduction

Approximately one-third of patients undergoing RP and 20–30% of patients treated with EBT and hormonal treatment show local recurrence or biochemical failures [1, 2].

Prostate-specific antigen (PSA) is secreted by prostatic acinar and ductal epithelial cells into the seminal fluid. High PSA levels may indicate prostatic intraepithelial neoplasia, prostate cancer, or some benign conditions [3]. It is a very important tool for the primary diagnosis and posttreatment surveillance. Sequential measurements

F. Akyol, M.D. • M. Gultekin, M.D. • G. Yazici, M.D. • P. Hurmuz, M.D. • S.Y. Sari, M.D.
G. Ozyigit, M.D. (✉)
Department of Radiation Oncology, Hacettepe University, Ankara, Turkey
e-mail: gozyigit@hacettepe.edu.tr

G. Ozyigit, U. Selek (eds.), *Principles and Practice of Urooncology*,
DOI 10.1007/978-3-319-56114-1_23

are routinely required for early detection of recurrent disease after definitive treatment in patients with localized disease.

PSA concentration after RT is frequently in detectable level since residual prostatic epithelial cells produce PSA under androgenic stimulation [4]. PSA after treatment is decreased to the minimum level steadily but then can be increased. In the evaluation of tumor activity, PSA level is therefore accepted as unreliable for cases treated with RT against those undergoing RP.

After RT, PSA monitoring is the primary tool for measuring treatment success. The lowest PSA level during follow-up period is called as "PSA nadir." It takes years to reach a PSA nadir and stabile level after three sequential measurements is essential to define the PSA nadir [5]. If PSA nadir is low than 0.1 ng/mL, the presence of complete biochemical remission can be defined [6]. Rising trend in PSA level over time depends on either tumor recurrence or recovery of prostate parenchyma (PSA bounce) [7].

23.2 PSA Bounce Phenomenon

"PSA bounce" is the temporary benign rise in PSA within the first 3 years after RT [8, 9]. This phenomenon is firstly called as "spike" by Wallner et al. in 1997 [10]. It is defined as PSA bounce in the following period [11]. The first PSA bounce value is above the PSA nadir and a subsequent PSA level is equal to or lower than PSA nadir (Fig. 23.1). PSA bounce is observed in 24–50% of patients after BRT using cutoff value ≥0.2 ng/mL [11–16]. The etiology of PSA bounce remains unclear, but

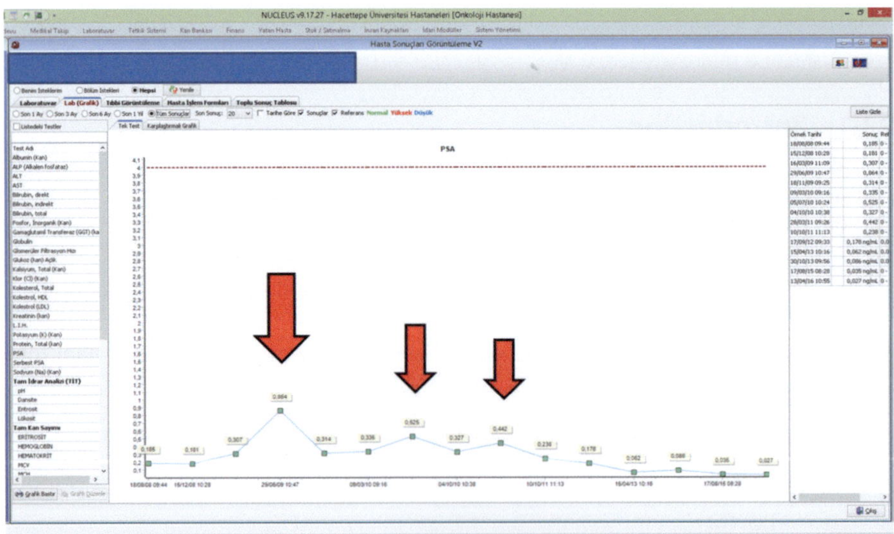

Fig. 23.1 Illustration of PSA bounce phenomenon in a patient treated with CyberKnife™. Patient did not receive androgen blockage. Patient had three PSA bounces after PSA nadir level during his routine follow-up (*red arrows*)

there are some theories; late lethal or sublethal radiation damage on prostate tissue, fluctuations in testosterone kinetics after short-term androgen deprivation treatment (ADT), recent ejaculation, testosterone effect on residual normal prostate tissue, bacterial prostatitis, and instrumentation [7, 17]. Antibiotic treatment or sequential PSA follow-up without any treatment can be applied [18].

Most commonly PSA bounce is defined as a minimum 0.2 ng/mL increase in PSA nadir and a subsequent decrease in PSA levels to PSA nadir or below without treatment [17]. Median time to PSA bounce is 21 months after RT and median value is 0.7 ng/mL [19]. Fifteen percent of PSA bounce values can be >2 ng/mL and sometimes exceed pretreatment PSA level [5]. This situation can be worrying for patients and clinicians, but these values frequently return to normal level within 1 year without any treatment.

PSA bounce can be observed after any RT modalities but significantly less frequent with EBT than BRT [7, 20, 21]. The literature related to PSA bounce is mainly based on permanent seed LDR-BRT studies. However, PSA bounce is also observed after HDR-BRT. Cell death mechanisms are also different depending on different dose rates, and therefore PSA kinetics after treatment is not expected to be the same. McGrath et al. reported higher rates of PSA bounce after HDR monotherapy compared to cases treated with LDR monotherapy or HDR boost treatment (40, 25, 29%, respectively, $p = 0.04$). Increased inflammatory response due to high BED after HDR may result in this observation.

Even though biochemical mechanism is not yet known fully, it is believed that PSA bounce is developed by sudden PSA secretion into the blood stream after conversion of sublethal damage to lethal damage [22]. Better biochemical disease-free survival (bDFS) in some patients with PSA bounce can be explained by this mechanism. However, the relationship between PSA bounce and bDFS is not clear. There are also publications showing no or worse effect on bDFS [13, 15, 22–24]. Hinnen et al. reported that the prostate cancer specific mortality rate for patients who experienced a PSA bounce after I-125 BRT was 0.3%, and those without bounce was 6.1% [15]. Engeler et al. showed that the biochemical failure rate was 3.9% and PSA bounce rate was 24.3% for 713 patients with minimum 2 years of follow-up after I-125 BRT [22]. Biochemical failure occurred 1.7% of the cases with PSA bounce and 4.6% of those without PSA bounce ($p < 0.05$).

PSA bounce is often associated with patient, tumor, and treatment characteristics [25]. In several studies, young age (≤60 yaş) is the most significant predictor for PSA bounce [12, 13, 21]. Besides, more bounces are observed in patients with lower Gleason score [24, 26]. Contradictory results regarding the RT dose have been reported in the literature [27].

23.3 Biochemical Failure

Different definitions of biochemical failures exist after EBT [3, 28–31]. These differences may cause different biochemical failure rates in literature. During the consensus conference by American Society for Therapeutic Radiology and Oncology (ASTRO) in 1997, biochemical failure was defined as three consecutive PSA rises after nadir, spaced 3–6 months apart [31]. On the other hand, the date of biochemical failure is defined as mid-interval between the PSA nadir and the first rise in PSA. The disadvantages of this definition are becoming a retrospective evaluation and extensive period of time required to observe three consecutive rises in PSA level. For this reason, the second ASTRO and RTOG consensus conference was held at Arizona in 2005, and "Phoenix" definition was designed. According to this definition, a rise by ≥2 ng/mL (nadir + 2) above the nadir PSA is called as biochemical failure after EBT independent of whether patients receiving hormonal therapy. The date of failure is defined as the time of the PSA rise [3]. A Phoenix criterion is the most commonly accepted definition for biochemical failure [3, 32]. In the original ASTRO definition, alternative RT techniques such as permanent or temporary BRT and neoadjuvant or adjuvant hormonal treatment have not been considered. Although the Phoenix criteria are developed for cases treated with EBT, this concept is also frequently used in patients receiving BRT. It should be considered that these definitions are used for populations instead of individuals and biochemical failure definition should be performed for each patient individually (Table 23.1).

All of these definitions originally developed by considering PSA kinetics after EBT. Date of positive biopsy or initiation of salvage treatment is accepted as failure for patients treated with salvage therapy options including hormonal therapy, prostatectomy, BRT, or cryosurgery which are not suitable to Phoenix criteria. The sensitivity, specificity, positive predictive value (PPV), and negative predictive value (NPV) of the original ASTRO definition were 51, 78, 52, and 88%, respectively [3, 33]. On the other hand, in Phoenix definition, sensitivity of 64%, specificity of 78%, PPV of 36%, and NPV of 92%, respectively.

When ASTRO definition used, biochemical failure rates reach to 40% in literature [34–36]. Biochemical recurrence is frequently identified before patients experience clinical symptoms of recurrent disease. Kuban et al. reported that only 4% of the cases showed clinical progression before detecting any biochemical failure [35].

Poor prognostic factors for PSA failure include Gleason score at diagnosis (≥8), clinical stage (T3, N1), PSA level at diagnosis (>20 ng/mL), the duration between the first treatment and biochemical failure (≤2 years) and absence of biochemical control after local treatment [1, 2]. Pretreatment PSA level is one of the most important predictive factor for biochemical failure [37, 38]. Zagars et al. reported a significant relationship between pretreatment PSA level and clinical or biochemical relapse after RT [37]. In 6-year follow-up period, the risk of PSA relapse for patients with PSA ≤4, 4.1–10.0, 10.1–20 or >20 ng/mL were 16, 34, 51, and 89%, respectively.

Table 23.1 The definitions of biochemical failure

ASTRO definition [31]	Three consecutive PSA rises after PSA nadir, spaced 3–6 months apart
Vancouver definition [28, 29]	At least two consecutive PSA rises with at least one >1.5 ng/mL over the PSA nadir
ASTRO-Phoenix criteria [3]	A rise by ≥2 ng/mL (nadir + 2) over PSA nadir
Kamat definition [30]	A rise by ≥1.5 ng/mL over PSA nadir at least 24 months over EBT

The date of PSA failure after treatment is also relevant with the survival. If PSA rise (nadir + 2) is detected within 18 months after treatment, the risk of prostate cancer specific mortality is significantly high [39]. Another prognostic factor for the development of biochemical failure is posttreatment PSA doubling time (PSADT) [40, 41]. Local recurrences are more common in cases with the long PSADT (median, 12–14 months) whereas distant metastases are more common in cases with short PSADT (median, 4–6 months) [42]. Prostate cancer specific mortality is 20 times higher in patients with PSADT <3 months compared to PSADT ≥3 months [43]. Gleason score with PSADT is the best prognostic indicators for prostate cancer specific mortality in cases have rising PSA after RT [41]. Patients with short PSADT (<3 ay) and Gleason score ≥8 are at increased risk of prostate cancer mortality, and long-term disease control cannot be achieved only with the local salvage treatments.

PSA nadir after RT is an independent predictive factor which is correlated with biochemical or clinical relapse and local or metastatic disease. Pretreatment PSA level is correlated with tumor grade and clinical T stage. Several studies showed that better clinical results were obtained in cases with PSA nadir <0.5 ng/mL [6, 44]. Alcantara et al. reported that 10-year distant metastases-free rate is 4% for 12-month PSA nadir ≤2 ng/mL and is 19% for >2 ng/mL ($p < 0.0001$) [45]. Although low PSA nadir is associated with favorable clinical outcomes, there is no absolute level to distinguish treatment success from treatment failure [46].

Several prognostic models including factors such as pretreatment variables, RT dose and posttreatment PSA levels have recently tried to estimate clinical relapse risk after RT. However, none of them has been implemented in routine clinical practice [47].

23.4 The Distinguishing PSA Bounce from Biochemical Failure

PSA is not a reliable indicator to evaluate effectiveness of treatment due to benign PSA bounce in first 3 years after RT. PSA monitoring is recommended following RT but PSA fluctuations especially during the first 2 years should not be considered as biochemical failure without any clinical symptoms [48]. Several factors including time to PSA rise, PSADT and PSA velocity have been evaluated in the literature in order to distinguish PSA bounce from biochemical failure [5, 11–13, 16]. However, there is no definitive method to distinguish a benign PSA bounce from biochemical failure. In approximately 10% of cases with PSA bounce, PSA level exceed nadir + 2 which is defined as a biochemical failure [5]. In these cases, consecutive measurements are recommended to distinguish PSA bounce.

The time from the end of RT to PSA rise is an important parameter to distinguish PSA bounce from biochemical failure [16, 18, 26]. In general, PSA rise during early follow-up period is correlated with PSA bounce [5, 12, 16]. The median time to first PSA bounce was 17 months, in contrast the median time to biochemical failure was 41 months after RT [5, 13, 14, 24]. Caloglu et al. reported that PSA bounce was observed in 15–18 months after treatment whereas biochemical failure was observed in 34 months after treatment (16). Similarly, Crook et al. reported that the median time to PSA bounce was 15 months, in contrast to the median time to biochemical failure was 30 months [5]. In the studies related to PSADT, no significant difference was reported in terms of PSA failure or PSA bounce [13, 49].

PSA velocity is another investigated parameter to distinguish PSA failure from PSA bounce. One article in literature reported that PSA velocity was 0.28 ng/mL/month for cases with PSA failure and 0.08 ng/mL/month for those with PSA bounce [50].

PSA elevation after neoadjuvant or adjuvant androgen deprivation therapy (ADT) should be interpreted with caution. PSA rise may be observed when the testosterone returns to normal level after completeness of ADT, and it could not be related with biochemical recurrence [51].

Any medical attempt should not be taken only by detecting an increase in PSA (even it is above nadir + 2) in the first 3 years following RT. PSA monitoring at 3 months interval is suggested for those cases. It is necessary to avoid from unnecessary investigations and salvage treatments especially for patients with low and medium risks but clinician must be more careful for those with high risk. If PSA rises rapidly within 24–30 months after treatment, posttreatment PSA rise after 3 years and PSA >10 ng/mL are mostly correlated with recurrent prostate cancer [11, 18]. Diagnostic and therapeutic approaches should be done in these cases [5, 18, 26].

In patients with biochemical failure, firstly the recurrence pattern (local vs. metastatic disease) should be investigated. In this situation several imaging techniques can be performed, but none of them has sufficient sensitivity or specificity for diagnostic purposes [52]. The recurrence should be firstly confirmed by biopsy after ruled out distant metastases [53]. Posttreatment biopsy should be performed at least 24 months later to assure evaluability [54]. In patients with negative biopsy result, the recommended approach is follow-up [55].

After biochemical failure, bone scintigraphy or computed tomography (CT) is recommended for cases with PSA >20 ng/mL, PSADT <10–12 months or high risk factors at diagnosis [55]. Dynamic contrast-enhanced magnetic resonance imaging (MRI) is recommended for cases treated with EBT or BRT to detect local recurrence after biochemical failure. Choline positron-emission tomography (PET)-CT is the current gold standard in detecting local recurrences after biochemical failure in those were treated with EBRT or BRT. A recent meta-analysis showed that choline PET-CT is superior to CT, MRI, or bone scintigraphy in detecting recurrences in lymph nodes, bones, and the prostate gland [56].

Salvage treatment after biochemical recurrence depends on primary treatment, clinical features of patients and tumor characteristics at presentation or relapse. Salvage treatment is only applied to 16–35% of patients with biochemical failure. It is important to determine which relapsing patients benefit from salvage treatment because of high risk of death from prostate cancer for cases with metastases only and mortality from other causes for cases with biochemical recurrence.

Ideal patient group for local salvage treatment after RT should meet all of the following characteristics: age <70 years, life expectancy >10 years, diagnosis of low or intermediate-risk cancer before initial treatment, PSADT ≥10–12 months, progression or relapse-free interval ≥2 years, PSA value during recurrence ≤10 ng/mL, and no serious intestinal or urinary comorbidities causing contraindications to treatment [57]. Otherwise, treatment decision should be made individually.

RP, BRT, cryosurgery, EBT, or high-intensity focused ultrasound (HIFU) can be performed as a salvage treatment [58–61]. In patients who are not eligible for local treatment, early ADT may be useful [62]. There is no randomized study comparing different salvage treatment options.

23.5 PSA Kinetics After SBRT

Early PSA response is observed in patients treated with SBRT compared to other RT modalities [63–65]. Initially after treatment, PSA levels decline rapidly and then more slowly. The decrease in PSA levels continues during 3-year follow-up period. It means that lower PSA nadir will be detected in case of longer follow-up.

Anwar et al. evaluated posttreatment PSA kinetics of patients with localized prostate cancer after SBRT and compared the results with those after conventional fractionation of dose-escalated IMRT [66]. The significantly lower PSA nadir was observed in the SBRT group. The median slope for SBRT was −0.09 ng/mL/mo, −0.06 ng/mL/mo ve −0.05 ng/mL/mo, respectively, for durations of 1–3 years. Furthermore, the incidence of PSA bounce was more frequent in patients treated with SBRT. Kole et al. studied posttreatment PSA kinetics of 175 patients with localized prostate cancer after SBRT without ADT [67]. The prescription dose was 35–36.5 Gy in five fractions. The median PSA nadir was 0.3 ng/mL for SBRT, and it was lower when compared to conventional fractionated RT. PSA bounce was observed in 36.2% of patients. It was observed that the patients with PSA bounce had mostly high PSA nadir values. In another study, PSA bounce was observed in 28% of patients and correlated with young age [68].

Kim et al. investigated the treatment results of SBRT as a monotherapy or boost treatment in 61 patients with prostate cancer [69]. They were not treated with ADT. SBRT dose was 36.25 Gy in five fractions for monotherapy and 21 Gy in three fractions for boost treatment after 45 Gy whole-pelvic RT. With a median follow-up of 52.4 months, the median PSA nadir was 0.31 ng/mL for the cases treated with SBRT monotherapy. The maximum decline in PSA was observed in the first year and slower decline thereafter. PSA slope for the first year, the second year, the third year, and the fourth year was −0.41, −0.17, −0.12, and −0.09 ng/mL/month, respectively. PSA bounce was observed in 30.4% of cases. The median time to PSA bounce was 12 months. Pretreatment PSA level, Gleason score, and low-risk group were associated with PSA bounce.

We evaluated the long-term results of two different fractionation schemes and PSA bounce phenomenon in our patients treated with robotic SBRT (CyberKnife™). D'Amico risk classification system was used to group patients [70]. In the low-risk (LR) group (n = 54), 20 patients received androgen blockade (AB). In the intermediate-risk (IR) group (n = 52), 42 patients received neoadjuvant/adjuvant

AB. SBRT was delivered in five fractions to a total dose of 36.5 Gy either sequentially ($n = 58$) or every other day ($n = 48$). PSA bounce phenomenon (≥0.2 ng/mL) was observed in 17 patients (16%), and among them only one patient had PSA relapse. We did not find a relation between PSA bounce and biochemical relapse. Five-year BRFS rate was 89% in patients with PSA bounce phenomenon compared to 94.2% in patients without bounce ($p = 0.9$). There was no difference in the incidence of PSA bounce for different treatment schemes [71].

Conclusion

Approximately one-third of patients undergoing RP and 20–30% of patients treated with EBT and hormonal treatment show local recurrence or biochemical failures. *After RT, PSA monitoring is the primary tool for measuring treatment success. The lowest PSA level during follow-up period is called as "PSA nadir." It takes years to reach a PSA nadir, and stabile level after three sequential measurements is essential to define the PSA nadir*. Salvage treatment after biochemical recurrence depends on primary treatment, clinical features of patients, and tumor characteristics at presentation or relapse. Salvage treatment is only applied to 16–35% of patients with biochemical failure. It is important to determine which relapsing patients benefit from salvage treatment because of high risk of death from prostate cancer for cases with metastases only and mortality from other causes for cases with biochemical recurrence.

"PSA bounce" is the temporary benign rise in PSA within the first 3 years after RT. The etiology of PSA bounce remains unclear, but there are some theories; late lethal or sublethal radiation damage on prostate tissue, fluctuations in testosterone kinetics after short-term androgen deprivation treatment (ADT), recent ejaculation, testosterone effect on residual normal prostate tissue, bacterial prostatitis, and instrumentation.

References

1. Heidenreich A, Bastian PJ, Bellmunt J, Bolla M, Joniau S, van der Kwast T, et al. EAU guidelines on prostate cancer. Part II: treatment of advanced, relapsing, and castration-resistant prostate cancer. Eur Urol. 2014;65(2):467–79.
2. Keto CJ, Aronson WJ, Terris MK, Presti JC, Kane CJ, Amling CL, et al. Detectable prostate-specific antigen Nadir during androgen-deprivation therapy predicts adverse prostate cancer-specific outcomes: results from the SEARCH database. Eur Urol. 2014;65(3):620–7.
3. Roach M 3rd, Hanks G, Thames H Jr, Schellhammer P, Shipley WU, Sokol GH, et al. Defining biochemical failure following radiotherapy with or without hormonal therapy in men with clinically localized prostate cancer: recommendations of the RTOG-ASTRO Phoenix Consensus Conference. Int J Radiat Oncol Biol Phys. 2006;65(4):965–74.
4. Willett CG, Zietman AL, Shipley WU, Coen JJ. The effect of pelvic radiation therapy on serum levels of prostate specific antigen. J Urol. 1994;151(6):1579–81.
5. Crook J, Gillan C, Yeung I, Austen L, McLean M, Lockwood G. PSA kinetics and PSA bounce following permanent seed prostate brachytherapy. Int J Radiat Oncol Biol Phys. 2007;69(2):426–33.

6. Ray ME, Thames HD, Levy LB, Horwitz EM, Kupelian PA, Martinez AA, et al. PSA nadir predicts biochemical and distant failures after external beam radiotherapy for prostate cancer: a multi-institutional analysis. Int J Radiat Oncol Biol Phys. 2006;64(4):1140–50.
7. Pickles T. British Columbia cancer agency prostate cohort outcomes I. Prostate-specific antigen (PSA) bounce and other fluctuations: which biochemical relapse definition is least prone to PSA false calls? An analysis of 2030 men treated for prostate cancer with external beam or brachytherapy with or without adjuvant androgen deprivation therapy. Int J Radiat Oncol Biol Phys. 2006;64(5):1355–9.
8. Zietman AL, Christodouleas JP, Shipley WU. PSA bounces after neoadjuvant androgen deprivation and external beam radiation: impact on definitions of failure. Int J Radiat Oncol Biol Phys. 2005;62(3):714–8.
9. Rosser CJ, Kuban DA, Levy LB, Chichakli R, Pollack A, Lee AK, et al. Prostate specific antigen bounce phenomenon after external beam radiation for clinically localized prostate cancer. J Urol. 2002;168(5):2001–5.
10. Wallner KE, Dattoli MJ. Prostate brachytherapy made complicated. Seattle, WA: Smart Medicine Press; 1997.
11. Critz FA, Williams WH, Benton JB, Levinson AK, Holladay CT, Holladay DA. Prostate specific antigen bounce after radioactive seed implantation followed by external beam radiation for prostate cancer. J Urol. 2000;163(4):1085–9.
12. Zwahlen DR, Smith R, Andrianopoulos N, Matheson B, Royce P, Millar JL. Prostate-specific antigen bounce after permanent iodine-125 prostate brachytherapy – an Australian analysis. Int J Radiat Oncol Biol Phys. 2011;79(1):179–87.
13. Ciezki JP, Reddy CA, Garcia J, Angermeier K, Ulchaker J, Mahadevan A, et al. PSA kinetics after prostate brachytherapy: PSA bounce phenomenon and its implications for PSA doubling time. Int J Radiat Oncol Biol Phys. 2006;64(2):512–7.
14. Toledano A, Chauveinc L, Flam T, Thiounn N, Solignac S, Timbert M, et al. PSA bounce after permanent implant prostate brachytherapy may mimic a biochemical failure: a study of 295 patients with a minimum 3-year follow-up. Brachytherapy. 2006;5(2):122–6.
15. Hinnen KA, Monninkhof EM, Battermann JJ, van Roermund JG, Frank SJ, van Vulpen M. Prostate specific antigen bounce is related to overall survival in prostate brachytherapy. Int J Radiat Oncol Biol Phys. 2012;82(2):883–8.
16. Caloglu M, Ciezki JP, Reddy CA, Angermeier K, Ulchaker J, Chehade N, et al. PSA bounce and biochemical failure after brachytherapy for prostate cancer: a study of 820 patients with a minimum of 3 years of follow-up. Int J Radiat Oncol Biol Phys. 2011;80(3):735–41.
17. Cavanagh W, Blasko JC, Grimm PD, Sylvester JE. Transient elevation of serum prostate-specific antigen following (125)I/(103)Pd brachytherapy for localized prostate cancer. Semin Urol Oncol. 2000;18(2):160–5.
18. Gaztanaga M, Crook J. Interpreting a rising prostate-specific antigen after brachytherapy for prostate cancer. Int J Urol. 2013;20(2):142–7.
19. Thames H, Kuban D, Levy L, Horwitz EM, Kupelian P, Martinez A, et al. Comparison of alternative biochemical failure definitions based on clinical outcome in 4839 prostate cancer patients treated by external beam radiotherapy between 1986 and 1995. Int J Radiat Oncol Biol Phys. 2003;57(4):929–43.
20. Hanlon AL, Pinover WH, Horwitz EM, Hanks GE. Patterns and fate of PSA bouncing following 3D-CRT. Int J Radiat Oncol Biol Phys. 2001;50(4):845–9.
21. Sheinbein C, Teh BS, Mai WY, Grant W, Paulino A, Butler EB. Prostate-specific antigen bounce after intensity-modulated radiotherapy for prostate cancer. Urology. 2010;76(3):728–33.
22. Rosser CJ, Kamat AM, Wang X, Do KA, Sanchez-Ortiz RF, Kuban DA, et al. Is patient age a factor in the occurrence of prostate-specific antigen bounce phenomenon after external beam radiotherapy for prostate cancer? Urology. 2005;66(2):327–31.
23. Akyol F, Ozyigit G, Selek U, Karabulut E. PSA bouncing after short term androgen deprivation and 3D-conformal radiotherapy for localized prostate adenocarcinoma and the relationship with the kinetics of testosterone. Eur Urol. 2005;48(1):40–5.

24. Naghavi AO, Strom TJ, Nethers K, Cruz AA, Figura NB, Shrinath K, et al. Clinical implications of a prostate-specific antigen bounce after radiation therapy for prostate cancer. Int J Clin Oncol. 2015;20(3):598–604.
25. Reis LO, Sanches BC, Zani EL, Castilho LN, Monti CR. PSA-nadir at 1 year as a sound contemporary prognostic factor for low-dose-rate iodine-125 seeds brachytherapy. World J Urol. 2014;32(3):753–9.
26. Mehta NH, Kamrava M, Wang PC, Steinberg M, Demanes J. Prostate-specific antigen bounce after high-dose-rate monotherapy for prostate cancer. Int J Radiat Oncol Biol Phys. 2013;86(4):729–33.
27. Merrick GS, Butler WM, Wallner KE, Lief JH, Hinerman-Mulroy A, Galbreath RW. Prostate-specific antigen (PSA) velocity and benign prostate hypertrophy predict for PSA spikes following prostate brachytherapy. Brachytherapy. 2003;2(3):181–8.
28. Pickles T, Duncan GG, Kim-sing C, McKenzie MR, Morris WJ. PSA relapse definitions – the vancouver rules show superior predictive power. Int J Radiat Oncol Biol Phys. 1999;43(3):699–700.
29. Hanlon AL, Hanks GE. Scrutiny of the ASTRO consensus definition of biochemical failure in irradiated prostate cancer patients demonstrates its usefulness and robustness. American society for therapeutic radiology and oncology. Int J Radiat Oncol Biol Phys. 2000;46(3):559–66.
30. Kamat AM, Rosser CJ, Levy LB, Chichakli R, Lee AK, Cheung MR, et al. Rise in serum PSA of 1.5 ng/mL above 24-month nadir after external beam radiotherapy is predictive of biochemical failure. Urology. 2004;63(6):1132–7.
31. American Society for Therapeutic Radiology and Oncology Consensus Panel. Consensus statement: guidelines for PSA following radiation therapy. Int J Radiat Oncol Biol Phys. 1997;37(5):1035–41.
32. Buyyounouski MK, Pickles T, Kestin LL, Allison R, Williams SG. Validating the interval to biochemical failure for the identification of potentially lethal prostate cancer. J Clin Oncol. 2012;30(15):1857–63.
33. Kestin LL, Vicini FA, Martinez AA. Practical application of biochemical failure definitions: what to do and when to do it. Int J Radiat Oncol Biol Phys. 2002;53(2):304–15.
34. Sandler HM, Dunn RL, McLaughlin PW, Hayman JA, Sullivan MA, Taylor JM. Overall survival after prostate-specific-antigen-detected recurrence following conformal radiation therapy. Int J Radiat Oncol Biol Phys. 2000;48(3):629–33.
35. Kuban DA, Thames HD, Levy LB, Horwitz EM, Kupelian PA, Martinez AA, et al. Long-term multi-institutional analysis of stage T1-T2 prostate cancer treated with radiotherapy in the PSA era. Int J Radiat Oncol Biol Phys. 2003;57(4):915–28.
36. Khuntia D, Reddy CA, Mahadevan A, Klein EA, Kupelian PA. Recurrence-free survival rates after external-beam radiotherapy for patients with clinical T1-T3 prostate carcinoma in the prostate-specific antigen era: what should we expect? Cancer. 2004;100(6):1283–92.
37. Zagars GK, Pollack A, von Eschenbach AC. Prognostic factors for clinically localized prostate carcinoma: analysis of 938 patients irradiated in the prostate specific antigen era. Cancer. 1997;79(7):1370–80.
38. Potters L, Morgenstern C, Calugaru E, Fearn P, Jassal A, Presser J, et al. 12-year outcomes following permanent prostate brachytherapy in patients with clinically localized prostate cancer. J Urol. 2005;173(5):1562–6.
39. Harrell FE Jr, Lee KL, Mark DB. Multivariable prognostic models: issues in developing models, evaluating assumptions and adequacy, and measuring and reducing errors. Stat Med. 1996;15(4):361–87.
40. Zelefsky MJ, Ben-Porat L, Scher HI, Chan HM, Fearn PA, Fuks ZY, et al. Outcome predictors for the increasing PSA state after definitive external-beam radiotherapy for prostate cancer. J Clin Oncol. 2005;23(4):826–31.
41. Zhou P, Chen MH, McLeod D, Carroll PR, Moul JW, D'Amico AV. Predictors of prostate cancer-specific mortality after radical prostatectomy or radiation therapy. J Clin Oncol. 2005;23(28):6992–8.

42. Zagars GK, Pollack A, Kavadi VS, von Eschenbach AC. Prostate-specific antigen and radiation therapy for clinically localized prostate cancer. Int J Radiat Oncol Biol Phys. 1995;32(2):293–306.
43. D'Amico AV, Moul JW, Carroll PR, Sun L, Lubeck D, Chen MH. Surrogate end point for prostate cancer-specific mortality after radical prostatectomy or radiation therapy. J Natl Cancer Inst. 2003;95(18):1376–83.
44. Zietman AL, Tibbs MK, Dallow KC, Smith CT, Althausen AF, Zlotecki RA, et al. Use of PSA nadir to predict subsequent biochemical outcome following external beam radiation therapy for T1-2 adenocarcinoma of the prostate. Radiother Oncol. 1996;40(2):159–62.
45. Alcantara P, Hanlon A, Buyyounouski MK, Horwitz EM, Pollack A. Prostate-specific antigen nadir within 12 months of prostate cancer radiotherapy predicts metastasis and death. Cancer. 2007;109(1):41–7.
46. Crook JM, Choan E, Perry GA, Robertson S, Esche BA. Serum prostate-specific antigen profile following radiotherapy for prostate cancer: implications for patterns of failure and definition of cure. Urology. 1998;51(4):566–72.
47. Taylor JM, Yu M, Sandler HM. Individualized predictions of disease progression following radiation therapy for prostate cancer. J Clin Oncol. 2005;23(4):816–25.
48. Vigna-Taglianti R, Russi EG, Boriano A, Gianello L, Denaro N, Lucio F, et al. Reliability of prostate-specific antigen-marker in determining biochemical failure during the first 2 years after external beam radiation therapy and hormone therapy in patients with non-operated prostate cancer. Urol Oncol. 2014;32(1):30 e1–7.
49. Thompson A, Keyes M, Pickles T, Palma D, Moravan V, Spadinger I, et al. Evaluating the Phoenix definition of biochemical failure after (125)I prostate brachytherapy: can PSA kinetics distinguish PSA failures from PSA bounces? Int J Radiat Oncol Biol Phys. 2010;78(2):415–21.
50. Mitchell DM, Swindell R, Elliott T, Wylie JP, Taylor CM, Logue JP. Analysis of prostate-specific antigen bounce after I(125) permanent seed implant for localised prostate cancer. Radiother Oncol. 2008;88(1):102–7.
51. Stone NN. Editorial Comment from Dr Stone to interpreting a rising prostate-specific antigen after brachytherapy for prostate cancer. Int J Urol. 2013;20(2):148.
52. Zaorsky NG, Yamoah K, Thakur ML, Trabulsi EJ, Showalter TN, Hurwitz MD, et al. A paradigm shift from anatomic to functional and molecular imaging in the detection of recurrent prostate cancer. Future Oncol. 2014;10(3):457–74.
53. Casalino DD, Remer EM, Arellano RS, Bishoff JT, Coursey CA, Dighe M, et al. ACR Appropriateness Criteria(R) posttreatment follow-up of prostate cancer. J Am Coll Radiol. 2011;8(12):863–71.
54. Crook J, Malone S, Perry G, Bahadur Y, Robertson S, Abdolell M. Postradiotherapy prostate biopsies: what do they really mean? Results for 498 patients. Int J Radiat Oncol Biol Phys. 2000;48(2):355–67.
55. Punnen S, Cooperberg MR, D'Amico AV, Karakiewicz PI, Moul JW, Scher HI, et al. Management of biochemical recurrence after primary treatment of prostate cancer: a systematic review of the literature. Eur Urol. 2013;64(6):905–15.
56. Umbehr MH, Muntener M, Hany T, Sulser T, Bachmann LM. The role of 11C-choline and 18F-fluorocholine positron emission tomography (PET) and PET/CT in prostate cancer: a systematic review and meta-analysis. Eur Urol. 2013;64(1):106–17.
57. Lopez Torrecilla J, Hervas A, Zapatero A, Gomez Caamano A, Macias V, Herruzo I, et al. Uroncor consensus statement: management of biochemical recurrence after radical radiotherapy for prostate cancer: from biochemical failure to castration resistance. Rep Pract Oncol Radiother. 2015;20(4):259–72.
58. Gomez-Veiga F, Marino A, Alvarez L, Rodriguez I, Fernandez C, Pertega S, et al. Brachytherapy for the treatment of recurrent prostate cancer after radiotherapy or radical prostatectomy. BJU Int. 2012;109(Suppl 1):17–21.
59. Pisters LL, Leibovici D, Blute M, Zincke H, Sebo TJ, Slezak JM, et al. Locally recurrent prostate cancer after initial radiation therapy: a comparison of salvage radical prostatectomy versus cryotherapy. J Urol. 2009;182(2):517–25; discussion 25–7.

60. Darwish OM, Raj GV. Management of biochemical recurrence after primary localized therapy for prostate cancer. Front Oncol. 2012;2:48.
61. Ismail M, Ahmed S, Kastner C, Davies J. Salvage cryotherapy for recurrent prostate cancer after radiation failure: a prospective case series of the first 100 patients. BJU Int. 2007;100(4):760–4.
62. Studer UE, Whelan P, Albrecht W, Casselman J, de Reijke T, Hauri D, et al. Immediate or deferred androgen deprivation for patients with prostate cancer not suitable for local treatment with curative intent: European Organisation for Research and Treatment of Cancer (EORTC) Trial 30891. J Clin Oncol. 2006;24(12):1868–76.
63. Chen LN, Suy S, Uhm S, Oermann EK, Ju AW, Chen V, et al. Stereotactic body radiation therapy (SBRT) for clinically localized prostate cancer: the Georgetown University experience. Radiat Oncol. 2013;8:58.
64. Katz AJ, Santoro M, Diblasio F, Ashley R. Stereotactic body radiotherapy for localized prostate cancer: disease control and quality of life at 6 years. Radiat Oncol. 2013;8:118.
65. King CR, Brooks JD, Gill H, Presti JC Jr. Long-term outcomes from a prospective trial of stereotactic body radiotherapy for low-risk prostate cancer. Int J Radiat Oncol Biol Phys. 2012;82(2):877–82.
66. Anwar M, Weinberg V, Chang AJ, Hsu IC, Roach M 3rd, Gottschalk A. Hypofractionated SBRT versus conventionally fractionated EBRT for prostate cancer: comparison of PSA slope and nadir. Radiat Oncol. 2014;9:42.
67. Kole TP, Chen LN, Obayomi-Davies O, Kim JS, Lei S, Suy S, et al. Prostate specific antigen kinetics following robotic stereotactic body radiotherapy for localized prostate cancer. Acta Oncol. 2015;54(6):832–8.
68. CC V, Haas JA, Katz AE, Witten MR. Prostate-specific antigen bounce following stereotactic body radiation therapy for prostate cancer. Front Oncol. 2014;4:8.
69. Kim HJ, Phak JH, Kim WC. Prostate-specific antigen kinetics after stereotactic body radiotherapy as monotherapy or boost after whole pelvic radiotherapy for localized prostate cancer. Prostate Int. 2015;3(4):118–22.
70. D'Amico AV, Whittington R, Malkowicz SB, Schultz D, Blank K, Broderick GA, et al. Biochemical outcome after radical prostatectomy, external beam radiation therapy, or interstitial radiation therapy for clinically localized prostate cancer. JAMA. 1998;280(11):969–74.
71. Ozyigit G, Hurmuz P, Akyol F. Comparison of two fractionation schemes in prostate cancer patients treated with robotic SBRT. Proceedings of ESTRO 36; 2017 May 5–9; Vienna, Austria.

Re-irradiation in Prostate Cancer

24

Cem Onal

Abstract

Selection of appropriate patients for consideration of salvage treatment depends on whether the patient is still potentially curable. For this purpose, the key issue is to differentiate isolated local recurrence from systemic spread. Additionally, the risk of potential harm from re-treatment against the risk of progression to clinically important symptoms within that patient's lifetime must be also evaluated.

24.1 Introduction

External beam radiotherapy (EBRT) is one of the standard options for definitive treatment of clinically localized or locally advanced prostate cancer. However, approximately 20–50% of patients will have biochemical failure within 10 years, even with image guidance and dose escalation [1, 2]. Local failure still occurs in one-third of patients after 78 Gy ERT, and the original intraprostatic lesion site is the most frequent location of relapse [3]. Without further treatment, progression to clinical symptoms with urinary obstruction, hematuria, or chronic pain would negatively affect the patients' quality of life. Moreover, local recurrence is a potential source of systemic dissemination [4, 5]. However, despite the potential benefits of local treatment, salvage therapies are rarely offered, because of advanced patient age, existing comorbidities and especially concerns about potential toxicity from local salvage procedures.

C. Onal, M.D.
Department of Radiation Oncology, Adana Dr. Turgut Noyan Research and Treatment Center, Başkent University, Adana, Turkey
e-mail: hcemonal@hotmail.com

G. Ozyigit, U. Selek (eds.), *Principles and Practice of Urooncology*,
DOI 10.1007/978-3-319-56114-1_24

Both the American national dataset (CaPSURE) and the British Columbia Tumour Registry show marked underuse of salvage options, in which 25% of patients with biochemical failure are managed with observation, whereas 70% are offered androgen deprivation therapy (ADT), while less than 5% of patients with recurrence undergo potentially curative local salvage treatment [6, 7]. Although conservative approaches are adequate for most of the patients, in selected cases, salvage local treatment with curative intent may be beneficial. Local salvage treatment options include salvage prostatectomy, brachytherapy, cryotherapy, high-intensity focused ultrasound (HIFU), and stereotactic body radiotherapy (SBRT).

In this chapter, we only focus on re-irradiation procedures including brachytherapy and EBRT with discussion of the procedures, oncologic outcomes, and potential toxicity.

24.2 Patient Selection

Selection of appropriate patients for consideration of salvage treatment depends on whether the patient is still potentially curable. For this purpose, the key issue is to differentiate isolated local recurrence from systemic spread. Additionally, the risk of potential harm from re-treatment against the risk of progression to clinically important symptoms within that patient's lifetime must be also evaluated. Approximately 25% of biochemical failures would become clinical failures within 10 years [8].

24.2.1 Biochemical Failure

A rising PSA within 2 years of definitive RT should not be considered indicative of isolated local failure [9, 10]. Most of the patients with local recurrence may also have clinical or subclinical systemic disease. Such patients usually also have a higher PSA nadir after RT and a more rapid PSA doubling time, all of which are predictors of the likely ineffectiveness of local salvage. PSA nadir ≥2 ng/mL, PSA doubling time ≤6 months, and an interval to biochemical failure ≤18 months are all strongly associated with occurrence of distant metastasis [9–11].

Transrectal ultrasound (TRUS)-guided biopsies have been traditionally the first step to evaluate true local recurrence. However, locally recurrent disease can be rarely visualized with TRUS. For better defining local recurrence multiparametric magnetic resonance imaging (mpMRI) is highly sensitive than TRUS. Diffusion-weighted MRI image is altered throughout the irradiated gland. On the contrary, dynamic contrast enhancement, with an infusion of gadolinium, is especially useful in demonstrating recurrent disease, because of the neovascularity of the tumor seen against the background of a relatively avascular irradiated prostate [12]. The use of mpMRI or (dynamic contrast enhancement) MRI have shown better accuracy in identifying recurrent disease (Fig. 24.1) [13, 14]. The TRUS-guided biopsies should follow for confirmation of the MR findings.

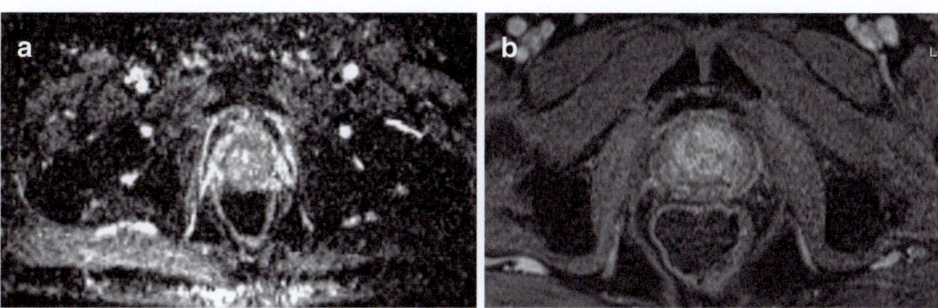

Fig. 24.1 Diffusion-weighted magnetic resonance images demonstrating (**a**) locally recurrent disease at central part and right posterolateral part of prostate and (**b**) basal anterior fibromuscular stroma

Histopathologic resolution of prostate cancer after RT takes approximately 2–3 years. It has been demonstrated that one-third of biopsies showing tumor at 12 months after radiation would become negative by 24–30 months [15, 16]. Biopsies performed before this time are not helpful in determining the success or failure of local treatment, and arising PSA earlier than this interval is generally indicative of systemic disease.

Radiation change alters the gland morphology such that cellular drop out often leaves isolated cells or nests of cells with no residual recognizable gland formation. This mimics high-grade disease, when indeed it represents severe radiation effect. The hallmarks of radiation change include nuclear and cytoplasmic changes such as smudged and distorted chromatin, large bizarre or pyknotic nuclei, microvesicular or macrovesicular changes, ruptured cytoplasm, and scarce or no glandular formation. These biopsies cannot be assigned a Gleason score. Before considering any local salvage treatment, residual tumor with minimal or no radiation change must be demonstrated on histopathology.

Once local recurrence has been proven, further effort should be made to rule out distant metastases. For this purpose, pelvic computed tomography (CT) or MRI and bone scan has been used to assess both regional and bone metastases. Perhaps, the most promising imaging tool for evaluation of biochemical recurrence after definitive RT is functional imaging using a small-molecule ligand of prostate membrane-specific antigen (PSMA) (Fig. 24.2). PSMA is a type II membrane glycoprotein with an extracellular, transmembrane, and intracellular component. It is overexpressed in 90–100% of localized prostate cancer. Gallium-68 PSMA PET/CT has excellent tumor penetration, a high tumor to normal tissue ratio and ideal pharmacokinetics [17].

24.2.2 Prognostic Factors

The risk of micrometastases was estimated by reviewing the prognostic factors at initial treatment, as well as at the time of recurrence. Zelefsky et al. [1] studied 1650 patients with T1–T3 prostate cancer treated with median dose of

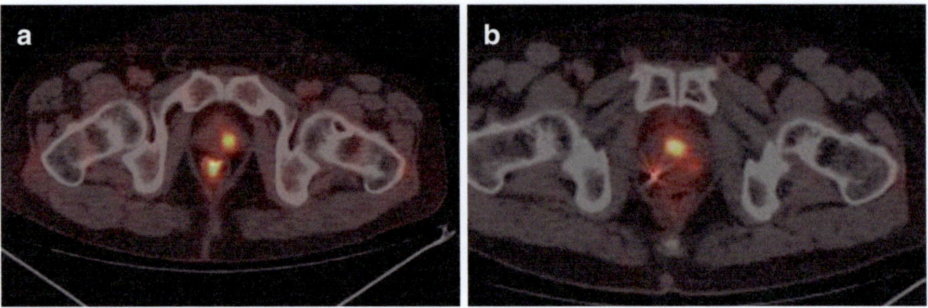

Fig. 24.2 Increased 68 Ga-PSMA ligand uptake (*yellow area*) representing tumors in patients with localized prostate cancer

75.6 Gy EBRT, and the authors reported that the predictors for distant metastasis are PSA doubling time, Gleason score, and T-stage. Patients with a PSA doubling time of less than 6 months are least likely to benefit from local salvage treatment and may more appropriately be offered upfront systemic treatment. Nguyen et al. [18] suggested that patients most likely to benefit from local salvage are those with an initial favorable presentation (cT1c–T2a disease, Gleason score ≤6, PSA level <10 ng/mL), initial PSA velocity <2 ng/mL/year, time to biochemical failure >3 years, PSA doubling time >12 months, and PSA at the time of salvage <10 ng/mL.

24.3 Salvage Brachytherapy

Local recurrence after definitive RT is often owing to insufficient irradiation dose. The dose–response relationship for EBRT has been demonstrated in multiple mature randomized clinical trials and the optimal effective dose from EBRT has not still been reached yet [19–23]. Studies comparing EBRT to brachytherapy, or to combinations both, has demonstrated the superiority of brachytherapy in effective long-term outcomes [24–26].

24.3.1 LDR Brachytherapy

Brachytherapy is an ablative local approach appropriate for salvage local therapy, delivering a very high and conformal radiation dose to the prostate, while reducing exposure to the surrounding normal organs. However, re-irradiation increases the side effects significantly. For this reason, patients considered for salvage brachytherapy should have lower side effects at initial EBRT. The outcomes from salvage low-dose brachytherapy series are summarized in Table 24.1.

After salvage brachytherapy, the 5-year BCR-free survival rate is around 50% (range: 34–77%) [27–32]. However, more recent series show higher BCR-free survival rates approximately 70–75%, because of more appropriate patient selection. For patients with poor prognostic factors, such as prolonged prior hormonotherapy use, or castrate resistance, outcomes are not so favorable [33, 34].

Table 24.1 Salvage low-dose rate brachytherapy series

Study (year)	Patient no	Median follow-up (months)	BCR-free survival	CSS
Burri et al. (2010)	37	86	5 years 65% 10 years 54%	10 years 96%
Grado et al. (1999)	49	64	5 years 34%	5 years 79%
Moman et al. (2010)	31	108	5 years 20%	6 years 65%
Nguyen et al. (2007)	25	47	4 years 70%	
Vargas et al. (2014)	69	60	5 years 74%	5 years 96%
Henriquez et al. (2014)	56	48	5 years 77%	

The optimal prescription dose and critical organ constraints have not been established for salvage low-dose rate brachytherapy after prior EBRT. However, the prescribed dose ranged from 110 to 145 Gy for 125-iodine implants and from 100 to 120 Gy for 103-Paladium implants. The planned volume receiving 100% of the prescribed dose was 90–99%. The RTOG-0526 phase II trial on salvage low-dose rate brachytherapy after EBRT has completed accrual of 96 patients and will soon be reported. Although the planning target volume, V100 ≥98%, D90 ≤125%, and prescribed dose of 140 Gy with 125-I or 120 Gy with 103-Pd, were not dissimilar to prescription for a de novo implant, dose homogeneity requirements were very conservative, aiming to keep the implants "cool." The volume of the prostate receiving 150% of the prescribed dose (V150) was kept <45% and V200 <10%.

Acute side effects after low-dose rate salvage brachytherapy are comparable in nature to those after primary treatment. The genitourinary system toxicities, such as frequency and urgency, are the most common and return to baseline can take up to 24–27 months [34, 35]. However, late toxicities are more frequently seen, late grade 3 toxicities are observed in 10–25% of the cases [28, 30, 31]. Most commonly seen late toxicities include urethral strictures requiring dilatation or transurethral resection and less frequently, persistent hematuria. Although less frequent, late rectal toxicity may lead to greater morbidity. Grades 3 and 4 rectal toxicities are seen in 2–6% after salvage brachytherapy and mostly require colostomy [28, 30, 31, 36, 37].

Accurate spatial localization of recurrences enables focal salvage treatment, with the potential to reduce toxicity compared with whole-prostate salvage. Hsu et al. [38] performed focal salvage brachytherapy treatments using MRI, magnetic resonance spectroscopy, and TRUS images for evaluation of the target volume in 15 patients. Full dose was delivered to sites of recurrent disease without implanting the entire gland. This limited the dose to the remaining prostate, urethra, and rectum. After a median 24-month follow-up, there were two local failures, and the 3-year BCR-free survival rate was 71%. There were no ≥grade 3 gastrointestinal and genitourinary toxicities, but 33% experienced grade 2 genitourinary toxicities. Peters et al. [39] reported results of mpMRI fused focal brachytherapy with a total of 144 Gy prescribed to the gross tumor volume on MRI and dose constraints for the organs at risk were same as first brachytherapy application. The 3-year BCR-free survival rate was 60%, and no patients developed ≥grade 3 gastrointestinal system toxicity. Consequently, when compared with whole-prostate salvage, focal salvage brachytherapy has the potential to limit the rectal, urethral, and bladder doses and thereby reduce severe toxicity.

Table 24.2 Salvage high-dose rate brachytherapy series

Study (year)	Patient no	Median follow-up (months)	BCR-free survival	CSS
Lee et al. (2007)	52	60	5 years 51%	
Jo et al. (2012)	11	29	2 years 64%	
Tharp et al. (2008)	7	58	71%	71%
Yamada et al. (2014)	42	36	5 years 69%	5 years 90%

24.3.2 HDR Brachytherapy

High-dose rate brachytherapy involves the implantation of an array of treatment needles into the prostate under TRUS guidance. A single high-activity iridium-192 source then negotiates each treatment catheter in turn, pausing at 3 mm intervals to deliver the required dose to target volumes with fraction sizes up to 19 Gy delivered in 15–20 min. This allows elegant control of the dose to both the target volume and to critical structures. Furthermore, treatment catheters can also be placed to include seminal vesicles and also any extracapsular extension. Although few series on high-dose rate brachytherapy series were reported, the efficacy seems to be equivalent to low-dose rate brachytherapy series, with less toxicities (Table 24.2).

Lee et al. [40] reported an estimated 2-year BCR-free survival rate of 89% in 21 patients, and the authors reported a 14% grade 3 genitourinary toxicity, but no ≥grade 2 gastrointestinal toxicity. Two other small series presented similar outcomes with BCR-free survival rate of 65–71% without ≥grade 3 genitourinary and gastrointestinal toxicity [41, 42]. In a phase II study, Yamada et al. [43] reported a 5-year BCR-free survival rate of 69% with single implant used in 42 patients to deliver 32 Gy in 4 fractions. Only three patients developed urethral stricture requiring dilatation, and one patient developed urinary incontinence. A French group presented the results of focal high-dose rate salvage brachytherapy with "real-time transperineal ultrasound-targeted MRI/choline PET-guided brachytherapy." They delivered 20 Gy in 2 fractions, with median prostate D90 value of 5.3 Gy and the median CTV D90 of 18.7 Gy. Among 15 patients treated, only one patient had BCR, but none developed acute ≥grade 2 gastrointestinal or genitourinary toxicity. However, median follow-up was only 11 months, so further follow-up is required to corroborate the outcomes.

With the growing interest in high-dose rate brachytherapy salvage, there are some phase I and phase II ongoing trials. The inverse treatment-planning optimization algorithm used for high-dose rate brachytherapy treatment planning allows a very high conformal dose and limits the dose to surrounding organs. Guidelines for dose, fractionation, and organs-at-risk constraints need to be further established.

24.4 Salvage Stereotactic Radiotherapy

Stereotactic body RT (SBRT) is another technique that is being investigated for local or locoregional salvage with its main advantage being a noninvasive procedure (Figs. 24.3 and 24.4). Image guidance is used for localization before delivery of a

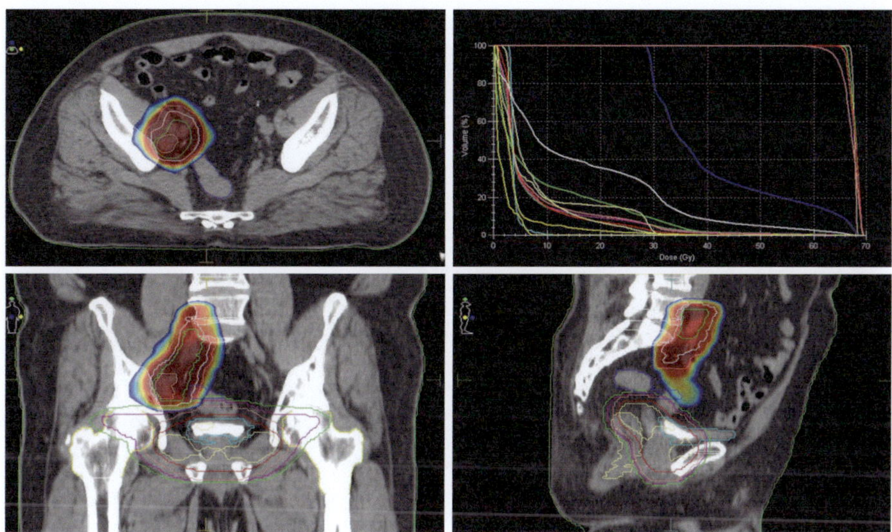

Fig. 24.3 Regional pelvic lymphatic recurrence 2 years after completion of primary prostate radiotherapy. The 40 Gy dose distribution delivered in five fractions encompassing left iliac lymphatics (*orange-red area*)

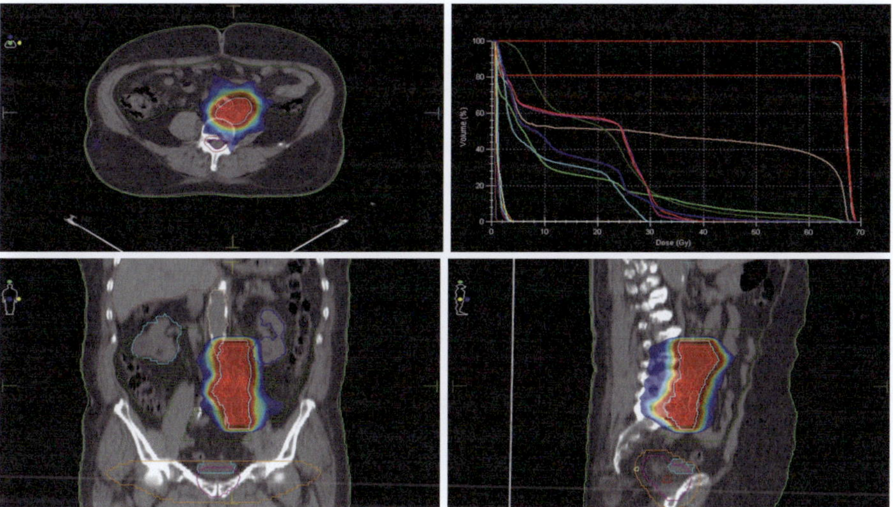

Fig. 24.4 Para-aortic lymphatic recurrence 36 months after completion of primary prostate radiotherapy. The 36 Gy dose distribution delivered in 6 fractions encompassing left iliac lymphatics (*orange-red area*)

highly conformal dose to the prostate (Fig. 24.5). In a phase II study, Fuller et al. [44] reported the outcomes of 29 patients treated with salvage SBRT, delivering 34 Gy in five fractions with prostate coverage and organs-at-risk constraints similar to those used for high-dose rate brachytherapy, using fiducial-based image guidance

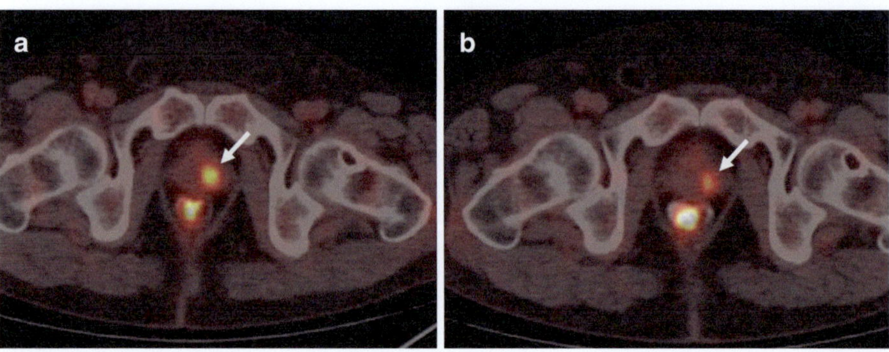

Fig. 24.5 (**a**) Ga-68 PSMA PET demonstrating local recurrence after definitive radiotherapy (*arrow*). (**b**) A decrease in Ga-68 PSMA enhancement after local salvage stereotactic radiotherapy

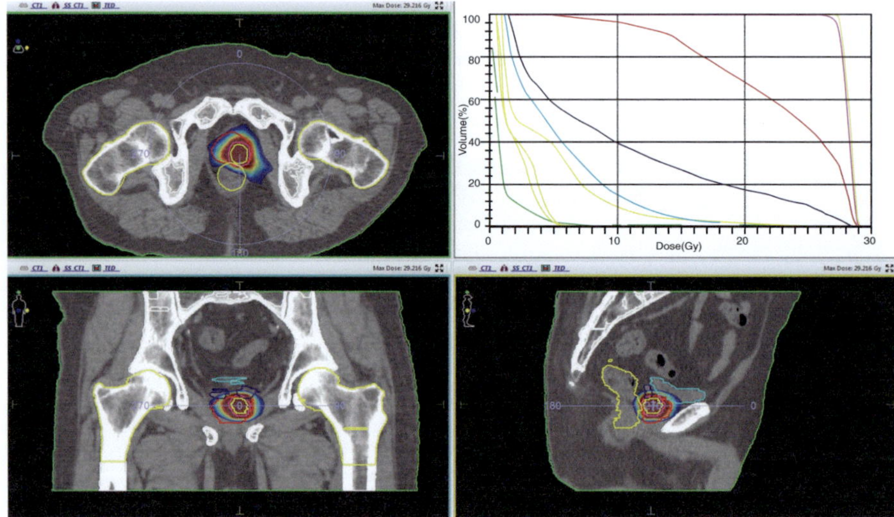

Fig. 24.6 Dose distribution of local recurrent tumor treated with a total dose of 35 Gy delivered in seven fractions using stereotactic radiotherapy

(Fig. 24.6). With a median 24-month follow-up, the 2-year BCR-free survival was 82%, and ≥grade 2 genitourinary toxicity rate of 18%. Although still preliminary, these results suggest the possibility of PSA control with this noninvasive technique. However, particular attention should be paid to the accuracy of the SBRT methodology, the dosimetric parameters, and the inevitable higher integral dose compared with brachytherapy.

Table 24.3 Recommended criteria for salvage local therapy

Patient characteristics
Life expectancy ≥10 years
Tumor characteristics
Biopsy proven local recurrence
No distant metastasis
PSA doubling time >6–12 months
Gleason score <7
PSA at recurrence <10 ng/mL
Interval to re-irradiation >3 years

Conclusions

Management of isolated asymptomatic local failure after definitive RT remains challenging. Although the most frequently used option is androgen deprivation therapy, local salvage options should be considered for highly selected patients with a reasonable chance of cure and sufficient life expectancy to appreciate the benefits. None of the available salvage treatments stands out as superior; the efficacies fall within the same range with 5-year BCR-free survival approximately 50%, with different toxicity profiles. Most published series were reported from single center, and only a few studies have mature follow-up. Furthermore, there are no randomized trials comparing different modalities. The ideal candidate for local salvage is one with a local recurrence that is aggressive enough to require treatment but is still potentially curable (Table 24.3). Among nonsurgical alternatives for salvage, the side effect profile can potentially be improved by adopting a focal-targeted treatment approach. With early detection and more sensitive functional imaging for tumor localization and staging, the role for local salvage of RT failures would expand.

References

1. Zelefsky MJ, Ben-Porat L, Scher HI, Chan HM, Fearn PA, Fuks ZY, et al. Outcome predictors for the increasing PSA state after definitive external-beam radiotherapy for prostate cancer. J Clin Oncol. 2005;23(4):826–31. doi:10.1200/JCO.2005.02.111.
2. Kuban DA, Thames HD, Levy LB, Horwitz EM, Kupelian PA, Martinez AA, et al. Long-term multi-institutional analysis of stage T1–T2 prostate cancer treated with radiotherapy in the PSA era. Int J Radiat Oncol Biol Phys. 2003;57(4):915–28.
3. Cellini N, Morganti AG, Mattiucci GC, Valentini V, Leone M, Luzi S, et al. Analysis of intraprostatic failures in patients treated with hormonal therapy and radiotherapy: implications for conformal therapy planning. Int J Radiat Oncol Biol Phys. 2002;53(3):595–9.
4. Grossfeld GD, Olumi AF, Connolly JA, Chew K, Gibney J, Bhargava V, et al. Locally recurrent prostate tumors following either radiation therapy or radical prostatectomy have changes in Ki-67 labeling index, p53 and bcl-2 immunoreactivity. J Urol. 1998;159(5):1437–43. doi:10.1097/00005392-199805000-00004.
5. Crook JM, Malone S, Perry G, Eapen L, Owen J, Robertson S, et al. Twenty-four-month postradiation prostate biopsies are strongly predictive of 7-year disease-free survival: results from a Canadian randomized trial. Cancer. 2009;115(3):673–9. doi:10.1002/cncr.24020.

6. Agarwal PK, Sadetsky N, Konety BR, Resnick MI, Carroll PR. Cancer of the Prostate Strategic Urological Research E. Treatment failure after primary and salvage therapy for prostate cancer: likelihood, patterns of care, and outcomes. Cancer. 2008;112(2):307–14. doi:10.1002/cncr.23161.
7. Tran H, Kwok J, Pickles T, Tyldesley S, Black PC. Underutilization of local salvage therapy after radiation therapy for prostate cancer. Urol Oncol. 2014;32(5):701–6. doi:10.1016/j.urolonc.2013.12.014.
8. Heidenreich A, Bastian PJ, Bellmunt J, Bolla M, Joniau S, van der Kwast T, et al. EAU guidelines on prostate cancer. Part 1: screening, diagnosis, and local treatment with curative intent-update 2013. Eur Urol. 2014;65(1):124–37. doi:10.1016/j.eururo.2013.09.046.
9. Kapadia NS, Olson K, Sandler HM, Feng FY, Hamstra DA. Interval to biochemical failure as a biomarker for cause-specific and overall survival after dose-escalated external beam radiation therapy for prostate cancer. Cancer. 2012;118(8):2059–68. doi:10.1002/cncr.26498.
10. Shilkrut M, McLaughlin PW, Merrick GS, Vainshtein JM, Feng FY, Hamstra DA. Interval to biochemical failure predicts clinical outcomes in patients with high-risk prostate cancer treated by combined-modality radiation therapy. Int J Radiat Oncol Biol Phys. 2013;86(4):721–8. doi:10.1016/j.ijrobp.2013.03.028.
11. Buyyounouski MK, Hanlon AL, Horwitz EM, Pollack A. Interval to biochemical failure highly prognostic for distant metastasis and prostate cancer-specific mortality after radiotherapy. Int J Radiat Oncol Biol Phys. 2008;70(1):59–66. doi:10.1016/j.ijrobp.2007.05.047.
12. Rothke MC, Afshar-Oromieh A, Schlemmer HP. [Potential of PET/MRI for diagnosis of prostate cancer]. Radiologe. 2013;53(8):676–81. doi:10.1007/s00117-013-2499-0.
13. Arumainayagam N, Kumaar S, Ahmed HU, Moore CM, Payne H, Freeman A, et al. Accuracy of multiparametric magnetic resonance imaging in detecting recurrent prostate cancer after radiotherapy. BJU Int. 2010;106(7):991–7. doi:10.1111/j.1464-410X.2010.09291.x.
14. Kara T, Akata D, Akyol F, Karcaaltincaba M, Ozmen M. The value of dynamic contrast-enhanced MRI in the detection of recurrent prostate cancer after external beam radiotherapy: correlation with transrectal ultrasound and pathological findings. Diagn Interv Radiol. 2011;17(1):38–43. doi:10.4261/1305-3825.DIR.3079-09.1.
15. Crook J, Malone S, Perry G, Bahadur Y, Robertson S, Abdolell M. Postradiotherapy prostate biopsies: what do they really mean? Results for 498 patients. Int J Radiat Oncol Biol Phys. 2000;48(2):355–67.
16. Scardino PT, Frankel JM, Wheeler TM, Meacham RB, Hoffman GS, Seale C, et al. The prognostic significance of post-irradiation biopsy results in patients with prostatic cancer. J Urol. 1986;135(3):510–6.
17. Eiber M, Maurer T, Souvatzoglou M, Beer AJ, Ruffani A, Haller B, et al. Evaluation of hybrid ^{68}Ga-PSMA ligand PET/CT in 248 patients with biochemical recurrence after radical prostatectomy. J Nucl Med. 2015;56(5):668–74. doi:10.2967/jnumed.115.154153.
18. Nguyen PL, D'Amico AV, Lee AK, Suh WW. Patient selection, cancer control, and complications after salvage local therapy for postradiation prostate-specific antigen failure: a systematic review of the literature. Cancer. 2007;110(7):1417–28. doi:10.1002/cncr.22941.
19. Beckendorf V, Guerif S, Le Prise E, Cosset JM, Bougnoux A, Chauvet B, et al. 70 Gy versus 80 Gy in localized prostate cancer: 5-year results of GETUG 06 randomized trial. Int J Radiat Oncol Biol Phys. 2011;80(4):1056–63. doi:10.1016/j.ijrobp.2010.03.049.
20. Dearnaley DP, Sydes MR, Graham JD, Aird EG, Bottomley D, Cowan RA, et al. Escalated-dose versus standard-dose conformal radiotherapy in prostate cancer: first results from the MRC RT01 randomised controlled trial. Lancet Oncol. 2007;8(6):475–87. doi:10.1016/S1470-2045(07)70143-2.
21. Kuban DA, Tucker SL, Dong L, Starkschall G, Huang EH, Cheung MR, et al. Long-term results of the M. D. Anderson randomized dose-escalation trial for prostate cancer. Int J Radiat Oncol Biol Phys. 2008;70(1):67–74. doi:10.1016/j.ijrobp.2007.06.054.
22. Peeters ST, Heemsbergen WD, Koper PC, van Putten WL, Slot A, Dielwart MF, et al. Dose-response in radiotherapy for localized prostate cancer: results of the Dutch multicenter randomized phase III trial comparing 68 Gy of radiotherapy with 78 Gy. J Clin Oncol. 2006;24(13):1990–6. doi:10.1200/JCO.2005.05.2530.

23. Zietman AL, Bae K, Slater JD, Shipley WU, Efstathiou JA, Coen JJ, et al. Randomized trial comparing conventional-dose with high-dose conformal radiation therapy in early-stage adenocarcinoma of the prostate: long-term results from proton radiation oncology group/American college of radiology 95-09. J Clin Oncol. 2010;28(7):1106–11. doi:10.1200/JCO.2009.25.8475.
24. Hoskin PJ, Rojas AM, Bownes PJ, Lowe GJ, Ostler PJ, Bryant L. Randomised trial of external beam radiotherapy alone or combined with high-dose-rate brachytherapy boost for localised prostate cancer. Radiother Oncol. 2012;103(2):217–22. doi:10.1016/j.radonc.2012.01.007.
25. Zelefsky MJ, Yamada Y, Pei X, Hunt M, Cohen G, Zhang Z, et al. Comparison of tumor control and toxicity outcomes of high-dose intensity-modulated radiotherapy and brachytherapy for patients with favorable risk prostate cancer. Urology. 2011;77(4):986–90. doi:10.1016/j.urology.2010.07.539.
26. Deutsch I, Zelefsky MJ, Zhang Z, Mo Q, Zaider M, Cohen G, et al. Comparison of PSA relapse-free survival in patients treated with ultra-high-dose IMRT versus combination HDR brachytherapy and IMRT. Brachytherapy. 2010;9(4):313–8. doi:10.1016/j.brachy.2010.02.196.
27. Beyer DC. Salvage brachytherapy after external-beam irradiation for prostate cancer. Oncology (Williston Park). 2004;18(2):151–8; discussion 158–60, 163–4.
28. Burri RJ, Stone NN, Unger P, Stock RG. Long-term outcome and toxicity of salvage brachytherapy for local failure after initial radiotherapy for prostate cancer. Int J Radiat Oncol Biol Phys. 2010;77(5):1338–44. doi:10.1016/j.ijrobp.2009.06.061.
29. Chen CP, Weinberg V, Shinohara K, Roach M 3rd, Nash M, Gottschalk A, et al. Salvage HDR brachytherapy for recurrent prostate cancer after previous definitive radiation therapy: 5-year outcomes. Int J Radiat Oncol Biol Phys. 2013;86(2):324–9. doi:10.1016/j.ijrobp.2013.01.027.
30. Grado GL, Collins JM, Kriegshauser JS, Balch CS, Grado MM, Swanson GP, et al. Salvage brachytherapy for localized prostate cancer after radiotherapy failure. Urology. 1999;53(1):2–10.
31. Henriquez I, Sancho G, Hervas A, Guix B, Pera J, Gutierrez C, et al. Salvage brachytherapy in prostate local recurrence after radiation therapy: predicting factors for control and toxicity. Radiat Oncol. 2014;9:102. doi:10.1186/1748-717X-9-102.
32. Lee HK, Adams MT, Motta J. Salvage prostate brachytherapy for localized prostate cancer failure after external beam radiation therapy. Brachytherapy. 2008;7(1):17–21. doi:10.1016/j.brachy.2007.11.002.
33. Vargas C, Swartz D, Vashi A, Blasser M, Kasraeian A, Cesaretti J, et al. Salvage brachytherapy for recurrent prostate cancer. Brachytherapy. 2014;13(1):53–8. doi:10.1016/j.brachy.2013.10.012.
34. Rose JN, Crook JM, Pickles T, Keyes M, Morris WJ. Salvage low-dose-rate permanent seed brachytherapy for locally recurrent prostate cancer: association between dose and late toxicity. Brachytherapy. 2015;14(3):342–9. doi:10.1016/j.brachy.2015.01.002.
35. Nguyen PL, Chen MH, D'Amico AV, Tempany CM, Steele GS, Albert M, et al. Magnetic resonance image-guided salvage brachytherapy after radiation in select men who initially presented with favorable-risk prostate cancer: a prospective phase 2 study. Cancer. 2007;110(7):1485–92. doi:10.1002/cncr.22934.
36. Moman MR, van der Poel HG, Battermann JJ, Moerland MA, van Vulpen M. Treatment outcome and toxicity after salvage 125-I implantation for prostate cancer recurrences after primary 125-I implantation and external beam radiotherapy. Brachytherapy. 2010;9(2):119–25. doi:10.1016/j.brachy.2009.06.007.
37. Mahal BA, Ziehr DR, Hyatt AS, Neubauer-Sugar EH, O'Farrell DA, O'Leary MP, et al. Use of a rectal spacer with low-dose-rate brachytherapy for treatment of prostate cancer in previously irradiated patients: initial experience and short-term results. Brachytherapy. 2014;13(5):442–9. doi:10.1016/j.brachy.2014.05.001.
38. Hsu CC, Hsu H, Pickett B, Crehange G, Hsu IC, Dea R, et al. Feasibility of MR imaging/MR spectroscopy-planned focal partial salvage permanent prostate implant (PPI) for localized recurrence after initial PPI for prostate cancer. Int J Radiat Oncol Biol Phys. 2013;85(2):370–7. doi:10.1016/j.ijrobp.2012.04.028.

39. Peters M, Maenhout M, van der Voort van Zyp JR, Moerland MA, Moman MR, Steuten LM, et al. Focal salvage iodine-125 brachytherapy for prostate cancer recurrences after primary radiotherapy: a retrospective study regarding toxicity, biochemical outcome and quality of life. Radiother Oncol. 2014;112(1):77–82. doi:10.1016/j.radonc.2014.06.013.
40. Lee B, Shinohara K, Weinberg V, Gottschalk AR, Pouliot J, Roach M 3rd, et al. Feasibility of high-dose-rate brachytherapy salvage for local prostate cancer recurrence after radiotherapy: the University of California-San Francisco experience. Int J Radiat Oncol Biol Phys. 2007;67(4):1106–12. doi:10.1016/j.ijrobp.2006.10.012.
41. Jo Y, Fujii T, Hara R, Yokoyama T, Miyaji Y, Yoden E, et al. Salvage high-dose-rate brachytherapy for local prostate cancer recurrence after radiotherapy—preliminary results. BJU Int. 2012;109(6):835–9. doi:10.1111/j.1464-410X.2011.10519.x.
42. Tharp M, Hardacre M, Bennett R, Jones WT, Stuhldreher D, Vaught J. Prostate high-dose-rate brachytherapy as salvage treatment of local failure after previous external or permanent seed irradiation for prostate cancer. Brachytherapy. 2008;7(3):231–6. doi:10.1016/j.brachy.2008.03.003.
43. Yamada Y, Kollmeier MA, Pei X, Kan CC, Cohen GN, Donat SM, et al. A phase II study of salvage high-dose-rate brachytherapy for the treatment of locally recurrent prostate cancer after definitive external beam radiotherapy. Brachytherapy. 2014;13(2):111–6. doi:10.1016/j.brachy.2013.11.005.
44. Fuller DB, Wurzer J, Shirazi R, Bridge SS, Law J, Mardirossian G. High-dose-rate stereotactic body radiation therapy for postradiation therapy locally recurrent prostatic carcinoma: preliminary prostate-specific antigen response, disease-free survival, and toxicity assessment. Pract Radiat Oncol. 2015;5(6):e615–23. doi:10.1016/j.prro.2015.04.009.

Functional Imaging-Guided Radiotherapy and Radiolabelled Targeted Therapies in Prostate Cancer

25

Gokhan Ozyigit, Sezin Yuce Sari, Pervin Hurmuz, and Ugur Selek

Abstract

Positron emission tomography (PET) imaging using PSMA ligand is a promising radiotracer in prostate cancer. Recent trials suggest its potential role in accurate staging of high-risk prostate cancer and detecting metastases and local-regional relapses during biochemical recurrence with 68Ga-PSMA positron emission tomography/computed tomography (PET/CT). However, the data related with its role in radiotherapy are still lacking. Therefore, we summarized our experience with 68Ga-PSMA PET/CT guided hypofractionated stereotactic radiotherapy in patients with oligometastatic disease after biochemical recurrence. Radiolabelled targeted therapies gains popularity in the management metastatic bone disease in prostate cancer. We particularly review the applications of radium-223 chloride in prostate cancer patients in the light of available clinically relevant data.

25.1 Ga-68 PSMA PET/CT in Prostate Cancer

Positron emission tomography/computed tomography (PET/CT) is a hybrid imaging technique combining functional and morphological data. Several radiotracers have been used for functional imaging of prostate cancer such as 18F-choline or 11C-choline, 11C-acetate, and 18F-FACBC. However, most of them were found to have low sensitivity and specificity [1–5].

G. Ozyigit, M.D. (✉) • S.Y. Sari, M.D. • P. Hurmuz, M.D.
Department of Radiation Oncology, Hacettepe University, Ankara, Turkey
e-mail: gozyigit@hacettepe.edu.tr

U. Selek, M.D.
Department of Radiation Oncology, Koc University, Istanbul, Turkey

G. Ozyigit, U. Selek (eds.), *Principles and Practice of Urooncology*,
DOI 10.1007/978-3-319-56114-1_25

Prostate cancer cells have significantly elevated expression of specific transmembrane protein called prostate-specific membrane antigen (PSMA). Several retrospective trials demonstrated its diagnostic value compared to other tracers (e.g., 18F-choline, 11C-choline) [1, 6–9]. Ga-68 PSMA PET/CT was found to be superior in staging of particularly intermediate-high-risk prostate cancer [7]. The ability of Ga-68 PSMA to detect early regional lymph node metastases makes possible the application of salvage therapeutic approaches such as salvage lymphadenectomy, functional imaging-guided radiotherapy with a potentially curative intent [10].

On the other hand, Ga-68 PSMA are not fully specific for prostate cancer, and some selected reports showed its increased uptake in thyroid adenoma, Paget's disease, schwannoma, tuberculosis, adrenal adenoma, or sarcoidosis [11–14]. Additionally, celiac ganglia may show a significant Ga-68 PSMA uptake, which may be misinterpreted as lymph node metastases [15]. PSMA overexpression has also been reported in glioblastoma, hepatocellular carcinoma, lung cancer, renal cell carcinoma, and thyroid cancer [16–20].

25.2 Ga-68 PSMA-Guided Stereotactic Body Radiotherapy for Oligometastatic or Recurrent Prostate Cancer: Hacettepe Experience

We retrospectively evaluated the treatment results of 15 prostate cancer patients with oligometastatic disease (Unpublished data). The term oligometastasis encompassed the presence of five or less metastases. RT was delivered to the metastatic sites in the form of either SBRT or IGRT. Median age of the patients was 67 years (range, 58–79). At the time of initial diagnosis, median vPSA level was 15.3 ng/mL (range, 5–101 ng/mL) and median total Gleason score was 8 (range, 6–9). Most of the patients (86%) had T3 disease, two patients (13%) had LN, and one patient had bone metastases. As a primary treatment nine patients (60%) had surgery. Thirteen patients received local RT. Primary local RT doses were 70–76 Gy in the definitive setting and 64–70 Gy in the adjuvant setting. Metastases were detected with gallium-68 PSMA in all patients after the evidence of rising PSA in the follow-up. Median number of metastatic lesions was 2 (range, 1–4); six in regional LN's (40%), four in bone (27%), and three in non-regional LN's (20%). All the patients received ADT. Only one patient received chemotherapy. Most frequently used dose schedules were 5 × 6 Gy (47%) and 5 × 7 Gy (33%). With a median follow-up of 9.5 months, all of our patients are alive. No treatment-related acute or late toxicities were observed. Although the number of patients is small and the follow-up time is short, aggressive treatment of oligometastatic prostate cancer patients seems to be effective and safe.

We have presented our three selected cases treated with SBRT as follows:

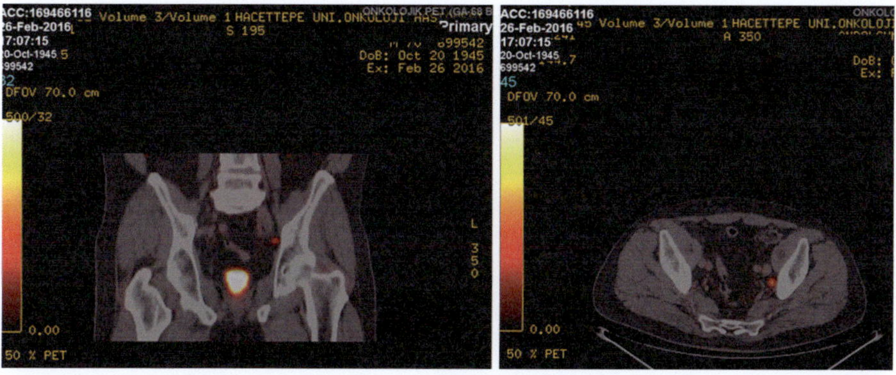

Fig. 25.1 Ga-68 PSMA PET/CT revealed a left parailiac lymph node (LN) of 16 × 19 mm (SUVmax: 5.85)

25.2.1 Case 1

A 65-year-old male was diagnosed with prostate cancer in 2010, when he had a PSA level of 9.6. Pathologic specimen after robotic prostatectomy revealed a T3aN0M0 adenocarcinoma with a Gleason score (GS) of 4 + 4 = 8. Perineural invasion was present, and surgical margins were positive. No adjuvant treatment was administered at that time. He was admitted to us with a rising PSA. The PSA level was increased to 0.3 in July 2013, and we applied 66 Gy of intensity modulated radiation therapy (IMRT) in 33 fractions was administered via Novalis followed by 1-year androgen deprivation therapy (ADT). His PSA was 1.31 in January 2016. His Ga-68 PSMA PET/CT revealed a left parailiac lymph node (LN) of 16 × 19 mm (SUVmax: 5.85) (Fig. 25.1). In March 2016, 35 Gy (7 Gy/day in five fractions) stereotactic body radiotherapy (SBRT) was administered to the left parailiac LN via Novalis (Fig. 25.2). On his last control in September 2016, his PSA was <0.005 ng/mL, and there was no evidence of disease. We observed no acute or late toxicity.

25.2.2 Case 2

A 59-year-old male patient with a PSA level of 38 ng/mL was diagnosed with prostate cancer in 2007. His transrectal biopsy of prostate gland revealed an adenocarcinoma with a GS of 3 + 3 = 6 with perineural invasion. His stage was cT3bN0M0. After 9 months of ADT, his PSA decreased to 0.19 ng/mL. Between April 2008 and May 2008, 70 Gy of 3D conformal RT was administered in 35 fractions. ADT was completed to 2 years. In October 2014, his PSA level increased to 4.3 ng/mL, and Ga-68 PSMA PET/CT revealed a pathologic right parailiac lymph node (LN) (SUVmax: 10.5) (Fig. 25.3). Between March 2015 and April 2015, 30 Gy in 5

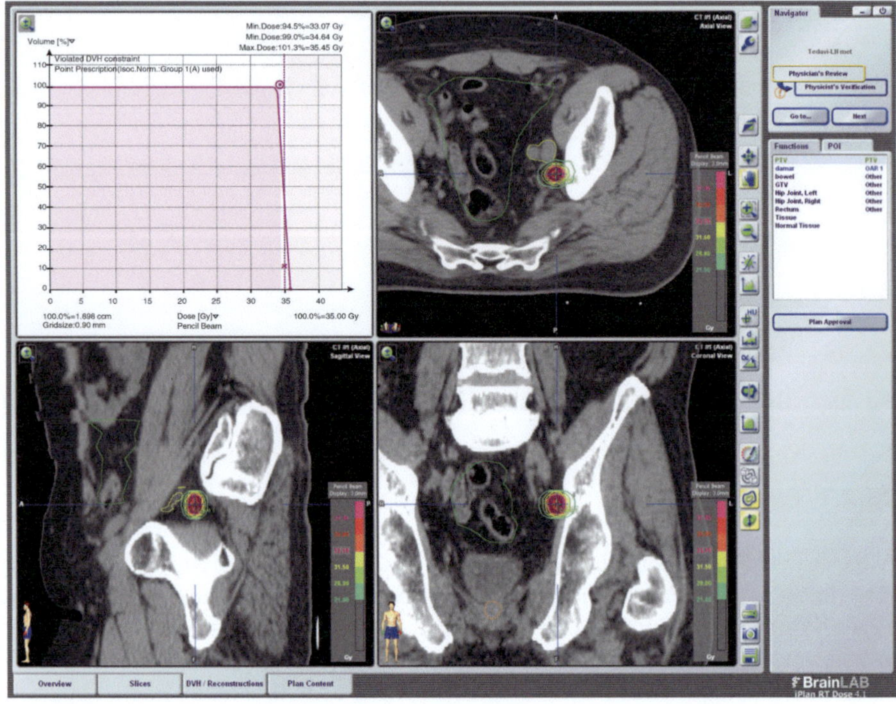

Fig. 25.2 SBRT Plan of Case 1: 35 Gy (7 Gy/day in 5 fractions) stereotactic body radiotherapy (SBRT) was administered to the left parailiac LN via Novalis

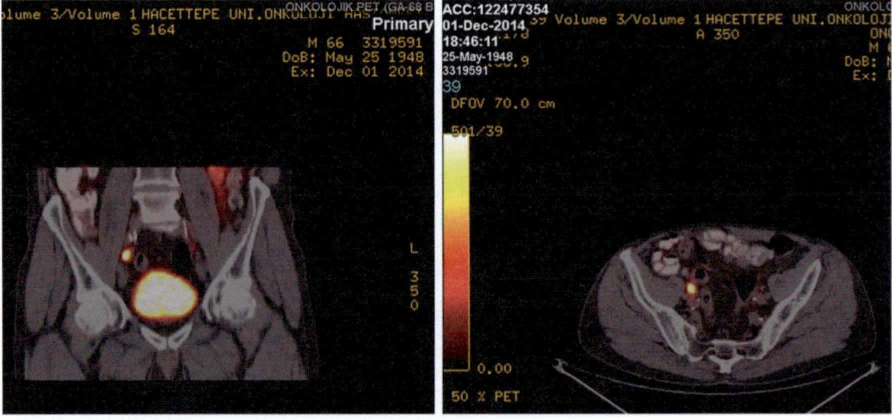

Fig. 25.3 Ga-68 PSMA PET/CT revealed a pathologic right parailiac lymph node (LN) (SUVmax: 10.5)

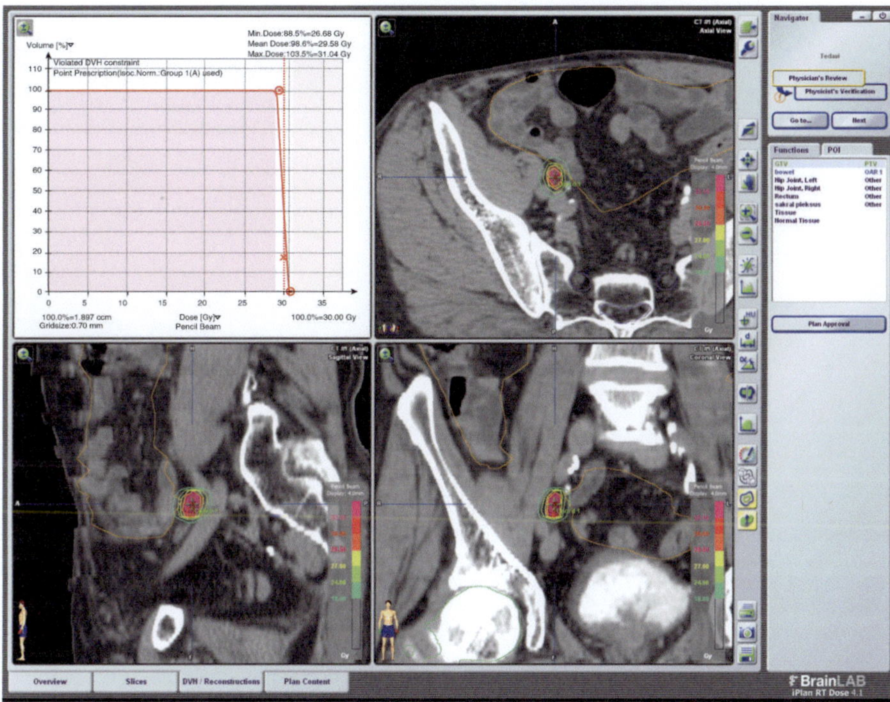

Fig. 25.4 SBRT Plan of Case 2: 30 Gy in 5 fractions SBRT was administered to the right external iliac LN via Novalis

fractions SBRT was administered to the right external iliac LN via Novalis (Fig. 25.4). In his last follow-up, his PSA level was 0.3 ng/mL on January 2017 with no evidence of disease. We observed no acute or late toxicity.

25.2.3 Case 3

A 76-year-old male was diagnosed with prostate cancer after his PSA level was found to be 10 ng/mL in 2011. Prostatic biopsy revealed an adenocarcinoma with a GS of 4 + 3 = 7. His stage was cT3bN0M0. After 3 months of ADT, 74 Gy IMRT was administered to the prostate and proximal seminal vesicles between June 2011 and August 2011.

In February 2016, his PSA level increased to 5 ng/mL, and Ga-68 PSMA PET/CT revealed recurrence in left external iliac LN (SUVmax: 5.4) (Fig. 25.5). On February 2016, he received 35 Gy in five fractions SBRT to the recurrent area (Fig. 25.6). While prostate cancer-free, he was succumbed to brain metastasis of small cell lung cancer in November 2016.

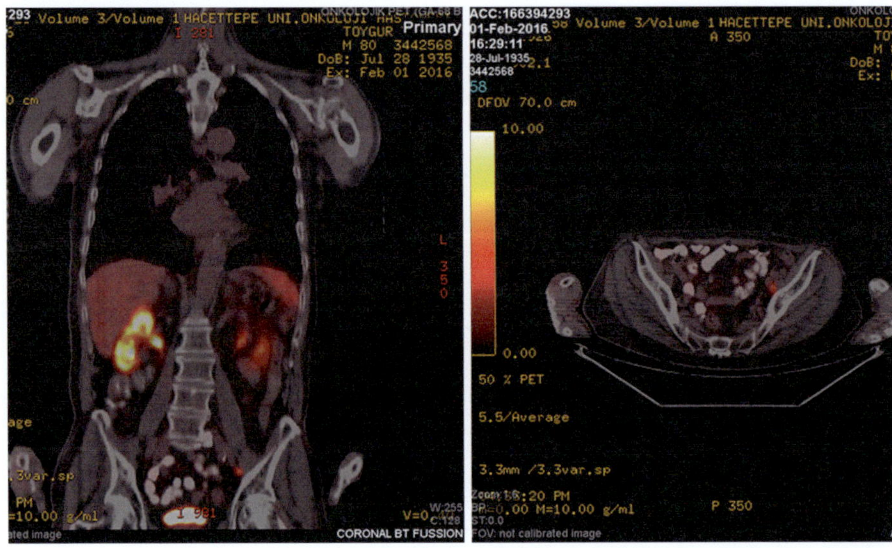

Fig. 25.5 Ga-68 PSMA PET/CT revealed recurrence in left external iliac LN (SUVmax: 5.4)

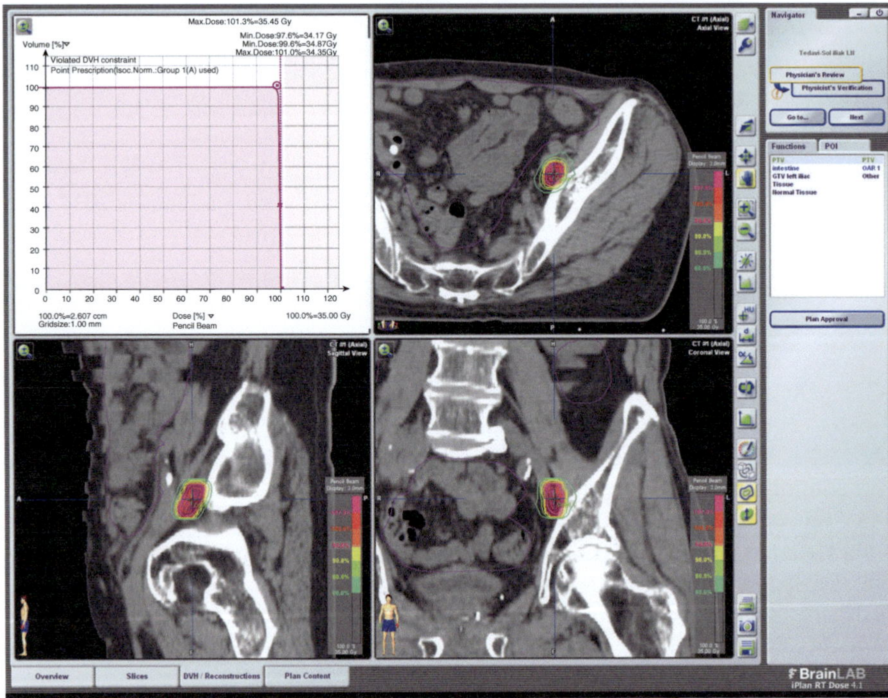

Fig. 25.6 SBRT Plan of Case 3: 35 Gy in five fractions SBRT delivered to the recurrent area

25.3 Radiolabelled Targetted Therapy with Radium-223 Dichloride

Radium-223 dichloride, an alpha-particle emitting radiotherapeutic drug, acts mimicking calcium at bone metastases with increased bone turnover in order to form complexes with hydroxyapatite. The Food and Drug Administration (FDA) has first approved radium-223 dichloride treatment, provided by Bayer HealthCare Pharmaceuticals Inc. (Xofigo Injection), on May 15, 2013 for the castration-resistant prostate cancer patients who have symptomatic bone metastases without any visceral metastasis. FDA approval was due to the randomized, double-blind, placebo-controlled trial randomly enrolling 541 patients to receive intravenous 50 kBq/kg radium-223 dichloride (1.35 μCi/kg) per month prescribed for six cycles plus best standard of care (local external radiotherapy, corticosteroids, antiandrogens, estrogens, estramustine, or ketoconazole) versus 268 patients to receive a placebo plus best standard of care. The interim analysis demonstrated statistically significant overall survival improvement with radium-223 dichloride (14 vs 11.2 months; hazard ratio: 0.70; $p = 0.00185$) in addition to a delay benefit in time-to-first symptomatic skeletal event [21–25].

Radium-223 dichloride is recommended to be prescribed at a dose of 50 kBq/kg by a relatively slow intravenous injection approximately over 1 min administered every 4 weeks to a total of six doses [21–25]. The intravenous access line or cannula needs to be flushed with isotonic saline before and after injection. The product radioactivity concentration (1000 kBq/mL; 27 μCi/mL) at the reference date (single-use vials containing 6 mL of solution in market) is important in dose calculation as well as decay correction factor for physical decay of radium-223. Typical activity of a treatment is below 8000 kBq with low external radiation exposure due to handling of patient doses. As radium-223 primarily emits 95.3% of its energy as alpha-particles, fractions emitted as beta particles and gamma radiation are 3.6% and 1.1%, respectively. The gamma radiation and its daughters allow for the accurate radioactivity measurement of radium-223 dichloride as well as the detection of contamination.

The major organs with highest expected absorbed radiation doses are bone (mainly osteogenic cells), red marrow, and upper & lower large intestine walls [21]. Therefore, the clinician should be aware of most common (≥10%) adverse reactions of nausea, vomiting, diarrhea, and peripheral edema, in addition to anemia, neutropenia, lymphocytopenia, leukopenia, and thrombocytopenia; while risk of bone marrow failure or continuing pancytopenia risks are around 2%. Hematologic evaluation at baseline and prior to every dose of radium-223 dichloride must be performed; ensuring mandatory counts of absolute neutrophil $\geq 1.5 \times 10^9$/L, platelet $\geq 100 \times 10^9$/L and hemoglobin ≥10 g/dL at first injection, and absolute neutrophil $\geq 1 \times 10^9$/L, the platelet $\geq 50 \times 10^9$/L at subsequent administrations [22–25]. Though no inadvertent overdosing has been reported during clinical trials, it is necessary to know that there is no specific antidote. If there is an unfortunate inadvertent overdosing happens, medical counter measures such as aluminum hydroxide, barium sulfate, calcium carbonate, calcium gluconate, calcium phosphate, or sodium alginate can be considered in addition to general supportive measures [21–24].

Sartor et al. documented the randomized phase 3, double-blind, ALSYMPCA trial, which enrolled patients to receive either six intravenous injections of 50 kBq/kg radium-223 (614 patients) or matching placebo (307 patients) [24]. Symptomatic skeletal events happened in 33% of radium-223 group and 38% of placebo group with longer time to first symptomatic event with radium-223 (median: 15.6 vs 9.8 months; hazard ratio: 0.66; $p = 0.00037$). The requirement of external radiotherapy for bone pain and spinal cord compression decreased with radium-223 in comparison to placebo; however, radium-223 did not significantly reduce symptomatic pathological bone fracture risks or tumor-related orthopedic surgical intervention [25]. Therefore, radium-223 should be considered one of viable options for symptomatic bone metastases in case of castration-resistant prostate cancer patients.

Conclusion

Prostate cancer cells have significantly elevated expression of specific transmembrane protein called prostate-specific membrane antigen (PSMA). Several retrospective trials demonstrated its diagnostic value compared to other tracers. Ga-68 PSMA PET/CT is superior in staging of particularly intermediate-high-risk prostate cancer. On the other hand, it should be kept in mind that Ga-68 PSMA are not fully specific for prostate cancer, and some selected reports showed its increased uptake in some benign conditions. The ability of Ga-68 PSMA to detect early regional lymph node metastases makes possible the application of salvage therapeutic approaches such as salvage lymphadenectomy, functional imaging-guided radiotherapy with a potentially curative intent. Radium-223 dichloride, an alpha-particle emitting radiotherapeutic drug, acts mimicking calcium at bone metastases with increased bone turnover in order to form complexes with hydroxyapatite. The Food and Drug Administration (FDA) has first approved radium-223 dichloride treatment, provided by Bayer HealthCare Pharmaceuticals Inc. (Xofigo Injection), on May 15, 2013 for the castration-resistant prostate cancer patients who have symptomatic bone metastases without any visceral metastasis. Radium-223 should be considered one of viable options for symptomatic bone metastases in case of castration-resistant prostate cancer patients.

References

1. Afshar-Oromieh A, Zechmann CM, Malcher A, et al. Comparison of PET imaging with a (68)Ga-labelled PSMA ligand and (18)F-choline-based PET/CT for the diagnosis of recurrent prostate cancer. Eur J Nucl Med Mol Imaging. 2014;41(1):11–20.
2. Schmid DT, John H, Zweifel R, et al. Fluorocholine PET/CT in patients with prostate cancer: initial experience. Radiology. 2005;235(2):623–8.
3. Krause BJ, Souvatzoglou M, Tuncel M, et al. The detection rate of [11C]choline-PET/CT depends on the serum PSA-value in patients with biochemical recurrence of prostate cancer. Eur J Nucl Med Mol Imaging. 2008;35(1):18–23.

4. Castellucci P, Picchio M. 11C-choline PET/CT and PSA kinetics. Eur J Nucl Med Mol Imaging. 2013;40(Suppl 1):S36–40.
5. Beer AJ, Eiber M, Souvatzoglou M, et al. Radionuclide and hybrid imaging of recurrent prostate cancer. Lancet Oncol. 2011;12(2):181–91.
6. Eiber M, Weirich G, Holzapfel K, et al. Simultaneous 68Ga-PSMA HBED-CC PET/MRI improves the localization of primary prostate cancer. Eur Urol. 2016;70(5):829–36.
7. Maurer T, Gschwend JE, Rauscher I, et al. Diagnostic efficacy of (68)gallium-PSMA positron emission tomography compared to conventional imaging in lymph node staging of 130 consecutive patients with intermediate to high risk prostate cancer. J Urol. 2016;195(5):1436–43.
8. Eiber M, Maurer T, Souvatzoglou M, et al. Evaluation of hybrid ^{68}Ga-PSMA ligand PET/CT in 248 patients with biochemical recurrence after radical prostatectomy. J Nucl Med. 2015;56(5):668–74.
9. Afshar-Oromieh A, Avtzi E, Giesel FL, et al. The diagnostic value of PET/CT imaging with the (68)Ga-labelled PSMA ligand HBED-CC in the diagnosis of recurrent prostate cancer. Eur J Nucl Med Mol Imaging. 2015;42(2):197–209.
10. Maurer T, Weirich G, Schottelius M, et al. Prostate-specific membrane antigen-radioguided surgery for metastatic lymph nodes in prostate cancer. Eur Urol. 2015;68(3):530–4.
11. Artigas C, Alexiou J, Garcia C, et al. Paget bone disease demonstrated on (68)Ga-PSMA ligand PET/CT. Eur J Nucl Med Mol Imaging. 2016;43(1):195–6.
12. Kanthan GL, Drummond J, Schembri GP, et al. Follicular thyroid adenoma showing avid uptake on 68Ga PSMA-HBED-CC PET/CT. Clin Nucl Med. 2016;41(4):331–2.
13. Kobe C, Maintz D, Fischer T, et al. Prostate-specific membrane antigen PET/CT in splenic sarcoidosis. Clin Nucl Med. 2015;40(11):897–8.
14. Rischpler C, Maurer T, Schwaiger M, et al. Intense PSMA-expression using (68)Ga-PSMA PET/CT in a paravertebral schwannoma mimicking prostate cancer metastasis. Eur J Nucl Med Mol Imaging. 2016;43(1):193–4.
15. Krohn T, Verburg FA, Pufe T, et al. [(68)Ga]PSMA-HBED uptake mimicking lymph node metastasis in coeliac ganglia: an important pitfall in clinical practice. Eur J Nucl Med Mol Imaging. 2015;42(2):210–4.
16. Schwenck J, Tabatabai G, Skardelly M, et al. vivo visualization of prostate-specific membrane antigen in glioblastoma. Eur J Nucl Med Mol Imaging. 2015;42(1):170–1.
17. Verburg FA, Krohn T, Heinzel A, et al. First evidence of PSMA expression in differentiated thyroid cancer using [^{68}Ga]PSMA-HBED-CC PET/CT. Eur J Nucl Med Mol Imaging. 2015;42(10):1622–3.
18. Rowe SP, Gorin MA, Hammers HJ, et al. Imaging of metastatic clear cell renal cell carcinoma with PSMA-targeted (18)F-DCFPyL PET/CT. Ann Nucl Med. 2015;29(10):877–82.
19. Pyka T, Weirich G, Einspieler I, et al. 68Ga-PSMA-HBED-CC PET for differential diagnosis of suspicious lung lesions in patients with prostate cancer. J Nucl Med. 2016;57(3):367–71.
20. Sasikumar A, Joy A, Nanabala R, et al. (68)Ga-PSMA PET/CT imaging in primary hepatocellular carcinoma. Eur J Nucl Med Mol Imaging. 2016;43(4):795–6.
21. Kluetz PG, Pierce W, Maher VE, Zhang H, Tang S, Song P, Liu Q, Haber MT, Leutzinger EE, Al-Hakim A, Chen W, Palmby T, Alebachew E, Sridhara R, Ibrahim A, Justice R, Pazdur R. Radium Ra 223 dichloride injection: U.S. Food and Drug Administration drug approval summary. Clin Cancer Res. 2014 Jan 1;20(1):9–14. doi:10.1158/1078-0432.CCR-13-2665. PMID: 24190979. Free Article.
22. Parker C, Nilsson S, Heinrich D, Helle SI, O'Sullivan JM, Fosså SD, Chodacki A, Wiechno P, Logue J, Seke M, Widmark A, Johannessen DC, Hoskin P, Bottomley D, James ND, Solberg A, Syndikus I, Kliment J, Wedel S, Boehmer S, Dall'Oglio M, Franzén L, Coleman R, Vogelzang NJ, O'Bryan-Tear CG, Staudacher K, Garcia-Vargas J, Shan M, Bruland ØS, Sartor O, ALSYMPCA Investigators. Alpha emitter radium-223 and survival in metastatic prostate cancer. N Engl J Med. 2013 Jul 18;369(3):213–23. doi:10.1056/NEJMoa1213755. PMID: 23863050.

23. Parker CC, Pascoe S, Chodacki A, O'Sullivan JM, Germá JR, O'Bryan-Tear CG, Haider T, Hoskin P. A randomized, double-blind, dose-finding, multicenter, phase 2 study of radium chloride (Ra 223) in patients with bone metastases and castration-resistant prostate cancer. Eur Urol. 2013 Feb;63(2):189–97. doi:10.1016/j.eururo.2012.09.008. PMID: 23000088.
24. Hoskin P, Sartor O, O'Sullivan JM, Johannessen DC, Helle SI, Logue J, Bottomley D, Nilsson S, Vogelzang NJ, Fang F, Wahba M, Aksnes AK, Parker C. Efficacy and safety of radium-223 dichloride in patients with castration-resistant prostate cancer and symptomatic bone metastases, with or without previous docetaxel use: a prespecified subgroup analysis from the randomised, double-blind, phase 3 ALSYMPCA trial. Lancet Oncol. 2014 Nov;15(12):1397–406. doi:10.1016/S1470-2045(14)70474-7. PMID: 25439694.
25. Sartor O, Coleman R, Nilsson S, Heinrich D, Helle SI, O'Sullivan JM, Fosså SD, Chodacki A, Wiechno P, Logue J, Widmark A, Johannessen DC, Hoskin P, James ND, Solberg A, Syndikus I, Vogelzang NJ, O'Bryan-Tear CG, Shan M, Bruland ØS, Parker C. Effect of radium-223 dichloride on symptomatic skeletal events in patients with castration-resistant prostate cancer and bone metastases: results from a phase 3, double-blind, randomised trial. Lancet Oncol. 2014 Jun;15(7):738–46. doi:10.1016/S1470-2045(14)70183-4. PMID: 24836273.

26 Quality Assurance of Modern Radiotherapy Techniques in Prostate Cancer Treatment

Vildan Alpan, Yücel Sağlam, and Steven Kirsner

Abstract

Prostate cancer is one of the most prevalent malignant diseases that occur among men with a new case diagnosed every 2.2 min, affecting one in six men their lifetime. Radiotherapy has been a vital part of the treatment of prostate cancer with three-dimensional conformal radiotherapy (3DCRT) as the historical standard. By utilizing techniques such as intensity-modulated radiation therapy (IMRT) or volumetric modulated arc therapy (VMAT) with image-guided radiotherapy (IGRT), the amount of normal tissue treated can be reduced and thus limit this increased toxicity. These types of treatments use the multi-leaf collimator to create a sequence of small apertures to deliver a high dose to the tumor. The treatment plans are created so that a high dose is given to the target while keeping dose to organs at risk low. This requires a treatment planning system (TPS) that has the capabilities of inverse planning to generate such treatment fields. The inverse planning engine uses as input contours of the targets and OARs to generate an optimal plan. With new technologies comes a new set of quality assurance (QA) tasks that need to be performed to ensure that what is being planned in the TPS is actually what is delivered to the patient. In this chapter, we will encompass the simulation, planning, and treatment of tumors located in the prostate region. In addition we will discuss the QA methods of each component of the radiation therapy process when treating tumors in the prostate region.

V. Alpan, M.Sc. (✉) • Y. Sağlam, M.Sc.
Department of Radiation Oncology, American Hospital Texas MD Anderson Cancer Center, Istanbul, Turkey
e-mail: vildana@amerikanhastanesi.org

S. Kirsner, M.Sc.
Department of Radiation Oncology, The University of Texas MD Anderson Cancer Center, Houston, TX, USA

G. Ozyigit, U. Selek (eds.), *Principles and Practice of Urooncology*,
DOI 10.1007/978-3-319-56114-1_26

26.1 Patient Simulation

26.1.1 Setup and Immobilization

Prior to beginning radiation treatment, all patients undergo a 3DCT simulation. A few days before CT simulation, several marker seeds are be inserted into prostate tumor volume. These markers help to more precisely locate prostate during each radiation treatment session. CT simulation allows us to visualize the tumor and other anatomy in 3D. CT numbers are proportional to electron density, which is necessary in heterogeneous dose calculation algorithms. Patients are brought to the simulator and positioned on the CT couch. At this point, immobilization devices are created to make sure that the patient can be set up in a reproducible position for treatment. Patient immobilization is a key component to the radiation treatment process. Complex treatments are good only if they are treating the area that is intended. That includes setting the patient up in an accurate, reproducible, and comfortable manner for the patient so that they can be positioned in the exact same way each day they come for treatment. Patients are simulated with CT in supine position on a flat tabletop. A custom-formed Vak-Loc bag is utilized to ensure consistent setup and stabilization. The bladder at time of simulation is filled to a degree that are maintainable and reproducible for daily treatment [1]. These immobilization devices must comfortably allow the patient to be positioned reproducibly each day during the course of radiation therapy [2–4].

26.2 Patient Planning

Historically prostate tumors were treated, with either an AP/PA beam arrangement and/or a series of oblique beams. Treatment plans were run utilizing manually collected single contours and calculations were performed with the use of heterogeneity corrections. As technology has evolved, so have the treatment planning strategies. Complex treatment plans using intensity-modulated radiation therapy techniques (IMRT) and volumetric-modulated arc therapy (VMAT) with full heterogeneity corrections has now become the standard [5–7]. The advances in imaging techniques and delivery techniques have aided in supporting the evolvement of treatment of tumors in the pelvic region. The advances in technology of imaging have been complemented by the improvements and advanced technology in treatment delivery. The primary focus on this improved technology has been the advent and development of the multi-leaf collimator (MLC). IMRT and VMAT utilize the MLC on the linear accelerator to create small and complex beam apertures to deliver a high dose to the target while minimizing dose to surrounding tissues. These delivery methods are now standard of care for patients with prostate cancer and other pelvic malignancies. All of these advanced delivery techniques require a treatment planning system that can perform accurate dose calculations utilizing full heterogeneity corrections.

26.3 Consideration of Tumor Margins During the Planning Process

The type of imaging modality used at simulation, the treatment method to be used, the amount of tumor motion, and setup uncertainties should dictate the size of the margins placed on the tumor volume when generating the treatment plan. These margins are necessary to account for the fact that the tumor is not in the *exact* position it was at simulation for the reasons described above. Accounting for these uncertainties and/or tumor motion will ensure that the tumor will receive the full prescribed dose. ICRU 62 [8] describes a series of target volumes that are generated during the planning process. The first of which is the gross tumor volume (GTV), which is the gross disease visible on the CT data set. The clinical target volume (CTV) is generated by adding a margin around the GTV to account for microscopic disease that is not visible on the CT scan. An internal margin (IM) is added to the CTV to account for tumor and physiological motion to generate the internal target volume (ITV). Finally, expanding the ITV by a margin to account for geometric uncertainties in treatment generates the planning target volume (PTV).

Similar to the imaging process, the type of treatment and the immobilization devices used will also play a role in how treatment margins will be used to generate the PTV [9–11]. If margins are going to be reduced during the planning process, an increase in the imaging used to verify this reduced margin. The use of daily setup verification images will become necessary.

26.4 Practice of Plan Quality Evaluation

It is the physician's responsibility to make clinical decisions regarding plan generation and plan evaluation. Upon completion of the treatment planning process, it is the physicist's responsibility to ensure the overall quality of the treatment plan [12]. This involves several tasks, (1) overall physics evaluation of the treatment plan, (2) evaluation of planning criteria and dose volume constraints, and (3) independent verification of the dose calculation.

To evaluate the plan from a physics perspective, one must understand the limitations of the dose calculation algorithm. While this is not a comprehensive list of questions to ask for each treatment plan, the following provide examples of what should be evaluated as part of a physics plan check. Is the proper dose prescribed by the physician displayed on the CT slices in the treatment plan? Is the proper dose per fraction and number of fractions correct along with the correct energy? Is the dose normalization point located within the beam apertures and positioned where there is electronic equilibrium? Are the beams entering the patient on an overly sloped surface? Are the beam apertures sufficiently sized or overmodulated to ensure an accurate dose calculation? Was the correct CT data set used for dose computation? Were heterogeneous dose calculations used? These by no means are a complete list of items to look for, but it is the physicist's responsibility to ensure that what is generated by the TPS accurately depicts the intentions of the directives given by the physician. Published DVH criteria are available for reference [13]; however, an institution may wish to develop and implement their own set of DVH criteria. In this case these criteria must be spelled out in the treatment planning directives. While there are circumstances where the DVH criteria may not be met, good clinical practice should include a review of the DVH constraints of each plan that is generated. If a DVH criteria is outside of those used in clinical practice, this should be discussed with the physician before the initiation of treatment.

26.5 TPS Dose Calculation Verification

Generating a treatment plan that is an accurate representation of what the linear accelerator can actually deliver first requires accurate imaging information and secondly requires accurate beam modeling. Validating the treatment planning system's beam model is a critical component to the radiotherapy process [14, 15]. This task is completed prior to the release of the treatment planning for use in the clinical environment. A major component of the beam model verification and commissioning involves the verification of the dose computation algorithm [16, 17]. For static beams, common practice is to perform a hand calculation of the monitor unit settings based on basic machine parameters, percent depth doses (PDDs) or tissue-maximum ratios (TMRs), output factors, inverse square correction, etc. This can be done either manually or with the use of automated software to perform such tasks. For more complex delivery techniques such as IMRT or VMAT deliveries where many irregularly shaped beam apertures are used in the patient's treatment, measurements should be performed by delivering actual treatments planned with the linear accelerator. Several software vendors make products that can compute dose for IMRT and VMAT fields as a second check on the MU settings and the dose delivered. Once the commissioning of the beam modeling process is complete a routine QA program should be implemented. This comprehensive QA program should verify that the treatment planning system continues to perform as it did at the time of acceptance and commissioning of the system. The initial commissioning of the system as well as the QA program should include the following: (1) verification that the CT to density table is generated properly, (2) the TPS is able to accurately compute dose to simple and complex geometry fields as compared with measured data, (3) output factors generated by the TPS are accurate, (4) the contouring tools still perform accurately, (5) DVH generation remains accurate, and (6) data transfer to the record and verify system maintains the integrity of the intended treatment fields. These tests should be performed on a routine basis and are particularly important after an upgrade to the TPS software is made. Finally, in all cases, every patient and independent check of the treatment plan should be performed. This can be done with simple manual calculations of MU settings for simple cases. These manual calculations are prone to errors in that a typical photon beam in the prostate cavity traverses different areas of density often traveling between areas having different densities. In addition, irregularly shaped, small fields will lead to in accurate hand calculation of MU settings. Recently, secondary check software programs have been developed that are capable of a full 3D heterogeneous dose calculation. Such systems similar to the TPS will perform a full 3D dose calculation and independently compute the MU settings. These systems can provide information on both MU and dose calculations as well as DVH information. Such comprehensive systems are a valuable tool in verifying the TPS dose calculation [18, 19].

26.6 Patient-Specific QA

One of the most important part of prostate treatment with IMRT or VMAT is patient-specific QA. IMRT and VMAT treatment techniques have highly conformal dose distributions though MLC shape, gantry speed, and dose rate. Patient-specific QA is required to deliver the actual dose with accuracy [20]. There are several methods for patient-specific QA. Generally routine QA method for plan verification is done on a LINAC in a specific phantom using small volume ion chamber and an electrometer to measure the absolute dose or film dosimetry for relative dose [21]. Also two dimensional array (2D) and electronic portal imaging devices (EPID) which is known as portal dosimetry are used for performing patient-specific QA. New-generation EPID systems has amorphous silicon detectors. This system uses the portal imager to acquire fluence patterns of the patient treatment fields [22]. This data can be used to compute the dose and compare it to the TPS [23]. Recently, three-dimensional (3D) verification system which provide patient anatomical structure information is being start to use for patient-specific QA. These system captures the log files generated from the treatment machine and compute dose to the patient CT data set, which can be compared to the dose computed in the TPS.

These systems have advantage and disadvantage. Single-ion chamber is advantageous in terms of availability in different shapes and sizes, good dosimetric response, absolute dose measurement and easy calibration. It is a disadvantage in terms of measurement in a single-point measurement. Generally, single-ion chamber is used with film measurement. Films advantages are excellent spatial resolution and cheaper than other dosimetric systems. But it depends on the film processor and storage conditions. Also it may vary from one batch of film to another. EPID can be accounted for at different gantry angles and needs no processor, and data acquisition takes less time. EPID provides good spatial resolution like film. But its resolution depends upon MV detector which needs to be properly calibrated [22].

Ion chamber, film, and 2D diode array measurements are direct measurement methods [24]. Log file in order to 3D QA methods is not direct measurement method. Log file-based IMRT and VMAT QA systems take the log files of the treatment machine [25–27]. These systems compute dose using an independent computed algorithm. These systems provide 3D dose comparison as computed on a heterogeneous data set. Also IMRT and VMAT QA can detect data transfer errors or data errors comes from the TPS to the treatment machine.

26.7 Patient Setup and Delivery

26.7.1 Setup and Pretreatment Imaging

We can deliver higher radiation doses than conventional radiation treatment methods to the prostate treatment with IMRT or VMAT. (The margin given to planning target volume can be reduced while significantly minimizing dose to normal structures.)

The prostate gland's position is affected by changes in the bladder or rectum. Its position may change depending on whether bladder is full or empty or rectum filling with gas. Changes of the prostate gland's localization causes to geographic miss.

To reduce the risk of geographic miss, we make sure that the patient position on the couch is the same as that in the simulation and planning process to guarantee that dose is delivered accurately. An image guidance system is used to reduce setup uncertainties and allows correcting the target localization.

Image guidance radiotherapy systems are used cone beam computer tomography (CBCT), MV imaging (EPID), transabdominal ultrasound, tracking of implanted gold fiducial markers, and orthogonal planar KV imaging for verify the prostate daily before treatment [28–30].

Electronic portal imaging modality uses low-energy photon beam to image the patient in the treatment position. The electronic portal imaging panel used to take the image from the transmission photons through the patient. Open field and treatment fields images combination is used to verify the patient positioning before the treatment.

For kV imaging, a kilovoltage (kV) X-ray and detector are mounted to the linear accelerator. For verification, AP and lateral images are taken with kV tube and used to verify patient setup before the treatment. Same time, kV imaging systems is used to acquire a cone beam CT (CBCT). CBCT images are taken using a flat panel detector by rotation of a kV source mounted on the linear accelerator. Obtained 3D images is used for verification of patient setup. CBCT is good choice for IGRT because it is taken high-resolution images of the target. Also CBCT provides information about the shape and location of organs at risk such as the bladder and rectum. However, it takes longer time than (2D) portal imaging (EPID) or orthogonal planar kV imaging.

Prostate localization using fiducial markers is increasing. Gold fiducial markers are placed inside the prostate before the simulation process. It is contoured on the planning system. After cone beam CT (CBCT), the fiducial markers are matched to a reference CT [31–33].

Ultrasound (US) imaging for prostate radiation therapy localization was used in the late 1990s. Its advantages are its ability to detect soft tissue targets, low cost, noninvasive process, and portability [9, 10]. But image quality depends on the user's experience, and the differences in localization can be sown by different users [34–37].

Electromagnetic transponders are the first localization system to provide objective localization. Electromagnetic transponders implanted within the prostate is used for prostate localization. Three transponders implanted in the prostate are detected as electromagnetic. Monitoring of the prostate position follows after radiation therapy. Electromagnetic transponders provide user-independent method of localizing the prostate gland in patients. However, it gives no information about the target or organs at risk [38].

26.8 End-to-end Testing of the Treatment Process

End-to-end test of the system should be done before starting treatment of the prostate. Each component of the treatment process should be checked. All imaging system, treatment planning, and recording and verification systems should be checked if working. For this purpose, phantom images are acquired from the CT scan, sent to treatment planning system, planned, and sent to recording and verification system. Before the treatment, phantom is placed on the treatment couch, CBCT and kV images are taken, and the phantom setup and treatment delivery are verified. If all system works, second end-to-end system should be created independently to evaluate the treatment process. Phantom sent from independent center is simulated, generated plan and treatment delivery. Then, phantom is sent back to the independent center, and it is evaluated and final result is sent back to the site.

Conclusion

One of the most important part of prostate treatment with IMRT or VMAT is patient-specific QA. IMRT and VMAT treatment techniques have highly conformal dose distributions though MLC shape, gantry speed, and dose rate. To be able to deliver the actual dose with the planned accuracy, patient-specific QA is required. There are several methods for patient-specific QA. Generally routine QA method for plan verification is done on a LINAC in a specific phantom using small volume ion chamber and an electrometer to measure the absolute dose or film dosimetry for relative dose. Also two-dimensional array (2D) and electronic portal imaging devices (EPID) which is known as portal dosimetry are used for performing patient-specific QA. New-generation EPID systems have amorphous silicon detectors. This system uses the portal imager to acquire fluence patterns of the patient treatment fields. This data can be used to compute the dose and compare it to the TPS. Recently, three-dimensional (3D) verification system which provide patient anatomical structure information is being start to use for patient-specific QA. These systems capture the log files generated from the treatment machine and compute dose to the patient CT data set, which can be compared to the dose computed in the TPS.

References

1. O'Doherty ÚM, McNair HA, Norman AR, Miles E, Hooper S, Davies M, Lincoln N, Balyckyi J, Childs P, Dearnaley DP, Huddart RA. Variability of bladder filling in patients receiving radical radiotherapy to the prostate. Radiother Oncol. 2006;79:335–40.
2. Malone S, Szanto J, Perry G, Gerig L, Manion S, Dahrouge S, Crook J. A prospective comparison of three systems of patient immobilization for prostate radiotherapy. Int J Radiat Oncol Biol Phys. 2000;48:657–65.
3. White P, Yee CK, Shan LC, Chung LW, Man NH, Cheung YS. A comparison of two systems of patient immobilization for prostate radiotherapy. Radiat Oncol. 2014;9:29.
4. Fiorino C, Reni M, Bolognesi A, Bonini A, Cattaneo GM, Calandrino R. Set-up error in supine-positioned patients immobilized with two different modalities during conformal radiotherapy of prostate cancer. Radiother Oncol. 1998;49:133–41.
5. Ezzell GA, Galvin JM, Low D, Palta JR, Rosen I, Sharpe MB, et al. Guidance document on delivery, treatment planning, and clinical implementation of IMRT: report of the IMRT Subcommittee of the AAPM Radiation Therapy Committee. Med Phys. 2003;30:2089–115.
6. Palma D, Vollans E, James K, Nakano S, Moiseenko V, Shaffer R, et al. Volumetric modulated arc therapy for delivery of prostate radiotherapy: comparison with intensity-modulated radiotherapy and three-dimensional conformal radiotherapy. Int J Radiat Oncol Biol Phys. 2008;72(4):996–1001.
7. Zhang P, Happersett L, Hunt M, Jackson A, Zelefsky M, Mageras G. Volumetric modulated arc therapy: planning and evaluation for prostate cancer cases. Int J Radiat Oncol Biol Phys. 2010;76(5):1456–62.
8. ICRU. ICRU Report 62: Prescribing, recording and reporting photon beam therapy (Supplement to ICRU Report 50). Bethesda, MD: International Commission on Radiation Units and Measurements; 1999.
9. Oh YK, et al. Assessment of setup uncertainties for various tumor sites when using daily CBCT for more than 2200 VMAT treatments. J Appl Clin Med Phys. 2014;15(2):85–99.
10. Schmidhalter D, et al. Assessment of patient setup errors in IGRT in combination with a six degrees of freedom couch. Z Med Phys. 2014;24(2):112–22.
11. Huang CY, et al. Six degrees-of-freedom prostate and lung tumor motion measurements using kilovoltage intrafraction monitoring. Int J Radiat Oncol Biol Phys. 2015;91(2):368–75.
12. Fraass B, et al. American Association of Physicists in Medicine Radiation Therapy Committee Task Group 53: quality assurance for clinical radiotherapy treatment planning. Med Phys. 1998;25(10):1773–829.
13. Lee TF, Fang FM. Quantitative analysis of normal tissue effects in the clinic (QUANTEC) guideline validation using quality of life questionnaire datasets for parotid gland constraints to avoid causing xerostomia during head-and-neck radiotherapy. Radiother Oncol. 2013;106(3):352–8.
14. Van Dyk J, et al. Commissioning and quality assurance of treatment planning computers. Int J Radiat Oncol Biol Phys. 1993;26(2):261–73.
15. Ten Haken RK, Fraass BA. Quality assurance in 3-D treatment planning. Front Radiat Ther Oncol. 1996;29:104–14.
16. Stern RL, et al. Verification of monitor unit calculations for non-IMRT clinical radiotherapy: report of AAPM Task Group 114. Med Phys. 2011;38(1):504–30.
17. Gibbons JP, et al. Monitor unit calculations for external photon and electron beams: report of the AAPM Therapy Physics Committee Task Group No. 71. Med Phys. 2014;41(3):031501.
18. Butts JR, Foster AE. Comparison of commercially available three-dimensional treatment planning algorithms for monitor unit calculations in the presence of heterogeneities. J Appl Clin Med Phys. 2001;2(1):32–41.
19. Chan J, et al. Comparison of monitor unit calculations performed with a 3D computerized planning system and independent "hand" calculations: results of three years clinical experience. J Appl Clin Med Phys. 2002;3(4):293–301.

20. Elith CA, Dempsey SE, Cao F, Farshadi A, Warren-Forward HM. The quality assurance of volumetric modulated arc therapy (VMAT) plans for early stage prostate cancer: a technical note. J Med Radiat Sci. 2014;61(4):261–6.
21. Pimthong J, Kakanaporn C, Tuntipumiamorn L, Laojunun P, Iampongpaiboon P. Commissioning and validation of COMPASS system for VMAT patient specific quality assurance. J Phys Conf Ser. 2016;694:012025.
22. Grządziel A, Smolińska B, Rutkowski R, Ślosarek K. EPID dosimetry—configuration and pre-treatment IMRT verification. Rep Pract Oncol Radiother. 2007;12(6):307–12.
23. Antonuk LE. Electronic portal imaging devices: a review and historical perspective of contemporary technologies and research. Phys Med Biol. 2002;47(31):1–65.
24. Schreibmann E, Dhabaan A, Elder E, Fox T. Patient-specific quality assurance method for VMAT treatment delivery. Med Phys. 2009;36(10):4530–5.
25. Calvo-Ortega JF, et al. A Varian DynaLog file-based procedure for patient dose-volume histogram-based IMRT QA. J Appl Clin Med Phys. 2014;15(2):100–9.
26. Rangaraj D, et al. Catching errors with patient-specific pretreatment machine log file analysis. Pract Radiat Oncol. 2013;3(2):80–90.
27. Litzenberg DW, Moran JM, Fraass BA. Verification of dynamic and segmental IMRT delivery by dynamic log file analysis. J Appl Clin Med Phys. 2002;3(2):63–72.
28. Low DA, et al. Dosimetry tools and techniques for IMRT. Med Phys. 2011;38(3):1313–38.
29. Ravichandran R, et al. Need of patient-specific quality assurance and pre-treatment verification program for special plans in radiotherapy. J Med Phys. 2011;36(3):181–3.
30. O'Daniel J, et al. Volumetric-modulated arc therapy: effective and efficient end-to-end patient-specific quality assurance. Int J Radiat Oncol Biol Phys. 2012;82(5):1567–74.
31. Nederveen AJ, Dehnad H, van der Heide UA, van Moorselaar RJ, Hofman P, Lagendijk JJ. Comparison of megavoltage position verification for prostate irradiation based on bony anatomy and implanted fiducials. Radiother Oncol. 2003;68(1):81–8.
32. Scarbrough TJ, Golden NM, Ting JY, Fuller CD, Wong A, Kupelian PA, Thomas CR. Comparison of ultrasound and implanted seed marker prostate localization methods: implications for image-guided radiotherapy. Int J Radiat Oncol Biol Phys. 2006;65(2):378–87.
33. Gayou O, Miften M. Comparison of mega-voltage cone-beam computed tomography prostate localization with online ultrasound and fiducial markers methods. Med Phys. 2008;35(2):531–8.
34. Kuban D, Dong L, Cheung R, Strom E, De Crevoiseir R. Ultrasound-based localization. Semin Radiat Oncol. 2005;15(3):180–91.
35. Fung AYC, Ayyangar KM, Djajaputra D, Nehru RM, Enke CA. Ultrasound-based guidance of intensity modulated radiation therapy. Med Dosim. 2006;31(1):20–9.
36. Orton NP, Jaradat HA, Tomé WA. Clinical assessment of three-dimensional ultrasound prostate localization for external beam radiotherapy. Med Phys. 2006;33(12):4710–7.
37. Fuss M, Cavanaugh SX, Fuss C, Cheek DA, Salter BJ. Daily stereotactic ultrasound prostate targeting: inter-user variability. Technol Cancer Res Treat. 2003;2(2):161–70.
38. Foster RD, Pistenmaa DA, Solberg TD. A comparison of radiographic techniques and electromagnetic transponders for localization of the prostate. Radiat Oncol. 2012;7:101.

Radiation-Induced Toxicity and Related Management Strategies in Urological Malignancies

27

Sezin Yuce Sari, Melis Gultekin, Pervin Hurmuz,
Gozde Yazici, Fadil Akyol, and Gokhan Ozyigit

Abstract

The lower abdomen and pelvis encompass several organs at risk (OAR), some of which are vital and are inevitably affected during radiotherapy (RT). In this chapter, the contouring recommendations and dose-volume constraints of the rectum, bowel bag (i.e., the whole small and large bowel together with their meso), urinary bladder, penile bulb, proximal femurs, and sacral plexus will be discussed in order to spare these OARs as much as possible during the RT of urological malignancies. Among these OARs, the bowel bag, penile bulb, and sacral plexus are serial organs in which the maximum point dose affects the function of the whole organ. On the other hand, the rectum, bladder, and femurs are in a parallel structure for which the mean dose to a specific volume is more important than the maximum dose. In order to interpret the dose-volume histograms (DVH) precisely, the accurate delineation of OARs is crucial.

27.1 Rectum and Sigmoid Colon

Dose-volume constraints in this chapter have been derived from the studies of Emami, Radiation Therapy Oncology Group (RTOG) protocols and guidelines, and the reviews of Quantitative Analyses of Normal Tissue Effects in the Clinic (QUANTEC). The most commonly used scoring systems for toxicity are the RTOG scoring criteria and the Common Terminology Criteria for Adverse Events (CTCAE) (Cox et al., Int J Radiat Oncol Biol Phys 31:1341–6, 1995; Program CTE. Common Terminology Criteria for Adverse Events. Version 4.0. Washington, DC: Division of

S.Y. Sari, M.D. (✉) • M. Gultekin, M.D. • P. Hurmuz, M.D. • G. Yazici, M.D. • F. Akyol, M.D.
G. Ozyigit, M.D.
Department of Radiation Oncology, Hacettepe University, Ankara, Turkey
e-mail: sezin_yuce@hotmail.com

G. Ozyigit, U. Selek (eds.), *Principles and Practice of Urooncology*,
DOI 10.1007/978-3-319-56114-1_27

Cancer Treatment and Diagnosis, National Cancer Institute, National Institutes of Health, Department of Health and Human Services, 2009).

27.1.1 Contouring

The RTOG has reported recommendations on the delineation of the anorectum and sigmoid colon in their "Pelvis Normal Tissue Consensus Contouring Guidelines" [3]. They recommend marking the anal verge with a radiopaque marker at the time of simulation and delineating the anorectum from this point at the inferior until the rectum loses its round shape in axial images at the superior and becomes elongated where it is connected to the sigmoid at the anterior. However, the rectum is usually delineated alone while treating genitourinary (GU) tumors (Fig. 27.1). In this case, the authors define the inferior border of the rectum as the level where the levator muscles fuse with the external sphincter muscles or where the mesorectal fat/space can no longer be seen. When the rectum is present in the bowel bag in axial slices, it should be included into the bowel bag as a part of it. Otherwise, it should be excluded from the bowel bag. The sigmoid colon ends before it connects to the ascending colon laterally.

The QUANTEC data also recommend the superior border as the rectosigmoid flexure and inferior border as the level of the anal verge, the level of or 2 cm below the ischial tuberosities or above the anus which is the caudal 3-cm part of the intestines [4]. The authors start the delineation of the rectum from the superior portion of the anal verge at the inferior until the sigmoid colon curve moving anteriorly is seen at the superior. In some studies, the superior and inferior border of the rectum was recommended to be 1 cm below and above the target volume or treatment fields, respectively. The rectum should be empty at the simulation process in order to prevent systematic errors in the planning target volume (PTV) coverage. The whole anorectal wall should be outlined in the OAR contouring [5]. Some authors delineate the rectum together with its perirectal contents [6, 7]. In the study of Peeters et al. [8], it was shown that the DVH of the anorectal wall reflected the risk for rectal bleeding and high stool frequency, whereas the DVH of distal 3 cm of the anal canal wall was better associated with the risk of fecal incontinence. It should not be forgotten that the rectum can move inter- and intra-fractionally due to rectal filling, intestinal gas, and bladder filling.

27.1.2 Dose-Volume Constraints and Toxicity

Acute rectal toxicity can occur during or soon after RT presenting as pain, diarrhea, rectal distention, cramping, and superficial ulceration. Late toxicity generally occurs years after RT and is presented with rectal stricture, diminished compliance, frequent bowel movements, and even fecal incontinence in case of anal musculature damage. The severity of these toxicities varies and somewhat affects the quality of life (QOL) of the patient.

It should be kept in mind that elder patients with comorbidities such as diabetes, inflammatory bowel disease, or prior abdominal surgery are at increased risk of

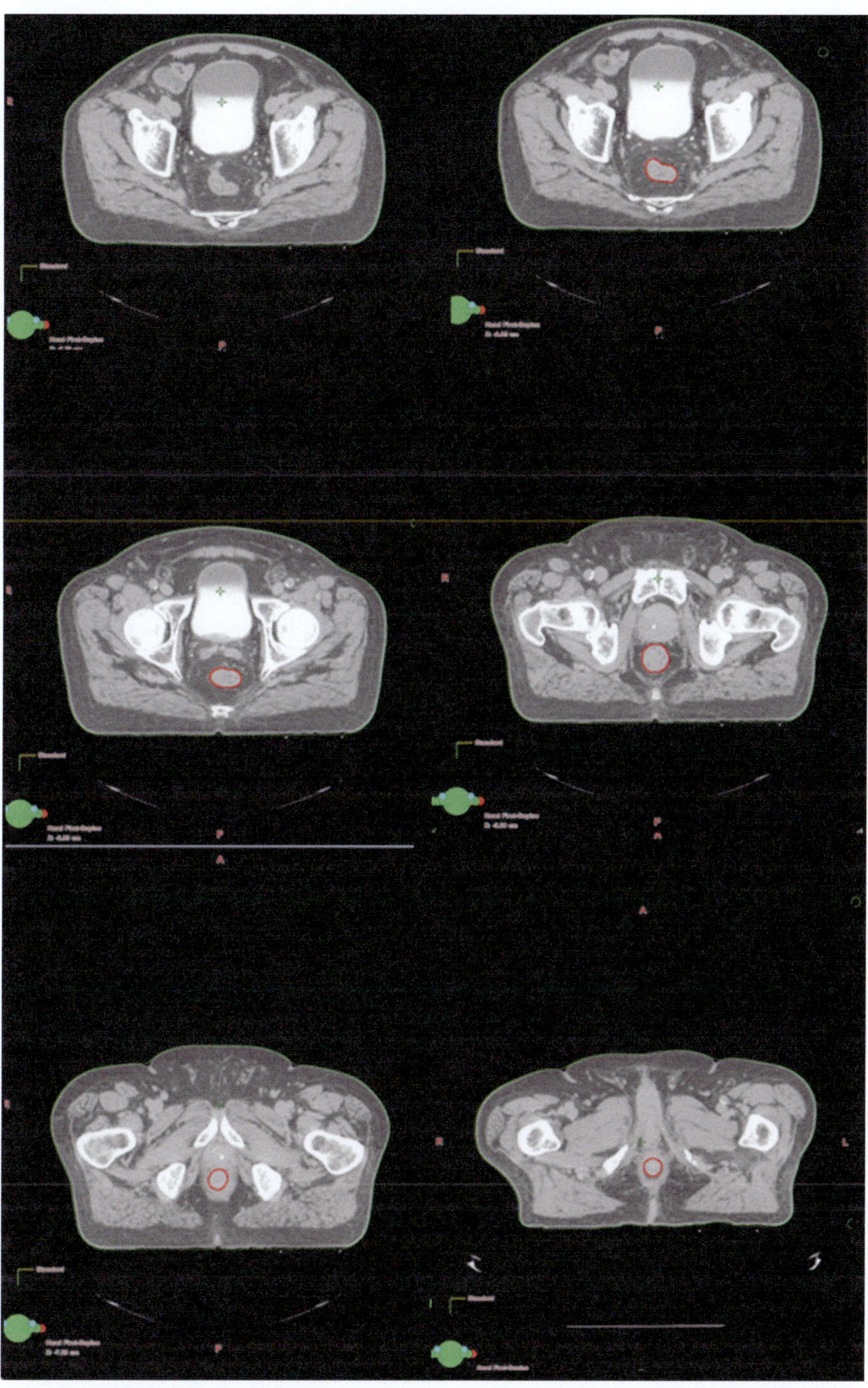

Fig. 27.1 Delineation of the rectum

rectal toxicity [9–12]. Furthermore, in the RTOG 9406 trial, the rate of rectal toxicity was reported to increase with larger PTV [13]. Additionally, patients that observe severe acute rectal toxicity are also more susceptible to late toxicity [12, 14]. Therefore, managing the symptoms of acute rectal toxicity can decrease the rate of late toxicity.

Studies mostly reported late grade ≥2 rectal toxicity with doses over 60 Gy to the full length of the rectum, and it is rare with doses ≤45 Gy in conventional fractions. The routinely recommended volumes for the rectum as an OAR for three-dimensional (3D) treatment planning are V_{50} <50%, V_{60} <35%, V_{65} <25%, V_{70} <20%, and V_{75} <15%. These constraints decrease the risk of grade ≥2 late rectal toxicity to <15% and grade ≥3 late rectal toxicity to <10% for prescriptions up to 79.2 Gy in conventional fractions [4]. Higher doses are more related to the development of rectal toxicity; therefore, decreasing the V_{70} and V_{75} is more efficient than decreasing the V_{50} or V_{60}. In IMRT treatment, low to intermediate dose-volume constraints are better achieved, and the rectal toxicity is expected to be lower [15].

The RTOG keeps the 50% volume of the rectum <55 Gy in the ongoing 0712 trial on bladder cancer; 50% <50 Gy and 25% <66.6 Gy in the ongoing 0621 trial on prostate cancer; 50% <60 Gy, 35% <65 Gy, 25% <70 Gy, and 15% <75 Gy in the ongoing 0415 trial on prostate cancer; and 55% <40 Gy and 35% <65 Gy in the ongoing 0534 trial on prostate cancer. In the RTOG 0631 trial on spine stereotactic body RT (SBRT), the maximum dose to the rectum is recommended 18.4 Gy and 20 cc <14.3 Gy with a single fraction of 16 Gy [16].

Higher doses to a large volume of the rectal wall increase the toxicity risk. Storey et al. [17] reported 37% risk of grade ≥2 rectal toxicity in prostate cancer patients that received at least 70 Gy to >25% of the rectal wall, whereas the risk was reduced to 13% in patients that received the same dose to <25% of the rectal wall. In the update of this study, the incidence of grade 2 rectal toxicity was 46% and 14% in the respective patients [18]. Zelefsky et al. [15] reported the 10-year rate of grade ≥2 rectal toxicity 9% in patients with prostate cancer. Although higher total doses were administered via intensity-modulated RT (IMRT), rectal toxicity was observed significantly lower in patients that received IMRT compared to patients that received 3D conformal RT (5% vs. 13%).

When rectal abnormalities are identified on endoscopic imaging in a patient that received RT, the cause is most likely this treatment. Biopsy should not be performed in this case because of the risk of chronic infection, delayed healing, and ulceration. It should also be kept in mind that colonoscopy should be postponed until 1 year after pelvic RT if there is no urgency for it. Acute rectal bleeding is usually self-limited. However, 3–10% of patients may require medical management with anti-inflammatory suppositories and antibiotics. In severe cases endoscopic coagulative therapies or even surgical diversion can be administered. Initial treatment for late radiation proctitis is the same as for acute proctitis. If the symptoms and rectal bleeding persist, laser treatment of rectal telangiectasis or ulcers is frequently beneficial. If conservation management fails, a colostomy may be required.

27.2 Bowel Bag

27.2.1 Contouring

The RTOG recommends delineating the bowel bag from the most inferior bowel loop at the inferior or above the rectum, whichever is most inferior [3]. If the rectum enters the bowel bag at any slice in axial images, it should be included into the bowel bag. Delineation of the bowel at each slice is strongly recommended as the bowel is highly mobile except for the duodenum and regions with postsurgical adhesions. A prone position with a belly board can reduce the volume of small bowel receiving high dose (Fig. 27.2) [19].

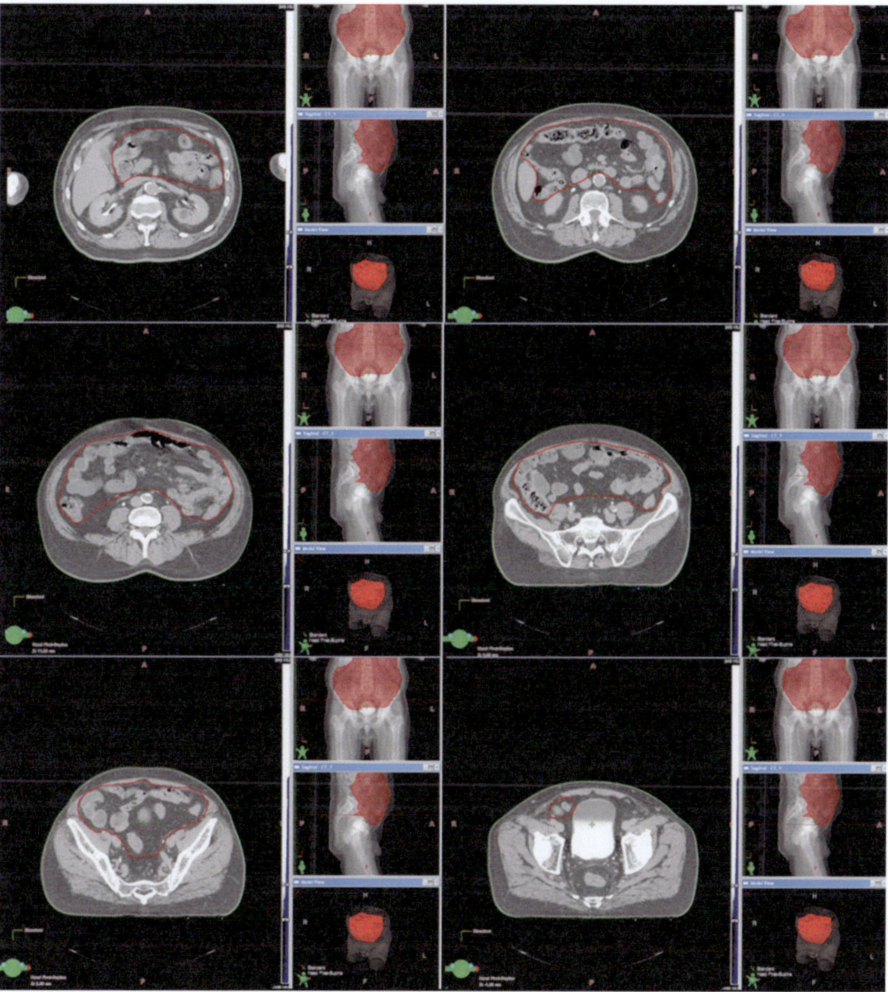

Fig. 27.2 Delineation of the bowel bag (intestines)

All muscles, bones, and other organs in the abdomen and pelvis should be excluded while delineating the bowels [3]. However, these organs can be left inside if the treatment planning system (TPS) does not allow subtraction. Using an oral contrast 30 min prior to scanning in order to distinguish the small bowel (i.e., the loops containing contrast) from the colon, vessels, and lymph nodes is also recommended.

27.2.2 Dose-Volume Constraints and Toxicity

Radiotherapy can cause mucositis in the small bowel in 1–2 weeks and can be presented as cramping and diarrhea. Late complications of RT often occur within 3 years and include persistent diarrhea, ulceration, obstruction, fistula, bleeding, and fibrosis which may require emergency surgery. Malabsorption of nutrients can also be observed in the long follow-up. Following the treatment of initial complications, patients are at risk for other complications for their whole life.

Emami et al. estimated the 5% risk of toxicity at 5 years ($TD_{5/5}$) and 50% risk at 5 years ($TD_{50/5}$) for 1/3 of the small-bowel irradiation 50 Gy and 60 Gy and for the whole organ 40 Gy and 55 Gy, respectively [20]. It has clearly been shown that concurrent chemotherapy significantly increases the risk of acute small-bowel toxicity [21–23]. Larger RT fields also negatively affect the rate of toxicity; para-aortic irradiation significantly increases the risk compared to pelvic irradiation [24]. Although some studies reported reduced toxicity rates with preoperative RT compared to postoperative RT, Birgisson et al. reported the opposite after a long follow-up [25–28]. As a conclusion, the rate of late severe small-bowel toxicity was reported 2–9% with 50 Gy in conventional fractionation and 25 Gy in 5 fractions to a partial volume.

The QUANTEC recommends keeping the volume of small bowel receiving ≥15 Gy <120 cc when bowel loops are delineated [29]. On the other hand, if the entire volume of peritoneal space is delineated, the volume receiving >45 Gy should be <195 cc. Keeping the volume of small bowel that receive higher doses as little as possible is also important. The RTOG recommends the percentage volume of the small bowel receiving ≥52 Gy should be 0 in the treatment of prostate cancer [30]. In RTOG 0529 for anal cancer and the ongoing RTOG 0822 for rectal cancer, the maximum dose to the small bowel is recommended <50 Gy [31]. RTOG 0529 also recommends keeping the 200 cc of the small bowel <30 Gy, 150 cc <35 Gy, and 20 cc <45 Gy.

When SBRT is to be applied, different constraints have been recommended for varying number of fractions. Three patients observed severe small-bowel toxicity in a SBRT study on liver metastasis, and all three patients received 30 Gy in 3 fractions [32]. The rate of duodenal ulcer was 12.5% in patients treated with 45 Gy conventional RT followed by a single fraction of 25 Gy SBRT for pancreatic cancer [33]. In another study on pancreatic cancer with 25 Gy in a single fraction, the rate of toxicity increased when the volume of small bowel receiving >12.5 Gy was >30 cc [34]. If SBRT is administered, QUANTEC recommends the volume receiving >12.5 Gy should be <30 cc in a single fraction, and the maximum point dose should be kept <30 Gy in 3–5 fractions [29].

27.3 Urinary Bladder

27.3.1 Contouring

The delineating of the urinary bladder as an OAR is the least challenging issue as it can easily be identified in the computed tomography (CT) images (Fig. 27.3). The RTOG recommends delineating the bladder "inferiorly from its base to superiorly to its dome" [3]. When there is contrast in both the bladder and small bowel, analyzing the coronal and sagittal views is recommended in order to distinguish the dome of the bladder from the bowel [3]. The trigone is more difficult to identify on CT images though. While some authors recommend delineating the entire bladder together with the urine inside, others only contour the bladder wall alone excluding the urine [35].

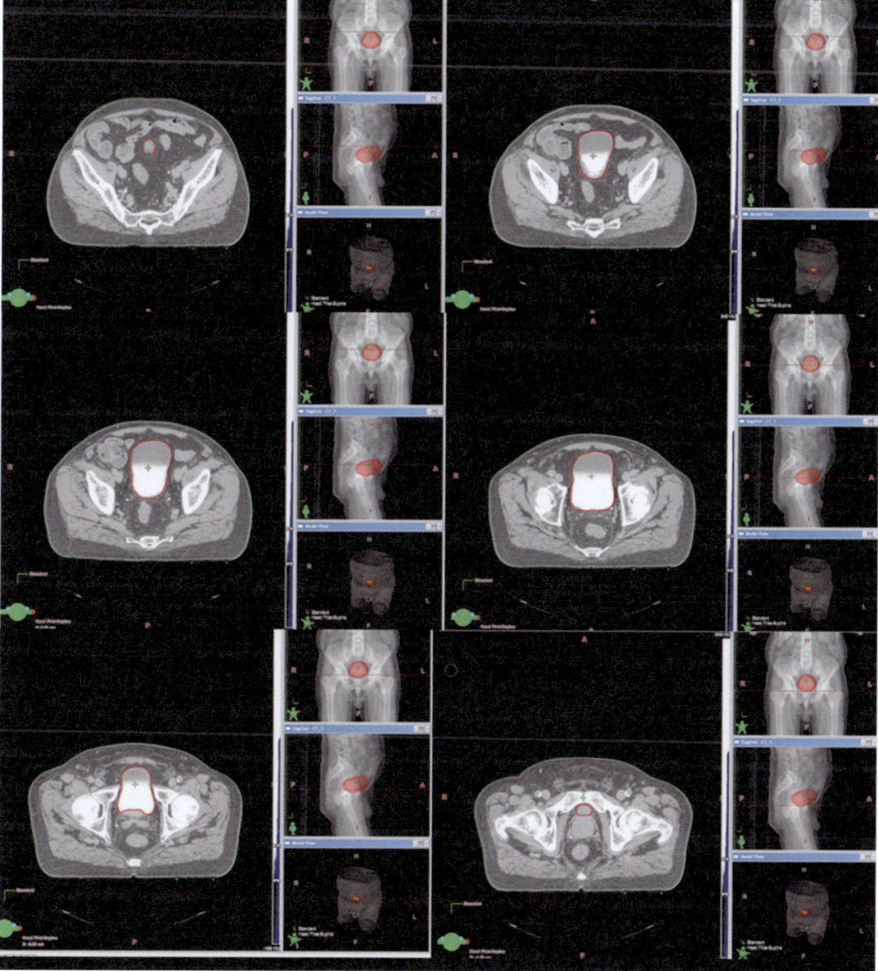

Fig. 27.3 Delineation of the urinary bladder

The most important problem about the delineation of the bladder is that it is highly distensible, and it can move with respiration, bowel filling, or positioning. Many patients cannot undergo RT with a constant bladder volume in every fraction. Studies reported that the bladder (and the tumor) can move up to 4 cm and its volume can vary up to 44% [36, 37]. The QUANTEC offers a "SimDVH" which is the bladder volume in a single CT image, to underline that a true dose distribution for the bladder cannot be obtained [35].

27.3.2 Dose-Volume Constraints and Toxicity

Radiotherapy-related acute toxicity such as dysuria, frequency, urgency, and hematuria usually resolves within a few months. Late toxicity includes long-term above-mentioned symptoms and may even be more severe with contracture, spasm, reduced flow, incontinence, fistula, obstruction, ulceration, and necrosis. These symptoms can also be originated from the urethra. Late toxicity occurs more frequently in patients that suffered acute toxicity during RT and that had GU morbidity or intervention prior to RT [38, 39]. Green et al. reported the incidence of incontinence 5% with transurethral prostate resection (TURP) before definitive RT compared to 1% in patients without TURP [40]. Hypofractionation, older age, hormonal therapy, and concurrent chemotherapy also increase the rate of grade ≥2 toxicity [41–43]. However, 65 Gy to the tumor concurrently with cisplatin was reported to not increase the rate of long-term urinary toxicity [44].

In patients with bladder cancer, the whole bladder dose varies between 40 and 69.4 Gy and the partial bladder dose 12–57.5 Gy leading to severe toxicity rate of 0–31% [43, 45–49]. In prostate cancer trials, on the other hand, severe toxicity rate was 13–20% after treatment doses of 78–81 Gy [15, 50]. The QUANTEC recommends the dose limits in the ongoing RTOG 0415 trial which are the volume receiving >80 Gy should be under 15%, >75 Gy under 25%, >70 Gy under 35%, and >65 Gy under 50% [35].

27.4 Penile Bulb

27.4.1 Contouring

The RTOG recommends delineating the portion of the bulbous spongiosum of the penis immediately inferior to the GU diaphragm, and not extending this structure anteriorly into the shaft or pendulous portion of the penis (Fig. 27.4) [3]. The authors state that the penile bulb is best visualized with T2 magnetic resonance imaging (MRI) or CT with contrast in the urethra as an oval-shaped structure posterior to it [51]. It is surrounded with the crura, corpus spongiosum, and the levator ani muscle. It is the most proximal portion of the penis just inferior to the prostate. Common errors in the delineation of the penile bulb include contouring it anterior to the urethra or symphysis pubis; too small in diameter; not round but triangular, trapezoidal, or rectangular in shape; too anteriorly; or too superior and close to the prostatic apex.

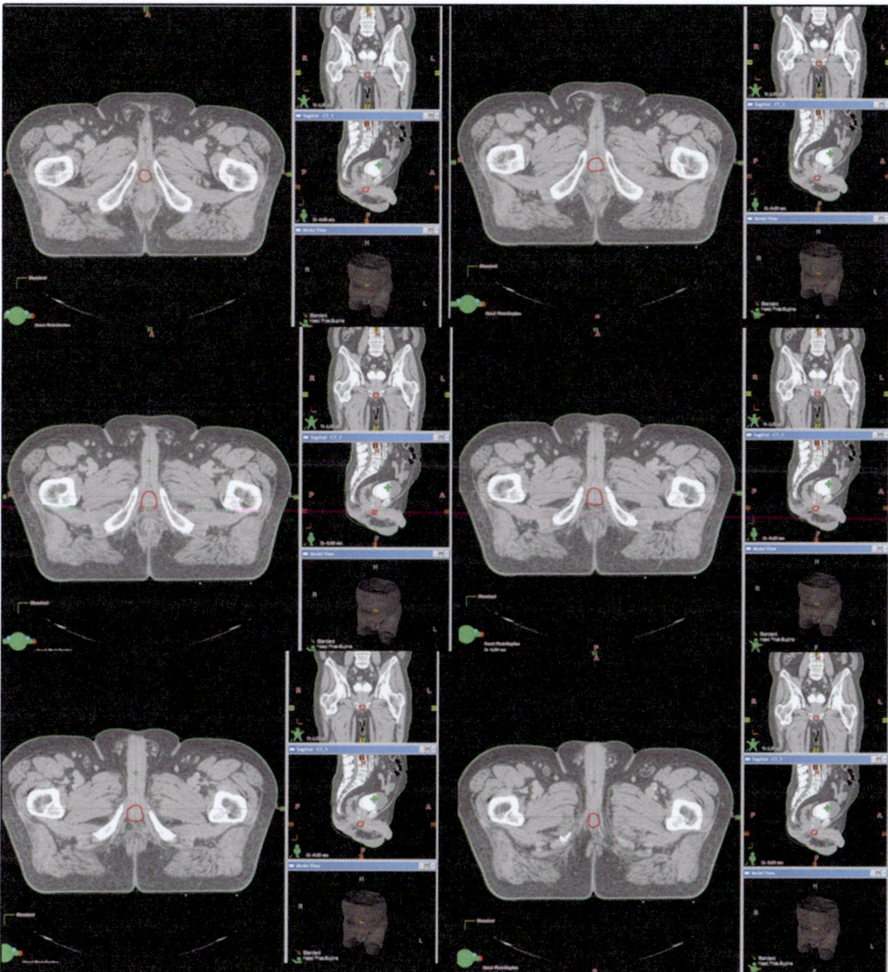

Fig. 27.4 Delineation of the penile bulb

27.4.2 Dose-Volume Constraints and Toxicity

The penile bulb itself is not a part of the erectile apparatus but an anatomic surrogate for periprostatic tissue likely to receive high doses of RT. Erectile dysfunction (ED) has an incidence of 24% after brachytherapy (BT), 40% after BT and external RT (ERT), and 45% after ERT alone [52]. However, it can also occur with increasing age, previous pelvic surgery, hormonal therapy, and comorbidities such as diabetes, hypertension, and atherosclerotic heart disease [39, 53, 54]. Therefore, it is not easy to attribute ED to RT alone. The RT dose and irradiated volume of the penile bulb are also effective in the development of ED [55]. The potency rate decreases gradually in time [56].

The International Index of Erectile Function (IIEF) can be used to assess ED [57]. Fisch et al. [58] reported the rate of ED 0%, 80%, and 100% in patients whose D_{70} is 0–40, 40–70, and >70 Gy, respectively. Mangar et al. [53] showed that the risk of ED significantly increases when the D_{90} is ≥50 Gy. Wernicke et al. [55], on the other hand, reported an increased risk of ED when the D_{30} is ≥67 Gy, D_{45} ≥63 Gy, D_{60} ≥42 Gy, and D_{75} ≥20 Gy. Roach et al. [59] found that a median dose of 52.5 Gy to the penile bulb significantly increased the rate of ED.

Based on the studies stated above, the QUANTEC recommends limiting the mean dose to 95% of the penile bulb volume <50 Gy [60]. They also offer keeping the D_{70} <70 Gy and D_{90} <50 Gy. In case of ED development after RT, sildenafil administration significantly improves erectile function [61].

27.5 Proximal Femurs

27.5.1 Contouring

The proximal femurs are contoured beginning at the lowest level of bilateral ischial tuberosities at the inferior to the top of the ball of the femur, including the trochanters at the superior (Fig. 27.5) [3]. Common errors in the delineation of proximal femurs include only contouring the ball of the femoral head, not contouring inferiorly to the lowest level of the ischial tuberosities, contouring unnecessarily below the ischial tuberosities, not contouring the trochanters, not conforming to the round shape of the ball of the femur or drawing it too large or small, and using the auto-threshold contouring tools in the TPS and not editing the resulting errors.

27.5.2 Dose-Volume Constraints and Toxicity

Increased dose to the femoral head and neck can result in fractures and even necrosis at a long-time follow-up. Patients usually complain about persistent low back pain. Cigarette smoking, osteoporosis, concurrent chemotherapy, and RT dose increase the risk of toxicity [62]. The per-patient incidence of femoral neck fracture was found 4.8% with a cumulative incidence of 11% at 5 years and 15% at 10 years in gynecological cancer patients that received 45–63 Gy pelvic and inguinal RT [62]. In another trial, the rate of insufficiency fracture was 1.7% in median 12 months in patients with cervical cancer that received 50.4–55.8 Gy ERT followed by 24 Gy BRT [63]. In the ongoing RTOG 0529 trial on anal cancer, 50% of the volume is recommended to be <30 Gy, 35% <40 Gy, and 5% <44 Gy. In the ongoing RTOG 0822 trial on locally advanced rectal cancer, 40% of the volume is kept <40 Gy and 25% <45 Gy, and mean dose <50 Gy. In the RTOG 0712 trial on bladder cancer, the mean dose is recommended <45 Gy. Another RTOG recommendation is also keeping the 5% volume <50 Gy [30].

It should be kept in mind that insufficiency fractures can be misdiagnosed as metastases on positron emission tomography (PET)/CT. If insufficiency fracture

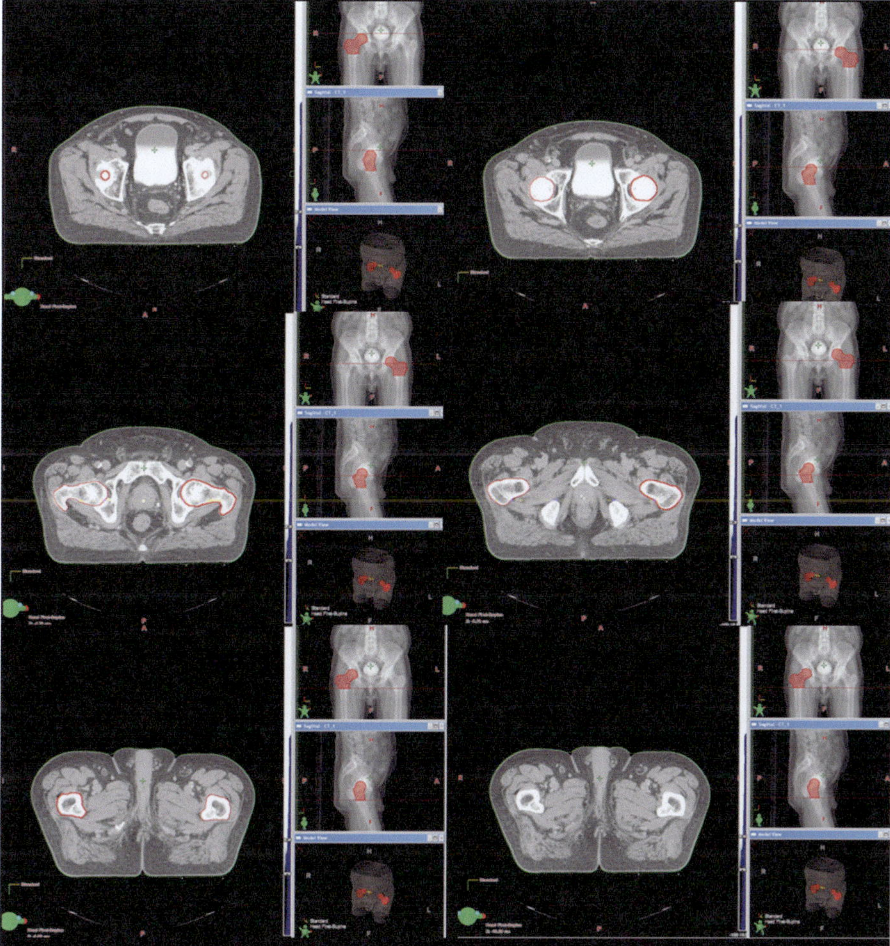

Fig. 27.5 Delineation of the proximal femurs

occurs, it usually resolves within a year with nonsteroidal anti-inflammatory drugs and rest. In unresponsive cases, sacroplasty can be applied.

27.6 Sacral Plexus

27.6.1 Contouring

Yi et al. published a study on the delineation and dose distribution of the lumbosacral plexus in patients with rectal and anal canal cancers treated with IMRT [64]. They recommended delineating the lumbosacral plexus (LSP) from L4-L5 vertebrae interspace at the superior to the level of the sciatic nerves at the inferior using the psoas, iliacus, piriformis, obturator internus and gluteus maximus muscles, common and internal iliac vessels, and adjacent vertebral bodies and sacral bones as landmarks. According to the authors, the entire lumbar foramina should be contoured at the L4 and L5 levels, the L4 root by including the space defined by the psoas muscle at the anterior and lateral and the facet joint/posterior vertebral body elements at the posterior, and the L5 root using the common iliac vein and psoas muscle at the anterior, the iliacus muscle at the lateral, and the vertebral body and sacrum at the posterior (Fig. 27.6). Below this level, they recommend the sacroiliac joint as the lateral border. When it comes to the sacral level, the borders are the iliac vessels at the anterior, the iliacus muscle and sacroiliac joint at the lateral, the sacral

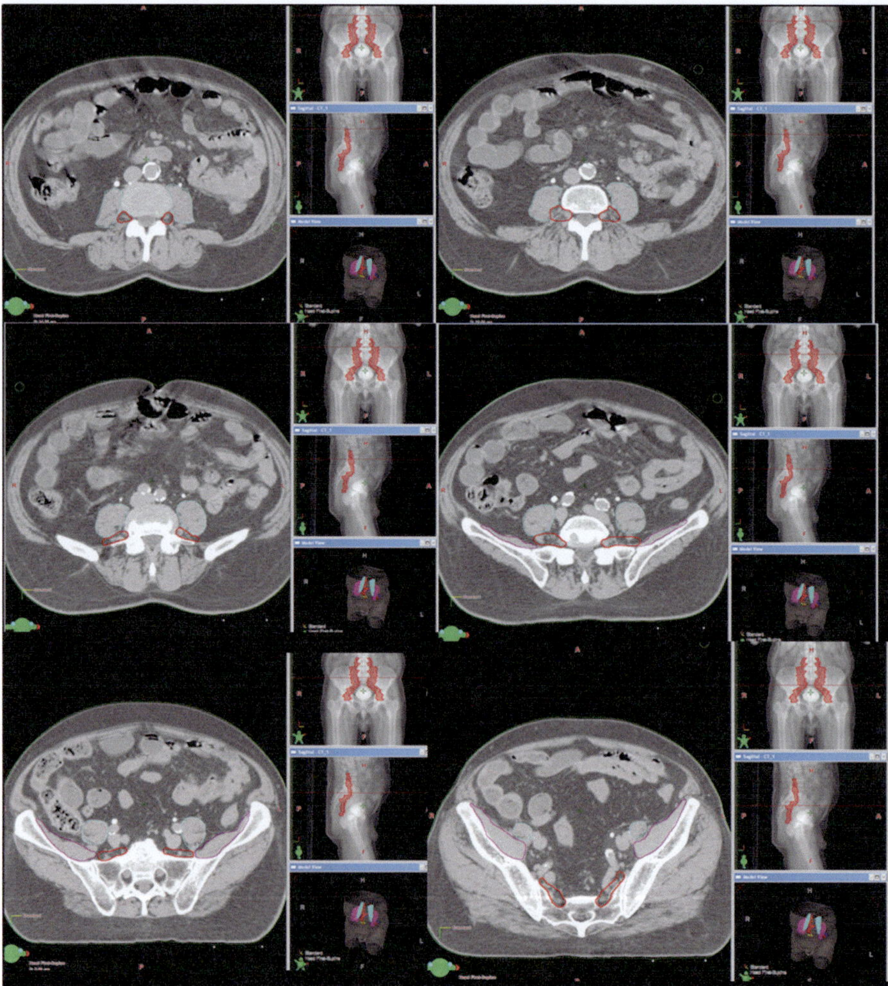

Fig. 27.6 Delineation of the sacral plexus (*cyan*: psoas muscle, *blue*: piriformis muscle, *magenta*: iliacus muscle)

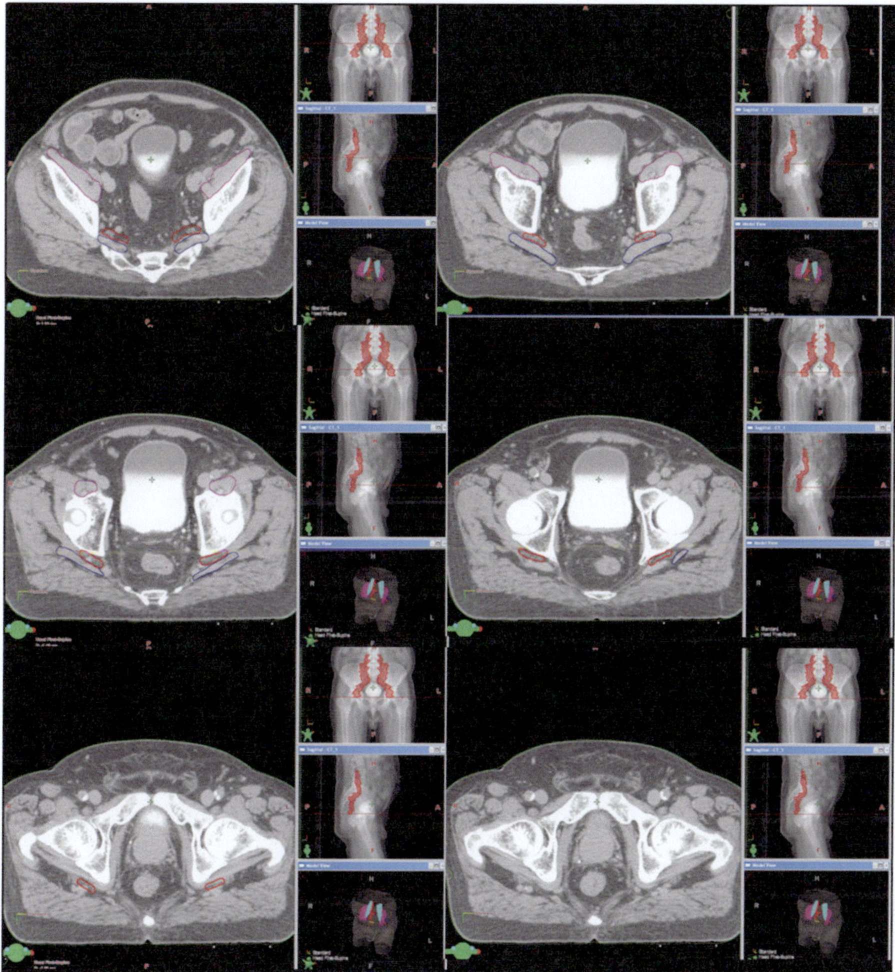

Fig. 27.6 (continued)

ala at the posterior, and the medial border of the S1 foramen at the medial. At the level of the origin of the piriformis muscle, the LSP should be delineated with borders of the iliac vessels at the anterior, the iliacus muscle and iliac wing at the lateral, and the piriformis muscle at the posterior. At the lower margin of the greater sciatic foramen, the borders of the LSP are the obturator internus muscle and ischial spine at the anterior, the piriformis muscle at the lateral, the gluteus maximus muscle at the posterior, and the medial border of the obturator internus muscle at the medial. Below the pirifomis muscle, they recommend delineating the space between the obturator internus muscle at the anterior and the gluteus maximus muscle at the posterior and extending the medial and lateral borders by 1–2 cm. They recommend ending the delineation of the LSP at the level of the superior border of the femoral neck at the inferior.

27.6.2 Dose-Volume Constraints and Toxicity

Radiation-induced lumbosacral plexopathy is a rare condition that can occur in patients treated for pelvic tumors with doses of 60–67.5 Gy with an incidence of 1–7% [65, 66]. It presents with lower extremity pain, weakness, dysesthesia, and numbness, and can lead to paresis, paralysis, and urinary and/or fecal incontinence [64]. The risk significantly increases when the LSP receives >70–79 Gy [67]. Tunio et al. [68] reported 8% incidence of lumbosacral plexopathy in cervical cancer patients treated with 50.4–59 Gy ERT with concurrent chemotherapy followed by 21 Gy BRT. They found the D_{mean} and D_{max} to be 52.9 Gy and 59.6 cGy and V_{40}, V_{50}, V_{55}, and V_{60} 61.8%, 44.4%, 8%, and 1.8% in patients with RT-induced plexopathy, respectively, and all these were significantly associated with the development of this toxicity, together with point doses >50 Gy. The ongoing RTOG 0631 trial on spine SBRT recommends the mean dose <18 Gy and 5 cc of the LSP <14.4 Gy with a single fraction of 16 Gy.

It is important to distinguish this toxicity from tumor recurrence. Thomas et al. [69] reported that while leg weakness occurs earlier in radiation-induced plexopathy, pain was the initial symptom in tumor recurrence. In parallel with this finding, electromyographic abnormalities are more frequently seen in patients with radiation-induced plexopathy. If neurologic deficit develops, it is irreversible and there is no effective therapy other than supportive care.

Conclusion

Most data in the literature of RT toxicity in GU cancers are based on conventional fractionation. Data on advanced RT techniques have been accumulated. It is important to apply the recommended dose-volume constraints in order to minimize toxicity.

References

1. Cox JD, Stetz J, Pajak TF. Toxicity criteria of the Radiation Therapy Oncology Group (RTOG) and the European Organization for Research and Treatment of Cancer (EORTC). Int J Radiat Oncol Biol Phys. 1995;31:1341–6.
2. Program CTE. Common terminology criteria for adverse events. Version 4.0. Washington, DC: Division of Cancer Treatment and Diagnosis, National Cancer Institute, National Institutes of Health, Department of Health and Human Services; 2009.
3. Gay HA, Barthold HJ, O'Meara E, et al. Pelvic normal tissue contouring guidelines for radiation therapy: a Radiation Therapy Oncology Group consensus panel atlas. Int J Radiat Oncol Biol Phys. 2012;83:e353–62.
4. Michalski JM, Gay H, Jackson A, et al. Radiation dose-volume effects in radiation-induced rectal injury. Int J Radiat Oncol Biol Phys. 2010;76:S123–9.
5. Meijer GJ, van den Brink M, Hoogeman MS, et al. Dose-wall histograms and normalized dose-surface histograms for the rectum: a new method to analyze the dose distribution over the rectum in conformal radiotherapy. Int J Radiat Oncol Biol Phys. 1999;45:1073–80.
6. Sohn M, Yan D, Liang J, et al. Incidence of late rectal bleeding in high-dose conformal radiotherapy of prostate cancer using equivalent uniform dose-based and dose-volume-based normal tissue complication probability models. Int J Radiat Oncol Biol Phys. 2007;67:1066–73.

7. Tucker SL, Dong L, Bosch W, et al. Fit of a generalized Lyman normal-tissue complication probability (NTCP) model to grade >2 late rectal toxicity data from patients treated on protocol RTOG 94–06. In: American Society for Therapeutic Radiology and Oncology 49th Annual Meeting. Los Angeles, CA. Int J Radiat Oncol Biol Phys. 2007;69:S8–9.
8. Peeters ST, Hoogeman MS, Heemsbergen WD, et al. Rectal bleeding, fecal incontinence, and high stool frequency after conformal radiotherapy for prostate cancer: normal tissue complication probability modeling. Int J Radiat Oncol Biol Phys. 2006;66:11–9.
9. Skwarchuk MW, Jackson A, Zelefsky MJ, et al. Late rectal toxicity after conformal radiotherapy of prostate cancer (I): multivariate analysis and dose-response. Int J Radiat Oncol Biol Phys. 2000;47:103–13.
10. Vavassori V, Fiorino C, Rancati T, et al. Predictors for rectal and intestinal acute toxicities during prostate cancer high-dose 3D-CRT: results of a prospective multicenter study. Int J Radiat Oncol Biol Phys. 2007;67:1401–10.
11. Willett CG, Ooi CJ, Zietman AL, et al. Acute and late toxicity of patients with inflammatory bowel disease undergoing irradiation for abdominal and pelvic neoplasms. Int J Radiat Oncol Biol Phys. 2000;46:995–8.
12. Peeters ST, Lebesque JV, Heemsbergen WD, et al. Localized volume effects for late rectal and anal toxicity after radiotherapy for prostate cancer. Int J Radiat Oncol Biol Phys. 2006;64:1151–61.
13. Michalski JM, Bae K, Roach M, et al. Long-term toxicity following 3D conformal radiation therapy for prostate cancer from the RTOG 9406 phase I/II dose escalation study. Int J Radiat Oncol Biol Phys. 2010;76:14–22.
14. Heemsbergen WD, Peeters ST, Koper PC, et al. Acute and late gastrointestinal toxicity after radiotherapy in prostate cancer patients: consequential late damage. Int J Radiat Oncol Biol Phys. 2006;66:3–10.
15. Zelefsky MJ, Levin EJ, Hunt M, et al. Incidence of late rectal and urinary toxicities after three-dimensional conformal radiotherapy and intensity-modulated radiotherapy for localized prostate cancer. Int J Radiat Oncol Biol Phys. 2008;70:1124–9.
16. Ryu S, Pugh SL, Gerszten PC, et al. RTOG 0631 phase 2/3 study of image guided stereotactic radiosurgery for localized (1–3) spine metastases: phase 2 results. Pract Radiat Oncol. 2014;4:76–81.
17. Storey MR, Pollack A, Zagars G, et al. Complications from radiotherapy dose escalation in prostate cancer: preliminary results of a randomized trial. Int J Radiat Oncol Biol Phys. 2000;48:635–42.
18. Kuban DA, Tucker SL, Dong L, et al. Long-term results of the M. D. Anderson randomized dose-escalation trial for prostate cancer. Int J Radiat Oncol Biol Phys. 2008;70:67–74.
19. Martin J, Fitzpatrick K, Horan G, et al. Treatment with a belly-board device significantly reduces the volume of small bowel irradiated and results in low acute toxicity in adjuvant radiotherapy for gynecologic cancer: results of a prospective study. Radiother Oncol. 2005;74:267–74.
20. Emami B, Lyman J, Brown A, et al. Tolerance of normal tissue to therapeutic irradiation. Int J Radiat Oncol Biol Phys. 1991;21:109–22.
21. Keys HM, Bundy BN, Stehman FB, et al. Cisplatin, radiation, and adjuvant hysterectomy compared with radiation and adjuvant hysterectomy for bulky stage IB cervical carcinoma. N Engl J Med. 1999;340:1154–61.
22. Macdonald JS, Smalley SR, Benedetti J, et al. Chemoradiotherapy after surgery compared with surgery alone for adenocarcinoma of the stomach or gastroesophageal junction. N Engl J Med. 2001;345:725–30.
23. Bosset JF, Collette L, Calais G, et al. Chemotherapy with preoperative radiotherapy in rectal cancer. N Engl J Med. 2006;355:1114–23.
24. Mak AC, Rich TA, Schultheiss TE, et al. Late complications of postoperative radiation therapy for cancer of the rectum and rectosigmoid. Int J Radiat Oncol Biol Phys. 1994;28:597–603.
25. Frykholm GJ, Glimelius B, Pahlman L. Preoperative or postoperative irradiation in adenocarcinoma of the rectum: final treatment results of a randomized trial and an evaluation of late secondary effects. Dis Colon Rectum. 1993;36:564–72.

26. Peeters KC, van de Velde CJ, Leer JW, et al. Late side effects of short-course preoperative radiotherapy combined with total mesorectal excision for rectal cancer: increased bowel dysfunction in irradiated patients—a Dutch colorectal cancer group study. J Clin Oncol. 2005;23:6199–206.
27. Bujko K, Nowacki MP, Nasierowska-Guttmejer A, et al. Long-term results of a randomized trial comparing preoperative short-course radiotherapy with preoperative conventionally fractionated chemoradiation for rectal cancer. Br J Surg. 2006;93:1215–23.
28. Birgisson H, Pahlman L, Gunnarsson U, Glimelius B. Late gastrointestinal disorders after rectal cancer surgery with and without preoperative radiation therapy. Br J Surg. 2008;95:206–13.
29. Kavanagh BD, Pan CC, Dawson LA, et al. Radiation dose-volume effects in the stomach and small bowel. Int J Radiat Oncol Biol Phys. 2010;76:S101–7.
30. Lawton CA, Michalski J, El-Naqa I, et al. RTOG GU radiation oncology specialists reach consensus on pelvic lymph node volumes for high-risk prostate cancer. Int J Radiat Oncol Biol Phys. 2009;74:383–7.
31. Kachnic LA, Winter K, Myerson RJ, et al. RTOG 0529: a phase 2 evaluation of dose-painted intensity modulated radiation therapy in combination with 5-fluorouracil and mitomycin-C for the reduction of acute morbidity in carcinoma of the anal canal. Int J Radiat Oncol Biol Phys. 2013;86:27–33.
32. Hoyer M, Roed H, Traberg Hansen A, et al. Phase II study on stereotactic body radiotherapy of colorectal metastases. Acta Oncol. 2006;45:823–30.
33. Koong AC, Christofferson E, Le QT, et al. Phase II study to assess the efficacy of conventionally fractionated radiotherapy followed by a stereotactic radiosurgery boost in patients with locally advanced pancreatic cancer. Int J Radiat Oncol Biol Phys. 2005;63:320–3.
34. Schellenberg D, Goodman KA, Lee F, et al. Gemcitabine chemotherapy and single-fraction stereotactic body radiotherapy for locally advanced pancreatic cancer. Int J Radiat Oncol Biol Phys. 2008;72:678–86.
35. Viswanathan AN, Yorke ED, Marks LB, et al. Radiation dose-volume effects of the urinary bladder. Int J Radiat Oncol Biol Phys. 2010;76:S116–22.
36. Muren LP, Smaaland R, Dahl O. Organ motion, set-up variation and treatment margins in radical radiotherapy of urinary bladder cancer. Radiother Oncol. 2003;69:291–304.
37. Turner SL, Swindell R, Bowl N, et al. Bladder movement during radiation therapy for bladder cancer: implications for treatment planning. Int J Radiat Oncol Biol Phys. 1997;39:355–60.
38. Peeters ST, Heemsbergen WD, van Putten WL, et al. Acute and late complications after radiotherapy for prostate cancer: results of a multicenter randomized trial comparing 68 Gy to 78 Gy. Int J Radiat Oncol Biol Phys. 2005;61:1019–34.
39. Cahlon O, Zelefsky MJ, Shippy A, et al. Ultra-high dose (86.4 Gy) IMRT for localized prostate cancer: toxicity and biochemical outcomes. Int J Radiat Oncol Biol Phys. 2008;71:330–7.
40. Green N, Treible D, Wallack H. Prostate cancer: post-irradiation incontinence. J Urol. 1990;144:307–9.
41. Peeters ST, Hoogeman MS, Heemsbergen WD, et al. Volume and hormonal effects for acute side effects of rectum and bladder during conformal radiotherapy for prostate cancer. Int J Radiat Oncol Biol Phys. 2005;63:1142–52.
42. Levine LA, Richie JP. Urological complications of cyclophosphamide. J Urol. 1989;141:1063–9.
43. Moonen L, van der Voet H, Horenblas S, Bartelink H. A feasibility study of accelerated fractionation in radiotherapy of carcinoma of the urinary bladder. Int J Radiat Oncol Biol Phys. 1997;37:537–42.
44. Shipley WU, Bae K, Efstathiou JA, et al. Late pelvic toxicity following bladder-sparing therapy in patients with invasive bladder cancer: Analysis of RTOG 89-03, 95-06, 97-06, 99-06. In: American Society for Therapeutic Radiology and Oncology 49th Annual Meeting. Los Angeles, CA. Int J Radiat Oncol Biol Phys. 2007;69:S38.
45. Pos FJ, van Tienhoven G, Hulshof MC, et al. Concomitant boost radiotherapy for muscle invasive bladder cancer. Radiother Oncol. 2003;68:75–80.
46. Rodel C, Grabenbauer GG, Kuhn R, et al. Combined-modality treatment and selective organ preservation in invasive bladder cancer: long-term results. J Clin Oncol. 2002;20:3061–71.

47. Mangar SA, Foo K, Norman A, et al. Evaluating the effect of reducing the high-dose volume on the toxicity of radiotherapy in the treatment of bladder cancer. Clin Oncol (R Coll Radiol). 2006;18:466–73.
48. Cowan RA, McBain CA, Ryder WD, et al. Radiotherapy for muscle-invasive carcinoma of the bladder: results of a randomized trial comparing conventional whole bladder with dose-escalated partial bladder radiotherapy. Int J Radiat Oncol Biol Phys. 2004;59:197–207.
49. Scholten AN, Leer JW, Collins CD, et al. Hypofractionated radiotherapy for invasive bladder cancer. Radiother Oncol. 1997;43:163–9.
50. Al-Mamgani A, van Putten WL, Heemsbergen WD, et al. Update of Dutch multicenter dose-escalation trial of radiotherapy for localized prostate cancer. Int J Radiat Oncol Biol Phys. 2008;72:980–8.
51. Wallner KE, Merrick GS, Benson ML, et al. Penile bulb imaging. Int J Radiat Oncol Biol Phys. 2002;53:928–33.
52. Robinson JW, Moritz S, Fung T. Meta-analysis of rates of erectile function after treatment of localized prostate carcinoma. Int J Radiat Oncol Biol Phys. 2002;54:1063–8.
53. Mangar SA, Sydes MR, Tucker HL, et al. Evaluating the relationship between erectile dysfunction and dose received by the penile bulb: using data from a randomised controlled trial of conformal radiotherapy in prostate cancer (MRC RT01, ISRCTN47772397). Radiother Oncol. 2006;80:355–62.
54. van der Wielen GJ, Hoogeman MS, Dohle GR, et al. Dose-volume parameters of the corpora cavernosa do not correlate with erectile dysfunction after external beam radiotherapy for prostate cancer: results from a dose-escalation trial. Int J Radiat Oncol Biol Phys. 2008;71:795–800.
55. Wernicke AG, Valicenti R, Dieva K, et al. Radiation dose delivered to the proximal penis as a predictor of the risk of erectile dysfunction after three-dimensional conformal radiotherapy for localized prostate cancer. Int J Radiat Oncol Biol Phys. 2004;60:1357–63.
56. Mantz CA, Nautiyal J, Awan A, et al. Potency preservation following conformal radiotherapy for localized prostate cancer: impact of neoadjuvant androgen blockade, treatment technique, and patient-related factors. Cancer J Sci Am. 1999;5:230–6.
57. Rosen RC, Riley A, Wagner G, et al. The international index of erectile function (IIEF): a multidimensional scale for assessment of erectile dysfunction. Urology. 1997;49:822–30.
58. Fisch BM, Pickett B, Weinberg V, Roach M. Dose of radiation received by the bulb of the penis correlates with risk of impotence after three-dimensional conformal radiotherapy for prostate cancer. Urology. 2001;57:955–9.
59. Roach M, Winter K, Michalski JM, et al. Penile bulb dose and impotence after three-dimensional conformal radiotherapy for prostate cancer on RTOG 9406: findings from a prospective, multi-institutional, phase I/II dose-escalation study. Int J Radiat Oncol Biol Phys. 2004;60:1351–6.
60. Roach M 3rd, Nam J, Gagliardi G, et al. Radiation dose-volume effects and the penile bulb. Int J Radiat Oncol Biol Phys. 2010;76:S130–4.
61. Zelefsky MJ, Eid JF. Elucidating the etiology of erectile dysfunction after definitive therapy for prostatic cancer. Int J Radiat Oncol Biol Phys. 1998;40:129–33.
62. Grigsby PW, Roberts HL, Perez CA. Femoral neck fracture following groin irradiation. Int J Radiat Oncol Biol Phys. 1995;32:63–7.
63. Huh SJ, Kim B, Kang MK, et al. Pelvic insufficiency fracture after pelvic irradiation in uterine cervix cancer. Gynecol Oncol. 2002;86:264–8.
64. Yi SK, Mak W, Yang CC, et al. Development of a standardized method for contouring the lumbosacral plexus: a preliminary dosimetric analysis of this organ at risk among 15 patients treated with intensity-modulated radiotherapy for lower gastrointestinal cancers and the incidence of radiation-induced lumbosacral plexopathy. Int J Radiat Oncol Biol Phys. 2012;84:376–82.
65. Dahele M, Davey P, Reingold S, Shun Wong C. Radiation-induced lumbo-sacral plexopathy (RILSP): an important enigma. Clin Oncol (R Coll Radiol). 2006;18:427–8.
66. Topkan E, Önal HC, Yavuz AA, Yavuz MN. Pathophysiology and management of radiation-induced lumbosacral plexopathy. Turk Onkoloji Dergisi. 2008;23:147–52.

67. Georgiou A, Grigsby PW, Perez CA. Radiation induced lumbosacral plexopathy in gynecologic tumors: clinical findings and dosimetric analysis. Int J Radiat Oncol Biol Phys. 1993;26:479–82.
68. Tunio M, Al Asiri M, Bayoumi Y, et al. Lumbosacral plexus delineation, dose distribution, and its correlation with radiation-induced lumbosacral plexopathy in cervical cancer patients. Onco Targets Ther. 2015;8:21–7.
69. Thomas JE, Cascino TL, Earle JD. Differential diagnosis between radiation and tumor plexopathy of the pelvis. Neurology. 1985;35:1–7.

Index

G. Ozyigit, U. Selek (eds.), *Principles and Practice of Urooncology*,
DOI 10.1007/978-3-319-56114-1

B

C

D

E

F

G

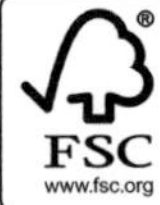

MIX
Papier aus verantwortungsvollen Quellen
Paper from responsible sources
FSC® C105338

If you have any concerns about our products, you can contact us on
ProductSafety@springernature.com

In case Publisher is established outside the EU, the EU authorized representative is:
Springer Nature Customer Service Center GmbH
Europaplatz 3, 69115 Heidelberg, Germany

Printed by Libri Plureos GmbH
in Hamburg, Germany